Psychosocial Factors in Arthritis

Perry M. Nicassio
Editor

Psychosocial Factors in Arthritis

Perspectives on Adjustment and Management

Springer

Editor
Perry M. Nicassio, PhD
Clinical Professor
Department of Psychiatry
School of Medicine
University of California, Los Angeles
Los Angeles, CA, USA

ISBN 978-3-319-22857-0 ISBN 978-3-319-22858-7 (eBook)
DOI 10.1007/978-3-319-22858-7

Library of Congress Control Number: 2015954172

Springer Cham Heidelberg New York Dordrecht London

Printed on acid-free paper

Springer International Publishing AG Switzerland is part of Springer Science+Business Media (www.springer.com)

Preface

The growing worldwide prevalence of arthritis has had a major impact on a range of populations across gender, different socioeconomic strata, ethnicities, and particularly among the elderly, who disproportionately are affected by the disability, role limitations, and deficits in quality of life that arthritis may cause. Arthritis has sparked considerable interest among psychologists, behavioral medicine specialists, and rheumatology health professionals in examining the adjustment of patients using an interdisciplinary lens. Their contributions have led not only to new insights about the plight of arthritis patients but also to new paradigms that are applicable to studying chronic illnesses in general. Importantly, much can be learned from examining processes of adjustment in arthritis that may be generalizable to other chronic illnesses. The pain, fatigue, and psychological distress that are hallmark features of arthritis are found in many other chronic conditions that create significant burdens for patients, challenge the expertise of clinicians, and place a strain on the capacity of health care systems to respond appropriately to patients' multifaceted health care needs. In many respects, arthritis can be viewed as a "model" chronic illness in which processes of adaptation can be examined that may enlighten our understanding of other medical conditions.

Most importantly, however, the harmful effects of arthritis have created a need for understanding the interplay between psychological, social, and biomedical factors in the adjustment of affected patients. Accordingly, the struggles of arthritis patients have created a heightened demand for novel and effective treatment approaches that complement medical treatments, mitigate the deleterious impact of arthritis, and improve patients' ability to cope with difficult symptoms and enhance functional adaptation. There is considerable evidence that a range of health professionals have embraced the challenge of researching and applying new treatment paradigms and approaches that can be translated into more effective and efficient models of care.

The major purposes of this book are to provide a synthesis of the empirical research that provides a foundation for the biopsychosocial care of arthritis patients and to highlight trends and developments in psychosocial treatment approaches. Specifically, this edited book addresses the following aims: (1) to increase understanding of the contribution of psychosocial variables and processes to health outcomes in arthritis, (2) to analyze mechanisms of arthritis pain, coping processes, and the role and efficacy of behavioral treatment approaches, (3) to address the role of socioeconomic status and health care disparities in the adjustment to arthritis, access to care, and quality of life, (4) to examine psychiatric comorbidities in arthritis such as depression and anxiety, and (5) to provide an overview of psychological and behavioral approaches to management.

The book is divided into two sections. The first section addresses theory and research on the adjustment to arthritis with a focus on psychosocial processes. Chapters provide an overview of such topics as arthritis pain, psychiatric comorbidity, the impact of arthritis on minority and disadvantaged populations, resilience, stress, disability, sleep, and the doctor–patient relationship. The second section specifically focuses on psychosocial management, with chapters addressing the need for psychological screening and evaluation, complementary treatments, self-help and community interventions, the role of physical activity, and challenges for behavioral interventions.

The book has an interdisciplinary focus that is reflected not only in its content but also in the expertise of the chapter contributors whose backgrounds span the fields of health psychology, behavioral medicine, rheumatology, epidemiology, nursing, and health services research. As such, the book is designed for an interdisciplinary audience that is involved in research on arthritis and health care professionals who provide service to arthritis patients across a range of clinical and community settings. The book also provides a theoretical and empirical foundation for researchers and clinicians of other chronic diseases and health problems.

Moreover, the book illustrates the importance of integrative care in arthritis, which represents a natural extension of the biopsychosocial model and the contribution of interdisciplinary research to health promotion and disease management. While the philosophy of integrative care has been increasingly embraced across the health professions over the last decade, its adoption in rheumatology practice has been limited. Integrative care focuses on patients and their needs, deemphasizes the effects of professional boundaries and rigid disciplinary frameworks, and fosters the importance of shared paradigms of understanding adjustment and treatment that include better teamwork on the part of health care professionals in clinical settings. Integrative care is a central and necessary component in the clinical application of the biopsychosocial model. It is hoped that this book will provide a framework for the expansion and dissemination of integrative care for the arthritis patient.

I would like to express my sincere appreciation to the chapter authors and coauthors who have demonstrated their scientific and clinical expertise in contributing to the book, and to the staff at Springer for their encouragement and efforts in developing the themes of the book and for its production. Importantly, I would like to acknowledge the efforts of arthritis patients for their cooperation in the research that has provided the foundation for this book, and their impressive resilience and courage in coping with the challenges that they face on a daily basis.

Los Angeles, CA Perry M. Nicassio

Contents

Part II Management

Contributors

Ana F. Abraido-Lanza, PhD Department of Sociomedical Science, Mailman School of Public Health, Columbia University, New York, NY, USA

Adria N. Armbrister, PhD Gender and Diversity Division, Social Sector, Inter-American Development Bank, Washington, DC, USA

Desiree R. Azizoddin, MA Department of Psychology, Loma Linda University, Loma Linda, CA, USA

Antoine R. Baldassari Thurston Arthritis Research Center, School of Medicine, University of North Carolina at Chapel Hill, Chapel Hill, NC, USA

Teresa J. Brady, PhD Arthritis Program, Centers for Disease Control and Prevention, Atlanta, GA, USA

Diana Taibi Buchanan, PhD, RN Department of Biobehavioral Nursing and Health Systems, School of Nursing, University of Washington, Seattle, WA, USA

Leigh F. Callahan, PhD Thurston Arthritis Research Center, School of Medicine, University of North Carolina at Chapel Hill, Chapel Hill, NC, USA

Department of Medicine and Social Medicine, University of North Carolina at Chapel Hill, Chapel Hill, NC, USA

Daniel J. Clauw, MD Department of Anesthesiology, University of Michigan Health System, Ann Arbor, MI, USA

Mary C. Davis, PhD Department of Psychology, Arizona State University, Tempe, AZ, USA

Hannah M. Fisher Department of Psychiatry and Behavioral Sciences, Duke University Medical Center, Durham, NC, USA

Melissa L. Harris, PhD Faculty of Health and Medicine, Research Centre for Gender, Health and Ageing, University of Newcastle, University Drive, Callaghan, NSW, Australia

M. Cameron Hay, PhD Department of Anthropology, Miami University, Oxford, OH, USA

Center for Culture and Health, Semel Institute for Neuroscience and Human Behavior, UCLA, Los Angeles, California, USA

Patricia Katz, PhD Department of Medicine, School of Medicine, University of California, San Francisco, San Francisco, CA, USA

Sarah A. Kelleher, PhD Department of Psychiatry and Behavioral Sciences, Duke University Medical Center, Durham, NC, USA

Dhwani J. Kothari, MA Department of Psychology, Arizona State University, Tempe, AZ, USA

Angelyna M. Lowe, MA Department of Psychology, Loma Linda University, Loma Linda, CA, USA

Faith S. Luyster, PhD School of Nursing, University of Pittsburgh, Pittsburgh, PA, USA

Perry M. Nicassio, PhD Department of Psychiatry, School of Medicine, University of California, Los Angeles, CA, USA

Kristine Phillips, MD, PhD Department of Internal Medicine (Rheumatology), University of Michigan Health System, Ann Arbor, MI, USA

Rebecca A. Shelby, PhD Department of Psychiatry and Behavioral Sciences, Duke University Medical Center, Durham, NC, USA

Tamara J. Somers, PhD Department of Psychiatry and Behavioral Sciences, Duke University Medical Center, Durham, NC, USA

John A. Sturgeon, PhD Department of Anesthesia, Perioperative, and Pain Medicine, Stanford University, Palo Alto, CA, USA

Lekeisha A. Sumner, PhD, ABPP Department of Psychology, Alliant International University, Los Angeles, CA, USA

Department of Psychiatry, University of California, Los Angeles, CA, USA

Kristina A. Theis, PhD Division of Population Health, Centers for Disease Control and Prevention, Atlanta, GA, USA

Kirti Thummala, MA Department of Psychology, Arizona State University, Tempe, AZ, USA

Cinnamon Westbrook, MA Department of Psychology, Loma Linda University, Loma Linda, CA, USA

David A. Williams, PhD Department of Anesthesiology, University of Michigan Health System, Ann Arbor, MI, USA

Alex J. Zautra, PhD Department of Psychology, Arizona State University, Tempe, AZ, USA

Part I

Psychosocial Factors

The Importance of the Biopsychosocial Model for Understanding the Adjustment to Arthritis

1

Lekeisha A. Sumner and Perry M. Nicassio

To be a prisoner held captive by one's own body is the ultimate betrayal. With chronic pain, one is not living. Only existing.

RA Patient

Introduction

The first cases of arthritis have been traced as far back as 4500 BC. Arthritis often causes severe pain and emotional suffering that may contribute to disability, interfere with physical mobility, and lead to declines in quality of life in many patients. Arthritic conditions account for some of the leading causes of years lived with disability worldwide, with elderly populations carrying a disproportionate share of the burden (Woolf & Pfleger, 2003). Due to medically related impairments, patients with arthritis may be unable to maintain gainful employment and, as a result, encounter significant financial losses. As such, treatment approaches today reflect the vast shifts in health and disease management seen in the health care system in recent decades that focus on prevention, management, and quality of life.

L.A. Sumner, PhD, ABPP (✉)
Department of Psychology, Alliant International University, Los Angeles, CA, USA

Department of Psychiatry, University of California, Los Angeles, CA, USA
e-mail: lsumner@mednet.ucla.edu

P.M. Nicassio, PhD
Department of Psychiatry, School of Medicine, University of California, Los Angeles, CA, USA
e-mail: pnicassio@mednet.ucla

Recognizing the global impact and scope of the devastation of arthritic conditions, the World Health Organization (WHO) and United Nations declared 2000–2010 The Bone and Joint Decade (WHO Scientific Group on the Burden of Musculoskeletal Conditions at the Start of the New Millennium, 2003). From these efforts, a number of global and national bone and joint initiatives have emerged with the goals of informing policy, raising public awareness, and advancing science to alleviate the physical and emotional suffering of those affected. Subsequently, scientific discovery in the understanding and treatment of arthritic conditions has grown substantially in the past several years, resulting in improved treatments to reduce disease activity, alleviate pain, and improve functioning. These discoveries were due, in part, to a growing appreciation for the heuristic and practical value of frameworks of disease and treatments that emphasize a decidedly comprehensive view of the patient and patient care. Yet, despite medical and technological advances in the detection, treatment, and management of arthritic conditions, challenges remain regarding how to translate this knowledge into clinical practice.

The biopsychosocial model, which ushered in a revolutionary paradigm of conceptualizing patient health and the way in which patients are treated, offers both a practical and holistic

P.M. Nicassio (ed.), *Psychosocial Factors in Arthritis*, DOI 10.1007/978-3-319-22858-7_1

perspective for addressing evaluation and treatment (Engel, 1977, 1980). For patients suffering from arthritic conditions, this is a particularly important and welcome change. However, greater awareness of the role of social, psychological, and behavioral factors in the trajectory of arthritis and treatment outcomes is needed. With the goal of facilitating a fuller understanding of the lived emotional and social experiences of patients affected by arthritis, clinicians become better equipped to demonstrate increased sensitivity to the needs of patients and develop tailored treatment interventions. A multidisciplinary approach is central to achieving these outcomes. Thus, this chapter seeks to achieve the following:

1. Provide a brief description of select arthritic conditions.
2. Discuss a conceptual overview of the biopsychosocial model of arthritic conditions, and how the model can be adopted to provide a clinically useful framework for facilitating adjustment and treatment.
3. Using rheumatoid arthritis as an exemplar, discuss empirical findings on the associations of psychological, social, behavioral, and cultural factors with health outcomes.
4. Highlight the utility of integrative approaches to the treatment and management of patients with arthritis.

Overview of Arthritic Conditions

Arthritic conditions are a group of approximately 110 diseases and syndromes associated with intense pain that usually worsens over time (Sangha, 2000). Prevalent and debilitating, they also contribute to the development of other medical comorbidities and, for many patients, significant functional impairments (Ang, Choi, Kroenke, & Wolfe, 2005; Joyce, Smith, Khandker, Melin, & Singh, 2009). Arthritis translates to mean "joint inflammation" and the word *rheuma* has been used to denote pain coursing through the bodily joints; hence, the unifying presentation of most musculoskeletal conditions includes inflammation and penetrating pain of the joints (Sangha, 2000).

Although rheumatic conditions can develop among individuals of any developmental stage, many of the most common forms afflict older adults. Of the 9.6 billion people expected to populate the earth by 2050, the percentage of individuals 60 years of age and over will increase from the current 11 % of the world's population to 20 % (UNFPA & HelpAge International, 2012). Subsequently, as individuals continue to live longer than ever and the aging population rises, the global prevalence of arthritic conditions is expected to increase (Woolf & Pfleger, 2003).

Osteoarthritis (OA) and rheumatoid arthritis (RA) are two of the most common forms of arthritis and have a high prevalence among elderly populations. Other frequently diagnosed arthritic conditions include juvenile arthritis, infectious arthritis, gout, and systemic lupus erythematosus (SLE or lupus). It is worth noting that definitions for many of these conditions vary considerably according to whether the patient is a child or adult. Historically, varying classifications of determining disease have also contributed to some inconsistency in definitions and prevalence estimates. The following section provides an overview of some of these common conditions.

Rheumatoid Arthritis

RA, one of the major musculoskeletal conditions and a systemic disease, is an inflammatory condition that is associated with increased risk for medical and psychiatric comorbidities, disability, and early mortality. Patients with RA experience chronic pain, fatigue, joint stiffness, and joint damage over many years that, without treatment, usually worsen over time (National Institutes of Health & National Institute of Arthritis and Musculoskeletal and Skin Diseases, 2014a, 2014b). While the etiology of RA remains largely unknown, genetic susceptibility is thought to play a role as a causal factor as the disease tends to run in families; however, research suggests that there is no single gene responsible for the onset of RA. Hormones related to the female gender have also been postulated to contribute to risk as women are disproportionately affected.

RA affects approximately 21 million individuals worldwide (UN World Population Database, 2004 revision). Many believe the first characterization of RA to occur in the Caraka Samhita, an ancient medical text from 123 AD, referring to bilateral joint pain in hands and feet that spreads through the body (Joshi, 2012). In 1859, as RA was starting to be seen and documented more frequently in western medicine, Dr. Alfred Garrod coined the term rheumatoid arthritis (Joshi, 2012). Many individuals with RA not only live with severe pain, fatigue, depression, and functional impairment but also encounter increased medical comorbidities and risk for early death (Ang et al., 2005; Joyce et al., 2009). Patients with RA tend to report lower levels of quality of life than patients with most other chronic diseases (Lundkvist, Kastäng, & Kobelt, 2008). Complicating treatment is determining a firm diagnosis early in the disease course as many symptoms of RA overlap with other conditions, such as SLE (Sangha, 2000). Although no cure exists, medical therapies and research have advanced considerably in recent decades and have been successful in reducing pain and disease activity. Yet, marked variability in treatment outcomes and subjective experiences of the condition persist, causing speculation on the part of health professionals regarding the factors that might account for such striking differences.

RA is a progressive and disabling autoimmune disease in which the immune system attacks the lining of joints and connective tissues, causing inflammation. There is a range of potentially debilitating symptoms: pain, inflammation at the joints, fatigue, limited movement around joints, swelling, and stiffness (National Rheumatoid Arthritis Society, n.d.). Worldwide, more than 20 million individuals are diagnosed with RA with rates expected to sharply increase as the population ages. Indeed, in the United States alone, more than a projected 67 million adults are expected to be diagnosed with RA by 2030 (Hootman & Helmick, 2006).

RA affects more women than men; likely as a result of sex hormones and other reproductive factors (Sangha, 2000). Its prevalence tends to rise with age, and obesity and smoking have been identified as risk factors (WHO Scientific Group on the Burden of Musculoskeletal Conditions at the Start of the New Millennium, 2003; Woolf & Pfleger, 2003). Although genetics are postulated to contribute to up to 60 % of the risk in developing RA, environmental factors, such as infections, chronic and extreme stress, trauma, and viruses are also believed to also play a role in the susceptibility to RA (MacGregor et al., 2000; National Rheumatoid Arthritis Society, n.d.). Interestingly, although precise estimates are difficult to formulate due to differences in classifications and methodology, available data indicate considerable variability regarding the incidence and prevalence of the disease, as well as life expectancy. For example, countries with low per capita income, such as Poland, have been observed to have an increased burden of RA (Lundkvist et al., 2008). Some Native American groups tend to have a higher prevalence than other ethnic groups while lower prevalence rates have been found in rural sub-Saharan Africa and Caribbean Blacks (Sangha, 2000; Silman & Hochberg, 1993). While the prevalence of RA is generally higher among persons from industrialized countries, it appears to be lower in developing nations and rural areas (Woolf & Pfleger, 2003).

Osteoarthritis (OA), the most common type of arthritis, is a degenerative joint disease that can affect any bodily joint but typically affects the hands, hips, knees, and spine. With the fastest growing prevalence among serious conditions worldwide, OA causes degradation of articular cartilage over time, resulting in bones rubbing up against one another leading to pain, joint swelling, tenderness, and limited mobility (Symmons, Mathers, & Pfleger, 2000; Wittenauer, Smith, & Aden, 2013). The Subcommittee on Osteoarthritis of the American College of Rheumatology Diagnostic and Therapeutic Criteria Committee (1986) defines OA as "A heterogeneous group of conditions that lead to joint symptoms and signs which are associated with defective integrity of articular cartilage, in addition to related changes in the underlying bone at the joint margins" (Altman et al., 1986).

An estimated 10 % of the world's population over age 60 experiences symptoms of OA. OA is more common among women above age 65 and more common among men below age 45. At least 10–15 % of individuals over 60 years of age are affected by OA globally (Lim & Lau, 2011). OA affects over 135 million people worldwide (WHO Scientific Group on the Burden of Musculoskeletal Conditions at the Start of the New Millennium, 2003). In addition to older age, obesity, inactivity, and joint injury are risk factors for OA (Felson, 1996; WHO Scientific Group on the Burden of Musculoskeletal Conditions at the Start of the New Millennium, 2003).

Juvenile Arthritis

Juvenile arthritis (JA) is a term used to describe a range of arthritic conditions occurring in children, ages 15 and below. Juvenile idiopathic arthritis (JIA), the most commonly occurring of these conditions affects approximately 1 in 1000 children, is an umbrella term used to characterize children with inflammatory arthritis whose etiology is unknown with a duration of at least 6 weeks (Manners & Bower, 2002). Patients with JA may experience deformity and destruction of the joints with intense and unpredictable pain resulting in short stature and psychological distress, especially depression. Interestingly, while as many as 60 % of those affected enter adulthood without active synovitis or functional limitations, adults commonly exhibit high levels of disability (Packham & Hall, 2002). As the condition progresses, the number of joints affected increases, resulting in restricted mobility in adulthood. Although there is some evidence for genetic vulnerability, the precise etiology of JA remains unknown (Manners & Bower, 2002).

Other Arthritic Conditions

Globally, gout is the most commonly occurring type of arthritis affecting 1–2 % of adults (Smith, az-Torne, Perez-Ruiz, & March, 2010). Gout was once believed to occur only among the wealthy as it was thought to have been caused by food and alcohol overconsumption, which only the wealthy could afford. It is now known that there is a genetic component in gout as the condition commonly occurs in families. Gout also is more prevalent in males between the ages of 40 and 50, individuals with metabolic disorders, and in those with medical conditions that cause renal insufficiency (e.g., hypertension, hypothyroidism). Substantial weight gain in early adulthood, obesity, exposure to toxins, diet, and alcohol consumption and renal insufficiency are all risk factors for developing gout. Certain foods, such as those containing high levels of sugar, red meats, and shellfish, as well as some medications and stress may trigger attacks, which typically occur at night. Common symptoms include acute join pain, swelling, usually in the knees, foot, and big toe that result from a buildup of uric acid crystals in the body. Unlike many other arthritic conditions, symptoms can go into and out of complete remission. As in other arthritic conditions, lifestyle changes, including weight management and nutrition, are essential to address in treatment. Individuals with gout are at increased risk for other medical conditions, such as Type 2 diabetes.

Infectious arthritis, also referred to as septic arthritis, is similar to most types of arthritis in that symptoms include swelling and pain in the joints, thereby restricting mobility (WHO Scientific Group on the Burden of Musculoskeletal Conditions at the Start of the New Millennium, 2003). However, it is also marked by damage of the cartilage and bone within the joint. Bacterial, viral, or fungal infections may trigger septic arthritis, especially those with staphylococcus aureus. Infants and older adults are most susceptible to this condition. Risk factors include having a chronic medical condition that affects the joints, such as RA, taking medications that suppress immune functioning such as those taken for RA, skin conditions, and a weakened immune system.

SLE is a chronic inflammatory condition in which the immune system attacks healthy tissues and cells throughout the body, which in turn, can affect skin, brain, joints, lungs, kidneys, blood vessels, and organs (National Institutes of Health & National Institute of Arthritis and Musculoskeletal and Skin Diseases, 2014a, 2014b). While there are many types of lupus, SLE is the most common type. Most patients affected by lupus experience periods of illness and remission. During times of illness, those impacted may report a range of symptoms, including debilitating levels of fatigue, swollen and painful joints and glands, fever, skin rashes, difficulty breathing and chest pains, sun sensitivity, swelling around the legs or eyes, oral ulcers, hair loss, color changes in fingers and toes, and renal problems. While anyone can develop lupus and the cause is unknown, women, and especially women of color, are at heightened risk for lupus. The diagnosis of lupus can take months and often years to make as a single test cannot determine a diagnosis. Thus, many laboratory tests (those that identify particular types of antibodies), patient history, and symptoms help to rule out other diagnoses and confirm a diagnosis of lupus.

The Biopsychosocial Model of Arthritis

Basic Tenets, Patient-Provider Interactions, and the Role of Culture/Ethnicity

Arthritic conditions affect individuals across every major life domain. While the etiology of many of the conditions remains unknown, lifestyle factors, genetic, and social–environmental factors all may play a role in disease onset, severity, and treatment response. Similarly, the potency of these factors, involving interrelationships among social, physiologic, biologic, environmental, and genetic systems can no longer be ignored by health care professions. Clinicians working with patients with arthritis conditions are often struck by the level of variability in patients' experiences, including role functioning, quality of life, and emotional adjustment. Variations in pain intensity and frequency, medial utilization, adjustment to illness, fragility to medical interventions, emotional distress, physical disability, and suffering are striking and common among patients with similar backgrounds and medical pathologies.

Over three decades ago, George Engel developed an integrated model of health that was in sharp contrast to the long-held views of the reductionist biomedical model based on Western science (Engel, 1977, 1980). Engel (1980) noted that bench scientists often rely on a dualistic mind-set and work in controlled circumstances where they are able to isolate components of disease. In contrast, he recognized that clinicians work in a dynamic and interactive system with humans in which many factors cannot be controlled or isolated, and acknowledged that optimal treatment outcomes must take into consideration patient-related processes. Thus, to understand variations in adjustment and treatment response, the biopsychosocial framework affirms the importance of a comprehensive paradigm that focuses on patients' experiences.

Engel (1977) postulated that in addition to the medical condition and biologic mechanisms of disease, greater attention to the complex and interactive role of a wide range of factors across multiple levels of patients' lives is needed in order to contextualize the impact of the condition and clinical outcomes. In the biopsychosocial model, there are subsystems within each larger system that can have ripple effects on other systems. Variables can affect health outcomes directly, or indirectly, through the influence of other variables. Accordingly, the model assumes that no single factor accounts for health outcomes. Rather, health outcomes are considered to be the product of the synergistic and sometimes reciprocal interaction of many factors. Importantly, the model offers clinicians a framework for gathering and organizing additional patient information. As opposed to the biomedical model which focuses only on biological, genetic, and physiological factors, the biopsychosocial framework addresses the effects of psychological, social, and cultural factors on health, and the associated potential feedback loops between both *disease* ("objective biological events," Turk & Monarch, 2002) and *illness* ("subjective experience of disease or self-attribution that a disease is present," Gatchel, Peng, Peters, Fuchs, & Turk, 2007). Not only does this approach situate the patient front and center in treatment, it represents a paradigm shift in which clinical awareness and knowledge play central roles in calibrating greater sensitivity to patient needs.

There is ample evidence supporting the associations of biological, social, and psychological domains in health and well-being in arthritis conditions. For example, in a large-scale observational study that relied on retrospective data from the World Mental Health Surveys of 18,309 adults, Von Korff et al. (2009) provided evidence of the association of childhood adversities, mental disorders, and risk for adult onset arthritis. After controlling for age, sex, and early onset mental disorders, results revealed that, relative to individuals with no childhood adversities, those with two childhood adversities had greater risk for adult-onset arthritis and those with three or more adversities had even greater risk. Moreover, after controlling for childhood adversities, early onset depression and anxiety disorders were associated with greater risk for adult-onset arthritis. While this research did not delineate causation among study variables, there is mounting evidence that adverse chronic psychological and environmental stress and adaptation to these stressors, genetic vulnerability, and health behaviors may all interact to modify the brain and physiological processes (sympathetic, neuroendocrine, and immune functioning), resulting in increased risk for diseases and mental disorders (Gatchel et al., 2007; Harris et al., 2013; McEwen, 2012).

Importantly, Engel envisioned a health care system that acknowledged the inherent dignity of patients and their active role in treatment. Moreover, the centrality of patient experiences and perspectives in diagnosis and treatment provide richly textured data to use in understanding patients' health and treatment planning. Empirical findings have confirmed the importance of considering patient perceptions about the quality of their health. Studies have shown health-related quality of life to be strikingly accurate in predicting health outcomes, and, in some populations (diabetes, arthritis), health care utilization and mortality (Mapes et al., 2003; Singh, Nelson, Fink, & Nichol, 2005).

Research has supported Engel's emphasis on the value of integrating a humanistic approach in health care as findings have consistently demonstrated that physician–patient interactions can affect adherence and have significant effects on patient health outcomes. In a landmark paper, Kaplan, Greenfield, and Ware (1989) examined the influence of physician–patient interactions on health outcomes across three domains in patients with chronic diseases: physiological (blood pressure or blood sugar), behavioral (functional status), and subjective (patient perception of overall health) in four clinical trials. The authors found the following to facilitate physician–patient interactions: more information provided to the patient by physicians, greater expression of emotion—either positive or negative—expressed by both physician and patient, more patient control, and greater conversation by the patient relative to the physician. These elements contributed to better functional and subjective health outcomes in patients. The authors concluded that control, communication, and affect are vital elements that affect the doctor–patient relationship.

Subsequent studies have confirmed that patients who trust their physicians have greater ease in disclosing information and adhering to treatment recommendations (Berrios-Rivera et al., 2006). In order to identify patient characteristics and components of the patient–doctor relationship associated with perceived trust in physicians, one U.S. study included an ethnically and socioeconomically diverse sample of patients diagnosed with inflammatory rheumatic diseases, rheumatoid arthritis, or SLE ($N=102$), all of whom had received care in publicly funded clinics by multiple physicians (Berrios-Rivera et al., 2006). Findings revealed that all components of the medical encounter (e.g., ethnicity, physician informativeness, physician sensitivity to patient concerns, patient-centered approach, disease activity, and patient trust in the health system) to contribute to patient trust in physicians. Results also indicated that severity of disease and patient perceptions of physician patient-centeredness were predictive of patient disclosure. Interestingly, gender and ethnicity appeared to influence patients' trust of physicians as African American and Latino men reported lower levels of trust in their physicians than African American women and Latina women, suggesting the need for health providers to demonstrate greater sensitivity to non-White patients. These findings illustrate the role of ethnicity and, likely cultural factors, in improving patient–provider communication.

Micro-level dimensions of the biopsychosocial framework also include interpersonal and systemic cultural insensitivity and discrimination, both deliberate and outside of conscious awareness. These factors account for considerable variance in outcomes and are reflective of broader societal problems that persist in the health care system (Institute of Medicine, 2002). Ethnic, gender, sexual, and other forms of bias and discrimination are not uncommon among health providers in the delivery of care and impede optimal outcomes in chronic pain populations. Even after symptom presentation and pain severity are controlled, gender and ethnicity of patients (e.g., women, African Americans) may adversely impact pain management decisions among physicians (Institute of Medicine, 2011). However, some studies have found that the significance of these findings is less pronounced among female physicians who demonstrate increased empathy in patient encounters relative to their male counterparts (Drwecki, Moore, Ward, & Prkachin, 2011; Weisse, Sorum, Sanders, & Syat, 2001).

Despite the burden and prevalence of pain conditions in ethnic minority communities, patients from these groups continue to receive inadequate health care, including undertreatment for pain (Institute of Medicine, 2002). For example, in the United States which has a significant history of ethnic discrimination, White Americans across the socioeconomic strata are more likely to receive higher quality of care relative to individuals from ethnically marginalized groups—even after controlling for confounding factors (Institute of Medicine, 2002, 2011; Mossey, 2011). Despite evidence that White Americans are at heightened risk of misusing pain prescription medications relative to ethnic minorities, White Americans have been found to receive better pain treatment, including prescriptions for higher dosages of pain and analgesic medications (Mossey, 2011). Negative stereotypes held by physicians based on which patients are most likely to overutilize and abuse pain medications, along with underreporting of pain intensity by the patients, have contributed to these findings. While African Americans and Latino chronic pain patients report higher levels of pain intensity and are at heightened risk for severe forms of pain than those from White populations in the United States, they are underprescribed opioid medications and receive worse quality of care (Anderson, Green, & Payne, 2009; Mossey, 2011; Reyes-Gibby, Aday, Todd, Cleeland, & Anderson, 2007). Given the preponderance of studies confirming bias and discrimination in health care, even the most well-intentioned and gifted providers will benefit from continued examination of their own biases and the impact of broader societal inequities and disparities in patients' presentations and delivery of care. Moreover, because these groups, along with women, are at heightened risk for incongruent physician–patient communication, they would benefit from an approach that emphasizes establishing trust.

In addition to the aforementioned examples illustrating the role of ethnic and gender discrimination in the delivery of care is the influence of cultural factors on other aspects of the disease experience. In an influential study on the role of cultural patterns in reactions to pain, anthropologist Zborowski (1952) interviewed 103 participants (87 patients in a VA hospitalization unit and 16 of their relatives or friends) from varying ethnic backgrounds—Irish Americans, Jewish Americans, Italian Americans, and Old Americans (those from white Protestant families who had been in the United States for at least three generations). Results showed both similarities and differences in the interpretation, meaning, and reactions to pain between ethnic groups. For instance, some ethnic groups viewed the ability to endure pain as a source of pride and strength while other groups ascribed meaning to the pain experience through a moral and religious prism (e.g., punishment from God, a test of faith). There was also variability in the groups in reference to how pain was expressed publicly (e.g., crying, stoicism, masking distress), preferences on social connections versus social withdrawal, and expectations for pain relief. In addition to variability by ethnicity, results also revealed some similarities in the implications of pain by social class. For example, substantial concern over loss of employment was reported from individuals from lower socioeconomic statuses. While the Zborowski study was criticized on methodological grounds (Kleinman, Brodwin, Good, & Good, 1992; Wolff & Langley, 1968), subsequent findings have confirmed the contributions of cultural norms in shaping the response to illness, including such factors as expressions of distress, coping, illness schemas, the meaning ascribed to illness, pain intensity and tolerance, and treatment-seeking (Bates, Edwards, & Anderson, 1993; Institute of Medicine, 2011).

It is important to remember that although cultural groups may vary in their response to the illness experience, stereotypes that reflect biases concerning how effective some groups function relative to others can interfere with treatment outcomes (Ludwig-Beymer, 2008). Therefore, clinicians are encouraged to be aware of the effect of cultural influences on how individual patients cope with illness, while being attentive to intragroup differences and similarities. From a macrolevel, inequities in health care are amplified by lack of insurance and access to quality care, particularly among low-income populations. A cohesive body of findings highlights the greater efficiency of care resulting in decreased need for referrals, better recovery, and improved emotional health when using a patient-centered approach, characterized by increased empathy and shared decision making in clinical encounters (Carr & Donovan, 1998; Stewart et al., 2000).

Building on the literature of patient outcomes, Borrell-Carrió, Suchman, and Epstein (2004) reviewed the biopsychosocial model from philosophical, scientific, and clinical perspectives. They concluded that the model would have greater utility for clinical practice by incorporating seven "pillars" of application. These pillars of clinical practice embrace a relational framework between health professionals and patients to sharpen diagnostic accuracy, treatment decisions, and greater collaboration between the practitioner and patient. The pillars include: (1) self-awareness; (2) active cultivation of trust; (3) an emotional style characterized by empathic curiosity; (4) self-calibration as a way to reduce bias; (5) educating the emotions to assist with diagnosis and forming therapeutic relationships (e.g., distress tolerance for ambiguity); (6) using informed intuition; and (7) communicating clinical evidence to foster dialogue, not just the mechanical application of protocol. They implore health professionals to consider patients' narratives of their condition as a method of understanding patients and their subjective experiences of pain, and gathering data to use for treatment planning. Moreover, health professionals are also to be mindful of the role of power in the patient–provider relationship and how this power is used to cope with the emotions of the patient and its influence on treatment options.

A convincing literature has emerged to support the heuristic value and clinical utility of the biopsychosocial model for the treatment of rheumatic conditions. As an illustration, Nicassio et al. (2011) examined the relationships between physical, psychological, and social factors and health-related quality of life and disability in a cross-sectional study that included a sample of 106 adults with RA. Using self-report measures that assessed disease activity by both patients and physicians, along with indicators of psychosocial functioning (e.g., coping, personal mastery, social network, perceived stress, illness beliefs, disability, and health-related quality of life), findings demonstrated that subjective personal resources were significantly associated with study outcomes. Specifically, lower self-reported disease activity was associated with higher levels of physical functioning, while higher disease activity and helplessness were associated with greater disability. Moreover, lower levels of self-reported disease activity, high personal mastery, and low perceived stress were significantly associated with better subjective mental health functioning. These findings underscore the independent and collective contributions of psychosocial variables to disability and health-related quality of life. Furthermore, the data also highlight the importance of assessing salient health outcomes from the patient's subjective perspective.

The Relevance of Other Psychosocial Factors

According to the WHO, "health is a state of complete physical, mental and social-wellbeing and not merely the absence of disease or infirmity" (Preamble to the Constitution of the WHO, 1946). The construct of health integrates social and emotional components and includes the subjective experiences of patients. Common to more recent conceptualizations of health, however, is an appreciation that health involves a dynamic process that occurs within a context that is significantly affected by emotional and social factors with increased emphasis on patients' ability to adapt (The Lancet Editorial, 2009; Üstün & Jakob, 2005). These recent conceptualizations are highly congruent with the major tenets of the biopsychosocial model.

Chronic medical illness has the potential to shatter patients' assumptions about the world, themselves, and their abilities, resulting in a decreased sense of self-worth and competence. Complicating adjustment to illness is the challenge of confronting the invisibility of suffering, disrupted autonomy, stigma, physical disability, job discrimination, and the chronicity and unpredictability of the condition. The adjustment to chronic illness occurs at the onset of symptoms and continues over time (Sharpe & Curran, 2006). The adjustment process involves the capacity of patients to accept their condition, cope with troublesome symptoms, and use personal and social resources to restore some balance to their lives. However, when patients find it difficult to perform even basic activities of daily living, such as bathing, dressing, walking, and traveling, personal coping and social resources become highly taxed, resulting in poorer quality of life. Adjustment to a chronic condition encompasses emotional, social, behavioral, cognitive, and physiological components (de Ridder, Geenen, Kuijer, & van Middendorp, 2008), all of which influence psychological morbidity and role functioning. Further, adjustment affects self-efficacy, referring to the belief of patients in their ability to complete goals and tasks, which in turn, predicts disease management via several pathways including treatment adherence, health beliefs and behaviors, motivation, health behaviors, and coping processes (Bandura, 1977, 1991).

Several domains influence the process of adjustment to chronic illness. A patient's cognitive schema of illness, usually influenced by pre-illness beliefs informed by social learning and attitudes, may play an important role. Patients are often faced with the challenge of reconciling discordant illness-related schemas with one's self-image and the reality of their prognosis. Adjustment requires that patients appraise the severity and meaning of the health threat that they confront. To achieve this, they must evaluate and mobilize their internal and external resources, calibrate the extent of personal control in managing the affective and physical components of illness, and ascribe meaning to salient changes in their health. As such, chronic conditions have a strong emotional component that has a bidirectional relationship with adjustment. Emotional and social factors can both influence, and be influenced by, disease course. Patients who struggle to adjust are likely to experience higher levels of stress and negative affective states. A biopsychosocial model of adjustment provides an organizing framework in which psychological variables are hypothesized to indirectly influence disease activity, pain, disability, and physical functioning, mediated through coping, appraisals, personality traits, and immune and neuroendocrine factors (Walker, Jackson, & Littlejohn, 2004). See Fig. 1.1 for a depiction of direct and indirect associations between these factors.

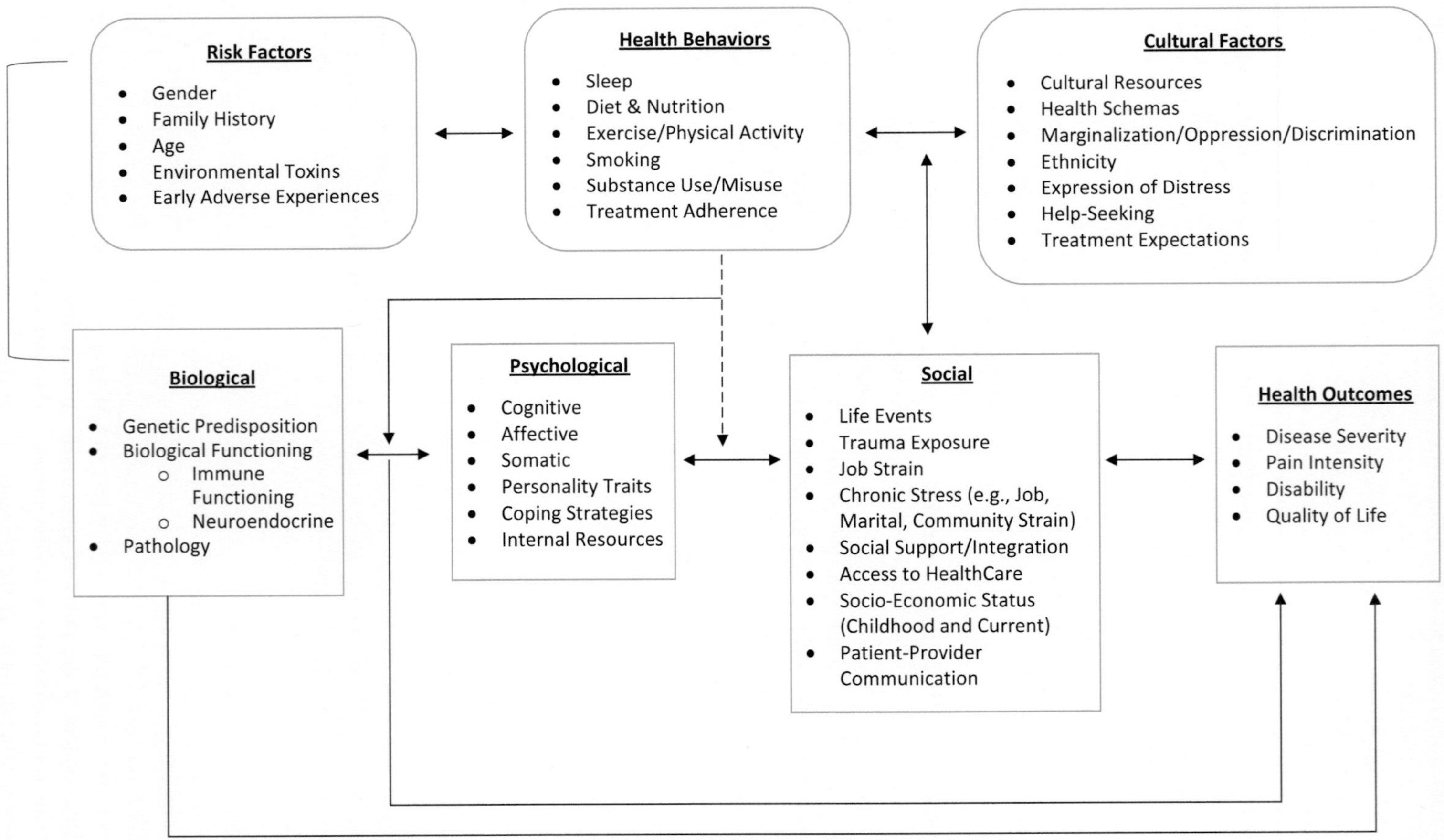

Fig. 1.1 Illustration of the conceptual model of the complex interaction between biological, psychological, social, and cultural processes contributing to health outcomes. These interactions are dynamic, often reciprocal and recursive, and shape outcomes over time

Interestingly, emerging evidence indicates that some individuals experience positive growth in dealing with the challenges of chronic illness. Some of the benefits patients have discovered include a renewed appreciation for relationships, and living a life with a deeper purpose, meaning, and sense of gratitude. There is some evidence that benefit finding among patients diagnosed with arthritis predicts positive affect and reduced disability (Danoff-Burg & Revenson, 2005; Evers et al., 2001). Although it is generally believed that the impact of benefit finding is most pronounced early in the course of disease, there is no known time frame for it to occur in order for patients to derive its salutary effects. These findings have important implications for the role of clinicians. In practice, this might entail a clinician embracing and querying existential factors in patients such as helping them explore and develop narratives centered on the *meaning* of their condition.

Taken together, research on the biopsychosocial framework on the adjustment to arthritis emphasizes the importance of the role of health care professionals in considering the time and processes needed for patients to adjust psychologically to their medical condition. This also entails considering the burden of treatments for patients and their capacity to fully engage in, and adhere, to treatment recommendations. The acknowledgement by clinicians that emotional distress is common among populations with arthritis also requires that emotional aspects of adjustment be addressed in order to optimize treatment outcomes. Psychological distress must be closely monitored and treated since it can interfere with social, behavioral, and biological mechanisms (e.g., sleep, fatigue, adherence, diet) that have significant effects on health outcomes, including premature death (Ang et al., 2005).

Psychosocial Resources, Stress, and Emotional Distress

Psychosocial resources, including coping style, self-efficacy, and cognitive schemas—influenced by cultural and social norms—contribute to emotional functioning. As an example, Covic, Adamson, Spence, and Howe (2003) used path analysis to determine whether physical disability, helplessness, and passive coping would predict pain and depression in a sample of 157 patients in both cross-sectional and longitudinal models. Findings revealed that helplessness and passive coping mediated the relationship between physical disability and future depression and pain. Both cross-sectional and longitudinal models accounted for significant variability in pain and depression, illustrating the central roles of illness beliefs and coping in depression among arthritis patients.

Chronic disease is a stressor that can leave patients feeling depleted cognitively, behaviorally, emotionally, and socially. Over a period of time, chronic stress strains the biological system and social relationships (Kiecolt-Glaser, 1999; Kiecolt-Glaser et al., 2003). For instance, in addition to the interruptions caused by medical difficulties, marriages and romantic partnerships become strained as a result of numerous changes in family and social systems, thereby amplifying the perception of stress and inducing feelings of social disconnectedness. For example, disability and health care costs create financial burdens for families: patients experience changes in sexual desire and functioning; and irritable mood and inability to complete household chores require other family members to take on additional responsibilities, thus, rearranging family dynamics. Chronic stress alters the sympathetic, neuroendocrine, and immune response to acute stress (Pike et al., 1997). Chronic psychological stress has been linked to negative affective states and clinical depression, along with increased disease risk and negative health-related outcomes in several diseases, including HIV/AIDS, cardiovascular disease, and cancer, which are likely the result of physiological and behavioral responses in adjusting to, and coping with, stress (Cohen et al., 2012; Cohen, Janicki-Deverts, & Miller, 2007). Moreover, disruptions in sleep, common among arthritis patients, further contribute to fatigue, inflammation, increased pain intensity, alterations in dietary habits, and depression (Irwin et al., 2012; Nicassio et al., 2012).

The Influence of Affective States, Coping, and Health Behaviors

Depression affects more than 350 million people worldwide and is an independent risk factor for early death and the second leading cause of disability (Symmons et al., 2000). Depression is usually recurrent and can present with somatic, behavioral, cognitive, and emotional symptoms. Individuals with early childhood adversities are more vulnerable to developing depression because early life experiences may interact with other psychological, biological, and environmental factors that diminish patients' resilience over the lifespan (McEwen, 2012).

Not surprisingly, depression exacerbates disease severity, interferes with medical adherence, nutrition, and quality of life, and compromises the response to medical treatments. Depression, along with ethnicity, has been found to significantly predict self-reported disease states among patients with SLE (Carr et al., 2011). Moreover, disease status among those with lupus predicts fatigue with helplessness and depression mediating the association (Tayer, Nicassio, Weisman, Schuman, & Daly, 2001). Overall, empirical data demonstrating that disease activity, health behaviors, and mood have direct and indirect associations with patient outcomes are robust and indicate the importance of assessment and treatment of these factors in clinical practice.

In addition to mood and immune factors, depression has molecular, genetic, social, and physiologic correlates and is associated with chronic exposure to stress (Slavich & Irwin, 2014). Patients at risk for depression may have some protective factors in reducing both risk and severity that can be targeted in treatment. For example, those with higher self-efficacy, social support, and social integration are less likely to become depressed than those who do not have these resources. However, perceived chronic stress heightens inflammation and may play a role in the onset of arthritis and depression (Slavich & Irwin, 2014).

What might explain the underlying mechanisms between psychosocial factors, especially depression and disease course? Recent theories on depression and inflammation integrate research findings on the social–environmental experiences to advance conceptualizations of the immunologic pathways and risk factors for depression. At the forefront of these theories is the social signal transduction theory of depression, which asserts that biological responses from social–environmental threats and lifelong exposure to stress in particular can result in changes in pro-inflammatory cytokines that can affect behavior, depression, and disease (Slavich & Irwin, 2014). Such changes further contribute to a patients' risk of withdrawing from their social network, which intensifies depressive symptoms (Eisenberger, Inagaki, Mashal, & Irwin, 2010). Relative to patients from upper socioeconomic backgrounds, those from socially and economically impoverished backgrounds, as well as those with histories of oppression and marginalization, are likelier to have had fewer educational and occupational opportunities for economic and social advancement, experience greater levels of chronic stress and trauma exposure, and reside in environments in which resources are lacking that could potentially act as stress buffers.

In addition to emotional distress and major depression, anxiety is common among populations afflicted with arthritis and may be even more prevalent than depression (Murphy, Sacks, Brady, Hootman, & Chapman, 2012). Negative affective states such as anxiety and depression are associated with increased pain severity, functional limitations, disrupted sleep cycles, maladaptive coping strategies (e.g., denying the severity of illness, smoking, alcohol, and sedentary lifestyle), decreased levels of self-efficacy and control of their medical condition, and increased utilization of health services. Unfortunately, despite the prevalence of depression and anxiety and their impact on health outcomes, most patients do not pursue treatment for these symptoms and they are not routinely assessed for these symptoms by their providers (Ang et al., 2005; Dickens, McGowan, Clark-Carter, & Francis, 2002; Gatchel, 2004; Matcham, Rayner, & Hotopf, 2013; Murphy et al., 2012; Nicassio, 2008). Thus, depression and anxiety often go undetected in clinical care.

Health behaviors and coping mechanisms may play important roles in immune function in arthritis.

Maladaptive coping and health behaviors, such as smoking, physical inactivity, overconsumption of alcohol, and high-fat processed foods have all been found to demonstrate direct and indirect relationships with disease risk, disability, pain sensitivity, and disease activity. For example, smoking causes inflammation and alters immune function (Arnson, Shoenfeld, & Amital, 2010). RA is substantially more common among smokers than nonsmokers, and individuals who smoke are at increased risk for developing a range of medical conditions, including rheumatoid arthritis, cancer, and cardiovascular disease (Costenbader, Feskanich, Mandl, & Karlson, 2006; U.S. Department of Health and Human Services, 2014). Recent findings indicate that smoking, along with genetic factors, increases vulnerability to developing arthritic conditions, exacerbates sleep problems, and also impairs the immune response (Arnson et al., 2010).

Lazarus and Folkman (1984) cite two major styles of coping when faced with a stressor, emotion-focused and problem-focused coping that can have a significant impact on psychosocial adjustment. People often choose which type of coping to use in response to a stressor based on several factors: the level of threat posed by the stressor, the type of stressor they are facing, level of arousal, the duration of the stressor, and perception of control of the stressor (Penley, Tomaka, & Wiebe, 2002). Emotion-focused coping is based on employing strategies, such as denial, distancing, avoidance, and wish-fulfillment fantasies, to minimize the deleterious effect of a stressor. While using these coping styles may be advantageous in minimizing emotional distress for a short period of time, the use of these strategies over the course of an illness can be maladaptive. For example, patients with arthritis who rely on denial may delay treatment seeking or fail to appreciate the severity of their condition.

Importantly, emotion-focused coping is associated with the development of depression and other forms of emotional distress and negative health outcomes (Penley et al., 2002). In problem-focused coping, individuals tend to acknowledge and confront a stressor directly before exploring its sources and ways of modifying the stressor. While problem-focused coping strategies may not always be feasible if the stressor is not controllable, in general, patients who adopt a problem-focused approach are likely to have better health outcomes (Penley et al., 2002).

Treatment Considerations

In addition to structural pathology and tissue damage, disease detection, assessment, management, and treatment outcomes may be further affected by numerous factors: individual material, and psychological resources, environmental exposure to toxins, patient–provider relationships, divergent perspectives of health and etiology of symptoms embedded through cultural and social norms, and medical knowledge and treatment expectations (Carr & Donovan, 1998; Felson, 1996; Kiecolt-Glaser, 1999; McEwen, 2012). Patients with arthritis often have comorbid medical problems such as diabetes, lung complications, and heart disease, all of which may be adversely impacted by emotional distress. Not surprisingly then, multidisciplinary approaches are needed to optimize treatment out comes. Even with the advent of increasingly effective medications that can slow deterioration of the joints and tissues and provide pain relief, the side effects of disease-modifying medications can be serious and create other health risks. Moreover, a considerable percentage of patients do not respond effectively to disease-modifying medications. This knowledge further underscores the complexities of arthritic conditions and the need to broaden traditional treatment approaches that rely solely on medication.

Because psychosocial (e.g., emotion, cognition), socio-demographic factors (e.g., socioeconomic status, ethnicity), and health behaviors (e.g., nutrition, physical activity, smoking, sleep) have both emotional and physiological consequences, the reliance on medication alone to treat depression and anxiety is insufficient. There is already compelling evidence that psychological and stress management interventions and other mind-body therapies can lead to improvements in both psychological well-being and health outcomes (Hewlett et al., 2011; Morgan, Irwin, Chung, & Wang, 2014; Nicassio, 2010).

Due to the high degree of psychiatric comorbidity in arthritis, it is important for clinicians to evaluate the psychosocial functioning of patients in the rheumatology setting during the first visit and on an ongoing basis thereafter (Harris et al., 2013). Even if symptom severity does not meet diagnostic criteria for a psychiatric disorder, screenings for sleep quality, sexual functioning, and levels of depression and emotional distress will highlight the need for potential psychological interventions and provide essential data for identifying barriers to effective medical treatment.

In conclusion, arthritic conditions have the potential to interfere with virtually every domain of patients' lives and exert a stressful impact on their families. The biopsychosocial model has advanced our ability to develop more sophisticated formulations of our patients, appreciate variability in their subjective experiences and outcomes, and increase awareness on the part of health professionals that transdisciplinary care is a vital component to restoring functioning, decreasing disability, and improving health outcomes. We recognize, more than ever, that medical treatments, while imperative, are insufficient to address all the factors that affect health outcomes in arthritis or the impact of having arthritis. In an effort to help patients maximize their functioning and lead productive lives, health professionals must embrace and investigate the interactions of biological, social, psychological, and cultural systems related to arthritis and identify factors within those systems that should be targeted for treatment through a multidisciplinary approach.

Key Points

- Arthritic conditions are highly prevalent and are among the leading causes of disability worldwide.
- The direct and indirect interrelationships among disease, immune functioning, brain functioning, mental distress, social functioning, and adherence are well established and modulate disease trajectories. Treatments must consider several systems concurrently to prevent and modulate changes within systems.
- Comorbid medical conditions, along with social and environmental factors, exacerbate chronic stress burden, emotional distress, and behavioral health risks.
- Pharmacological treatments alone are insufficient to treat arthritis. Applying the biopsychosocial model of care and management requires a transdisciplinary approach that may include care from a variety of health professionals.
- Behavioral and psychotherapeutic interventions have demonstrated effectiveness in improving health outcomes in patients with chronic disease and decreasing health costs.
- Health behaviors should be assessed as they may increase inflammation, impair treatment response, and affect health outcomes.

Additional Resources for Practitioners

- International Association for the Study of Pain
- www.isap-pain.org
- Bone and Joint Decade—Global Alliance for Musculoskeletal Health
- http://bjdonline.org
- Rheumatology News
- http://www.imng.com

References

Altman, R., Asch, E., Bloch, D., Bole, G., Borenstein, D., Brandt, K., … Wolfe, F. (1986). Development of criteria for the classification and reporting of osteoarthritis: Classification of osteoarthritis of the knee. *Arthritis & Rheumatism, 29*(8), 1039–1049. doi:10.1002/art.1780290816.

Anderson, K. O., Green, C. R., & Payne, R. (2009). Racial and ethnic disparities in pain: Causes and consequences of unequal care. *The Journal of Pain, 10*(12), 1187–1204. doi:10.1016/j.jpain.2009.10.002.

Ang, D. C., Choi, H., Kroenke, K., & Wolfe, F. (2005). Comorbid depression is an independent risk factor for mortality in patients with rheumatoid arthritis. *Journal of Rheumatology, 32*(6), 1013–1019. Retrieved from http://www.jrheum.org/.

Arnson, Y., Shoenfeld, Y., & Amital, H. (2010). Effects of tobacco smoke on immunity, inflammation and autoimmunity. *Journal of Autoimmunity, 34*(3), J258–J265. doi:10.1016/j.jaut.2009.12.003.

Bandura, A. (1977). Self-efficacy: Toward a unifying theory of behavioral change. *Psychological Review, 84*(2), 191–215. doi:10.1037//0033-295X.84.2.191.

Bandura, A. (1991). Self-efficacy mechanism in physiological activation and health-promoting behavior. In I. V. Madden (Ed.), *Neurobiology of learning, emotion and affect* (pp. 229–269). New York, NY: Raven.

Bates, M. S., Edwards, W. T., & Anderson, K. O. (1993). Ethnocultural influences on variation in chronic pain perception. *Pain, 52*, 101–112.

Berrios-Rivera, J. P., Street, R. L., Popa-Lisseanu M. G. G., Kallen, M. A., Richardson, M. N., Janssen, N. M., … Suarez-Almazor, M. E. (2006). Trust in physicians and elements of the medical interaction in patients with rheumatoid arthritis and systemic lupus erythematosus. *Arthritis and Rheumatism, 55*(3), 385–393. doi:10.1002/art.21988.

Borrell-Carrió, F., Suchman, A. L., & Epstein, R. M. (2004). The biopsychosocial model 25 years later: Principles, practice, and scientific inquiry. *Annals of Family Medicine, 2*(6), 576–582. doi:10.1370/afm.245.

Carr, A. J., & Donovan, J. L., (1998). Why doctors and patients disagree. *Rheumatology, 37*(1), 1a–a6. doi:10.1093/rheumatology/37.1.1a.

Carr, F. N., Nicassio, P. M., Ishimori, M. L., Moldovan, I., Katsaros, E., Torralba, K., … Weisman, M. H. (2011). Depression predicts self-reported disease activity in systemic lupus erythematosus. *Lupus, 20*(1), 80–84. doi:10.1177/0961203310378672.

Cohen, S., Janicki-Deverts, D., Doyle, W. J., Miller, G. E., Frank, E., Rabin, B. S., & Turner, R. B. (2012). Chronic stress, glucocorticoid receptor resistance, inflammation, and disease risk. *Proceedings of the National Academy of Sciences of the United States of America, 109*(16), 5995–5999. doi:10.1073/pnas.1118355109.

Cohen, S., Janicki-Deverts, D., & Miller, G. E. (2007). Psychological stress and disease. *Journal of the American Medical Association, 298*(14), 1685–1687. doi:10.1001/jama.298.14.1685.

Costenbader, K. H., Feskanich, D., Mandl, L. A., & Karlson, E. W. (2006). Smoking intensity, duration, and cessation, and the risk of rheumatoid arthritis in women. *The American Journal of Medicine, 119*(6), 503.e1–503.e9. doi:10.1016/j.amjmed.2005.09.053.

Covic, T., Adamson, B., Spence, D., & Howe, G. (2003). A biopsychosocial model of pain and depression in rheumatoid arthritis: A 12-month longitudinal study. *Rheumatology, 42*, 1287–1297. doi:10.1093/rheumatology/keg369.

Danoff-Burg, S., & Revenson, T. A. (2005). Benefit-finding among patients with rheumatoid arthritis: Positive effects on interpersonal relationships. *Journal of Behavioral Medicine, 28*(1), 91–103. Retrieved from http://www.springer.com/medicine/journal/10865.

de Ridder, D., Geenen, R., Kuijer, R., & van Middendorp, H. (2008). Psychological adjustment to chronic disease. *The Lancet, 372*(9634), 246–255. doi:10.1016/S0140-6736(08)61078-8.

Dickens, C., McGowan, L., Clark-Carter, D., & Francis, C. (2002). Depression in rheumatoid arthritis: A systematic review of the literature with meta-analysis. *Psychosomatic Medicine, 64*(1), 52–60.

Drwecki, B. B., Moore, C. F., Ward, S. E., & Prkachin, K. M. (2011). Reducing racial disparities in pain treatment: The role of empathy and perspective-taking. *Pain, 152*(5), 1001–1006. doi:10.1016/j.pain.2010.12.005.

Eisenberger, N. I., Inagaki, T. K., Mashal, N. M., & Irwin, M. R. (2010). Inflammation and social experience: An inflammatory challenge induces feelings of social disconnection in addition to depressed mood. *Brain, Behavior, and Immunity, 24*(4), 558–563. doi:10.1016/j.bbi.2009.12.009.

Engel, G. (1977). The need for a new medical model: A challenge for biomedicine. *Science, 196*, 129–136.

Engel, G. (1980). The clinical application of the biopsychosocial model. *The American Journal of Psychiatry, 137*(5), 535–544.

Evers, A. W., Kraaimaat, F. W., van Lankveld, W., Jongen, P. J., Jacobs, J. W., & Bijlsma, J. W. (2001). Beyond unfavorable thinking: The illness cognitive questionnaire for chronic diseases. *Journal of Consulting and Clinical Psychology, 69*(6), 1026–1036. doi:10.1037/0022-006X.69.6.1026.

Felson, D. T. (1996). Does excess weight cause osteoarthritis, and if so, why? *Annals of the Rheumatic Disease, 55*(1), 668–670. doi:10.1146/annurev.immunol.14.1.397.

Gatchel, R. J. (2004). Comorbidity of chronic pain and mental health disorders: The biopsychosocial perspective. *American Psychologist, 59*(8), 795–805. doi:10.1037/0003-066X.59.8.795.

Gatchel, R. J., Peng, Y. B., Peters, M. L., Fuchs, P. N., & Turk, D. C. (2007). The biopsychosocial approach to chronic pain: Scientific advances and future directions. *Psychological Bulletin, 133*(4), 581–624. doi:10.1037/0033-2909.133.4.4581.

Harris, M. H., Loxton, D., Sibbritt, D. W., & Byles, J. E. (2013). The influence of perceived stress on the onset of arthritis in women: Findings from the Australian Longitudinal Study on Women's Health. *Annals of Behavioral Medicine, 46*(1), 9–18. doi:10.1007/s12160-013-9478-6.

Hewlett, S., Ambler, N., Almeida, C., Cliss, A., Hammond, A., Kitchen, K., … Pollock, J. (2011). Self-management of fatigue in rheumatoid arthritis: A randomised controlled trial of group cognitive-behavioural therapy. *Annals of the Rheumatic Diseases, 70*(6), 1060–1067. doi:10.1136/ard.2010.144691.

Hootman, J. M., & Helmick, C. G. (2006). Projections of US prevalence of arthritis and associated activity limitations. *Arthritis & Rheumatism, 54*(1), 226–229. doi:10.1002/art.21562.

Institute of Medicine. (2002). *Unequal treatment: What healthcare providers need to know about racial and ethnic disparities in health care*. Washington, DC: National Academies Press.

Institute of Medicine. (2011). *Relieving pain in America: A blueprint for transforming prevention, care, education and research*. Washington, DC: National Academies Press.

Irwin, M. R., Olmstead, R., Carrillo, C., Sadeghi, N., FitzGerald, J. D., Ranganath, V. K., & Nicassio, P. M. (2012). Sleep loss exacerbates fatigue, depression, and pain in rheumatoid arthritis. *Sleep, 35*(4), 537–543. doi:10.5665/sleep.1742.

Joshi, V. R. (2012). Rheumatology, past, present and future. *The Journal of the Association of Physicians of India, 60*, 21–24.

Joyce, A. T., Smith, P., Khandker, R., Melin, J. M., & Singh, A. (2009). Hidden cost of rheumatoid arthritis (RA): Estimating cost of comorbid cardiovascular disease and depression among patients with RA. *The Journal of Rheumatology, 36*(4), 743–752. doi:10.3899/jrheum.08670.

Kaplan, S. H., Greenfield, S., & Ware, J. E. (1989). Assessing the effects of physician-patient interactions on the outcomes of chronic disease. *Medical Care, 27*(3), S110–S127.

Kiecolt-Glaser, J. (1999). Stress, personal relationships, and immune function: Health implications. *Brain, Behavior, and Immunity, 13*(1), 61–72. doi:10.1006/brbi.1999.0552.

Kiecolt-Glaser, J. K., Preacher, K. J., MacCallum, R. C., Atkinson, C., Malarkey, W. B., & Glaser, R. (2003). Chronic stress and age-related increases in the proinflammatory cytokine IL-6. *Proceedings of the National Academy of Sciences of the United States of America, 100*(15), 9090–9095. doi:10.1073/pnas.1531903100.

Kleinman, A., Brodwin, P. E., Good, B. J., & Good, M. D. V. (1992). Pain as human experience: An introduction. In M. D. V. Good, P. E. Brodwin, B. J. Good, & A. Kleinman (Eds.), *Pain as human experience: An anthropological perspective* (pp. 1–28). London, England: University of California Press.

Lazarus, R. S., & Folkman, S. (1984). *Stress, appraisal, and coping*. New York, NY: Springer.

Lim, K., & Lau, C. (2011). Perception is everything: OA is exciting. *International Journal of Rheumatic Diseases, 14*(2), 111–112. doi:10.1111/j.1756-185X.2011.01614.x.

Ludwig-Beymer, P. (2008). Transcultural aspects of pain. In M. M. Andrews & J. S. Boyle (Eds.), *Transcultural concepts in nursing care* (5th ed.). Philadelphia, PA: Lippincott Williams & Wilkins.

Lundkvist, J., Kastäng, F., & Kobelt, G. (2008). The burden of rheumatoid arthritis and access to treatment: Health burden and costs. *The European Journal of Health Economics, 8*(Suppl 2), S49–S60. doi:10.1007/s10198-007-0088-8.

MacGregor, A. J., Snieder, H., Rigby, A. S., Koskenvuo, M., Kaprio, J., Aho, K, & Silman, A. J. (2000). Characterizing the quantitative genetic contribution to rheumatoid arthritis using data from twins. *Arthritis and Rheumatism, 43*, 30–37.

Manners, P. J., & Bower, C. (2002). Worldwide prevalence of juvenile arthritis: Why does it vary so much? *Journal of Rheumatology, 29*(7), 1520–1530.

Mapes, D. L., Lopes, A. A., Satayathum, S., McCollough, K. P., Goodkin, D. A., Locatelli, F., … Port, F. K. (2003). Health-related quality of life as a predictor of mortality and hospitalization: The dialysis outcomes and practice patterns study (DOPPS). *Kidney International, 64*(1), 339–340. doi:10.1046/j.1523-1755.2003.00072.x.

Matcham, F., Rayner, S. S., & Hotopf, M. (2013). The prevalence of depression in rheumatoid arthritis: A systematic review and meta-analysis. *Rheumatology, 52*(12), 2136–2148. doi:10.1093/rheumatology/ket169.

McEwen, B. S. (2012). Brain on stress: How the social environment gets under the skin. *Proceedings of the National Academy of Sciences of the United States of America, 109*(Suppl 2), 17180–17185. doi:10.1073/pnas.1121254109.

Morgan, N., Irwin, M. R., Chung, M., & Wang, C. (2014). The effects of mind-body therapies on the immune system: Meta-analysis. *PLoS One, 9*(7), e100903. doi:10.1371/journal.pone.0100903.

Mossey, J. M. (2011). Defining racial and ethnic minorities in pain management. *Clinical Orthopaedics and Related Research, 469*(7), 1859–1870. doi:10.1007/s11999-011-1770-9.

Murphy, L. B., Sacks, J. J., Brady, T. J., Hootman, J. M., & Chapman, D. P. (2012). Anxiety and depression among US adults with arthritis: Prevalence and correlates. *Arthritis Care & Research, 647*(7), 968–976. doi:10.1002/acr.21685.

National Institutes of Health & National Institute of Arthritis and Musculoskeletal and Skin Diseases. (2014, August). *Rheumatoid arthritis: Handout on health* (NIH Publication No. 14-4179). Retrieved June 22, 2015, from http://www.niams.nih.gov/Health_Info/Rheumatic_Disease/default.asp

National Institutes of Health & National Institute of Arthritis and Musculoskeletal and Skin Diseases. (2014, August). *Handout on health: Systemic lupus erythematosus* (NIH Publication No. 14-4179). Retrieved June 22, 2015, from http://www.niams.nih.gov/Health_Info/Lupus/default.asp

National Rheumatoid Arthritis Society. (n.d.). *What is RA?* Retrieved from http://www.nras.org.uk/what-is-ra-article#symptoms

Nicassio, P. M. (2008). The problem of detecting and managing depression in the rheumatology clinic. *Arthritis and Rheumatism, 59*(2), 155–158. doi:10.1002/art.23348

Nicassio, P. M. (2010). Arthritis and psychiatric disorders: Disentangling the relationship. *Journal of Psychosomatic Research, 68*(2), 183–185. doi:10.1016/j.jpsychores.2009.09.008

Nicassio, P. M., Kay, M. A., Custodio, M. K., Irwin, M. R., Olmstead, R., & Weisman, M. H. (2011). An evaluation of a biopsychosocial framework for health-related quality of life and disability in rheumatoid arthritis. *Journal of Psychosomatic Research, 71*(2), 79–85. doi:10.1016/j.jpsychores.2011.01.008.

Nicassio, P. M., Ormseth, S. R., Custodio, M. K., Irwin, M. R., Olmstead, R., & Weisman, M. H. (2012). A multidimensional model of fatigue in patients with rheumatoid arthritis. *The Journal of Rheumatology, 39*(9), 1807–1813. doi:10.3899/jrheum.111068.

Packham, J. C., & Hall, M. A. (2002). Long-term follow-up of 246 adults with juvenile idiopath arthritis: Functional outcome. *Rheumatology (Oxford), 41*(12), 1428–1435. doi:10.1093/rheumatology/41.12.1428

Penley, J. A., Tomaka, J., & Wiebe, J. S. (2002). The association of coping to physical and psychological health outcomes: A meta-analytic review. *Journal of Behavioral Medicine, 25*(6), 551–603.

Pike, J. L., Smith, T. L., Hauger, R. L., Nicassio, P. M., Patterson T. L., McClintick, J., … Irwin, M. R. (1997). Chronic life stress alters sympathetic, neuroendocrine, and immune responsivity to an acute psychological stressor in humans. *Psychosomatic medicine, 59*(4), 447–457.

Preamble to the Constitution of the World Health Organization as adopted by the International Health Conference, New York, 19–22, 1946; signed on 22 July 1946 by the representatives of 61 States (Official Records of the World Health Organization, no. 2, p. 100) and entered into force on April 7, 1948. Retrieved from http://www.who.int/governance/eb/who_constitution_en.pdf

Reyes-Gibby, C. C., Aday, L. A., Todd, K. H., Cleeland, C. S., & Anderson, K. O. (2007). Pain in aging community-dwelling adults in the United States: Non-Hispanic whites, non-Hispanic blacks, and Hispanics. *The Journal of Pain, 8*, 75–84. doi:10.1016/j.jpain.2006.06.002.

Sangha, O. (2000). Epidemiology of rheumatic diseases. *Rheumatology, 39*(Suppl 2), 3–12.

Sharpe, L., & Curran, L. (2006). Understanding the process of adjustment to illness. *Social Science & Medicine, 62*(5), 1153–1166. doi:10.1016/j.socscimed.2005.07.010.

Silman, A. J., & Hochberg, M. C. (1993). *Epidemiology of the rheumatic diseases*. Oxford, England: Oxford University Press.

Singh, J. A., Nelson, D. B., Fink, H., & Nichol, K. L. (2005). Health-related quality of life predicts future health care utilization and mortality in veterans with self-reported physician-diagnosed arthritis: The veterans arthritis quality of life study. *Seminars in Arthritis and Rheumatism, 34*(5), 755–765. doi:10.1016/j.semarthrit.2004.08.001.

Slavich, G. M., & Irwin, M. R. (2014). From stress to inflammation and major depressive disorder: A social signal transduction theory of depression. *Psychological Bulletin, 140*(3), 774–815. doi:10.1037/a0035302.

Smith, E. U., az-Torne, C., Perez-Ruiz, F., & March, L. M. (2010). Epidemiology of gout: An update. *Best Practice & Research. Clinical Rheumatology, 24*, 811–827.

Stewart, M., Brown, J. B., Donner, A., McWhinney, I. R., Oates, J., Weston, W. W., & Jordan, J. (2000). The impact of patient-centered care on outcomes. *Journal of Family Practice, 49*(9), 796–804.

Symmons, D., Mathers, C., & Pfleger, B. (2000). The global burden of rheumatoid arthritis in the year 2000. Global burden of disease 2000. Geneva, Switzerland: World Health Organization.

Tayer, W. G., Nicassio, P. M., Weisman, M. H., Schuman, C., & Daly, J. (2001). Disease status predicts fatigue in systemic lupus erythematosus. *The Journal of Rheumatology, 28*(9), 1999–2007.

The Lancet Editorial. (2009). What is health? The ability to adapt. *The Lancet, 373*(9666), 781. doi:10.1016/S0140-6736(09)60456-6.

Turk, D. C., & Monarch, E. S. (2002). Biopsychosocial perspective on chronic pain. In D. C. Turk & R. J. Gatchel (Eds.), *Psychological approaches to pain management: A practitioner's handbook* (2nd ed., pp. 3–30). New York, NY: Guildford Press.

U.S. Department of Health and Human Services. (2014). *The health consequences of smoking—50 years of progress: A report of the Surgeon General.* Atlanta, GA: U.S. Department of Health and Human Services, Centers for Disease Control and Prevention, National Center for Chronic Disease Prevention and Health Promotion, Office on Smoking and Health. Retrieved May 8, 2015, from http://www.cdc.gov/tobacco/data_statistics/sgr/50th-anniversary/index.htm

UNFPA & HelpAge International. (2012). *Ageing in the twenty-first century: A celebration and a challenge.* Retrieved from http://unfpa.org/ageingreport/

Üstün, B., & Jakob, R. (2005). Re-defining 'Health.'. *Bulletin of the World Health Organization, 83*, 802.

Von Korff, M., Alonso, J., Ormel, A., Angermeyer, M., Bruffaerts, R., Fleiz, C., … Uda, H. (2009). Childhood psychosocial stressors and adult onset arthritis: Broad spectrum risk factors and allostatic load. *Pain, 143*(1–2), 76–83. doi:10.1016/j.pain.2009.01.034.

Walker, J. G., Jackson, H. J., & Littlejohn, G. O. (2004). Models of adjustment to chronic illness: Using the example of rheumatoid arthritis. *Clinical Psychology Review, 24*(4), 461–488. doi:10.1016/j.cpr.2004.03.001.

Weisse, C. S., Sorum, P. C., Sanders, K. N., & Syat, B. L. (2001). Do gender and race affect decisions about pain management? *Journal of General Internal Medicine, 16*(4), 211–217. doi:10.1046/j.1525-1497.2001.016004211.x.

WHO Scientific Group on the Burden of Musculoskeletal Conditions at the Start of the New Millennium. (2003). *Burden of musculoskeletal conditions at the start of the new millennium* (WHO Technical Report Series 919). Geneva, Switzerland: World Health Organization. Retrieved from http://whqlibdoc.who.int/trs/WHO_TRS_919.pdf

Wittenauer, R., Smith, L., & Aden, K. (2013). *Update on 2004 background paper, BP 6.12 osteoarthritis*. Retrieved from World Health Organization, http://www.who.int/medicines/areas/priority_medicines/BP6_12Osteo.pdf

Wolff, B. B., & Langley, S. (1968). Cultural factors and the response to pain: A review. *American Anthropologist, 70*, 494–501.

Woolf, A. D., & Pfleger, B. (2003). Burden of musculoskeletal conditions. *Bulletin of World Health Organization, 81*(9), 646–656. Retrieved from http://www.who.int/bulletin/volumes/81/9/Woolf.pdf

Zborowski, M. (1952). Cultural components in response to pain. *Journal of Social Issues, 8*(4), 16–30.

Mechanisms of Arthritis Pain

2

David A. Williams, Kristine Phillips, and Daniel J. Clauw

Abbreviations

5HTR2A	Serotonin receptor gene polymorphism
a.Insula	Anterior insula
ACC	Anterior cingulate cortex
ADRB2	Adrenoceptor beta-2 protein coding gene
CACNA2D3	Calcium channel, voltage-dependent, alpha 2/Delta subunit 3 gene
CBT	Cognitive behavioral therapy
CNS	Central nervous system
COMT	Catechol-*O*-methyltransferase gene
CPM	Conditioned pain modulation
DMARD	Disease-modifying antirheumatic drugs
DNIC	Diffuse noxious inhibitory controls
FM	Fibromyalgia
GCH1	GTP cyclohydrolase I gene
IASP	International Association for the Study of Pain
IBS	Irritable bowel syndrome
IC	Interstitial cystitis
IL-1	Interleukin-1
IL-6	Interleukin-6
KCNS1	Potassium voltage-gated channel delayed rectifier, subfamily S, member 1 gene
NSAID	Nonsteroidal anti-inflammatory drug
OA	Osteoarthritis
OPRM1	Opioid receptor, mu1 gene
p.Insula	Posterior insula
PAG	Periaqueductal gray
PFC	Prefrontal cortex
pH	Power of hydrogen (scale of acidity and alkalinity)
QST	Quantitative sensory testing
RA	Rheumatoid arthritis
S1	Somatosensory cortex 1
S2	Somatosensory cortex 2
SNRI	Serotonin norepinephrine reuptake inhibitor
TCA	Tricyclic antidepressant
TMD	Temporomandibular joint disorder
TNF	Tumor necrosis factor

D.A. Williams, PhD (✉) • D.J. Clauw, MD
Department of Anesthesiology, University of Michigan Health System, 24 Frank Lloyd Wright Drive, P.O. Box 385, Lobby M, Ann Arbor, MI 48106, USA
e-mail: daveawms@umich.edu

K. Phillips, MD, PhD
Department of Internal Medicine (Rheumatology), University of Michigan Health System, Ann Arbor, MI 48106, USA

P.M. Nicassio (ed.), *Psychosocial Factors in Arthritis*, DOI 10.1007/978-3-319-22858-7_2

Introduction

A survey by the Centers for Disease Control and Prevention conducted between 2007 and 2009 estimates that one in five U.S. adults has a diagnosis of arthritis (CDC, 2010). By age 65 and older, nearly half of adults will report having arthritis (CDC, 2013). Although there are over 100 types of arthritis, the two most common forms are osteoarthritis (OA) with an estimated 27 million afflicted (Lawrence et al., 2008) and rheumatoid arthritis (RA) with 1.5 million individuals (Myasoedova, Crowson, Kremers, Therneau, & Gabriel, 2010). Most patients and clinicians routinely suspect that the pain of arthritis is directly attributable to ongoing peripheral damage to joints/bone or to inflammation. It has been evident for some time however, that there are no chronic pain conditions in which the degree of tissue damage or inflammation alone (e.g., as measured by radiographs, neuroimaging techniques, or endoscopy) accurately predicts the presence or severity of pain (Phillips & Clauw, 2013). Thus, while peripheral factors such as damage or inflammation are certainly part of the equation, once this information is transferred to the central nervous system (CNS), other CNS-related factors influence the formation of the pain percept. The important interface between the periphery and the CNS make most forms of chronic pain "mixed" pain states where each system contributes in varying degrees to the overall perception of pain. For any given individual, the balance of peripheral and central influences is likely to be determined by genetic, individual, and environmental factors.

This chapter begins with a description of pain mechanisms and uses nociceptive pain as the model of pain that is most relevant for an initial understanding of arthritis pain. The chapter then describes the mechanisms of central pain augmentation that may further explain cases of arthritis pain where there is discordance between the degree of observable peripheral damage and the magnitude of pain. Finally, the chapter concludes with a brief discussion of treatment approaches that may be relevant in addressing CNS components of pain.

Mechanisms of Pain

Throughout history, pain has been attributed to various causes including tissue injury, spirits, magic, spells, punishment from gods, particles entering the body, unbalanced vital fluids, emotional upset, intense stimulation, firings of specific nerve fibers, nerve fibers firing in specific patterns, and structural/mechanical abnormalities in the body (Perl, 2011). The contemporary definition of pain comes from the International Association for the Study of Pain (IASP) which states that pain is "An unpleasant sensory and emotional experience associated with actual or potential tissue damage or described in terms of such damage" (IASP, 2015). Important to this definition are the notions that pain is more than just a sensory experience and that pain can be associated with but is separate from the actual bodily damage.

Modern biomedical practice tends to classify pain as being either acute (e.g., short term) or chronic (e.g., lasting 3 months or longer) and in accordance with body locations (e.g., foot pain, back pain, head pain, etc.) or by disease type (e.g., cancer pain, arthritis pain, etc.). An alternative method of classifying pain is by mechanism, of which there appear to be three types: nociceptive/inflammatory, neuropathic, and central. The first, nociceptive/inflammatory is thought to represent mechanisms associated with an unpleasant but adaptive warning of tissue injury (i.e., proper functioning of the body's pain system). The latter two, neuropathic and central, refer to damaged or aberrant functioning of the pain processing system itself that can result in the perception of pain that far exceeds actual tissue damage or that can occur in the absence of observable injury (Woolf, 2004, 2011).

Nociceptive and Inflammatory Pain Mechanisms

When functioning properly, nociceptive pain requires a three neuron relay: stimulation of nociceptors in the tissues (i.e., first-order neurons), transmission of the signal from the spinal cord to the brain (i.e., second-order neurons), and distributed communication to higher cortical pathways (i.e., third-order neurons) (Costigan, Scholz, & Woolf, 2009). At the first stage, there are several types of nociceptors designed to sense various types of damage. These nociceptors include those capable of detecting damage from chemicals (e.g., pH), heat (i.e., ≥45 °C), cold (i.e., ≤15 °C), and mechanical sources (e.g., pinch, pinprick, crush) (Purves et al., 2012). These first-order neurons can either be fast conducting myelinated A-delta neurons (e.g., 5–30 m/s) or slower unmyelinated C-fibers (e.g., <2 m/s). Both types of nociceptive fibers have afferents in tissue and terminate in the spinal cord for subsequent transmission to the brain via the second-order neurons (Purves et al., 2012). Most of the second-order neurons have terminals that include various aspects of the thalamus which then activate third-order neurons having projections to higher cortical areas responsible for encoding intensity and location (i.e., the lateral nociceptive system) and cortical areas responsible for affective and autonomic responses (i.e., the medial system) (Albe-Fessard, Berkley, Kruger, Ralston, & Willis, 1985). The lateral system is composed of areas such as the primary sensory cortex (S1), the secondary sensory cortex (S2), periaqueductal gray (PAG), and the posterior insula cortex (p.Insula). Again, this system is responsible for the sensory-discriminative aspects of nociception and of interest, lesions or damage to this system do not eliminate the ability to experience pain (Price, 2000). The medial system is composed of the anterior cingulate cortex (ACC), the prefrontal cortex (PFC), and the anterior insula cortex (a.insula). This system is responsible for limbic (e.g., affective) arousal, somatomotor and autonomic nervous system activation, as well as the evaluation of threat and/or perceived control (Price, 2000). Finally, a top-down pain inhibitory system operates to suppress nociception from lower sources. This system originates in higher cortical regions (e.g., PFC, amygdala), passes through the PAG and rostral ventromedial medulla, and acts to suppress or promote afferent nociceptive transmission within the spinal cord (Tracey & Mantyh, 2007). When functioning properly, each of these systems works together to detect damage or threat from the periphery and prepares the individual to respond appropriately (Lee & Tracey, 2013). This whole system can work in conjunction with the immune system and can be activated by either peripheral or central inflammation to again warn of damage and promote opportunities for healing (Fig. 2.1) (Lee, Nassikas, & Clauw, 2011).

Rheumatoid Arthritis

RA is characterized by systemic inflammation that can be related to pain, stiffness, and damage to joints. Referring to the model of pain just presented, there are a number of peripheral drivers associated with initiating and maintaining the nociceptive cascade in RA including mechanical stimulation (e.g., weight bearing and joint movement), nociceptive factors in the synovium or synovial fluids, inflammatory cytokines (e.g., IL-6, TNF), and growth factors (Walsh & McWilliams, 2014). Biomedical treatment of RA often includes direct-acting analgesic agents such as nonsteroidal anti-inflammatory agents (NSAIDs), agents that suppress inflammation such as glucocorticoids, DMARDs, and biologics (e.g., TNF blockers), and surgical approaches such as joint replacement (Walsh & McWilliams, 2014). For around 25 % of patients however, pain does not improve despite the use of anti-inflammatory agents and another 15 % are left with pain after completely removing and replacing the joint (e.g., 15 %) (Walsh & McWilliams, 2012). It is suspected that in these cases, while peripheral mechanisms are obviously active, there may be other centrally mediated aspects of nociception (e.g., higher cortical or descending modulatory influences) that are also contributing prominently to pain perception. For example, in studies of RA, subgroups of individuals with RA have been identified who have both lowered pain thresholds and impaired central descending analgesic activity (Gerecz-Simon, Tunks, Heale, Kean, & Buchanan, 1989; Hummel, Schiessl, Wendler, & Kobal, 2000), suggesting more involvement of the CNS in maintaining pain for these individuals.

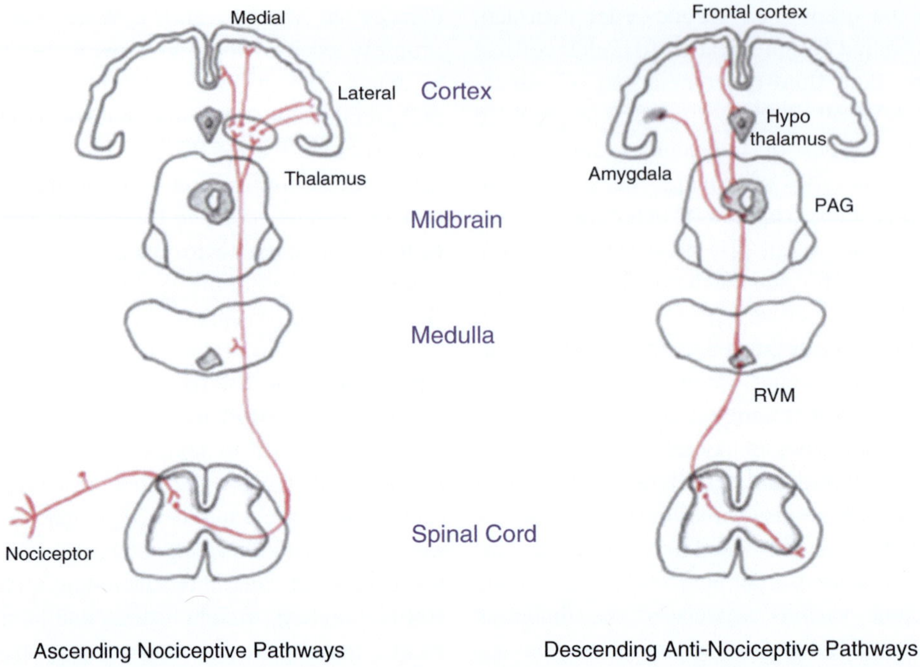

Fig. 2.1 Afferent nociceptive transmission utilizes a three neuron relay that involves nociceptors from the periphery that terminate in the dorsal horn of the spinal cord, get transmitted to higher centers including the thalamus, and then proceed to either the lateral or medial nociceptive pathways and structures. Descending pain modulation is initiated in the frontal cortex, amygdala, and hypothalamus, pass through the periaqueductal gray (PAG), and rostral ventromedial medulla (RVM) and terminates again in the spinal cord where it can influence subsequent ascending nociception

Osteoarthritis

OA, found predominantly in elderly individuals (Lee et al., 2013) is characterized by degradation to articular cartilage, bone, synovial joint lining, and adjacent connective tissue (Zhang, Ren, & Dubner, 2013).

Historically, OA has been considered a prototypic nociceptive pain condition with peripheral mechanical and inflammatory influences triggering the pain. As such, treatments for OA have historically been peripherally focused and based upon relieving symptoms through direct-acting analgesic agents (e.g., NSAIDs), anti-inflammatory (e.g., intra-articular glucocorticoid injections), and joint replacement surgery (Hassan & Walsh, 2014). As in the case of RA however, many individuals do not respond to these standard interventions (Zhang et al., 2013). For example, despite undergoing total knee replacement surgery, 44 % of OA patients still report pain 3–4 years after surgery, with 15 % reporting it as severe (Wylde, Hewlett, Learmonth, & Dieppe, 2011). Failure to respond to surgical or peripheral agents draws into question whether pain is a direct correlate of damage. Population-based studies suggest it is not. These studies report that 30–50 % of individuals with moderate to severe radiographic changes of OA can actually report no pain; whereas 10 % of individuals with normal radiographs report moderate to severe knee pain (Creamer & Hochberg, 1997; Hannan, Felson, & Pincus, 2000). As with RA, when peripherally directed therapies are ineffective with OA, pain might be best attributed to central pain mechanisms (Hassan & Walsh, 2014; McDougall & Linton, 2012).

Central Pain Augmentation: Terminology

The term "central pain" originally referred to pain from identifiable lesions to the CNS such as those following a stroke or spinal cord injury. The term "central" was used to differentiate this type of nerve damage from peripheral nerve damage (i.e., neuropathic pain—such as trauma or diseases like diabetic neuropathy). More recently, however, the meaning of the term "central pain" has been expanded to describe any CNS dysfunction or pathology that may be contributing to the development or maintenance of chronic pain (Williams & Clauw, 2009) and is perhaps better termed "centralized pain" to describe pain that is influenced predominantly by the CNS.

Another term that often shares a similar meaning to centralized pain is "central sensitization." Central sensitization originally referred to a very specific spinal mechanism that could account for pain perception exceeding what would be expected from peripheral tissue damage alone (Woolf & Thompson, 1991). In experimental studies, central sensitization has been characterized by the presence of tactile allodynia, secondary punctuate/pressure hyperalgesia, temporal summation, and sensory after effects (Woolf, 2011). Clinically, the hypersensitivity of central sensitization has been described as being disproportionate to the nature and extent of any injury (i.e., not nociceptive pain) and not being attributable to lesions or damage within the CNS (i.e., not neuropathic pain). Phenotypic characteristics of central sensitization include a widespread pain distribution, allodynia and/or hyperalgesia, and may include general hypersensitivity of all senses and perceptual systems (e.g., pressure, chemicals, heat/cold, stress, emotions, and mental load) (Nijs, Malfliet, Ickmans, Baert, & Meeus, 2014; Woolf, 2014).

CNS factors provide "gain" (using an electrophysical analogy) by which peripheral nociception is augmented or diminished in the determination of whether the nociceptive information is salient and subsequently painful (Legrain, Iannetti, Plaghki, & Mouraux, 2011). In nociceptive pain states, this gain appears to operate at a set point that facilitates a fairly good correspondence between the degree of tissue damage and the intensity of pain. In aberrant central pain states, this correspondence can be mismatched such that seemingly innocuous stimuli are experienced as being painful. A number of neurotransmitters and centrally mediated processes appear to be involved in determining this set point (Clauw, 2014).

In the next section of this chapter, we refer to pain arising from a predominance of CNS influences (e.g., set point, sensory augmentation, salience, and central sensitization) as "centralized pain." In referring to centralized pain mechanisms, we also acknowledge that most forms of arthritis pain will be "mixed pain states" (i.e., incorporating a balance of peripheral and central drivers) (Phillips & Clauw, 2013).

Centralized Pain: Characteristics and Mechanisms

Centralized pain, as defined here, was originally thought to be confined to individuals with idiopathic or functional pain syndromes, such as fibromyalgia (FM), headache, irritable bowel syndrome (IBS), temporomandibular joint disorder (TMD), and interstitial cystitis (IC) (Clauw et al., 1997; Hudson & Pope, 1994). These pain syndromes have been shown to be familial/genetic, as they strongly coaggregate within individuals and within families (Diatchenko, Nackley, Slade, Fillingim, & Maixner, 2006; Williams & Clauw, 2009). The symptoms experienced by individuals with centralized pain syndromes have been well characterized and consist of multifocal pain (with a high current and lifetime history of pain in many bodily regions), and a cluster of cooccurring somatic symptoms (i.e., fatigue, sleep disturbances, difficulties with thinking/memory) (Warren et al., 2009; Williams & Clauw, 2009). We know now that these central influences are not just limited to individuals with conditions like FM but can influence pain perception for a variety of chronic pain states under a "mixed-pain state" model.

Multifocal Pain and Cooccurring Somatic Symptoms

Being prone to pain augmentation via central influences (i.e., having a low set point for pain) is a lifelong condition usually beginning in young adulthood and manifested by multiple prolonged pain experiences occurring in many different body regions and over many different time periods (Tracey & Bushnell, 2009; Williams & Clauw, 2009; Woolf, 2011). Over a lifetime, such individuals tend to accumulate multiple diagnostic labels associated with various regions of the body; but in all likelihood, aberrant central pain mechanics underlie much of this symptomatology.

Multifocal pain is thought to be related to pathophysiologic excitatory neurotransmitter activity such as high substance P and high glutamate levels in cortical structures associated with afferent pain processing (i.e., part of the "gain" in determining the central pain set point). In addition, descending pain inhibitory pathways depend upon adequate levels of norepinephrine, GABA, or serotonin, which in centralized pain conditions tend to be low (i.e., also enhancing the "gain" that determines the set point for pain) (Clauw, 2014; Williams & Clauw, 2009).

While the aforementioned neurotransmitters are critical to pain perception, they also mediate the symptoms that can accompany multifocal pain such as fatigue, sleep difficulties (e.g., insomnia or nonrefreshing sleep), thinking and memory problems, and mood disturbances (Bannister, Bee, & Dickenson, 2009; Fukuda et al., 1997, 1998; Williams & Clauw, 2009). The broader role of these neurotransmitters in both multifocal pain and in these cooccurring symptoms is best supported by the fact that when centrally acting analgesics such as serotonin–norepinephrine reuptake inhibitors (SNRIs), gabapentinoids, tricyclics, or gamma-hydroxybutyrate are effective in patients suspected of having centralized pain involvement, these drugs also lead to improvements in one or more of these other symptom domains (Fishbain, Detke, Wernicke, Chappell, & Kajdasz, 2008; Russell et al., 2011; Tzellos et al., 2010). Thus, the assessment of these cooccurring symptoms is useful in identifying the presence of a centralized pain state and for identifying likely responders to pharmacological therapies targeting centralized pain states (Aaron, Burke, & Buchwald, 2000; Arnold et al., 2012; Williams & Clauw, 2009).

Hyperalgesia

Another hallmark characteristic of centralized pain conditions is the presence of diffuse hyperalgesia identifiable using quantitative sensory testing (QST) and corroborated by functional neuroimaging (Clauw, 2009; Diatchenko, Nackley, Slade, Fillingim, et al., 2006; Tracey & Bushnell, 2009; Woolf, 2011). Key to understanding the relevance of hyperalgesia in centralized pain states is the term "diffuse" which emphasizes the point that hyperalgesia is not confined to a location of injury per se; but rather, is present over noninjury sites as well.

Within both the general population and within chronic pain conditions, sensory sensitivity is normally distributed with some individuals having higher pain thresholds and others having lower pain thresholds. A low pain threshold is disproportionately seen in those individuals with a centralized pain condition (Coghill, McHaffie, & Yen, 2003; Diatchenko, Nackley, Slade, Fillingim, et al., 2006; Gibson, Littlejohn, Gorman, Helme, & Granges, 1994; Giesecke, Gracely, et al., 2004; Giesecke, Reed, et al., 2004; Gwilym et al., 2009; Kashima, Rahman, Sakoda, & Shiba, 1999; Kosek, Ekholm, & Hansson, 1995; Leffler, Hansson, & Kosek, 2002; Maixner, Fillingim, Booker, & Sigurdsson, 1995; Tracey & Bushnell, 2009; Whitehead et al., 1990; Williams & Clauw, 2009) but can occur in other pain states (e.g., OA and RA) where subgroups of individuals display more of a "mixed-pain state" presentation (Gerecz-Simon et al., 1989; Hummel et al., 2000).

The baseline presence of hyperalgesia has also been shown to be an important risk factor for a number of adverse pain outcomes, including predicting the subsequent intensity of an acute painful experience, predicting increased analgesic requirements following surgery, and the subsequent transition from an acute to a chronic pain state (Arendt-Nielsen & Yarnitsky, 2009; Granot et al., 2008; Yarnitsky et al., 2008). This latter phenomenon (i.e., the transition from an acute to chronic pain state) was first demonstrated in a study by Diatchenko and colleagues, who performed a longitudinal study of 202 young pain-free women, and followed them for 2 years with the outcome of interest being those who developed new onset TMD (Diatchenko et al., 2005). In this study, an individual's pain threshold at baseline (i.e., while completely asymptomatic) was a strong predictor of who would later develop TMD. In fact, those with a lower pain threshold while asymptomatic were three times more likely to develop TMD in the future than individuals with higher pain thresholds.

The above study raises the question of what might determine an asymptomatic baseline threshold for pain. In addition to demonstrating the importance of hyperalgesia in predicting the onset of new pain, this same TMD study was among the first to highlight the strong role that certain genes play in turning up the "gain" on pain processing (Diatchenko et al., 2005; Diatchenko, Nackley, Slade, Bhalang, et al., 2006; Diatchenko, Nackley, Slade, Fillingim, et al., 2006).

Genetics of Centralized Pain States

While several rare instances of single gene mutations associated with pain exist (Cox & Wood, 2013; Eijkelkamp et al., 2012), most instances of pain perception stem from polygenetic influences (Denk, McMahon, & Tracey, 2014). The genetic loci most associated with pain are those involving neurotransmitter systems (e.g., COMT, OPRM1, GCH1, 5HTR2A, ADRB2), ion channel functions (e.g., KCNS1, CACNA2D3), and immune functioning (IL1, TNF) (Denk et al., 2014; Mogil, 2012). In centralized pain states, genetic factors associated with metabolism or transport of monoamine compounds associated with sensory processing (e.g., heightened sensory sensitivity) and/or affective vulnerability and stress appear to be the most relevant in predicting the onset and maintenance of the condition (Buskila, 2007; Diatchenko, Nackley, Slade, Fillingim, et al., 2006).

A number of environmental "stressors" have also been associated with centralized pain states. These include early life trauma, physical trauma, certain infections such as Hepatitis C, Epstein–Barr virus, parvovirus, Lyme disease, emotional stress, and other regional pain or autoimmune disorders (Ablin & Clauw, 2009; Buskila, Neumann, Vaisberg, Alkalay, & Wolfe, 1997; Clauw & Chrousos, 1997). While these studies are informative, there does not appear to be any singular "cause" of centralized pain conditions; rather, in a genetically predisposed individual (i.e., someone predisposed to sensory hypersensitivity and/or affective vulnerability), any of these stressors can act as a temporary trigger for the subsequent development of the condition. The role of genetic predisposition is important given that in nonpredisposed individuals (i.e., 90 % of individuals), these same stressors tend to resolve and individuals regain their baseline state of health.

Conditioned Pain Modulation

As stated, there are central mechanisms that can influence the perception of pain. Conditioned pain modulation (CPM) or as it was previously labeled DNIC (i.e., diffuse noxious inhibitory controls) refers to studying the integrity of the descending endogenous analgesic pathways. CPM currently holds great promise as a means of "segmenting" individuals with chronic pain into those with and those without a central predominance to their pain.

The integrity of the pathway and the magnitude of pain inhibition can be tested experimentally by using two separate painful stimuli and observing how the experience of the first reduces the perceived intensity of the second. CPM is a powerful analgesic effect and is observed in 80–90 % of healthy individuals. It is attenuated or absent, however, in 60–80 % of individuals with centralized pain conditions (e.g., FM or IBS)

(Edwards, Ness, Weigent, & Fillingim, 2003; Julien, Goffaux, Arsenault, & Marchand, 2005; Kosek & Hansson, 1997; Le Bars, Villanueva, Bouhassira, & Willer, 1992; Pud, Granovsky, & Yarnitsky, 2009; Wilder-Smith & Robert-Yap, 2007). Both CPM (i.e., descending pain modulation) and hyperalgesia (i.e., ascending pain processing) appear to be unique characteristics of centralized pain and are not seen in other conditions that hold high comorbidities with chronic pain such as depression (Giesecke et al., 2005; Normand et al., 2011).

Neuroimaging Studies

Perhaps some of the strongest evidence pointing to aberrant central mechanisms playing a predominant role in centralized pain states comes from functional, chemical, and structural neuroimaging studies. To date, numerous studies have shown significantly increased neuronal activity in pain processing regions of the brain when individuals with central pain states are exposed to stimuli that healthy individuals find innocuous (Cook et al., 2004; Giesecke, Gracely, et al., 2004; Gracely, Petzke, Wolf, & Clauw, 2002; Naliboff et al., 2001). Such findings have been used to support the notion that patients' reports of pain to innocuous stimuli actually correspond with cortical pain processing activity rather than being attributable to biases in pain reporting or to hypervigilance on the part of the patient.

Neuroimaging studies have also helped to identify the separate but critical roles of both the sensory pathways and the affective pathways in creating a unified perception of pain. For example, within a single brain region such as the insula, the posterior insula is more involved in sensory processing whereas the anterior insula is more involved in affective processing. Even the left-to-right balance of insular activity may be associated with the emotional valence of pain (Craig, 2003). Recent studies also suggest that the balance between sensory and affective dimensions of pain do not remain stable even within the same individual, with the same injury, over time. For example, an initial injury may appear with the cortical signature of a sensory event; however with chronicity, pain can take on a cortical signature more closely resembling an emotion (Hashmi et al., 2013). This may be why attempts to treat chronic pain in the same way as acute pain (e.g., with peripherally acting agents) often fail (Lee et al., 2011).

Mechanism-Based Treatment

Historically, medical treatment of arthritis has focused upon treating the underlying disease process, which as stated, may or may not share a close relationship with pain. As such, the most common medical approach to arthritis pain is the use of nonsteroidal anti-inflammatory drugs (NSAIDs) or surgery. When patients with arthritis are nonresponsive to such pain treatment, they may have a stronger central driver of pain. This can be identified by the characteristics reviewed earlier in this chapter (e.g., chronic multifocal pain, multiple comorbid centrally mediated somatic symptoms, diffuse hyperalgesia, attenuated CPM, and ruling out nociceptive and neuropathic mechanisms). Given that central mechanisms act to enhance the gain on nociception, interventions that calm the CNS and/or restore balance within afferent and descending inhibitory pathways hold promise of being beneficial (Woolf, 2011). These treatments could be either biomedical or nonpharmacological in nature.

Examples of pharmacological interventions that have shown benefit in centralized pain conditions such as FM include tricyclic antidepressants (TCAs), SNRIs, and alpha-2 delta ligands. TCAs have many actions but are generally thought to exert their analgesic effects by inhibiting the reuptake of serotonin and norepinephrine. While a number of studies offer support for the use of TCAs in FM (Nishishinya et al., 2008), far fewer have examined their use in OA or RA. Those that have, however, tend to report significant reductions in pain (Ash, Dickens, Creed, Jayson, & Tomenson, 1999; Chuck, Swannell, House, & Pownall, 2000; Frank et al., 1988; Gringras, 1976; Macfarlane, Jalali, & Grace, 1986; Sarzi Puttini et al., 1988) that are independent of improvements in depression (Ash et al., 1999;

Macfarlane et al., 1986). A drawback of using this class of medication in arthritis patients, however, are the well-known side effects of this class of drugs which can include dizziness and sedation, blurred vision, constipation, and dryness of mouth. SNRIs act similarly to TCAs but tend to be more selective and have fewer side effects than TCAs. By selectively increasing the amount of available norepinephrine and serotonin, SNRIs are thought to help restore the functioning of the descending pain inhibitory pathway in centralized pain states (Lee et al., 2011). At least one clinical trial has supported the use of SNRIs in the management of OA pain (Chappell et al., 2009) but as of this writing, none have been conducted with RA pain. Finally, alpha-2 delta ligands are anticonvulsants and have been used successfully in the treatment of neuropathic pain conditions. This class of medication interferes with the release of pain-promoting neurotransmitters such as glutamate, noradrenaline, serotonin, and substance P. Clinical trials using this class of anticonvulsant in patients with central pain states have also demonstrated improvements in pain severity (Crofford et al., 2005, 2008).

The three most strongly supported nonpharmacological interventions for centralized pain states are education, cognitive-behavioral therapy (CBT), and exercise (Goldenberg, 2008; Goldenberg, Burckhardt, & Crofford, 2004). These nonpharmacological interventions tend to have treatment responses that equal or even exceed the magnitude of response found with pharmacological agents (Clauw, 2014). Over 80 studies support the use of exercise in central pain states with most showing improvements in pain intensity, improved functional status, and/or improvements in associated symptoms (Hassett & Williams, 2011). The type of exercise can vary (e.g., aerobic, strength training, flexibility training), with some evidence that pool-based exercise may be slightly more advantageous given reductions in weight bearing (Brosseau et al., 2008a, 2008b; Hauser et al., 2010). CBT has been used successfully with psychiatric conditions (e.g., anxiety and depression) (Hofmann & Smits, 2008; Twomey, O'Reilly, & Byrne, 2015) as well as in medical conditions such as cardiovascular disease (Lundgren, Andersson, & Johansson, 2015), diabetes (Pal et al., 2014), asthma (Creer, 2008), obesity (Van Dorsten & Lindley, 2011), tinnitus (McKenna, Handscomb, Hoare, & Hall, 2014), and insomnia (Wang, Wang, & Tsai, 2005). While the specific skills taught in each variation of CBT can differ, each version is grounded in shared psychological principles of behavioral change (e.g., operant and classical conditioning), social learning theory, and approaches for modifying thoughts, beliefs, and attributions about illness. This form of therapy, which incorporates elements of education, has been found to be beneficial in reducing pain and improving function in centralized pain conditions (Glombiewski et al., 2010; Rossy et al., 1999) as well as in OA and RA (Keefe & Caldwell, 1997; Keefe et al., 1991).

Conclusions

The diagnosis and treatment of arthritis has long assumed a 1:1 relationship between observable injury/damage and the magnitude of pain. More recently however, we have learned that CNS factors play an important role in determining how peripheral nociceptive stimuli are evaluated centrally with the resulting experience of pain either being in accordance with tissue damage (i.e., nociceptive pain) or augmented (i.e., predominance of CNS factors). Given that treatments need to be matched to active mechanisms, it is becoming increasingly clear that clinicians must recognize the balance of pain mechanisms that may accompany any given pain condition. Even in conditions such as OA and RA where the peripheral mechanisms are fairly well understood, there remains a sizable subset of individuals with prominent central drivers associated with their pain (Lee et al., 2014; Murphy, Lyden, Phillips, Clauw, & Williams, 2011). When central factors are present, both pharmacological and nonpharmacological interventions that calm the CNS (sensory, affective, and cognitive centers) need to be considered in order to optimally manage the condition. This integrated conceptualization of the factors that contribute to and maintain arthritis pain is apt to lead to a more insightful understanding of how pain is manifested in individual patients and to efficacious, biopsychosocial treatment interventions.

References

Aaron, L. A., Burke, M. M., & Buchwald, D. (2000). Overlapping conditions among patients with chronic fatigue syndrome, fibromyalgia, and temporomandibular disorder. *Archives of Internal Medicine, 160*(2), 221–227.

Ablin, K., & Clauw, D. J. (2009). From fibrositis to functional somatic syndromes to a bell-shaped curve of pain and sensory sensitivity: Evolution of a clinical construct. *Rheumatic Diseases Clinics of North America, 35*(2), 233–251.

Albe-Fessard, D., Berkley, K. J., Kruger, L., Ralston, H. J., III, & Willis, W. D., Jr. (1985). Diencephalic mechanisms of pain sensation. *Brain Research, 356*(3), 217–296.

Arendt-Nielsen, L., & Yarnitsky, D. (2009). Experimental and clinical applications of quantitative sensory testing applied to skin, muscles and viscera. *The Journal of Pain, 10*(6), 556–572.

Arnold, L. M., Williams, D. A., Hudson, J. I., Martin, S. A., Clauw, D. J., Crofford, L. J., Mease, P. J. (2012). Development of responder definitions for fibromyalgia clinical trials. *Arthritis and Rheumatism, 64*(3), 885–894.

Ash, G., Dickens, C. M., Creed, F. H., Jayson, M. I., & Tomenson, B. (1999). The effects of dothiepin on subjects with rheumatoid arthritis and depression. *Rheumatology, 38*(10), 959–967.

Bannister, K., Bee, L. A., & Dickenson, A. H. (2009). Preclinical and early clinical investigations related to monoaminergic pain modulation. *Neurotherapeutics, 6*(4), 703–712.

Brosseau, L., Wells, G. A., Tugwell, P., Egan, M., Wilson, K. G., Dubouloz, C. J., Veilleux, L. (2008a). Ottawa Panel evidence-based clinical practice guidelines for aerobic fitness exercises in the management of fibromyalgia: Part 1. *Physical Therapy, 88*(7), 857–871.

Brosseau, L., Wells, G. A., Tugwell, P., Egan, M., Wilson, K. G., Dubouloz, C. J., Veilleux, L. (2008b). Ottawa Panel evidence-based clinical practice guidelines for strengthening exercises in the management of fibromyalgia: Part 2. *Physical Therapy, 88*(7), 873–886.

Buskila, D. (2007). Genetics of chronic pain states. *Best Practice & Research. Clinical Rheumatology, 21*(3), 535–547.

Buskila, D., Neumann, L., Vaisberg, G., Alkalay, D., & Wolfe, F. (1997). Increased rates of fibromyalgia following cervical spine injury. A controlled study of 161 cases of traumatic injury [see comments]. *Arthritis and Rheumatism, 40*(3), 446–452.

CDC. (2010). Prevalence of doctor-diagnosed arthritis and arthritis-attributable activity limitation—United States, 2007-2009. *Morbidity and Mortality Weekly Report, 59*(39), 1261–1296.

CDC. (2013). Prevalence of doctor-diagnosed arthritis and arthritis-attributable activity limitation—United States, 2010-2012. *Morbidity and Mortality Weekly Report, 62*(44), 869–873.

Chappell, A. S., Ossanna, M. J., Liu-Seifert, H., Iyengar, S., Skljarevski, V., Li, L. C., Collins, H. (2009). Duloxetine, a centrally acting analgesic, in the treatment of patients with osteoarthritis knee pain: A 13-week, randomized, placebo-controlled trial. *Pain, 146*(3), 253–260.

Chuck, A. J., Swannell, A. J., House, A. O., & Pownall, R. (2000). The effects of dothiepin on subjects with rheumatoid arthritis and depression. *Rheumatology, 39*(12), 1425–1427.

Clauw, D. J. (2009). Fibromyalgia: An overview. *The American Journal of Medicine, 122*(12 Suppl), S3–S13.

Clauw, D. J. (2014). Fibromyalgia: A clinical review. *The Journal of the American Medical Association, 311*(15), 1547–1555.

Clauw, D. J., & Chrousos, G. P. (1997). Chronic pain and fatigue syndromes: Overlapping clinical and neuroendocrine features and potential pathogenic mechanisms. *Neuroimmunomodulation, 4*(3), 134–153.

Clauw, D. J., Schmidt, M., Radulovic, D., Singer, A., Katz, P., & Bresette, J. (1997). The relationship between fibromyalgia and interstitial cystitis. *Journal of Psychiatric Research, 31*(1), 125–131.

Coghill, R. C., McHaffie, J. G., & Yen, Y. F. (2003). Neural correlates of interindividual differences in the subjective experience of pain. *Proceedings of the National Academy of Sciences of the United States of America, 100*(14), 8538–8542.

Cook, D. B., Lange, G., Ciccone, D. S., Liu, W. C., Steffener, J., & Natelson, B. H. (2004). Functional imaging of pain in patients with primary fibromyalgia. *The Journal of Rheumatology, 31*(2), 364–378.

Costigan, M., Scholz, J., & Woolf, C. J. (2009). Neuropathic pain: A maladaptive response of the nervous system to damage. *Annual Review of Neuroscience, 32*, 1–32.

Cox, J. J., & Wood, J. N. (2013). No pain, more gain. *Nature Genetics, 45*(11), 1271–1272.

Craig, A. D. (2003). Interoception: The sense of the physiological condition of the body. *Current Opinion in Neurobiology, 13*(4), 500–505.

Creamer, P., & Hochberg, M. C. (1997). Why does osteoarthritis of the knee hurt—Sometimes? *British Journal of Rheumatology, 36*(7), 726–728.

Creer, T. L. (2008). Behavioral and cognitive processes in the self-management of asthma. *The Journal of Asthma, 45*(2), 81–94.

Crofford, L. J., Mease, P. J., Simpson, S. L., Young, J. P., Jr., Martin, S. A., Haig, G. M., Sharma, U. (2008). Fibromyalgia relapse evaluation and efficacy for durability of meaningful relief (FREEDOM): A 6-month, double-blind, placebo-controlled trial with pregabalin. *Pain, 136*(3), 419–431.

Crofford, L. J., Rowbotham, M. C., Mease, P. J., Russell, I. J., Dworkin, R. H., Corbin, A. E., Sharma, U. (2005). Pregabalin for the treatment of fibromyalgia syndrome: Results of a randomized, double-blind, placebo-controlled trial. *Arthritis and Rheumatism, 52*(4), 1264–1273.

Denk, F., McMahon, S. B., & Tracey, I. (2014). Pain vulnerability: A neurobiological perspective. *Nature Neuroscience, 17*(2), 192–200.

Diatchenko, L., Nackley, A. G., Slade, G. D., Bhalang, K., Belfer, I., Max, M. B., Maixner, W. (2006). Catechol-O-methyltransferase gene polymorphisms are associated with multiple pain-evoking stimuli. *Pain, 125*(3), 216–224.

Diatchenko, L., Nackley, A. G., Slade, G. D., Fillingim, R. B., & Maixner, W. (2006). Idiopathic pain disorders—Pathways of vulnerability. *Pain, 123*(3), 226–230.

Diatchenko, L., Slade, G. D., Nackley, A. G., Bhalang, K., Sigurdsson, A., Belfer, I., Maixner, W. (2005). Genetic basis for individual variations in pain perception and the development of a chronic pain condition. *Human Molecular Genetics, 14*(1), 135–143.

Edwards, R. R., Ness, T. J., Weigent, D. A., & Fillingim, R. B. (2003). Individual differences in diffuse noxious inhibitory controls (DNIC): Association with clinical variables. *Pain, 106*(3), 427–437.

Eijkelkamp, N., Linley, J. E., Baker, M. D., Minett, M. S., Cregg, R., Werdehausen, R., & Wood, J. N. (2012). Neurological perspectives on voltage-gated sodium channels. *Brain, 135*(Pt 9), 2585–2612.

Fishbain, D. A., Detke, M. J., Wernicke, J., Chappell, A. S., & Kajdasz, D. K. (2008). The relationship between antidepressant and analgesic responses: Findings from six placebo-controlled trials assessing the efficacy of duloxetine in patients with major depressive disorder. *Current Medical Research and Opinion, 24*(11), 3105–3115.

Frank, R. G., Kashani, J. H., Parker, J. C., Beck, N. C., Brownlee-Duffeck, M., Elliott, T. R., Kay, D. R. (1988). Antidepressant analgesia in rheumatoid arthritis. *Journal of Rheumatology, 15*(11), 1632–1638.

Fukuda, K., Dobbins, J. G., Wilson, L. J., Dunn, R. A., Wilcox, K., & Smallwood, D. (1997). An epidemiologic study of fatigue with relevance for the chronic fatigue syndrome. *Journal of Psychiatric Research, 31*(1), 19–29.

Fukuda, K., Nisenbaum, R., Stewart, G., Thompson, W. W., Robin, L., Washko, R. M., Reeves, W. C. (1998). Chronic multisymptom illness affecting Air Force veterans of the Gulf War. *Journal of the American Medical Association, 280*(11), 981–988.

Gerecz-Simon, E. M., Tunks, E. R., Heale, J. A., Kean, W. F., & Buchanan, W. W. (1989). Measurement of pain threshold in patients with rheumatoid arthritis, osteoarthritis, ankylosing spondylitis, and healthy controls [see comments]. *Clinical Rheumatology, 8*(4), 467–474.

Gibson, S. J., Littlejohn, G. O., Gorman, M. M., Helme, R. D., & Granges, G. (1994). Altered heat pain thresholds and cerebral event-related potentials following painful CO_2 laser stimulation in subjects with fibromyalgia syndrome. *Pain, 58*(2), 185–193.

Giesecke, T., Gracely, R. H., Grant, M. A., Nachemson, A., Petzke, F., Williams, D. A., & Clauw, D. J (2004). Evidence of augmented central pain processing in idiopathic chronic low back pain. *Arthritis and Rheumatism, 50*(2), 613–623.

Giesecke, T., Gracely, R. H., Williams, D. A., Geisser, M., Petzke, F., & Clauw, D. J. (2005). The relationship between depression, clinical pain, and experimental pain in a chronic pain cohort. *Arthritis and Rheumatism, 52*(5), 1577–1584.

Giesecke, J, Reed, B. D., Haefner, H. K., Giesecke, T., Clauw, D. J., & Gracely, R. H. (2004) Quantitative sensory testing in vulvodynia patients and increased peripheral pressure pain sensitivity. *Obstetrics and Gynecology, 104*(1), 126–133.

Glombiewski, J. A., Sawyer, A. T., Gutermann, J., Koenig, K., Rief, W., & Hofmann, S. G. (2010). Psychological treatments for fibromyalgia: A meta-analysis. *Pain, 151*(2), 280–295.

Goldenberg, D. L. (2008). Multidisciplinary modalities in the treatment of fibromyalgia. *Journal of Clinical Psychiatry, 69*(Suppl 2), 30–34.

Goldenberg, D. L., Burckhardt, C., & Crofford, L. (2004). Management of fibromyalgia syndrome. *The Journal of the American Medical Association, 292*(19), 2388–2395.

Gracely, R. H., Petzke, F., Wolf, J. M., & Clauw, D. J. (2002). Functional magnetic resonance imaging evidence of augmented pain processing in fibromyalgia. *Arthritis and Rheumatism, 46*(5), 1333–1343.

Granot, M., Weissman-Fogel, I., Crispel, Y., Pud, D., Granovsky, Y., Sprecher, E., & Yarnitsky, D. (2008). Determinants of endogenous analgesia magnitude in a diffuse noxious inhibitory control (DNIC) paradigm: Do conditioning stimulus painfulness, gender and personality variables matter? *Pain, 136*(1–2), 142–149.

Gringras, M. (1976). A clinical trial of Tofranil in rheumatic pain in general practice. *The Journal of International Medical Research, 4*(2 Suppl), 41–49.

Gwilym, S. E., Keltner, J. R., Warnaby, C. E., Carr, A. J., Chizh, B., Chessell, I., & Tracey, I. (2009). Psychophysical and functional imaging evidence supporting the presence of central sensitization in a cohort of osteoarthritis patients. *Arthritis and Rheumatism, 61*(9), 1226–1234.

Hannan, M. T., Felson, D. T., & Pincus, T. (2000). Analysis of the discordance between radiographic changes and knee pain in osteoarthritis of the knee. *The Journal of Rheumatology, 27*(6), 1513–1517.

Hashmi, J. A., Baliki, M. N., Huang, L., Baria, A. T., Torbey, S., Hermann, K. M., Apkarian, A. V. (2013). Shape shifting pain: Chronification of back pain shifts brain representation from nociceptive to emotional circuits. *Brain, 136*(Pt 9), 2751–2768.

Hassan, H., & Walsh, D. A. (2014). Central pain processing in osteoarthritis: Implications for treatment. *Pain Management, 4*(1), 45–56.

Hassett, A. L., & Williams, D. A. (2011). Non-pharmacological treatment of chronic widespread musculoskeletal pain. *Best Practice & Research. Clinical Rheumatology, 25*(2), 299–309.

Hauser, W., Klose, P., Langhorst, J., Moradi, B., Steinbach, M., Schiltenwolf, M., & Busch, A. (2010). Efficacy of different types of aerobic exercise in fibromyalgia syndrome: A systematic review and meta-analysis of randomised controlled trials. *Arthritis Research & Therapy, 12*(3), R79.

Hofmann, S. G., & Smits, J. A. (2008). Cognitive-behavioral therapy for adult anxiety disorders: A meta-analysis of randomized placebo-controlled trials. *The Journal of Clinical Psychiatry, 69*(4), 621–632.

Hudson, J. I., & Pope, H. G. (1994). The concept of affective spectrum disorder: Relationship to fibromyalgia and other syndromes of chronic fatigue and chronic muscle pain. *Baillieres Clinical Rheumatology, 8*(4), 839–856.

Hummel, T., Schiessl, C., Wendler, J., & Kobal, G. (2000). Peripheral and central nervous changes in patients with rheumatoid arthritis in response to repetitive painful stimulation. *International Journal of Psychophysiology, 37*(2), 177–183.

IASP. (2015). *IASP Taxonomy 2015*. Retrieved from www.IASP-Pain.org/taxonomy

Julien, N., Goffaux, P., Arsenault, P., & Marchand, S. (2005). Widespread pain in fibromyalgia is related to a deficit of endogenous pain inhibition. *Pain, 114*(1–2), 295–302.

Kashima, K., Rahman, O. I., Sakoda, S., & Shiba, R. (1999). Increased pain sensitivity of the upper extremities of TMD patients with myalgia to experimentally-evoked noxious stimulation: Possibility of worsened endogenous opioid systems. *Cranio, 17*(4), 241–246.

Keefe, F. J., & Caldwell, D. S. (1997). Cognitive behavioral control of arthritis pain. *Medical Clinics of North America, 81*(1), 277–290.

Keefe, F. J., Caldwell, D. S., Martinez, S., Nunley, J., Beckham, J., & Williams, D. A. (1991). Analyzing pain in rheumatoid arthritis patients. Pain coping strategies in patients who have had knee replacement surgery. *Pain, 46*(2), 153–160.

Kosek, E., Ekholm, J., & Hansson, P. (1995). Increased pressure pain sensibility in fibromyalgia patients is located deep to the skin but not restricted to muscle tissue [published erratum appears in Pain 1996 Mar;64(3):605]. *Pain, 63*(3), 335–339.

Kosek, E., & Hansson, P. (1997). Modulatory influence on somatosensory perception from vibration and heterotopic noxious conditioning stimulation (HNCS) in fibromyalgia patients and healthy subjects. *Pain, 70*(1), 41–51.

Lawrence, R. C., Felson, D. T., Helmick, C. G., Arnold, L. M., Choi, H., Deyo, R. A., Wolfe, F. (2008). Estimates of the prevalence of arthritis and other rheumatic conditions in the United States. Part II. *Arthritis and Rheumatism, 58*(1), 26–35.

Le Bars, D., Villanueva, L., Bouhassira, D., & Willer, J. C. (1992). Diffuse noxious inhibitory controls (DNIC) in animals and in man. *Patologicheskaia Fiziologiia i Eksperimentalnaia Terapiia, 4*, 55–65.

Lee, A. S., Ellman, M. B., Yan, D., Kroin, J. S., Cole, B. J., van Wijnen, A. J., & Im, H. J. (2013). A current review of molecular mechanisms regarding osteoarthritis and pain. *Gene, 527*(2), 440–447.

Lee, Y. C., Frits, M. L., Iannaccone, C. K., Weinblatt, M. E., Shadick, N. A., Williams, D. A., & Cui, J. (2014). Subgrouping of patients with rheumatoid arthritis based on pain, fatigue, inflammation, and psychosocial factors. *Arthritis and Rheumatism, 66*(8), 2006–2014.

Lee, Y. C., Nassikas, N. J., & Clauw, D. J. (2011). The role of the central nervous system in the generation and maintenance of chronic pain in rheumatoid arthritis, osteoarthritis and fibromyalgia. *Arthritis Research & Therapy, 13*(2), 211.

Lee, M. C., & Tracey, I. (2013). Imaging pain: A potent means for investigating pain mechanisms in patients. *British Journal of Anaesthesia, 111*(1), 64–72.

Leffler, A. S., Hansson, P., & Kosek, E. (2002). Somatosensory perception in a remote pain-free area and function of diffuse noxious inhibitory controls (DNIC) in patients suffering from long-term trapezius myalgia. *European Journal of Pain, 6*(2), 149–159.

Legrain, V., Iannetti, G. D., Plaghki, L., & Mouraux, A. (2011). The pain matrix reloaded: A salience detection system for the body. *Progress in Neurobiology, 93*(1), 111–124.

Lundgren, J., Andersson, G., & Johansson, P. (2015). Can cognitive behaviour therapy be beneficial for heart failure patients? *Current Heart Failure Reports, 12*(2), 166–172.

Macfarlane, J. G., Jalali, S., & Grace, E. M. (1986). Trimipramine in rheumatoid arthritis: A randomized double-blind trial in relieving pain and joint tenderness. *Current Medical Research and Opinion, 10*(2), 89–93.

Maixner, W., Fillingim, R., Booker, D., & Sigurdsson, A. (1995). Sensitivity of patients with painful temporomandibular disorders to experimentally evoked pain. *Pain, 63*(3), 341–351.

McDougall, J. J., & Linton, P. (2012). Neurophysiology of arthritis pain. *Current Pain and Headache Reports, 16*(6), 485–491.

McKenna, L., Handscomb, L., Hoare, D. J., & Hall, D. A. (2014). A scientific cognitive-behavioral model of tinnitus: Novel conceptualizations of tinnitus distress. *Frontiers in Neurology, 5*, 196.

Mogil, J. S. (2012). Pain genetics: Past, present and future. *Trends in Genetics, 28*(6), 258–266.

Murphy, S. L., Lyden, A. K., Phillips, K., Clauw, D. J., & Williams, D. A. (2011). Subgroups of older adults with osteoarthritis based upon differing comorbid symptom presentations and potential underlying pain mechanisms. *Arthritis Research & Therapy, 13*(4), R135.

Myasoedova, E., Crowson, C. S., Kremers, H. M., Therneau, T. M., & Gabriel, S. E. (2010). Is the incidence of rheumatoid arthritis rising?: Results from Olmsted County, Minnesota, 1955-2007. *Arthritis and Rheumatism, 62*(6), 1576–1582.

Naliboff, B. D., Derbyshire, S. W., Munakata, J., Berman, S., Mandelkern, M., Chang, L., & Mayer, E. A. (2001). Cerebral activation in patients with irritable bowel syndrome and control subjects during rectosigmoid stimulation. *Psychosomatic Medicine, 63*(3), 365–375.

Nijs, J., Malfliet, A., Ickmans, K., Baert, I., & Meeus, M. (2014). Treatment of central sensitization in patients with 'unexplained' chronic pain: An update. *Expert Opinion on Pharmacotherapy, 15*(12), 1671–1683.

Nishishinya, B., Urrutia, G., Walitt, B., Rodriguez, A., Bonfill, X., Alegre, C., & Darko, G. (2008). Amitriptyline in the treatment of fibromyalgia: A systematic review of its efficacy. *Rheumatology (Oxford), 47*(12), 1741–1746.

Normand, E., Potvin, S., Gaumond, I., Cloutier, G., Corbin, J. F., & Marchand, S. (2011). Pain inhibition is deficient in chronic widespread pain but normal in major depressive disorder. *The Journal of Clinical Psychiatry, 72*(2), 219–224.

Pal, K., Eastwood, S. V., Michie, S., Farmer, A., Barnard, M. L., Peacock, R., Murray, E. (2014). Computer-based interventions to improve self-management in adults with type 2 diabetes: A systematic review and meta-analysis. *Diabetes Care, 37*(6), 1759–1766.

Perl, E. R. (2011). Pain mechanisms: A commentary on concepts and issues. *Progress in Neurobiology, 94*(1), 20–38.

Phillips, K., & Clauw, D. J. (2013). Central pain mechanisms in the rheumatic diseases: Future directions. *Arthritis and Rheumatism, 65*(2), 291–302.

Price, D. D. (2000). Psychological and neural mechanism of the affective dimension of pain. *Science, 288*(5472), 1769–1772.

Pud, D., Granovsky, Y., & Yarnitsky, D. (2009). The methodology of experimentally induced diffuse noxious inhibitory control (DNIC)-like effect in humans. *Pain, 144*(1–2), 16–19.

Purves, D., Augustine, G. J., Fitzpatrick, D., Hall, W. C., LaMantia, A. S., & White, L. E. (2012). *Neuroscience* (5th ed.). Sunderland, MA: Sinauer Associates.

Rossy, L. A., Buckelew, S. P., Dorr, N., Hagglund, K. J., Thayer, J. F., McIntosh, M. J., Johnson, J. C. (1999). A meta-analysis of fibromyalgia treatment interventions. *Annals of Behavioral Medicine, 21*(2), 180–191.

Russell, I. J., Holman, A. J., Swick, T. J., Alvarez-Horine, S., Wang, Y. G., & Guinta, D. (2011). Sodium oxybate reduces pain, fatigue, and sleep disturbance and improves functionality in fibromyalgia: Results from a 14-week, randomized, double-blind, placebo-controlled study. *Pain, 152*(5), 1007–1017.

Sarzi Puttini, P., Cazzola, M., Boccassini, L., Ciniselli, G., Santandrea, S., Caruso, I., Benvenuti, C. (1988). A comparison of dothiepin versus placebo in the treatment of pain in rheumatoid arthritis and the association of pain with depression. *The Journal of International Medical Research, 16*(5), 331–337.

Tracey, I., & Bushnell, M. C. (2009). How neuroimaging studies have challenged us to rethink: Is chronic pain a disease? *The Journal of Pain, 10*(11), 1113–1120.

Tracey, I., & Mantyh, P. W. (2007). The cerebral signature for pain perception and its modulation. *Neuron, 55*(3), 377–391.

Twomey, C., O'Reilly, G., & Byrne, M. (2015). Effectiveness of cognitive behavioural therapy for anxiety and depression in primary care: A meta-analysis. *Family Practice, 32*(1), 3–15.

Tzellos, T. G., Toulis, K. A., Goulis, D. G., Papazisis, G., Zampeli, V. A., Vakfari, A., & Kouvelas, D. (2010). Gabapentin and pregabalin in the treatment of fibromyalgia: A systematic review and a meta-analysis. *Journal of Clinical Pharmacy and Therapeutics, 35*(6), 639–656.

Van Dorsten, B., & Lindley, E. M. (2011). Cognitive and behavioral approaches in the treatment of obesity. *The Medical Clinics of North America, 95*(5), 971–988.

Walsh, D. A., & McWilliams, D. F. (2012). Pain in rheumatoid arthritis. *Current Pain and Headache Reports, 16*(6), 509–517.

Walsh, D. A., & McWilliams, D. F. (2014). Mechanisms, impact and management of pain in rheumatoid arthritis. *Nature Reviews. Rheumatology, 10*(10), 581–592.

Wang, M. Y., Wang, S. Y., & Tsai, P. S. (2005). Cognitive behavioural therapy for primary insomnia: A systematic review. *Journal of Advanced Nursing, 50*(5), 553–564.

Warren, J. W., Howard, F. M., Cross, R. K., Good, J. L., Weissman, M. M., Wesselmann, U., Clauw, D. J. (2009). Antecedent nonbladder syndromes in case-control study of interstitial cystitis/painful bladder syndrome. *Urology, 73*(1), 52–57.

Whitehead, W. E., Holtkotter, B., Enck, P., Hoelzl, R., Holmes, K. D., Anthony, J., Schuster, M. M. (1990). Tolerance for rectosigmoid distention in irritable bowel syndrome. *Gastroenterology, 98*(5 Pt 1), 1187–1192.

Wilder-Smith, C. H., & Robert-Yap, J. (2007). Abnormal endogenous pain modulation and somatic and visceral hypersensitivity in female patients with irritable bowel syndrome. *World Journal of Gastroenterology, 13*(27), 3699–3704.

Williams, D. A., & Clauw, D. J. (2009). Understanding fibromyalgia: Lessons from the broader pain research community. *The Journal of Pain, 10*(8), 777–791.

Woolf, C. J. (2004). Pain: Moving from symptom control toward mechanism-specific pharmacologic management. *Annals of Internal Medicine, 140*(6), 441–451.

Woolf, C. J. (2011). Central sensitization: Implications for the diagnosis and treatment of pain. *Pain, 152*(3 Suppl), S2–S15.

Woolf, C. J. (2014). What to call the amplification of nociceptive signals in the central nervous system that contribute to widespread pain? *Pain, 155*(10), 1911–1912.

Woolf, C. J., & Thompson, S. W. (1991). The induction and maintenance of central sensitization is dependent on N-methyl-D-aspartic acid receptor activation: Implications for the treatment of post-injury pain hypersensitivity states. *Pain, 44*(3), 293–299.

Wylde, V., Hewlett, S., Learmonth, I. D., & Dieppe, P. (2011). Persistent pain after joint replacement: Prevalence, sensory qualities, and postoperative determinants. *Pain, 152*(3), 566–572.

Yarnitsky, D., Crispel, Y., Eisenberg, E., Granovsky, Y., Ben-Nun, A., Sprecher, E., Granot, M. (2008). Prediction of chronic post-operative pain: pre-operative DNIC testing identifies patients at risk. *Pain, 138*(1), 22–28.

Zhang, R. X., Ren, K., & Dubner, R. (2013). Osteoarthritis pain mechanisms: Basic studies in animal models. *Osteoarthritis and Cartilage/OARS, Osteoarthritis Research Society, 21*(9), 1308–1315.

Understanding and Enhancing Pain Coping in Patients with Arthritis Pain

3

Tamara J. Somers, Sarah A. Kelleher, Rebecca A. Shelby, and Hannah M. Fisher

Coping with Pain in Chronic Disease: Arthritis

When individuals are diagnosed with a chronic disease, they must learn new behaviors or strategies to cope with their disease and its symptoms. For optimal coping or management of chronic disease, new behaviors and strategies must become part of the individual's ongoing lifestyle and not just a temporary change. For many chronic diseases, persistent pain is a central or peripheral symptom that can have a major negative impact on one's quality of life. Arthritis is a chronic disease in which the hallmark symptom is pain that can be persistent and interfering (Keefe et al., 1987). The ability of patients to cope with their arthritis pain can have a significant impact, for better or worse, on their pain as well as their overall quality of life (Keefe et al., 1987).

Arthritis is inflammation of a joint or a number of joints and is the most common cause of disability in the United States. The main symptoms of arthritis are joint pain and stiffness. The information in this chapter will focus on the most common types of arthritis, which are osteoarthritis (OA) and rheumatoid arthritis (RA). Osteoarthritis affects over 27 million Americans (Hootman & Helmick, 2006; Murphy & Nagase, 2008). OA results from mechanical stresses on the joints and is most common in the hands, knees, and hips. RA is an autoimmune disease that causes pain stiffness, swelling, and limited range of motion; RA inflammation can also affect organs such as the eyes or lungs. It is estimated that more than 1.3 million Americans have RA (Hootman & Helmick, 2006). Both OA and RA are chronic diseases and most individuals diagnosed with OA or RA experience significant pain or at least intermittent pain due to their arthritis (Cojocaru et al., 2010).

While the most common treatment approach to arthritis and arthritis pain is biomedical, increasing evidence suggests that using an integrated biopsychosocial treatment approach may provide an individual with arthritis pain the highest likelihood of being able to positively cope with the disease's persistent pain and pain-related disability. The degree to which individuals can positively cope with arthritis pain can impact their overall quality of life. Individuals who have persistent arthritis pain can learn adaptive coping strategies (e.g., learn new behaviors such as pacing activity, modify expectations) or engage in maladaptive coping strategies (e.g., being sedentary, negative thinking, reliance on others); research has demonstrated that how individuals cope with

T.J. Somers, PhD (✉) • S.A. Kelleher, PhD
R.A. Shelby, PhD • H.M. Fisher
Department of Psychiatry and Behavioral Sciences, Duke University Medical Center, 2200 W. Main Street, Suite 340, Durham, NC, 27705, USA
e-mail: tamara.somers@dm.duke.edu; sarah.kelleher@dm.duke.edu; rebecca.shelby@duke.edu; hannah.fisher@dm.duke.edu

P.M. Nicassio (ed.), *Psychosocial Factors in Arthritis*, DOI 10.1007/978-3-319-22858-7_3

their arthritis pain can impact the intensity of their pain, the degree to which interferes with quality of life, and even their overall disease status (Affleck et al., 1992; Jensen, Turner, & Romano, 2001; Lame et al., 2005).

In this chapter, we will begin by describing arthritis pain coping within a biopsychosocial framework and examine biological, psychological, and social factors that have been related to an individual's ability to cope with arthritis pain. Next, we will describe psychosocial interventions that have been shown to improve individuals' abilities to cope with their arthritis pain. We will then discuss strategies for assessing coping with arthritis pain and when and how psychosocial interventions can be implemented to improve arthritis pain coping. Finally, we will suggest several areas that remain to be fully understood regarding coping with arthritis pain and pain-related disability.

Biopsychosocial Factors Related to Pain Coping

Understanding arthritis pain coping and the treatment of arthritis are increasingly guided by a biopsychosocial perspective due to growing evidence that a person's overall well-being is influenced by biological, psychological, and social factors. In fact, treating arthritis as only biological (or only psychological or social) in etiology is considered by many to be inadequate because arthritis symptoms are multifaceted in nature. Pain is the hallmark symptom of arthritic diseases, and while medications can be very helpful in managing pain, research suggests that analgesic therapies alone do not eliminate an individual's pain (Keefe, Shelby, & Somers, 2010; Kidd, Langford, & Wodehouse, 2007). A biopsychosocial approach to treatment is considered favorable because a person's psychological (e.g., depression, irritability) and social (e.g., social support) well-being can account for significant variance in the experience of pain and the degree to which pain interferes with daily functioning.

There is evidence of a strong relationship between biopsychosocial factors and the course of arthritis. Patients with arthritis who have increased physiological (e.g., joint deterioration) or biological markers (e.g., c-reactive protein (CRP) of disease, high levels of psychological distress, maladaptive coping, and/or low levels of social support) tend to have more persistent and intense physical symptoms and increased difficulty coping with arthritis. Moreover, living with a chronic disease such as arthritis can lead to feelings of depression and anxiety, and overall increased stress (Covic et al., 2012; Keefe et al., 2002; Lefebvre et al., 1999; Yelin & Callahan, 1995). Here we describe the prominent biological, psychological, and social factors related to pain coping in arthritis patients.

Biological Factors

The underlying biological factors that contribute to arthritis pain and individuals' abilities to cope are complex and can be difficult to treat. Chronic inflammation and degeneration of bone and cartilage can cause damage to joints, tendons, and ligaments. This swelling, stiffness, and joint deterioration result in immobility, discomfort, and persistent pain. The biomedical model is most commonly used to understand and treat arthritis pain symptoms (Keefe, Abernethy, & Campbell, 2005; Turk & Melzack, 2011). With a focus on pain and methods of pain relief, the biomedical model aims to manage pain symptoms by modifying biological mechanisms that contribute to pain (Keefe et al., 2005; Turk & Melzack, 2011).

From a biomedical perspective, blood tests (e.g., hematocrit and hemoglobin counts, white blood cell and platelet counts), X-rays, and magnetic resonance imaging (MRI) are often used in combination to diagnose and define arthritic conditions. Based on disease progression and symptom severity, results inform treatment decision-making and can also provide information on how well a patient may be responding to treatment.

Traditional biomedical treatments emphasize the use of pharmacologic and surgical interventions (Keefe et al., 2005; Turk & Melzack, 2011). Due to advances in its effectiveness, medication has become the mainstay of arthritis pain management as it reduces disease activity, eases pain, and increases mobility. Analgesic therapies, including acetaminophen and opioids, are the most common forms of medication prescribed to arthritis patients with persistent pain. Nonsteroidal anti-inflammatory drugs are also used to reduce swelling and stiffness and provide pain relief. Additional medication treatments include steroidal injections and topical pain relievers. Although a traditional method of pain management, these medications have side effects that can be burdensome and difficult for patients to tolerate, which increases arthritis patients' overall coping burden (Keefe et al., 2005; Turk & Melzack, 2011; van Laar et al., 2012). Biologic agents, such as Enbrel and Humira, are a new class of drugs that are genetically engineered to copy the effects of substances naturally made by the body's immune system. Given by injection under the skin or by intravenous infusion, biologics are designed to slow disease progression in patients with inflammatory arthritis conditions (Curtis & Singh, 2011). Although they work quickly to relieve symptoms and improve physical function, biologic agents are also associated with immunosuppressive effects creating risk for infections and other health problems (Curtis & Singh, 2011; Scheinfeld, 2005; Schiff et al., 2006). Surgical treatments for arthritis pain include joint replacement or stabilization to target pain and increase use and mobility. Similar to medication regimens, surgical treatments are not without risk. When deciding whether surgical treatment is an appropriate avenue, patients are encouraged to consider factors such as anesthesia, surgical risks, hospitalization, and the recovery phase, including the potential for physical therapy and rehabilitation (Keefe et al., 2005; Turk & Melzack, 2011).

Biological factors that influence pain coping include the disease process, physiological stress associated with chronic illness, and side effects of treatment (Gatchel et al., 2007; Keefe et al., 2002; Somers et al., 2009). Biological factors associated with the disease process include inflammation marked by CRP, cartilage damage, and joint degeneration (Keefe et al., 2002). CRP is a biological marker of arthritis disease activity—elevated levels of CRP reflect inflammation and pain flare up (Shadick et al., 2006). Higher levels of CRP have also been found to be associated with increased risk for psychological distress and depression (Wium-Andersen et al., 2013). Increases in tissue damage and joint inflammation lead to increased stiffness and discomfort, and decreased range of motion. These biological changes significantly interfere with one's ability to maintain an active lifestyle and engage in meaningful activities, ultimately leading to functional and social limitations. Due to the level of suffering and disability caused by the disease process, patients learn to adopt a more sedentary lifestyle in an attempt to minimize or avoid pain (Gatchel et al., 2007; Somers et al., 2009). Inactivity is a maladaptive coping strategy that is related to poor health outcomes and perpetuates difficulty coping; low levels of physical activity lead to weight gain and decreased muscle strength, two factors known to increase arthritis pain (Somers et al., 2009). Furthermore, the deconditioning (a biological response) that results from low levels of physical activity can exacerbate pain, muscle weakness, and difficulty tolerating activity (Keefe et al., 2002).

Treatment side effects are other biological factors that influence an individual's pain coping experience. For traditional analgesic treatments, common side effects can be difficult to tolerate, and prolonged use can have adverse effects, including gastrointestinal problems and weight gain, further impacting an individual's pain coping experience (Somers et al., 2009; van Laar et al., 2012). Issues with medication compliance may arise as a result of adverse side effects and have the potential to produce biological changes, which, in turn, influence pain symptoms (Keefe et al., 2002). Each of these biological and physical factors represents a stressor that challenges a person's ability to cope with pain, has the potential to lead to poor coping, and ultimately impacts social and psychological well-being, and overall quality of life (Irwin et al., 2012; Katz, 1998).

Psychological Factors

Depression and Anxiety

Individuals with arthritis may experience anxiety and depression symptoms due to persistent disease-related pain and other symptoms, ongoing medical appointments and treatment, lifestyle changes, and other factors associated with coping with a chronic illness (Katz & Yelin, 1993, 1995; Keefe et al., 2002). Many studies have identified a strong relationship between psychological and biological factors (Keefe et al., 2010). For example, pain and other increases in disease activity (e.g., inflammation) can influence the occurrence, frequency, and severity of anxiety and depression symptoms, which, in turn, can lead to increased pain and other disease-related symptoms (Keefe et al., 2010). Studies have found that pain is one of the strongest predictors of depression in RA patients (Covic et al., 2006; Isik et al., 2007; Wolfe & Michaud, 2009). Research has also shown that elevated levels of CRP are associated with increased risk for psychological distress and depression (Wium-Andersen et al., 2013). The prevalence of anxiety and depression in a group of RA patients was found to be up to 70 % compared to only 7 % in a healthy age- and sex-matched control group, suggesting psychological distress is highly prevalent among those with arthritis disorders (Isik et al., 2007). Anxiety and depression symptoms can negatively impact individuals' pain experiences and interfere with their abilities to cope effectively with pain. Individuals with chronic illness, such as arthritis, and comorbid anxiety and depression are more likely to experience increased symptom burden, functional impairment, decreased quality of life, and poor adherence to self-care regimens, all of which can lead to poor coping (Katon, 2011; Katz, 1998). Psychosocial interventions for patients with persistent disease-related pain target anxiety and depression symptoms with the goal of reducing these symptoms and their impact on pain, overall psychosocial functioning, disease management, and pain coping (Somers et al., 2009).

Self-Efficacy for Pain Management

Self-efficacy has been consistently shown to be an important factor in shaping an arthritis patient's pain coping experience. Self-efficacy is broadly conceptualized as having a sense of mastery in a specific domain. As defined by Bandura, perceived self-efficacy refers to individuals' beliefs about their capabilities to produce effects; self-efficacy is thought to be domain-specific rather than a general construct (Bandura et al., 1988). Self-efficacy for pain control refers specifically to the confidence of individuals in their ability to control pain related to their disease (Somers, Kurakula, Criscione-Schreiber, Keefe, & Clowse, 2012; Somers, Wren, & Shelby, 2012). Arthritis patients who have low levels of self-efficacy for pain control report higher levels of pain and functional impairment (Somers et al., 2009). Self-efficacy for managing pain and other symptoms may be especially important for individuals coping with arthritis diseases because self-efficacy can markedly influence whether patients attempt to self-manage their disease and whether they persist in their self-management efforts in the face of challenges (Somers, Kurakula, et al., 2012; Somers, Wren, et al., 2012).

In a study of RA patients, researchers found that even when controlling for disease severity, patients with higher self-efficacy for pain and other arthritis symptoms were more likely to experience less pain and better physical functioning (Somers et al., 2010). Another study found that for RA patients, the magnitude of treatment-related improvements in pain and joint inflammation, and psychosocial functioning, was correlated with the degree of self-efficacy enhancement and that perceived self-efficacy was accompanied by reductions in negative affect (O'Leary et al., 1988). This study also showed that self-efficacy to manage pain was positively related to objective biomarkers including levels of function immunity (i.e., suppressor/cytotoxic T cells and negatively to helper:suppressor T-cell ratios) (O'Leary et al., 1988). Research has also shown that higher levels of self-efficacy are associated with lower health care utilization (physician and ER visits) (Barlow, Wright, & Lorig, 2001).

Findings across studies show that self-efficacy is critical to an individual's ability to cope with arthritis pain (Somers et al., 2010). As we conceptualize arthritis in a biopsychosocial framework, it is evident that higher levels of self-efficacy are associated with healthy coping and lead to improvements in pain and function (Barlow et al., 2001; O'Leary et al., 1988; Somers et al., 2009, 2010).

Pain Catastrophizing

Research has shown that pain catastrophizing is a critical psychological variable that negatively impacts the pain experience of individuals coping with arthritic diseases. Pain catastrophizing is a maladaptive coping strategy that is most commonly described as the tendency to focus on and magnify pain sensations and to feel helpless and pessimistic in the face of pain (Edwards et al., 2010). More specifically, high levels of pain catastrophizing in arthritis patients have been associated with maladaptive coping behaviors (e.g., use of fewer active coping strategies like relaxation and distraction, more frequent visits to healthcare professionals, less effective use of medication, reduced likelihood of health-promoting behaviors like exercise), emotional difficulties (e.g., depression, anxiety), changes in other cognitive processes (e.g., skewed appraisal of pain), and poor physiological outcomes (e.g., impaired neuroendocrine functioning) (Dessein, Joffe, & Stanwix, 2004; Edwards et al., 2006, 2011; Quartana, Campbell, & Edwards, 2009). Pain catastrophizing is a key risk factor for a poor pain prognosis in patients with arthritis, in both the short- and long-term progression of their disease (Edwards et al., 2006, 2011; Quartana et al., 2009). In a study of OA and RA patients, higher baseline catastrophizing scores prospectively predicted more intense pain at follow-up. In addition, perceptions of helplessness (one component of catastrophizing) have been linked to increased systemic inflammation, early mortality, psychological distress, and poorer physical functioning in arthritis patients (Dessein et al., 2004; Edwards et al., 2006, 2010, 2011). In sum, pain catastrophizing is a maladaptive coping strategy that is highly correlated with pain, poor physical outcomes, and low levels of psychological functioning (Keefe et al., 1989).

Social Context Factors

Arthritis pain can influence and be influenced by an individual's social context (Keefe et al., 2010). Social and environmental factors, such as stressful life circumstances (e.g., work, family responsibilities), sleep patterns, exercise, diet, alcohol, toxins, and hormonal fluctuations, are multidimensional and interact to shape a person's pain coping experience (Turk & Melzack, 2011). Individuals with arthritis may experience changes in social role functioning, including difficulty fulfilling responsibilities as a parent or spouse (Aggarwal, Chandran, & Misra, 2006; Doeglas et al., 1994; Katz, Morris, & Yelin, 2006; Keefe, Somers, & Martire, 2008; Somers et al., 2009). Job-related problems may arise as a result of missed work due to frequent medical appointments, difficulty managing symptoms, and impaired physical functioning (Katz, 1998). Cultural (e.g., race and ethnicity) and socioeconomic factors also influence pain coping. Low socioeconomic status has been linked to poor health outcomes and low levels of coping self-efficacy among individuals with RA (Brekke et al., 1999; Somers et al., 2009). This may be attributed to social, economic, and cultural factors, such as low literacy, minority status, environmental stress, unemployment, low access to quality healthcare, cultural beliefs about illness, and poor health behaviors (Somers et al., 2009). Social context factors interact with biological and psychological factors; for example, someone who is unable to continue working may become depressed and adopt an overly sedentary lifestyle that contributes to physical deconditioning, increasing pain, and disability. Viewing arthritis pain through a biopsychosocial lens is critical to understanding the unique and complex issues associated with an individual's pain coping experience.

Social support, including perceived support, is closely related to an individual's ability to adjust to persistent pain and often serves as a buffer against depression and other psychosocial problems (Penninx et al., 1997). Evidence suggests that RA patients who receive higher levels of daily emotional support are less likely to be depressed and more likely to report high levels of psychological functioning (Doeglas et al., 1994). In a study of RA patients, researchers found that social network characteristics were associated with patients' self-reported functional status (Evers et al., 1998). Study results showed that RA patients with smaller social networks are at risk of decline in functional mobility within the first year of the disease (Evers et al., 1998). Results also showed better functional status (i.e., mobility and self-care) among RA patients who perceived a greater availability of support (Evers et al., 1998).

Patients with arthritis are likely to benefit from various forms of support, including social and familial, emotional, informational, behavioral, and tangible sources of support (Reese et al., 2010). Familial support and pain-related communication have received considerable attention in the arthritis pain coping literature because disease-related pain is not only a burden for the patient but can also impact one's partner. Partners may have difficulty judging and/or understanding the patient's pain experience and consequently struggle to provide adequate or appropriate support (Martire et al., 2006; Reese et al., 2010). When a partner misjudges the patient's pain experience, communication about pain can be strained or ineffective, which can lead to increased patient and caregiver burden and poor coping (Martire et al., 2006; Reese et al., 2010). For example, if the patient and/or partner intentionally hold back (also known as protective buffering, holding back is a hesitancy to fully communicate) with regard to discussing pain-related concerns, the patient may be more likely to respond to pain in a negative way. As a result, couples-, caregiver-, and group-based psychosocial interventions have been developed to target social context variables such as familial and social support and pain-related communication. Enhancing patients' social contexts by providing increased support can improve patients' coping experience, interpersonal functioning, and overall quality of life.

Psychosocial Intervention Strategies for Coping with Arthritis Pain

Psychosocial interventions have shown efficacy for decreasing burdensome symptoms of chronic disease. Several psychosocial interventions have been developed and tested that can help individuals with arthritis pain learn to manage or cope with their pain to decrease the negative impact of arthritis on their life. Psychosocial interventions for individuals with arthritis have been shown to decrease pain and have a positive impact on biological, psychological, and social factors related to arthritis and overall quality of life. Psychosocial interventions for arthritis pain have been designed for the patient with arthritis, for both patient and caregiver, and for the patient and other supportive persons in the patient's life. A newer area of work has been on psychosocial interventions for arthritis pain that also target comorbid medical problems that interfere with the management of arthritis pain (e.g., obesity). There is increasing acknowledgement of the comorbid disorders that individuals with arthritis must manage and that the challenges of comorbidities must be addressed to most effectively cope with arthritis pain (Somers et al., 2014). Below we present information on different psychosocial intervention approaches to arthritis pain management and empirical evidence for each approach.

Cognitive Behavioral Therapy for Pain Management

Cognitive behavioral therapy (CBT) for pain management is one of the most commonly developed, applied, and tested approaches for psychosocial pain interventions. CBT for pain management protocols systematically teach patients cognitive and behavioral strategies for managing psychological and social factors that negatively impact their pain. The main tenet of CBT for pain management is that learning skills to cope with pain is possible and that skills can be applied by patients in everyday life. CBT pain management interventions are generally taught with a series of in-person individual or groups sessions that last about 1 h each. Protocols have included as few as a single session to many sessions over several months; common protocols are 4–10 sessions in length. CBT protocols provide an educational rationale for why learning ways to enhance one's pain coping skills can be beneficial, including the premise that pain can be impacted by thoughts, feelings, and behaviors. Patients are then taught a series of coping skills such as relaxation, imagery, activity pacing, pleasant activity planning, cognitive restructuring, goal setting, and problem solving. Generally, therapists provide a rationale for each skill, teach each skill, model the skill, and then ask the participant to practice the skill in session and during the time in between sessions. Home practice of skills is an integral part of CBT for pain management. Most CBT-based pain management protocols conclude with the development of a pain coping skills maintenance plan that outlines the patient's goals for ongoing practice and pain management after the intervention period. An important overall goal of CBT for pain management is to increase patients' self-confidence (i.e., self-efficacy) in their ability to cope with their pain in a way that minimizes the negative impact of pain on their functioning and quality of life.

An early study examining the efficacy of CBT for pain management was conducted by Bradley et al. and examined a 15-session protocol applied to patients with RA ($N=53$) (Bradley et al., 1987). The CBT protocol included training in relaxation, biofeedback, goal setting, and self-rewards and was compared to a control condition that included 15 sessions of structured social support. This study found that the CBT protocol produced significant reductions in pain behavior, disease activity, and trait anxiety compared to the control condition. Other work has also examined CBT in patients having OA knee pain; Keefe et al. examined the efficacy of a 10-week group-based CBT protocol in 99 patients with OA (Keefe et al., 1996). In this study, the CBT protocol was compared to a 10-week group-based arthritis education condition and a standard care control condition. The findings were robust for the CBT condition, showing significant improvements in pain, psychological disability, and physical disability compared to the education and control conditions. Impressively, a 6-month follow-up study found that when compared to participants in the arthritis education group, participants in the CBT group maintained their improvements in psychological disability and showed a strong trend toward improvements in physical disability.

There is growing interest in translating CBT for pain management protocols to Internet interventions and to mobile health technologies (Rini et al., 2014). While CBT for pain management in arthritis has shown efficacy in several trials, many individuals with arthritis pain do not have access to such interventions—particularly when they are in-person and delivered at a major medical center. Internet interventions are likely to improve access to interventions for arthritis patients that may benefit from CBT for pain management. In a recent study by Rini et al. (2015), the investigators used a randomized controlled trial to examine the efficacy of an automated, Internet-based CBT intervention for OA pain (Rini et al., 2014, 2015). This group of investigators developed the automated, Internet program, paying particular attention to retaining critical in-person therapeutic elements of a CBT pain management program. The Internet-based program (PainCOACH) included eight modules completed in a self-directed manner (i.e., without therapist contact) at the rate of one module per week. Each module took 35–45 min to complete and provided interactive training in a cognitive-behavioral pain coping skill (e.g., progressive muscle relaxation, problem solving). As with in-person protocols, participants were encouraged to practice their new skills after learning them.

Participants in this study were 113 men and women with hip or knee OA pain. They were randomized to either PainCOACH or an assessment-only control group. Investigators were interested in the feasibility of this program as well as the effects of the program on the outcomes of pain, pain-related interference, pain-related anxiety, self-efficacy for pain management, and positive and negative affect. PainCOACH was found to be feasible with 91 % of participants completing the protocol in 8–10 weeks. Women were particularly likely to benefit from participating in the program; women who participated in PainCOACH had significantly lower postintervention levels of pain compared to women in the control group. Both men and women who participated in PainCOACH demonstrated increases in their self-efficacy from baseline to postintervention. The investigators also reported that smaller beneficial effects of PainCOACH were found for pain anxiety, pain-related interference with functioning, negative affect, and positive affect. This study is one of the first, if not the first, to report feasibility and initial efficacy of an automated, Internet-based CBT intervention to focus specifically on OA pain. The methods used in the development and testing will be valuable as work in Internet and technology-based interventions continues to advance.

Mindfulness for Pain Management

Mindfulness for pain management is emerging as a viable intervention for enhancing pain coping and is receiving increasing empirical support for use in arthritis (Day et al., 2014; Fjorback et al., 2011). Mindfulness for pain management, explained simply, is encouraging an individual with chronic pain to cope with their pain by attending to it with curiosity and without judgment instead of ruminating about how bad the pain is and ways to eliminate the pain. An important part of mindfulness for pain management is to accept the pain. This means learning to let go of goals and expectancies about pain and to instead work on doing the best one can with the pain just as it is. Jon Kabat-Zinn, the founder of an empirically supported program titled Mindfulness-Based Stress Reduction (MBSR), encourages individuals who use mindfulness for pain management to accept that nothing needs to be fixed, forced to stop, changed, or to go away (Kabat-Zinn, 2005).

The practice of mindfulness for pain management includes several exercises that are taught to an individual and then are recommended for regular, most often daily, practice. In the most traditional way, training in mindfulness for pain management would include a 1-day intensive practice and then 8 weeks of 2–2.5 h sessions to learn the exercises. Typically, the first exercise taught is a body scan. A body scan teaches an individual with pain to be aware of each part of the body, bring attention to that part of the body, and just experience the sensations with curiosity, even if the sensation is pain. During a body scan, one might be encouraged to really explore the pain—for example, the patient might be encouraged to notice which part of the back (e.g., lower or upper back) has the most sensation and which parts do not. A body scan meditation should be done in a quiet place and practice can last from 20 to 45 min. Another common exercise in mindfulness meditation for pain management is sitting meditation with a focus on the breath. These two exercises can be followed by a series of other exercises such as mindful movement, walking meditation, and/or meditation with yoga positions. Individuals who learn mindfulness for pain management are encouraged to bring mindfulness into their everyday lives and tasks.

In a study of 133 patients with arthritis and other persistent pain conditions, investigators examined the impact of an 8-week MBSR protocol on changes in bodily pain, health-related quality of life, and psychological symptoms (Rosenzweig et al., 2010). This study aimed to compare the intervention effects on subgroups of patients with different persistent pain conditions. Techniques used in this mindfulness intervention included body scan, awareness of breathing, awareness of emotions, mindful yoga and walking, mindful eating, and mindful listening. Participants were instructed to practice 20–25 min a day, 6 days each week. Participants with arthritis and other persistent pain conditions experienced significant pre- to postintervention changes in pain intensity and functional limitations due to pain. Interestingly, when compared to participants with headaches or fibromyalgia, participants with arthritis demonstrated the largest intervention effects for health-related quality of life and psychological distress. This finding is significant because it indicates that mindfulness-based meditation is a particularly viable intervention strategy for improving coping in patients with arthritis pain.

Davis et al. (2015) recently compared the impact of three intervention protocols on arthritis pain and other arthritis outcomes in a sample of 143 RA patients: (1) CBT for pain management, (2) pain focused mindful awareness and acceptance, and (3) pain arthritis education (Davis et al., 2015). The investigators used a daily diary approach to evaluate changes in pain and other outcomes. This particular study found that participants in the mindful awareness and acceptance condition were more likely to experience decreased pain catastrophizing, morning disability, fatigue, and daily stress than the other two conditions.

Psychosocial Interventions for Arthritis Patients and Caregivers'

Arthritis pain and coping with arthritis pain are prominent issues for patients with arthritis that also heavily impact patients' family and other loved ones (Kiecolt-Glaser & Newton, 2001). The biopsychosocial model of arthritis coping emphasizes the role of the patient's social context that includes the caregiver and/or significant other. There is evidence that caregivers of patients with arthritis can experience psychological distress and/or low levels of emotional well-being. Caregivers of patients with arthritis report that watching their loved one in pain or experiencing other arthritis-related difficulties is distressing and that they feel it is important to be able to assist their loved one as needed. Partners of arthritis patients may also have a harder time with their own health and health behaviors. For instance, a recent study found partners of arthritis patients with greater knee pain during the day report poorer overall sleep quality that night and feel less refreshed the following day (Martire et al., 2013).

Psychological interventions for arthritis pain and related disability have been developed and tested that include both the patient and their partner/caregiver. Two general approaches have been used when integrating partners/caregivers into psychological interventions for arthritis pain (Epstein & Baucom, 2002). There is the partner-assisted approach where the partner's role is that of an encourager or coach in helping patients learn to cope with arthritis pain. The second is a couples-based approach where the patient and partner are equal participants in the intervention and the goal is to increase pain coping in both members. Often, in a couples-based approach an additional goal is to improve the interactions between the patient and partner related to arthritis pain and other arthritis-related challenges.

An early study of partner-assisted pain coping skills training (PCST) randomized 88 patients to receive either: PCST (i.e., a CBT pain coping approach) without a partner, PCST with partner involvement, or arthritis education–partner support as a control condition (Keefe et al., 1996). Patients in the conventional PCST received a 10-week protocol that included a rationale for training, attention diversion, activity pacing, and cognitive coping strategies for pain control. In the partner-assisted PCST, the couple received these same skills plus training in patient–partner pain communication. Data from this study showed a consistent pattern in which patients in the partner-assisted protocol showed the best outcomes, the patients in pain coping skills without a partner showed the next best outcomes, and patients in the education condition showed the weakest outcomes. In another randomized controlled trial, Keefe et al. tested the separate and combined effects of a partner-assisted PCST along with exercise training in OA patients with knee pain (Keefe et al., 2004). Patients in this study were randomly assigned to either partner-assisted PCST alone, partner-assisted PCST plus exercise, exercise alone, or standard care. Results of this study found that an intervention that combines partner-assisted coping skills training and exercise training can improve pain coping, physical fitness, strength, and self-efficacy in patients with OA pain.

Psychosocial Interventions for Arthritis Pain and Comorbid Conditions

Arthritis is a very common disease and many individuals with arthritis also have at least one comorbid medical condition (e.g., heart disease, fatigue, obesity) (Briggs et al., 2009; Murphy et al., 2011). There is growing recognition that patients with arthritis pain may receive greater benefit from psychological interventions that enhance their arthritis pain coping and their ability to cope with comorbid medical conditions. Obesity is a comorbid medical condition that is highly prevalent in patients with arthritis and interferes with patients' abilities to learn to cope with their pain. Obese patients having arthritis pain are often advised to lose weight to improve their pain and pain-related disability. However, there is evidence that higher levels of arthritis pain challenge patients' ability to decrease their eating (Choi et al., 2014) and increase their activity (Der Ananian et al., 2008)—both key behaviors for weight management.

A recent study examined a psychosocial intervention that combined PCST with behavioral weight management (BWM) for patients with pain due to knee OA (Somers, Blumenthal, et al., 2012). Participants in this study were randomized to one of four conditions: PCST only, behavioral weight loss only (BWL only), and PCST+BWL, or a standard care control condition. The outcomes of interest in this work were pain, physical disability, psychological disability, and weight. Patients randomized to PCST+BWM demonstrated significantly better treatment outcomes in terms of pain, physical disability, stiffness, activity, and weight compared to the other three conditions. These results remained for up to 12 months following the intervention. This study is important because it emphasized the potential importance of learning to cope with both pain and weight for patients with arthritis working toward improving their pain and other medical conditions.

Other work has examined the comorbid problems of OA pain and insomnia. Individuals with arthritis-related pain commonly report problems with sleep and daytime fatigue. Vitiello et al. compared the benefits of three conditions in a randomized controlled trial: a cognitive-behavioral intervention for pain and insomnia, a cognitive-behavioral intervention for pain only, or an education-only condition (Vitiello et al., 2013). Primary outcomes of interest in this study were insomnia severity and pain severity; secondary outcomes of interest were actigraph-measured sleep efficiency and arthritis symptoms. The investigators found that participants who were randomized to the intervention targeting the comorbid problems of arthritis pain and insomnia had reduced insomnia compared to the education-only condition and the cognitive-behavioral intervention for pain only. The participants in the combined group reported improved sleep efficiency compared to the education-only group. Interestingly, changes in pain severity and arthritis symptoms did not differ between the three conditions. CBT for pain only improved sleep efficiency but not insomnia more than the education-only control group. The investigators conclude that the combined intervention—that is, adding insomnia-specific therapy to a cognitive-behavioral pain therapy—improves outcomes and that the combined intervention is effective in improving both self-report and objective sleep quality in persons with OA pain (Vitiello et al., 2013).

Assessment of Pain Coping

For individuals with arthritis pain, appropriate assessment is essential for successful treatment. Routine assessment often includes clarifying pain locations, intensity or severity, frequency, and duration. However, adjustment to persistent pain varies widely across individuals, and well-being among individuals suffering with arthritis pain is likely to be influenced by cognitive, affective, and behavioral processes (Reyes-Gibby, Aday, & Cleeland, 2002; Somers et al., 2009). Assessing pain coping efforts and related psychosocial factors can provide valuable insight into impacts on adjustment and targets for intervention among those with chronic arthritis pain (Jensen et al., 2001).

Measures of Pain Coping

Assessments of pain coping can be used to develop treatment plans that target the most critical beliefs, behaviors, and coping strategies for a particular patient. In contrast to more general measures of coping (e.g., Brief COPE Inventory), measures of pain coping specifically assess individuals' cognitive and behavioral efforts to manage pain (Carver, 1997). Examples of cognitive coping strategies include counting numbers and focusing on distracting features of the environment. Examples of behavioral coping strategies include activities such as walking or talking to other individuals. In selecting a pain coping measure, it is important to consider the nature and source of pain involved. For individuals with arthritis pain, the pain coping strategies used may differ from those commonly used by individuals with cancer-related pain or disease-related painful neuropathy (Parmelee, 2005). For example, pain coping among those with arthritis may be heavily influenced by the activity limitations caused by arthritis pain.

The Coping Strategies Questionnaire (CSQ) was developed in 1983 and is one of the most widely used measures of pain coping (Riley & Robinson, 1997; Robinson et al., 1997; Rosenstiel & Keefe, 1983). This pain coping measure has been successfully used in clinic and research settings for individuals with arthritis (Rapp, Rejeski, & Miller, 2000; Riddle & Jensen, 2013). The CSQ is a process rather than trait-oriented measure. For this measure, the process of coping with chronic pain is conceptualized as a complex and ongoing one. As the intensity of chronic pain varies, individuals may rely on different coping strategies. Thus, pain coping strategies assessed by the CSQ are viewed as part of a dynamic process rather than as enduring traits (Rosenstiel & Keefe, 1983).

The CSQ includes 42 items that assess the following coping strategies: diverting attention (e.g., counting numbers), reinterpreting pain sensations (e.g., thinking of pain as another sensation such as numbness), coping self-statements (e.g., telling myself to carry on despite the pain), ignoring pain (e.g., pretending it is not there), praying and hoping (e.g., praying that the pain will not last long), increasing behavioral activities (e.g., try to be around other people), and catastrophizing (e.g., worry all the time about whether pain will end). Using a 7-point scale for each item, individuals indicate how often they use each strategy when they experience pain (where 0 = never, 3 = sometimes, and 6 = always). Each domain of coping is scored separately by summing the responses for questions in that particular domain, with higher scores indicating greater use of the coping strategy. The CSQ scales have demonstrated excellent psychometric properties (i.e., internal consistency, test–retest reliability, convergent validity) (Main & Waddell, 1991; Robinson et al., 1997; Rosenstiel & Keefe, 1983).

Shorter versions of the CSQ have also been developed for use in clinic and research settings. The 27-item CSQ-Revised assesses distraction, catastrophizing, ignoring pain sensations, distancing from pain, coping self-statements, and praying and hoping (Riley & Robinson, 1997; Robinson et al., 1997). The CSQ-Revised has been well validated, takes approximately 10 min to complete, and has been translated for use in multiple languages (Irachabal et al., 2008; Monticone et al., 2014). A brief 14-item version of the CSQ has also been developed and has been widely used in the clinic setting (Jensen et al., 2003). This brief version includes 2-item scales for each of the coping domains assessed in the longer 42-item version of the CSQ. The brief 14-item CSQ has demonstrated excellent psychometric properties as well as construct and criterion-based validity for individuals with chronic OA pain (Jensen et al., 2003; Riddle & Jensen, 2013). The brief 14-item CSQ offers a rapid tool for capturing the use of multiple pain coping domains.

Another commonly used measure of pain coping is the Chronic Pain Coping Inventory (CPCI). The CPCI was first developed in 1995 as a 65-question pain coping measure, and a shorter 42-item version of the CPCI was developed in 2003 (Jensen et al., 1995; Romano, Jensen, & Turner, 2003). The CPCI was developed to assess behavioral and cognitive pain coping strategies that are often targets of pain management programs (e.g., exercise, guarding, resting, coping self-statements). When compared to the CSQ, the CPCI is more heavily weighted toward behavioral rather than cognitive aspects of coping and places a stronger emphasis on specific coping behaviors (e.g., lay down on a bed) (Monticone et al., 2013).

The 42-item CPCI assesses the following eight coping strategies: guarding (e.g., avoided using part of my body), resting (e.g., lay down on a sofa), asking for assistance (e.g., asked someone to do something for me), relaxation (e.g., focused on relaxing my muscles), task persistence (e.g., ignored the pain), exercise/stretching (e.g., engaged in aerobic exercise), seeking social support (e.g., got support from a friend), and coping self-statements (e.g., told myself things will get better). Individuals are asked to indicate how many days each strategy was used (at least once in the day) to cope with pain over the past week. Thus, each strategy is rated on a 0 (no days) to 7 (every day) scale. For each scale, the responses to items are summed and then divided by the number of items completed to obtain an average score, with higher scores indicating more frequent use of the strategy. The CPCI scales have been widely used, demonstrate excellent psychometric properties (i.e., internal consistency, test–retest reliability, convergent validity), and have been translated for use in multiple languages (Ektor-Andersen, Orbaek, & Isacsson, 2002; Garcia-Campayo et al., 2007; Jensen et al., 1995; Ko, Park, & Lim, 2010; Monticone et al., 2013; Romano et al., 2003; Truchon, Cote, & Irachabal, 2006; Wong et al., 2010).

A shorter 16-item version of the CPCI has been developed for use in busy clinics and research settings (Jensen et al., 2003). The brief 16-item version includes two items for each of the eight coping strategy scales of the CPCI. Each of the two-item CPCI scales has demonstrated strong correlations with the longer parent scales and has demonstrated sensitivity to change (Jensen et al., 2003).

Incorporating Assessments of Other Important Psychosocial Factors

Because the experience and impact of arthritis pain are best conceptualized using a biopsychosocial framework, any effort to comprehensively assess individuals with chronic arthritis pain requires evaluation of other psychosocial processes alongside pain coping (Parmelee, 2005). A comprehensive assessment should also include evaluations of anxiety and depression, pain catastrophizing, and self-efficacy for pain management. Pain catastrophizing is by far one of the most widely measured and relevant cognitive constructs for individuals with chronic pain (Burns et al., 2015; Rayahin et al., 2014; Sturgeon, Zautra, & Arewasikporn, 2014). Pain catastrophizing is conceptualized as a maladaptive pain coping strategy and all versions of the CSQ include a pain catastrophizing scale (Jensen et al., 2003; Robinson et al., 1997; Rosenstiel & Keefe, 1983). However, other measures of pain coping do not include scales specifically designed to assess pain catastrophizing. When using other pain coping measures, incorporating the CSQ pain catastrophizing scale or the longer Pain Catastrophizing Scale should be considered (Sullivan, Bishop, & Pivik, 1995).

The Less Known: Directions for Future Work

Over the last several years there has been increasing acknowledgement of the importance of approaching pain coping in arthritis patients from the biopsychosocial model. The biopsychosocial model of arthritis pain coping explains that biological factors, psychological factors, and social factors have direct and interacting influences on how an individual learns to cope with their arthritis pain. As this area of work in coping with arthritis pain continues to advance, there are several areas of importance to be considered.

Influence of Coping on Biological Markers of Disease

An individual's ability to cope with arthritis pain has been consistently related to subjective measurements of physical functioning, daily activity, and physical disability (Keefe et al., 2002).

Increasing evidence shows that pain coping is also related to more objective physiological and biological markers of arthritis; this relationship is critical to fully understand the biopsychosocial relationship of pain coping. In a study examining the relationship between pain and biomarkers in a healthy sample of participants, pain catastrophizing—a maladaptive coping strategy—was associated with changes in cortisol during an experimental pain induction (i.e., cold pressor task) (Cruz-Almeida et al., 2012). This suggests that engaging in pain catastrophizing can have a negative impact on biomarkers of the stress response. In arthritis patients who experience persistent pain and engage in pain catastrophizing, this relationship may suggest consistently high levels of stress hormones, which are associated with negative physiological outcomes (Keefe et al., 2002, 2010). Little work has been done to understand how improved pain coping might lead to changes in such biomarkers. In a secondary study to Somers et al., investigators examined the effects of PCST and BWM combined or alone on pain, function, and inflammatory biomarkers. Findings from this work showed that important biological markers of inflammation were related to reductions in pain as well as overall weight and body mass index (BMI) in the OA patients who received both PCST and BWM. These findings are particularly important because the relationships between inflammatory biomarkers (i.e., hsCRP, IL-6) of arthritis and reductions in pain, weight, and BMI were *only* found in the combined PCST and BMW group and not the groups that received either treatment alone. This work begins to show that improved pain coping may, in fact, have a unique, important influence on biomarkers of inflammation. Future work should purposefully begin to explore this potentially critical relationship.

Comorbid Medical Disorders

Many patients with arthritis must learn to cope with their arthritis pain and pain-related disability as well as pain and symptoms related to other comorbid medical problems. Patients with arthritis and other medical problems are significantly more likely to report a lower overall quality of life than patients with just arthritis and have more trouble learning to cope (Michaud, Wallenstein, & Wolfe, 2011; Mujica-Mota et al., 2015). Evidence from a study of obese RA patients with pain found that patients who had higher levels of positive coping related to each specific medical challenge, in this case RA pain and obesity, were more likely to have better outcomes related to the specific medical outcome (Somers et al., 2014). For instance, pain catastrophizing was uniquely associated with pain severity, and self-efficacy for weight management was uniquely related to weight-management behaviors. This suggests that when patients have arthritis pain and comorbid disorders, unique coping strategies or skills may be necessary to address challenges related to each condition (i.e., pain and obesity). Further work in the area of psychosocial interventions targeting coping with arthritis pain will need to consider the multiple comorbid medical problems that patients with arthritis may have and integrate coping with comorbidities into intervention protocols.

Geriatrics

Arthritis is common among elderly men and women and a significant cause of physical disability and decline. Although researchers have long studied arthritis in adult populations, research is needed to better understand arthritis pain and pain coping in elderly populations. Despite its high prevalence, evidence suggests pain is underreported and undertreated in elderly individuals (Bruera & Portenoy, 2010; Moore, 2009). Older patients may expect to experience pain as a natural part of the aging process, think treatments for pain are worse than dealing with the symptom, including concern about tolerating treatment side effects, or feel fearful of its underlying cause (Bruera & Portenoy, 2010; Moore, 2009). Psycho-education for elderly patients and training for healthcare professionals in developmental pain issues is needed to target misconceptions and deficits in knowledge to reduce barriers to adequate pain management in the elderly. Future research should focus on improving the validity of diagnostic and treatment tools for use with the elderly. Data are also needed to understand the mechanisms of age-related changes in arthritis pain and the effectiveness of pain management strategies in older adults. Also important and not well understood is the interaction of arthritis pain and biopsychosocial factors unique to the elderly (e.g., comorbid medical disorders, depression, life satisfaction, risk for falls). There is an urgent need to explore these gaps in knowledge and doing so will allow researchers and clinicians to better understand and address the unique needs related to pain coping of the elderly.

Psychosocial Interventions and Underserved and Ethnic Minorities

Arthritis affects men and women of varying racial and ethnic backgrounds and evidence suggests minority and underserved populations may experience unique risk factors and vulnerabilities in health and quality of life outcomes (Cross et al., 2014; McIlvane et al., 2008). Although arthritis prevalence rates are higher for Caucasian and American Indians/Alaska Natives, research has shown a greater negative impact for minority populations, including African Americans, Hispanics, and Asians/Pacific Islanders (Bolen et al., 2010; Green et al., 2003). For example, studies have documented higher pain severity ratings, greater functional disability and activity/work limitations, and lower utilization of surgical treatments and self-management programs among African Americans with arthritis (Casanova Vivas & Centers for Disease, and Prevention, 2005; Kreuter et al., 2003; McIlvane et al., 2008). Despite these findings, limited work has examined the impact of psychosocial pain coping interventions for ethnic minorities and underserved populations (McIlvane et al., 2008). Additionally, current protocols which have been developed and tested in mostly Caucasian samples may not be appropriate for minority patients due to cultural issues and language barriers; other barriers include acceptability, accessibility, and costs/reimbursement (Norris & Agodoa, 2005). Future research should prioritize investigating the effectiveness of psychosocial pain coping interventions in ethnically and culturally diverse arthritis patient populations. This research should focus not only on increasing minority participation, but also designing and tailoring culturally sensitive treatment protocols to meet the unique needs of minority and underserved arthritis patients.

Dissemination of Psychosocial Interventions to Improve Pain Coping

There is increasing evidence of the efficacy of several psychosocial interventions to enhance pain coping for patients with arthritis to manage their pain and pain-related disability. However, many patients that could benefit from such interventions do not have access to these interventions or face significant barriers to participating in such an intervention. This is particularly true for patients who live in rural areas or in areas with limited socioeconomic resources. Access barriers to psychosocial pain management interventions are often related to proximity to a medical center with psychosocial resources, availability of trained therapists to deliver psychosocial interventions, and healthcare providers' unawareness of the benefit of psychosocial pain management interventions. Patient-related barriers to accessing psychosocial interventions for pain management include such factors as financial resources, physical and psychological burden, travel, transportation, and time. Rini et al. (2015) provide a plausible model of a CBT pain management intervention (i.e., automated, self-directed Internet intervention) that may reduce some of these barriers for some people (Rini et al., 2015). More work is needed in the area of psychosocial interventions for pain management in arthritis that can be disseminated more widely with the use of a combination of the Internet and mobile health technologies.

References

Affleck G, Urrows S, Tennen H, Higgins P. Daily coping with pain from rheumatoid arthritis: patterns and correlates. Pain. 1992;51(2):221–9.

Aggarwal, A., Chandran, S., & Misra, R. (2006). Physical, psychosocial and economic impact of rheumatoid arthritis: A pilot study of patients seen at a tertiary care referral centre. *The National Medical Journal of India, 19*(4), 187–191.

Bandura A, Cioffi D, Taylor CB, Brouillard ME. Perceived self-efficacy in coping with cognitive stressors and opioid activation. J Pers Soc Psychol. 1988;55(3):479–88.

Barlow, J. H., Wright, C. C., & Lorig, K. (2001). The perils and pitfalls of comparing UK and US samples of people enrolled in an Arthritis Self-Management Program: The case of the Center for Epidemiological Studies-Depression (CES-D) Scale. *Arthritis and Rheumatism, 45*(1), 77–80.

Bolen J, Schieb L, Hootman JM, Helmick CG, Theis K, Murphy LB, et al. Differences in the prevalence and severity of arthritis among racial/ethnic groups in the United States, National Health Interview Survey, 2002, 2003, and 2006. Prev Chronic Dis. 2010;7(3):A64.

Bradley LA, Young LD, Anderson KO, Turner RA, Agudelo CA, McDaniel LK, et al. Effects of psychological therapy on pain behavior of rheumatoid arthritis patients. Treatment outcome and six-month followup. Arthritis Rheum. 1987;30(10):1105–14.

Brekke M, Hjortdahl P, Thelle DS, Kvien TK. Disease activity and severity in patients with rheumatoid arthritis: relations to socioeconomic inequality. Soc Sci Med. 1999;48(12):1743–50.

Briggs AM, March L, Lassere M, Reid C, Henderson L, Murphy B, et al. Baseline comorbidities in a population-based cohort of rheumatoid arthritis patients receiving biological therapy: data from the Australian rheumatology association database. Int J Rheumatol. 2009;2009:861481. doi:10.1155/2009/861481.

Bruera, E. D., & Portenoy, R. K. (Eds.). (2010). Cancer pain: Assessment and management (2nd ed.). New York, NY: Cambridge University Press.

Burns LC, Ritvo SE, Ferguson MK, Clarke H, Seltzer Z, Katz J. Pain catastrophizing as a risk factor for chronic pain after total knee arthroplasty: a systematic review. [Review]. J Pain Res. 2015;8:21–32. doi:10.2147/JPR.S64730.

Carver CS. You want to measure coping but your protocol's too long: Consider the brief COPE. International Journal of Behavioral Medicine. 1997;4(1):92–100.

Casanova Vivas, S., & Centers for Disease, and Prevention. (2005). CDC recommendations: Centers for Disease Control and Prevention of infectious diseases in the United States. *Revista de Enfermagem 28*(11):13–16

Choi KW, Somers TJ, Babyak MA, Sikkema KJ, Blumenthal JA, Keefe FJ. The relationship between pain and eating among overweight and obese individuals with osteoarthritis: an ecological momentary study. Pain Res Manag. 2014;19(6):e159–163.

Cojocaru M, Cojocaru IM, Silosi I, Vrabie CD, Tanasescu R. Extra-articular Manifestations in Rheumatoid Arthritis. Maedica (Buchar). 2010;5(4):286–91.

Covic T, Cumming SR, Pallant JF, Manolios N, Emery P, Conaghan PG, et al. Depression and anxiety in patients with rheumatoid arthritis: prevalence rates based on a comparison of the Depression, Anxiety and Stress Scale (DASS) and the hospital, Anxiety and Depression Scale (HADS). BMC Psychiatry. 2012;12:6. doi:10.1186/1471-244X-12-6.

Covic T, Tyson G, Spencer D, Howe G. Depression in rheumatoid arthritis patients: demographic, clinical, and psychological predictors. J Psychosom Res. 2006;60(5):469–76. doi:10.1016/j.jpsychores.2005.09.011.

Cross M, Smith E, Hoy D, Carmona L, Wolfe F, Vos T, et al. The global burden of rheumatoid arthritis: estimates from the global burden of disease 2010 study. Ann Rheum Dis. 2014;73(7):1316–22. doi:10.1136/annrheumdis-2013-204627.

Cruz-Almeida Y, King CD, Wallet SM, Riley 3rd JL. Immune biomarker response depends on choice of experimental pain stimulus in healthy adults: a preliminary study. Pain Res Treat. 2012;2012:538739. doi:10.1155/2012/538739.

Curtis, J. R., & Singh, J. A. (2011). Use of biologics in rheumatoid arthritis: Current and emerging paradigms of care. *Clinical Therapeutics, 33*(6), 679–707.

Davis MC, Zautra AJ, Wolf LD, Tennen H, Yeung EW. Mindfulness and cognitive-behavioral interventions for chronic pain: Differential effects on daily pain reactivity and stress reactivity. J Consult Clin Psychol. 2015;83(1):24–35. doi:10.1037/a0038200.

Day MA, Jensen MP, Ehde DM, Thorn BE. Toward a theoretical model for mindfulness-based pain management. J Pain. 2014;15(7):691–703. doi:10.1016/j.jpain.2014.03.003.

Der Ananian C, Wilcox S, Watkins K, Saunders R, Evans AE. Factors associated with exercise participation in adults with arthritis. J Aging Phys Act. 2008;16(2):125–43.

Dessein, P. H., Joffe, B. I., & Stanwix, A. E. (2004). High sensitivity C-reactive protein as a disease activity marker in rheumatoid arthritis. *The Journal of Rheumatology, 31*(6), 1095–1097.

Doeglas D, Suurmeijer T, Krol B, Sanderman R, van Rijswijk M, van Leeuwen M. Social support, social disability, and psychological well-being in rheumatoid arthritis. Arthritis Care Res. 1994;7(1):10–5.

Edwards RR, Bingham 3rd CO, Bathon J, Haythornthwaite JA. Catastrophizing and pain in arthritis, fibromyalgia, and other rheumatic diseases. Arthritis Rheum. 2006;55(2):325–32. doi:10.1002/art.21865.

Edwards RR, Cahalan C, Mensing G, Smith M, Haythornthwaite JA. Pain, catastrophizing, and depression in the rheumatic diseases. Nat Rev Rheumatol. 2011;7(4):216–24. doi:10.1038/nrrheum.2011.2.

Edwards RR, Giles J, Bingham 3rd CO, Campbell C, Haythornthwaite JA, Bathon J. Moderators of the negative effects of catastrophizing in arthritis. Pain

Med. 2010;11(4):591–9. doi:10.1111/j.1526-4637.2010.00804.x.

Ektor-Andersen J, Orbaek P, Isacsson SO. Behaviour-focused pain coping: consistency and convergence to work capability of the swedish version of the chronic pain coping inventory. [Research Support, Non-U.S. Gov't]. J Rehabil Med. 2002;34(1):33–9.

Epstein NB, Baucom DH. Enhanced cognitive-behavioral therapy for couples: A contextual approach. Washington, D.C.: American Psychological Association; 2002.

Evers AW, Kraaimaat FW, Geenen R, Bijlsma JW. Psychosocial predictors of functional change in recently diagnosed rheumatoid arthritis patients. Behav Res Ther. 1998;36(2):179–93.

Fjorback LO, Arendt M, Ornbol E, Fink P, Walach H. Mindfulness-based stress reduction and mindfulness-based cognitive therapy: a systematic review of randomized controlled trials. Acta Psychiatr Scand. 2011;124(2):102–19. doi:10.1111/j.1600-0447.2011.01704.x.

Garcia-Campayo, J., Pascual, A., Alda, M., & Gonzalez Ramirez, M. T. (2007). Coping with fibromialgia: usefulness of the Chronic Pain Coping Inventory-42. [Research Support, Non-U.S. Gov't

Gatchel RJ, Peng YB, Peters ML, Fuchs PN, Turk DC. The biopsychosocial approach to chronic pain: scientific advances and future directions. Psychol Bull. 2007;133(4):581–624. doi:10.1037/0033-2909.133.4.581.

Green MJ, Gough AK, Devlin J, Smith J, Astin P, Taylor D, et al. Serum MMP-3 and MMP-1 and progression of joint damage in early rheumatoid arthritis. Rheumatology (Oxford). 2003;42(1):83–8.

Hootman JM, Helmick CG. Projections of US prevalence of arthritis and associated activity limitations. Arthritis Rheum. 2006;54(1):226–9. doi:10.1002/art.21562.

Irachabal S, Koleck M, Rascle N, Bruchon-Schweitzer M. Pain coping strategies: French adaptation of the coping strategies questionnaire (CSQ-F). Encephale. 2008;34(1):47–53. doi:10.1016/j.encep.2006.11.002.

Irwin MR, Olmstead R, Carrillo C, Sadeghi N, Fitzgerald JD, Ranganath VK, et al. Sleep loss exacerbates fatigue, depression, and pain in rheumatoid arthritis. Sleep. 2012;35(4):537–43. doi:10.5665/sleep.1742.

Isik A, Koca SS, Ozturk A, Mermi O. Anxiety and depression in patients with rheumatoid arthritis. Clin Rheumatol. 2007;26(6):872–8. doi:10.1007/s10067-006-0407-y.

Jensen MP, Keefe FJ, Lefebvre JC, Romano JM, Turner JA. One- and two-item measures of pain beliefs and coping strategies. [Multicenter StudyResearch Support, Non-U.S. Gov't Research Support, U.S. Gov't, P.H.S.]. Pain. 2003;104(3):453–69.

Jensen MP, Turner JA, Romano JM. Changes in beliefs, catastrophizing, and coping are associated with improvement in multidisciplinary pain treatment. [Research Support, U.S. Gov't, P.H.S.]. J Consult Clin Psychol. 2001;69(4):655–62.

Jensen MP, Turner JA, Romano JM, Strom SE. The Chronic Pain Coping Inventory: development and preliminary validation. [Research Support, Non-U.S. Gov't]. Pain. 1995;60(2):203–16.

Kabat-Zinn, J., & University of Massachusetts Medical Center/Worcester Stress Reduction Clinic. (2005). *Full catastrophe living: Using the wisdom of your body and mind to face stress, pain, and illness* (xxxiii, 471 p.). Delta trade pbk (reissued). New York, NY: Delta Trade Paperbacks.

Katon, W. J. (2011). Epidemiology and treatment of depression in patients with chronic medical illness. *Dialogues in Clinical Neuroscience, 13*(1), 7–23.

Katz, P. P. (1998). The stresses of rheumatoid arthritis: Appraisals of perceived impact and coping efficacy. *Arthritis Care & Research, 11*(1), 9–22.

Katz, P. P., Morris, A., & Yelin, E. H. (2006). Prevalence and predictors of disability in valued life activities among individuals with rheumatoid arthritis. *Annals of the Rheumatic Diseases, 65*(6), 763–769.

Katz, P. P., & Yelin, E. H. (1993). Prevalence and correlates of depressive symptoms among persons with rheumatoid arthritis. *The Journal of Rheumatology, 20*(5), 790–796.

Katz, P. P., & Yelin, E. H. (1995). The development of depressive symptoms among women with rheumatoid arthritis. The role of function. *Arthritis and Rheumatism, 38*(1), 49–56.

Keefe, F. J., Abernethy, A. P., & L, C. Campbell. (2005). Psychological approaches to understanding and treating disease-related pain. Annu Rev Psychol, 56, 601-630. doi: 10.1146/annurev.psych.56.091103.070302

Keefe, F. J., Blumenthal, J., Baucom, D., Affleck, G., Waugh, R., Caldwell, D. S., Beaupre, P., Kashikar-Zuck, S., Wright, K., Egert, J., & Lefebvre, J. (2004). Effects of spouse-assisted coping skills training and exercise training in patients with osteoarthritic knee pain: a randomized controlled study. Pain, 110(3), 539–549. doi:10.1016/j.pain.2004.03.022

Keefe FJ, Brown GK, Wallston KA, Caldwell DS. Coping with rheumatoid arthritis pain: catastrophizing as a maladaptive strategy. Pain. 1989;37(1):51–6.

Keefe FJ, Caldwell DS, Baucom D, Salley A, Robinson E, Timmons K, et al. Spouse-assisted coping skills training in the management of osteoarthritic knee pain. Arthritis Care Res. 1996;9(4):279–91.

Keefe FJ, Caldwell DS, Queen KT, Gil KM, Martinez S, Crisson JE, et al. Pain coping strategies in osteoarthritis patients. J Consult Clin Psychol. 1987;55(2):208–12.

Keefe FJ, Shelby RA, Somers TJ. Catastrophizing and pain coping: moving forward. Pain. 2010;149(2):165–6. doi:10.1016/j.pain.2010.02.030.

Keefe FJ, Smith SJ, Buffington AL, Gibson J, Studts JL, Caldwell DS. Recent advances and future directions in the biopsychosocial assessment and treatment of arthritis. J Consult Clin Psychol. 2002;70(3):640–55.

Keefe FJ, Somers TJ, Martire LM. Psychologic interventions and lifestyle modifications for arthritis pain management. Rheum Dis Clin North Am. 2008;34(2):351–68. doi:10.1016/j.rdc.2008.03.001.

Kidd, B. L., Langford, R. M., & Wodehouse, T. (2007). Arthritis and pain. Current approaches in the treatment of arthritic pain. *Arthritis Research & Therapy, 9*(3), 214.

Kiecolt-Glaser, J. K., & Newton, T. L. (2001). Marriage and health: His and hers. *Psychological Bulletin, 127*(4), 472–503.

Ko, Y. M., Park, W. B., & Lim, J. Y. (2010). Cross-cultural adaptation and clinimetric property of Korean version of the Chronic Pain Coping Inventory-42 in patients with chronic low back pain. *Spine (Phila Pa 1976), 35*(6), 666–671.

Kreuter MW, Steger-May K, Bobra S, Booker A, Holt CL, Lukwago SN, et al. Sociocultural characteristics and responses to cancer education materials among African American women. Cancer Control. 2003;10(5 Suppl):69–80.

Lame IE, Peters ML, Vlaeyen JW, Kleef M, Patijn J. Quality of life in chronic pain is more associated with beliefs about pain, than with pain intensity. Eur J Pain. 2005;9(1):15–24. doi:10.1016/j.ejpain.2004.02.006.

Lefebvre JC, Keefe FJ, Affleck G, Raezer LB, Starr K, Caldwell DS, et al. The relationship of arthritis self-efficacy to daily pain, daily mood, and daily pain coping in rheumatoid arthritis patients. Pain. 1999;80(1-2):425–35.

Main, C. J., & Waddell, G. (1991). A comparison of cognitive measures in low back pain: Statistical structure and clinical validity at initial assessment. *Pain, 46*(3), 287–298.

Martire LM, Keefe FJ, Schulz R, Parris Stephens MA, Mogle JA. The impact of daily arthritis pain on spouse sleep. Pain. 2013;154(9):1725–31. doi:10.1016/j.pain.2013.05.020.

Martire LM, Keefe FJ, Schulz R, Ready R, Beach SR, Rudy TE, et al. Older spouses' perceptions of partners' chronic arthritis pain: implications for spousal responses, support provision, and caregiving experiences.PsycholAging.2006;21(2):222–30.doi:10.1037/0882-7974.21.2.222.

McIlvane JM, Baker TA, Mingo CA, Haley WE. Are behavioral interventions for arthritis effective with minorities? Addressing racial and ethnic diversity in disability and rehabilitation. Arthritis Rheum. 2008;59(10):1512–8. doi:10.1002/art.24117.

Michaud, K., Wallenstein, G., & Wolfe, F. (2011). Treatment and nontreatment predictors of health assessment questionnaire disability progression in rheumatoid arthritis: A longitudinal study of 18,485 patients. *Arthritis Care & Research, 63*(3), 366–372.

Monticone M, Ferrante S, Giorgi I, Galandra C, Rocca B, Foti C. Development of the Italian version of the 42-item Chronic Pain Coping Inventory, CPCI-I: cross-cultural adaptation, factor analysis, reliability and validity. Qual Life Res. 2013;22(6):1459–65. doi:10.1007/s11136-012-0271-y.

Monticone M, Ferrante S, Giorgi I, Galandra C, Rocca B, Foti C. The 27-item coping strategies questionnaire-revised: confirmatory factor analysis, reliability and validity in Italian-speaking subjects with chronic pain. Pain Res Manag. 2014;19(3):153–8.

Moore, R. J. (2009). Biobehavioral approaches to pain. New York, NY: Springer.

Mujica-Mota RE, Roberts M, Abel G, Elliott M, Lyratzopoulos G, Roland M, et al. Common patterns of morbidity and multi-morbidity and their impact on health-related quality of life: evidence from a national survey. Qual Life Res. 2014. doi:10.1007/s11136-014-0820-7.

Murphy, G., & Nagase, H. (2008). Reappraising metalloproteinases in rheumatoid arthritis and osteoarthritis: Destruction or repair? *Nature Clinical Practice Rheumatology, 4*(3), 128–135.

Murphy SL, Lyden AK, Phillips K, Clauw DJ, Williams DA. Subgroups of older adults with osteoarthritis based upon differing comorbid symptom presentations and potential underlying pain mechanisms. Arthritis Res Ther. 2011;13(4):R135. doi:10.1186/ar3449.

Norris, K. C., & Agodoa, L. Y. (2005). The need for health professionals and scientists from underrepresented minority and disadvantaged communities. *Ethnicity & Disease, 15*(3 Suppl 4), 1–2.

O'Leary A, Shoor S, Lorig K, Holman HR. A cognitive-behavioral treatment for rheumatoid arthritis. Health Psychol. 1988;7(6):527–44.

Parmelee, P. A. (2005). Measuring mood and psychosocial function associated with pain in late life. In S. J. Gibson & D. K. Weiner (Eds.), *Pain in older persons, progress in pain research and management* (pp. 175–202). Seattle, WA: IASP Press.

Penninx BW, van Tilburg T, Deeg DJ, Kriegsman DM, Boeke AJ, van Eijk JT. Direct and buffer effects of social support and personal coping resources in individuals with arthritis. Soc Sci Med. 1997;44(3):393–402.

Quartana, P. J., Campbell, C. M., & Edwards, R. R. (2009). Pain catastrophizing: A critical review. *Expert Review of Neurotherapeutics, 9*(5), 745–758.

Rapp, S. R., Rejeski, W. J., & Miller, M. E. (2000). Physical function among older adults with knee pain: The role of pain coping skills. *Arthritis Care & Research, 13*(5), 270–279.

Rayahin JE, Chmiel JS, Hayes KW, Almagor O, Belisle L, Chang AH, et al. Factors associated with pain experience outcome in knee osteoarthritis. [Research Support, N.I.H., Extramural]. Arthritis Care Res (Hoboken). 2014;66(12):1828–35. doi:10.1002/acr.22402.

Reese JB, Somers TJ, Keefe FJ, Mosley-Williams A, Lumley MA. Pain and functioning of rheumatoid arthritis patients based on marital status: is a distressed marriage preferable to no marriage? J Pain. 2010;11(10):958–64. doi:10.1016/j.jpain.2010.01.003.

Reyes-Gibby, C. C., Aday, L., & Cleeland, C. (2002). Impact of pain on self-rated health in the community-dwelling older adults. *Pain, 95*(1–2), 75–82.

Riddle, D. L., & Jensen, M. P. (2013). Construct and criterion-based validity of brief pain coping scales in persons with chronic knee osteoarthritis pain. *Pain Medicine, 14*(2), 265–275.

Riley, J. L., III, & Robinson, M. E. (1997). CSQ: Five factors or fiction? *The Clinical Journal of Pain, 13*(2), 156–162.

Rini C, Porter LS, Somers TJ, McKee DC, Keefe FJ. Retaining critical therapeutic elements of behavioral interventions translated for delivery via the Internet: recommendations and an example using pain coping skills training. J Med Internet Res. 2014;16(12), e245. doi:10.2196/jmir.3374.

Rini, C., Porter, L. S., Somers, T. J., McKee, D., Devellis, R.F., Smith, M., Winkel, G., Ahern, D.K., Goldman,

R., Stiller, J.L., Mariani, C., Pattterson, C., Jordan, J.M., Caldwell, D., & Keefe, F.J. (in press). Automated, Internet-based Pain Coping Skills Training to Manage Osteoarthritis Pain: A Randomized Controlled Trial. Pain.

Robinson ME, Riley 3rd JL, Myers CD, Sadler IJ, Kvaal SA, Geisser ME, et al. The Coping Strategies Questionnaire: a large sample, item level factor analysis. [Clinical Trial]. Clin J Pain. 1997;13(1):43–9.

Romano, J. M., Jensen, M. P., & Turner, J. A. (2003). The Chronic Pain Coping Inventory-42: Reliability and validity. *Pain, 104*(1–2), 65–73.

Rosenstiel, A. K., & Keefe, F. J. (1983). The use of coping strategies in chronic low back pain patients: Relationship to patient characteristics and current adjustment. *Pain, 17*(1), 33–44.

Rosenzweig S, Greeson JM, Reibel DK, Green JS, Jasser SA, Beasley D. Mindfulness-based stress reduction for chronic pain conditions: variation in treatment outcomes and role of home meditation practice. J Psychosom Res. 2010;68(1):29–36. doi:10.1016/j.jpsychores.2009.03.010.

Scheinfeld, N. (2005). Adalimumab: A review of side effects. *Expert Opinion on Drug Safety, 4*(4), 637–641.

Schiff MH, Burmester GR, Kent JD, Pangan AL, Kupper H, Fitzpatrick SB, et al. Safety analyses of adalimumab (HUMIRA) in global clinical trials and US postmarketing surveillance of patients with rheumatoid arthritis. Ann Rheum Dis. 2006;65(7):889–94. doi:10.1136/ard.2005.043166.

Shadick NA, Cook NR, Karlson EW, Ridker PM, Maher NE, Manson JE, et al. C-reactive protein in the prediction of rheumatoid arthritis in women. Arch Intern Med. 2006;166(22):2490–4. doi:10.1001/archinte.166.22.2490.

Somers TJ, Blumenthal JA, Guilak F, Kraus VB, Schmitt DO, Babyak MA, et al. Pain coping skills training and lifestyle behavioral weight management in patients with knee osteoarthritis: a randomized controlled study. Pain. 2012a;153(6):1199–209. doi:10.1016/j.pain.2012.02.023.

Somers TJ, Keefe FJ, Godiwala N, Hoyler GH. Psychosocial factors and the pain experience of osteoarthritis patients: new findings and new directions. Curr Opin Rheumatol. 2009;21(5):501–6. doi:10.1097/BOR.0b013e32832ed704.

Somers TJ, Kurakula PC, Criscione-Schreiber L, Keefe FJ, Clowse ME. Self-efficacy and pain catastrophizing in systemic lupus erythematosus: relationship to pain, stiffness, fatigue, and psychological distress. Arthritis Care Res (Hoboken). 2012b;64(9):1334–40. doi:10.1002/acr.21686.

Somers TJ, Shelby RA, Keefe FJ, Godiwala N, Lumley MA, Mosley-Williams A, et al. Disease severity and domain-specific arthritis self-efficacy: relationships to pain and functioning in patients with rheumatoid arthritis. Arthritis Care Res (Hoboken). 2010;62(6):848–56. doi:10.1002/acr.20127.

Somers TJ, Wren AA, Blumenthal JA, Caldwell D, Huffman KM, Keefe FJ. Pain, physical functioning, and overeating in obese rheumatoid arthritis patients: do thoughts about pain and eating matter? J Clin Rheumatol. 2014;20(5):244–50. doi:10.1097/RHU.0000000000000124.

Somers TJ, Wren AA, Shelby RA. The context of pain in arthritis: self-efficacy for managing pain and other symptoms. Curr Pain Headache Rep. 2012c;16(6):502–8. doi:10.1007/s11916-012-0298-3.

Sturgeon, J. A., Zautra, A. J., & Arewasikporn, A. (2014). A multilevel structural equation modeling analysis of vulnerabilities and resilience resources influencing affective adaptation to chronic pain. *Pain, 155*(2), 292–298.

Sullivan, M. J. L., Bishop, S. R., & Pivik, J. (1995). The Pain Catastrophizing Scale: Development and validation. *Psychological Assessment, 7*, 524–532.

Truchon, M., Cote, D., & Irachabal, S. (2006). The Chronic Pain Coping Inventory: Confirmatory factor analysis of the French version. *BMC Musculoskeletal Disorders, 7*, 13..

Turk, D. C., & Melzack, R. (2011). Handbook of pain assessment. New York, NY: Guilford Press.

van Laar M, Pergolizzi Jr JV, Mellinghoff HU, Merchante IM, Nalamachu S, O'Brien J, et al. Pain treatment in arthritis-related pain: beyond NSAIDs. Open Rheumatol J. 2012;6:320–30. doi:10.2174/1874312901206010320.

Vitiello MV, McCurry SM, Shortreed SM, Balderson BH, Baker LD, Keefe FJ, et al. Cognitive-behavioral treatment for comorbid insomnia and osteoarthritis pain in primary care: the lifestyles randomized controlled trial. J Am Geriatr Soc. 2013;61(6):947–56. doi:10.1111/jgs.12275.

Wium-Andersen MK, Orsted DD, Nielsen SF, Nordestgaard BG. Elevated C-reactive protein levels, psychological distress, and depression in 73, 131 individuals. JAMA Psychiatry. 2013;70(2):176–84. doi:10.1001/2013.jamapsychiatry.102.

Wolfe, F., & Michaud, K. (2009). Predicting depression in rheumatoid arthritis: The signal importance of pain extent and fatigue, and comorbidity. *Arthritis and Rheumatism, 61*(5), 667–673.

Wong, W. S., Jensen, M. P., Mak, K. H., Tam, B. K., & Fielding, R. (2010). Preliminary psychometric properties of the Chinese version of the Chronic Pain Coping Inventory (ChCPCI) in a Hong Kong Chinese population. [Research Support, Non-U.S. Gov't

Yelin, E., & Callahan, L. F. (1995). The economic cost and social and psychological impact of musculoskeletal conditions. National Arthritis Data Work Groups. *Arthritis and Rheumatism, 38*(10), 1351–1362.

Psychological Factors in Arthritis: Cause or Consequence?

4

Melissa L. Harris

Abbreviations

AIMS	Arthritis Impact Measurement Scale
CES-D	Center for Epidemiological Studies-Depression
CRP	C-reactive protein
DAS28 joints	Disease Activity Score in 28 joints
ESR	Erythrocyte sedimentation rate
HPA	Hypothalamic–pituitary–adrenal
OA	Osteoarthritis
RA	Rheumatoid arthritis
SAM	Sympathetic-adrenal-medullary
SF-36	Medical Outcomes Study Short Form-36
VAS	Visual Analog Scale
WOMAC	Western Ontario and McMaster osteoarthritis index

M.L. Harris, PhD (✉)
Faculty of Health and Medicine, Research Centre for Gender, Health and Ageing, University of Newcastle, University Drive, Callaghan, NSW 2308, Australia
e-mail: Melissa.Harris@newcastle.edu.au

Introduction: From Psychology to Biology

Chronic illness represents an ongoing public health challenge. It contributes significantly to global healthcare expenditure and burden of disease in terms of health service use, hospitalizations, as well as costs associated with treatment regimens (Australian Institute of Health and Welfare, 2006; World Health Organization, 2002). Arthritis, in particular, is considered one of the most insidious and pervasive chronic conditions affecting middle-aged and older adults (Andrianakos et al., 2005; Ehrlich, 2003). It is a major cause of disability, limited mobility, and chronic pain (Buckwalter, Saltzman, & Brown, 2004). Understanding the intersection between psychology and biology in arthritis has become a key priority for health professionals. This chapter will provide a brief overview of the change in perception regarding psychological factors and chronic disease. Attention will then be paid to describing the contribution of psychological factors (namely, depression and anxiety) to arthritis burden and their potential role in disease onset. A further focus will be to explore the mechanisms by which these psychological factors may influence arthritis, including dysregulation of the hypothalamic–pituitary–adrenal (HPA) axis. Although 'arthritis' is a collective term used to describe a subset of 100 diseases or conditions

P.M. Nicassio (ed.), *Psychosocial Factors in Arthritis*, DOI 10.1007/978-3-319-22858-7_4

characterized by inflammation in or around a joint, osteoarthritis (OA) and rheumatoid arthritis (RA) are the most prevalent forms (Australian Institute of Health and Welfare, 2005). Therefore, the following chapter will primarily focus on research relating to these two conditions.

Chronic Disease and the Paradigm Shift: The Psychological Influence

Chronic disease has traditionally been viewed within a biomedical framework based upon the seventeenth-century notion of '*Cartesian dualism*' (Descartes, 1968) which emphasizes the disparate nature of mind and body. While this model of health and illness has been influential in facilitating attempts to understand disease pathology and current treatment regimes, Jung proposed that this separation of psychology and biology is '*purely artificial*' as the '*human psyche lives in dissoluble union with the body*' (Jung, 1972). The current paradigm shift within the disciplines of medicine and public health involves a movement away from the mechanistic, reductionist perspective driven by the biomedical model to a 'holistic' model of health and illness. This notion was driven by the redefinition of health by the World Health Organization (1948) which suggested that '*health is a state of complete physical, mental and social well-being and not merely the absence of disease or infirmity*. This approach applies a systems philosophy, with health and disease influenced by biological, psychological, and social systems, thereby acknowledging the active interaction between the individual and environment in the process (Adler, Abraham, van Teijlinga, & Potter, 2009). In line with this thinking, Engel (1977) proposed a biopsychosocial model which does not replace the biomedical model but expands upon it (see Fig. 4.1).

Considerable interest has been generated around understanding the role psychological factors may play in influencing disease trajectories, including susceptibility, progression, and adjustment. In addition to influencing health-related quality of life (Adams et al., 2004; Olson, Trevino, Islam, & Denner, 2010; Thomten, Soares, & Sundin, 2011), as well as disease progression and relapse (Leserman et al., 1999; Pembroke, Rasul, Hart, Davey Smith, & Stansfeld, 2006; Porcelli, Zaka, Centonze, & Sisto, 1994), psychological factors have been related to early mortality in some chronic conditions (Rasul, Stansfeld, Smith, Shlomo, & Gallacher, 2007; Watson, Homewood, Haviland, & Bliss, 2005). Psychological factors are also now beginning to be considered in concert with traditional risk factors such as obesity, poor nutrition, and smoking for the development of some chronic diseases (Clarke & Currie, 2009).

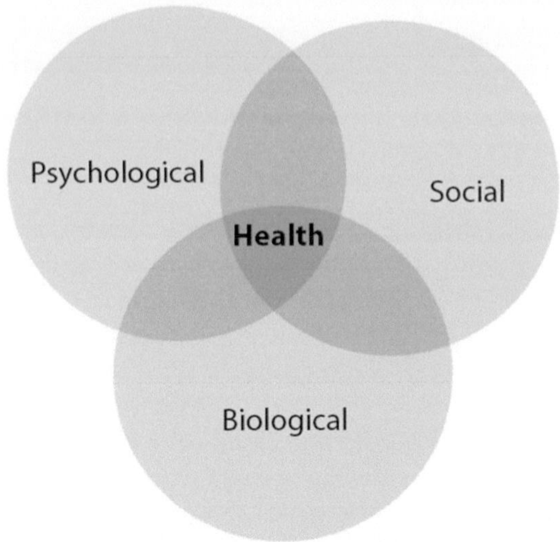

Fig. 4.1 Venn diagram of Engel's biopsychosocial model of health

Importantly, there is an increasing body of evidence to suggest that psychological disorders and arthritis are intimately intertwined (Murphy, Sacks, Brady, Hootman, & Chapman, 2012; Shih, Hootman, Strine, Chapman, & Brady, 2006; Soderlin, Hakala, & Nieminen, 2000). Depression is the most commonly examined psychological construct in arthritis research. While anxiety has been examined to a lesser extent, depression and anxiety co-occur in some individuals (Axford et al., 2010). Models of depression and anxiety (e.g., The Tripartite Model) suggest that conceptually these constructs contain shared and specific components (Clark & Watson, 1991). Explicitly, it suggests that anxiety and depression overlap through a general, non-specific factor related to negative affectivity, or more generally, psychological distress. Therefore, depression, and, by extension, anxiety have been found to result in deleterious health-related effects for individuals with arthritis. In particular, depression and anxiety are known to complicate disease management, thereby increasing health care utilization, costs (McLaughlin, Khandker, Kruzikas, & Tummala, 2006), and risk of early mortality (Ang, Choi, Kroenke, & Wolfe, 2005).

The Psychological Burden of Arthritis

The existence of a chronic illness is a strong risk factor for poor psychological health (Moussavi et al., 2007; Sareen, Cox, Clara, & Asmundson, 2005). Although the adaptation to chronic disease is highly individualistic, the debilitating pain and limitations associated with arthritis have been found to have a significant impact on psychological functioning. The following section describes the prevalence of depression and anxiety (including its more general derivative, psychological distress) in arthritis, changes in psychological functioning over the disease course, and the factors that contribute to poor psychological functioning in arthritis.

Prevalence

Depression

Analyses from a state-based telephone survey of noninstitutionalized US adults found that 13.4 % of individuals aged 45 and over with self-reported arthritis experienced more than 14 mentally unhealthy days in the past month (Strine et al., 2004). Other studies have demonstrated that individuals with arthritis have around a 2–3-fold increase in the odds of reporting depressive and anxiety symptoms when compared with the general population (Murphy et al., 2012; Shih et al., 2006). Dunlop, Lyons, Manheim, Song, and Chang (2004), using data from a population-based cohort of men and women aged 54–65 ($n=7825$), have suggested that as much as 18 % of experienced major depression may be attributed to having arthritis. However, these figures are dependent upon the populations studied and the measures utilized.

Specifically, in RA, prevalence of depression ranges from 13 to 20 % when focused on psychiatric assessment or clinical diagnosis (Dickens, McGowan, Clark-Carter, & Creed, 2002; Hyrich et al., 2006) and exceeds 50 % when based on self-report screening tools (El-Miedany & El-Rasheed, 2002). Particularly, a study of 238 Norwegian patients with clinically diagnosed early RA (≤4 years duration) found that 20 % had scores on the Arthritis Impact Measurement Scale (AIMS), indicating possible psychiatric disturbance (Smedstad, Moum, Vaglum, & Kvien, 1996). While less examined than that of RA, depression in OA has also been reported at elevated levels when compared to the general population. A 10-year study of 6153 consecutive RA outpatients found that 20 % fulfilled criteria for 'probable' depression, while 16.8 % of individuals with OA of the knee or hip, and 14.3 % with OA of the hand, were found to experience 'probable' mental distress (Hawley & Wolfe, 1993). However, slightly higher depression figures for men and women with OA (according to American College of Rheumatology criteria) were reported in a German primary care sample (19.4 %) (Rosemann, Laux, & Szecsenyi, 2007). Likewise, in a recent small clinical study ($n=86$), Marks found in men and women (≥60 years) with radiographic and clinical evidence of mild to moderate knee OA that approximately 28 % of the sample were classified as having 'possible depression' based on The Center for Epidemiological Studies-Depression (CES-D), while 21 % had nonclinically validated moderate to severe depression.

Anxiety

While anxiety has been less frequently studied in isolation from depression, current research suggests that between 21 and 70 % of individuals with arthritis experience heightened levels of anxiety (El-Miedany & El-Rasheed, 2002; Murphy, Creed, & Jayson, 1988). In particular, Lok, Mok, Cheng, and Cheung (2010), in their examination of rheumatology outpatients with median disease duration of 4 years, found the point prevalence of anxiety disorders (based on the Diagnostic and Statistical Manual of Mental Disorders Fourth Edition criteria) to be 13.0 %, with generalized anxiety disorder the most common.

The Relative Burden of Depression and Anxiety

Although considerable overlap between depression and anxiety has been noted in arthritis populations (Murphy et al., 2012), conjecture exists regarding the relative burden of depression compared to anxiety. While Isik, Koca, Ozturk, and Mermi (2007) reported a significantly higher prevalence of depression compared to anxiety in their small study ($n=82$) of consecutive RA patients (41.5 % with depression alone vs. 13.4 % with anxiety alone), Harris, Loxton, Sibbritt, and Byles (2012) argued that anxiety may be a primary and somewhat overlooked concern. In a representative sample of older Australian women, the diagnosis of an anxiety/nervous disorder was the only significant psychosocial factor associated with arthritis following the adjustment for demographic characteristics and health-related quality of life. This finding is supported by previous case–control and clinic-based research (El-Miedany & El-Rasheed, 2002; Hawley & Wolfe, 1988; Odegard, Finset, Mowinckel, Kvien, & Uhlig, 2007; Soderlin et al., 2000), in conjunction with the recent population-based study conducted by Murphy et al. (2012). While one-third of respondents with arthritis reported experiencing either anxiety or depression, the authors noted that anxiety was twice as common as depression (31 % vs. 18 %) and depression was contingent upon the presence of anxiety (84 %). Moreover, El-Miedany and El Rasheed (2002) noted in their Egyptian outpatient study ($n=80$) that 63.4 % of women with arthritis experienced depression, while an even greater proportion reported anxiety (66.2 %).

Taken together, these findings suggest that affective disturbance may have important implications over the disease course. It is important to note, however, that findings from a prospective study involving individuals with RA suggest that the prevalence or severity of depression is not dissimilar to individuals with other chronic diseases (Hawley & Wolfe, 1993) and, as such, may be related to reduced quality of life and not a function of the disease per se (Courvoisier et al., 2012; Hawley & Wolfe, 1993).

Psychological Functioning Over Time

Despite the increased reporting of psychological problems in individuals with arthritis, longitudinal studies have found that the process of psychological adjustment is complex with considerable variability in findings. Some studies have found a reduction in emotional distress over time (Crotty et al., 1994; Evers, Kraaimaat, Geenen, Jacobs, & Bijlsma, 2002; Persson, Larsson, Nived, & Eberhardt, 2005), while others have found that mental health remains relatively stable over the disease course (Smedstad, Vaglum, Moum, & Kvien, 1997; Uhlig et al., 2000). A longitudinal analysis of data from 158 Swedish primary care patients found that a latent effect may be associated with psychological adaptation in those newly diagnosed with RA. Improvements were not identified until the three-year follow-up (Persson et al., 2005). Meanwhile, in a 3-year prospective study of Hungarian and Austrian RA outpatients aged 40–75 years ($n=118$), it was found that compared to population norms, mild depressive symptoms were noted early in the RA disease process (Palkonyai et al., 2007). It has also been suggested that anxiety may present earlier, with the onset of depression occurring later (Wittchen, Kessler, Pfister, & Lieb, 2000).

However, findings from qualitative research suggest that arthritis involves a spectrum of emotions ranging from frustration and annoyance to fear, anger, resentment, misery, and helplessness (Baird, 2000; Lutze & Archenholtz, 2007; Melanson & Downe-Wamboldt, 2003). In one US study of older women ($n = 18$) with OA (aged 65–92 years), arthritis was described as an ever-present and unwelcomed entity which dominated their attention. This feeling was likened to 'wearing a heavy garment' (Baird, 2000). Norton, Sacker, Young, and Done (2011), using data from a large prospective cohort study of men and women with early RA, identified a non-linear change in distress over a 10-year period. Using latent growth mixture modeling techniques, the authors were able to demonstrate that while psychological distress remained relatively stable across the disease course (following an increase at the time of diagnosis), heterogeneity in psychological response was identified when individual trajectories were examined. While the majority experienced low levels of distress that remained relatively stable over time (68 %), 12 % demonstrated consistently high levels of distress. Meanwhile, a small proportion showed a decrease in psychological distress (9 %) with a further 11 % reporting increasing distress (see Fig. 4.2).

Predictors of Psychological Functioning in Arthritis

Given the variation in long-term psychological functioning identified above, it is important for health professionals to identify factors that differentiate between patients who do and do not successfully adjust psychologically to arthritis. At the extreme end of the spectrum, the coexistence of psychological disorders and chronic pain conditions (particularly RA) has been associated with increased risk of suicidal ideation and suicide completion (Timonen et al., 2003; Treharne, Lyons, & Kitas, 2000). Research has demonstrated that depression and anxiety in individuals with arthritis can result from a complex interaction between physical, clinical, and psychosocial factors (Covic, Tyson, Spencer, & Howe, 2006). Key factors are described below.

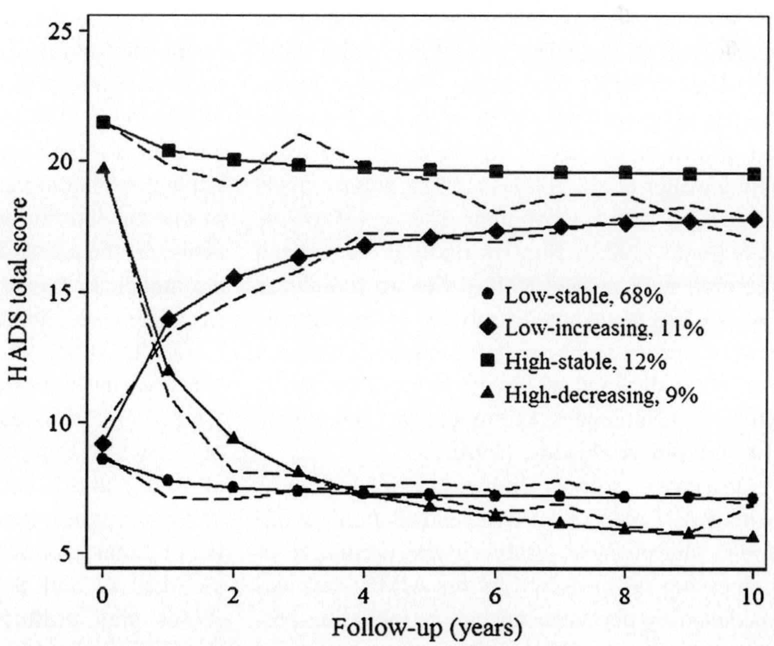

Fig. 4.2 Psychological distress trajectories of the 4-class growth mixture model. *Solid lines* are model-implied trajectories for each class and dashed lines are sample means weighted by class probabilities. Reprinted from Journal of Psychosomatic Research, 71(5), Norton S, Sacker A, Young A, Done J, Distinct psychological distress trajectories in rheumatoid arthritis: findings from an inception cohort, p. 293. Copyright (2011) with permission from Elsevier

Physical and Clinical Predictors

A number of studies have demonstrated an association between physical and clinical indicators of arthritis with reduced psychological functioning. Much of this research, however, has focused on depression or psychological distress as the outcome and has relied on data from RA subpopulations. Considerable conjecture exists regarding the relative importance of these factors.

Functional Impairment and Disability

Despite its slow development, arthritis is progressive in nature and eventually leads to joint destruction, significant loss of function, and reduced health-related quality of life in many patients (Hill et al., 2007; Peters, Sanders, Dieppe, & Donovan, 2005; van Dijk, Dekker, Veenhof, & van den Ende, 2006; Zochling, Stucki, Grill, & Braun, 2007). Findings from the Centers for Disease Control and Prevention (2005) in the USA have indicated that one in three individuals with arthritis report activity limitations as a result of their condition. Findings confined to OA populations have revealed that 80 % of people experience limitations in movement, with 25 % unable to perform major daily activities (WHO Scientific Group, 2003). Further, approximately 10 % of people aged over 60 are disabled as a result of the disease (Buckwalter et al., 2004), with increased levels associated with concomitant disease (Marks & Allegrante, 2002). Similar findings have been reported with respect to RA. Severe functional decline has been noted in 10 % of individuals within 2 years, and up to half of persons with RA are work- disabled within 10 years of diagnosis (Sokka, Kautiainen, Mottonen, & Hannonen, 1999; Wolfe & Hawley, 1998).

In a cross-sectional clinical study of 111 adults with RA, Covic, Adamson, and Hough (2000) found that physical disability was predictive of depression (as measured by the AIMS) and was mediated by psychosocial factors including passive coping and helplessness. Likewise, Margaretten et al. (2009) identified a significant relationship between physical disability and increased depressive symptomatology in their socioeconomic and ethnically diverse RA cohort ($n = 174$). Specifically, univariate analyses revealed no significant demographic differences between patients reporting depression (measured by the Patient Health Questionnaire 9) and those that did not. Of the clinical features, only physical functioning (measured by the Health Assessment Questionnaire; $p < 0.001$), disease activity (measured by RA-specific Disease Activity Score in 28 [DAS28] joints; $p = 0.04$), along with lower use of disease-modifying antirheumatic drugs ($p = 0.03$) were significant predictors. When these variables were entered into the multivariate model, however, only physical functioning remained significant ($p < 0.001$). In this multivariate model, a reduction in depressive symptoms was noted for individuals of Asian or Pacific Islander origin ($p = 0.02$). This finding is supported by another rheumatological outpatient study (El-Miedany & El-Rasheed, 2002). While it was found that functional disability was the only clinical predictor of depression, the authors were able to demonstrate disparate clinical profiles for depression and anxiety. Anxiety was associated with joint tenderness and stiffness, short disease duration, as well as rheumatoid factor and nodules. This finding however, contrasts with that of Ho, Fu, Chua, Cheak, and Mak (2011) who found that among consecutive patients at a University-based hospital ($n = 100$), while rheumatoid factor and biological indicators of disease activity were significant in univariate analyses, the effect disappeared in the multivariate model. In this study, rheumatoid factor was associated with depressive symptoms only.

On the other hand, a two-year longitudinal study of individuals ($n = 227$) with early stage RA (i.e., ≤4 years duration) examined predictors of change in depression and anxiety symptoms at both 1 and 2 years (Smedstad et al., 1997). With depression (measured using the AIMS) as the outcome, it was found in multivariate analyses that 1- and 2-year change in depression scores was predicted by level of disability. Serologic indicators of disease activity such as erythrocyte sedimentation rate (ESR), along with joint tenderness and pain levels, failed to predict the relationship. Importantly, previous depression scores also predicted depression. When cross-lagged analyses were conducted in an attempt to determine causality between the variables of interest, the only significant finding was related to depression at 1 year. High levels of disability at baseline predicted depression at time one. This effect, however, was not sustained at 2-year follow-up. In contrast, no disease-related factors were found to predict 1- and 2-year change in anxiety scores. Previous anxiety levels were the only predictor of future anxiety.

Moreover, in a nationally representative sample of US noninstitutionalized civilians, Godha, Shi, and Mavronicolas (2010) found a strong relationship between RA functional limitation severity and depression. In particular, after controlling for the confounding effects of age, physical activity, and comorbidities, patients belonging to Class II (i.e., able to perform usual self-care and vocational activities, but limited in avocational activities such as recreational activities and/or leisure; and activities related to work, school, and homemaking) were almost four times more likely to have a high tendency toward depression compared to Class I (i.e., completely able to perform usual activities of daily living such as self-care, vocational, and avocational). Meanwhile the odds of depression increased substantially (OR = 5.92) for those in Class III (i.e., able to perform self-care, but limited in vocational and avocational activities) compared to Class I. It is important to note that older age and level of physical activity were associated with a reduction in depression.

Pain and Disease Activity

While clinical expression and progression of arthritis are highly variable, particularly for RA, with the disease course marked by periods of exacerbations and remissions (Australian Institute of Health and Welfare, 2005), pain and joint stiffness have been identified as key indicators of arthritis. Pain, in particular, is often a common reason individuals seek medical attention (Gureje, Von Korff, Simon, & Gater, 1998).

In a longitudinal examination of clinically important predictors of self-reported depressive symptoms (evaluated using the mental health component score of the Medical Outcomes Study Short Form-36 [SF-36]) in 29,524 adults aged 18 and over with rheumatic disease, Wolfe and Michaud (2009) found that 9-year incidence of depression was in the vicinity of 40 %. When RA was specifically examined, those with depression were found to be characteristically different from those without depression on a range of sociodemographic, psychological, and disease-related indicators. Using Random Forest analyses, however, the authors identified factors associated with disease severity, that is, symptom intensity (measured as a combination of the fatigue component of the Visual Analog Scale [VAS] and Regional Pain Scale [i.e., painful nonarticular joint count]), pain and global severity (measured by the VAS), and fatigue, as well as disease comorbidity to classify patients with depressive symptoms. Despite this, when recursive partitioning was applied to the data, only symptom intensity was necessary to identify participants with depressive symptoms. In addition, the cumulative impact of this indicator of disease severity was found to contribute to mortality over the study period.

Further, in a longitudinal study of 15,282 patients with RA, pain was found to account for 44 % of the variance associated with psychological functioning (as measured by the mental health component of the SF-36) (Courvoisier et al., 2012). More specifically, multivariate analyses found that pain explained 60 % of the variance associated with the stable part of psychological functioning over the study period. In this analysis, disease activity and functional disability also contributed to psychological functioning. When the variable part of psychological functioning was assessed, only pain remained as the significant explanatory variable, explaining 5 % of the variance. Moreover, in the Norton study (described in the section above) (Norton et al., 2011), the four psychological trajectories over the 3-year study period were found to be related to self-reported disease severity. Those that had high levels of depression, either high stable or high decreasing, were found to have higher levels of disease severity at baseline compared to those with low-stable or low-increasing depression. Importantly, key serological markers of inflammation, ESR and C-reactive protein (CRP) failed to predict psychological functioning over time. Interestingly, disease severity indicators were also the difference between those with high levels of depression that remained stable over the course of the study compared to those that saw improvements in mental health.

Fatigue

The experience of fatigue is also common to both RA and OA. Although the prevalence has varied according to the measurement used and level of active disease present, it has been suggested that up to 93 % of individuals with OA or RA experience fatigue (Belza, 1995; Wolfe, Hawley, & Wilson, 1996). When clinically significant levels of fatigue have been investigated however, this figure approaches 50 % (Wolfe et al., 1996). Moreover, haematological manifestations have been found to be prominent in arthritis, particularly in RA subpopulations. The prevalence of mild anemia in RA has ranged from 33 to 60 % (Wilson, Yu, Goodnough, & Nissenson, 2004). Wolfe and Michaud (2006) found that mild anemia (as defined by the World Health Organization) was present in 31.5 % of participants with RA, with lifetime prevalence being in the vicinity of 50 %. Using discriminant analysis, Covic et al. (2006) identified 12 specific predictors that were able to correctly classify the majority of participants (80 %) in their rheumatological sample ($n=134$) based on depression status. Fatigue was found to be the strongest clinical predictor of depression (loading=0.57), followed by pain (loading=0.55) and physical disability (loading=0.44). Despite this, psychological factors, particularly tension and self-esteem, were the strongest overall predictors of the relationship (loadings=0.73). Likewise, in a large convenience community sample ($n=200$) of older adults with RA (mean age 66.7 years), Franklin and Harrell (2013) examined the unique effect of pain and fatigue on depression. In this study, functional impairment accounted for a significant amount of the variance associated with depressive symptoms ($\beta=0.47$; $r^2_{\text{part}}=0.18$). Importantly, pain did not contribute to the relationship between RA and depression following control for demographics and functional impairment. After controlling for demographics, functional impairment, and pain, fatigue was found to contribute 10 % unique variance to the RA–depression relationship.

Psychosocial Predictors

While the findings suggest that long-term disability, joint damage, and pain (to some extent) as opposed to RA disease activity (e.g., swollen joints, ESR, CRP) may contribute substantially to depression in arthritis, these findings are not conclusive. Psychosocial factors are increasingly being suggested as mediators or moderators of the relationship between arthritis and psychological functioning. Although the list of psychosocial factors implicated in psychological adaptation to arthritis is extensive, the following provides an overview of the role some of the key factors play.

Sociodemographics

Depending upon the variables included in the analyses, sociodemographic variables have been inconsistently linked to poor psychological adjustment to arthritis. In particular, various studies have suggested that age (particularly at diagnosis) (Patten, Williams, & Wang, 2006; Ramjeet, Koutantji, Barrett, & Scott, 2005), gender (Marks, 2013; Ramjeet et al., 2005; Theis, Helmick, & Hootman, 2007), education (Mella, Bertolo, & Dalgalarrondo, 2010), and marital status (Katz & Yelin, 1993; Strine et al., 2004) are important indicators. For instance, Strine et al. (2004), in their examination of Behavioral Risk Factor Surveillance System data, found that frequent mental distress in arthritis was associated with female gender, lower education (noncompletion of high school), marital status (previously married), younger age, ethnicity (Hispanic), and employment status. It is important to note, however, that disease-related and psychological factors were not controlled for in this study. Mella et al. (2010), on the other hand, found education to be the only demographic predictor of depressive symptoms, alongside levels of disease activity and functional impairment. In their longitudinal analysis of Swedish primary care patients ($n=158$) however, Persson et al. (2005) noted that higher risk of distress was associated with younger age, female gender, and a number of psychosocial factors, including lower social support and higher distress at baseline.

Psychological Vulnerability

Psychological vulnerability has been found to impact future levels of psychological distress. Importantly, previous levels of depression or anxiety have been found to be key predictors of short-term psychological functioning in arthritis (Smedstad et al., 1997). In a small study ($n=22$) of individuals with early RA, Sharpe and colleague found that initial levels of depression consistently predicted between 37 and 58 % of the variance attributed to psychological functioning over time. In this study, coping strategies were found to predict psychological functioning in the early stages of the disease, accounting for 9 % and 5 % of the variance at times two and three, respectively. Interestingly, while disability predicted psychological functioning at all follow-up time points (i.e., 2–6), joint function improved despite decreases in mood.

Additionally, in a 2-year longitudinal study of RA, Sinclair and Wallston (2010) identified that the construct psychological vulnerability (measured by Psychological Vulnerability Scale) added 9.3 % unique variance to concurrent depressive symptoms, beyond that of personal control factors such as helplessness and functional impairment. Meanwhile, lower psychological vulnerability contributed 5.6 % unique variance to depressive symptoms 1 year later. In this analysis, age and disease comorbidity failed to predict changes in depressive symptoms (measured by the CES-D). The authors argued that this suggests that these factors do not confound the relationship between psychological vulnerability and psychological distress in arthritis.

Further, while stress and its role in arthritis will be discussed in detail in Chap. 5, it is an important predictor of long-term psychological functioning in arthritis populations. In a study of Irish women ($n=59$) with established RA (mean age $=60$ years) attending an outpatient clinic, it was found that perceived stress was associated with affective disturbance at 1-year follow-up (Curtis, Groarke, Coughlan, & Gsel, 2004). Correlational and hierarchical regression analyses revealed that psychological stress was the best predictor of depression and was a better predictor than disease severity on measures of positive and negative emotionality. Treharne, Lyons, Booth, and Kitas (2007) provided additional support for the significant impact of perceived stress on mental health outcomes in arthritis. In their longitudinal study involving 134 U.K. outpatients with RA, the authors found that perceived stress had the strongest relationship with psychological well-being at baseline and perceived stress had an impact on anxiety levels at 6 month follow-up.

Coping Efforts

Coping efforts have been suggested as key factors in developing a sense of control and mastery over chronic illness (Dager, Kjeken, Fjerstad, & Hauge, 2012; Shaul, 1995). Studies focused on RA subpopulations have consistently demonstrated that coping strategies employed by an individual in response to arthritis-related symptoms such as pain have a significant impact on psychological and physical health outcomes (Brown, Nicassio, & Wallston, 1989; Covic, Adamson, Spencer, & Howe, 2003; Covic et al., 2006). The majority of this research has generally concentrated on assessing the way individuals manage chronic pain according to the dichotomous problem-focused and emotion-focused approaches (or variants thereof, e.g., active vs. passive coping) proposed by Lazarus and Folkman

(1987). Particularly, Curtis, Groarke, Coughlan, and Gsel (2005) found that although perceived stress was associated with affective disturbance and was the best predictor of depression in 59 Irish RA outpatients, the use of avoidant coping efforts (i.e., efforts to distract from, or avoid the stressor) contributed to the prediction of negative affect. These findings were supported in a 12-month follow-up study of this cohort of women (Curtis et al., 2004). Similarly, passive coping with pain has also been found to increase depression at 6-month follow-up. This finding, however, was specific to those with RA experiencing greater pain (Brown et al., 1989).

Previously, emotion or passive-based approaches to coping have generally been regarded as maladaptive. Snow-Turek, Norris, and Tan (1996) indicated that passive, maladaptive coping approaches have qualities that outweigh the benefits of active coping. These approaches have been previously associated with increased arthritis pain, disability, and depression in comparison to individuals who employ problem-based (or active) coping strategies (Brown, Wallston, & Nicassio, 1989; Covic et al., 2000, 2003; Evers, Kraaimaat, Geenen, Jacobs, & Bijlsma, 2003; van Lankveld, Naring, van't Pad Bosch, & van de Putte, 2000). However, a Canadian longitudinal qualitative study involving three time points (Melanson & Downe-Wamboldt, 2003) found that older men and women with RA ($n=39$) used a variety of strategies (i.e., confrontive, palliative, supportant, fatalistic, self-reliant, evasive, optimistic, and emotive) in order to adjust. Meanwhile, Gignac, Cott, and Badley (2000), using content analysis, noted that Canadian community-dwelling older adults with OA ($n=286$) employed 13 distinct behavioral efforts in order to adapt to their condition. These coping efforts concerning 'selection' (i.e., performing activities less often), 'optimization' (i.e., augmenting or enriching reserves to enable continued functioning), 'compensation' (i.e., substituting activities), and 'receiving help' were integral to perceptions of dependence (or independence) and facilitated psychological adjustment. Another study utilizing a narrative biographic approach, found that Austrian RA outpatients ($n=10$) described their experience as positive, with the disease seen as a challenge and facilitator of personal growth (Stamm et al., 2008).

Importantly, a recent systematic review examining the longitudinal association between coping and psychological adjustment in RA found limited evidence that passive or disengaging coping strategies such as helplessness, avoidance, and wishful thinking were prospectively associated with increased psychological distress (Vriezekolk, van Lankveld, Geenen, & van den Ende, 2011). It was also noted that there was no evidence for active or engagement-style coping (e.g., problem-solving, emotional regulation, distraction, and cognitive restructuring) playing a role in the improvement of psychological distress long-term. Therefore, coping strategies may play more of a role in understanding psychological functioning in the early stages of disease only.

Others (e.g., Gronning, Lomundal, Koksvik, & Steinsbekk, 2011) have suggested that adjusting to a chronic illness is a dynamic process, influenced not only by the disease but by the individual's life circumstances and personal resources. This finding is supported by a recent qualitative study of older Australian women with OA (Harris, Byles, Sibbritt, & Loxton, 2015). In this study it was found that psychological adjustment over time was similar to that of RA and was attributed primarily to cognitive and attitudinal factors such as stoicism, making downward comparisons, and cognitive reappraisal. This was a dynamic "day-to-day" process involving a constant struggle between grieving physical losses and increasing dependence amidst symptom management. Therefore, adopting a balanced or flexible coping approach may be the key to long-term psychological adjustment to chronic diseases such as arthritis (Masuda et al., 2011).

Social Support

Social support has been found to have direct and moderating effects (through the stress response) on the relationship between arthritis and psychological functioning (Brown et al., 1989; Dekkers et al., 2001; Evers, Kraaimaat, Geenen, & Bijlsma, 1997). Social support can be defined as the existence or perceived availability of people who care about an individual and whom they can rely on when needed (Ethgen et al., 2004). In a Dutch study of 229 randomly selected RA outpatients, the support of a spouse was found to be a significant predictor of lower depression and anxiety of individuals with RA (Kraaimaat, Van Dam-Baggen, & Bijlsma, 1995). Evers et al. (1997) found that recently diagnosed Dutch RA outpatients ($n=91$) who had smaller networks (i.e., quantity of social support) experienced greater psychological maladjustment in their first year after diagnosis compared to those with a larger network. An analysis of data from an international longitudinal cohort study (Demange et al., 2004) found that RA patients ($n=542$) who received more social support (i.e., perceived satisfaction with support given) or had a larger social network had better functional and psychological adjustment over time. However, it has been argued that the perceived availability and quality of the support received may be more important than the size of an individual's network (Leskela et al., 2006). Perceived social support, in particular, has been found to be beneficial for both physical and psychological outcomes in arthritis (Demange et al., 2004; Ethgen et al., 2004; Ferreira & Sherman, 2007; Sherman, 2003). Ferreira and Sherman (2007) and Sherman (2003) found that perceived social support was associated with reduced depressive symptoms in older adults with OA.

Personality

Personality-based characteristics have been found to influence the way in which individuals appraise a given situation and the selection of coping strategies (either adaptive or maladaptive) (Folkman & Greer, 2000). A longitudinal study of Dutch outpatients with early RA ($n=78$) found that neuroticism (i.e., the tendency to be relatively more tense and emotionally unstable) at diagnosis was the most consistent and effective predictor of increased psychological distress (depression and anxiety) at both 3- and 5-year follow-up (Evers et al., 2002). Further, Scheier and Carver (1987) and Scheier, Weintraub, and Carver (1986) have posited that an optimistic life approach may play a protective role in chronic disease, facilitating the choice of disease-related coping strategies and engagement in health behaviors. Optimism has been positively associated with psychological well-being (both cross-sectionally and prospectively) (Brenner, Melamed, & Panush, 1994; Fournier, de Ridder, & Bensing, 2002; Long & Sangster, 1993) and health-related quality of life (Allison, Guichard, & Gilain, 2000; Carver et al., 1994; Scheier et al., 1989) and inversely with symptom expression (Achat, Kawachi, Spiro, DeMolles, & Sparrow, 2000; Ferreira & Sherman, 2007; Scheier & Carver, 1985). Additionally, it is suggested that individuals with an optimistic outlook employ problem-based coping in response to situations appraised as controllable, and emotion-based strategies aimed at harm minimization in response to situations appraised as uncontrollable (Scheier et al., 1986). Similarly, a U.K. longitudinal study of 134 RA outpatients (predominantly women) identified pessimism as a predictor of increased anxiety at baseline and increased depression, anxiety, and decreased life satisfaction at 6-month follow-up (Treharne et al., 2007). Individuals who reported greater levels of optimism reported better adjustment in terms of anxiety at baseline and depression at 1-year follow-up.

The Contribution of Psychological Disorders to the Physical Burden of Arthritis

Management of arthritis has heavily focused on symptom relief, including the reduction of pain and inflammation (Branch, Lipsky, Nieman, & Lipsky, 1999). However, disease-related factors have been found to only modestly predict future arthritis disability (van der Heide, Jacobs, Haanen, & Bijlsma, 1995; Wolfe & Cathey, 1991). With significant variability associated with arthritis disability, it has been suggested that factors extraneous to the disease may play a key role in the burden of disease. Depression, when present in its clinical form, has been attributed to mortality in RA patients (Ang et al., 2005). However, with substantial discordance between objective disease indicators (including radiographic evidence and joint inspection) and the severity of symptomatology (Jones & Doherty, 1995; Kean, Kean, & Buchanan, 2004), a large focus has been on reduced health-related quality-of-life indicators. The link between psychological distress and pain has been suggested to be bidirectional (Kroenke et al., 2011). The following section describes the influence of psychological disorders (depression and anxiety) on physical functioning, pain, and other clinical indicators of arthritis.

Physical Functioning and Disability

With the exception of a few studies, research examining the impact of psychological disorders on physical functioning and disability has largely come from cross-sectional studies (see previous section). In particular, Strine et al. (2004), examining predictors of arthritis in the Behavioral Risk Factor Surveillance System cohort, found that frequent mental distress had a significant impact on physical health. Although a cross-sectional study, the authors noted that after controlling for important sociodemographic characteristics (age, ethnicity, gender, employment status, marital status, and educational attainment), those with frequent mental distress (i.e., reported ≥14 mental health days as not good) were found to have increased associations with reporting their general health as either fair or poor (adjusted OR = 3.1), had 14 or more physically unhealthy days in the past month (adjusted OR = 4.1), as well as increased inability to perform daily activities (adjusted OR = 2.2), and the need to use support aids (adjusted OR = 1.8).

In an earlier RA-focused study (n = 80), Murphy et al. (1988) found that psychiatric illness (depression and anxiety) was only associated with two of the assessed indicators of disease outcomes, grip strength, and functional grade. Psychiatric illness was also not related to disease duration. Using the SF-36 physical summary score as the outcome, Kojima et al. (2009) found that while psychological distress was associated with physical functioning in bivariate analyses, this association disappeared at a multivariate level with only current symptom and physical status predictive of SF-36 physical quality of life.

Similar findings have been obtained in OA. Using a publicly and privately funded prospective cohort study of adults aged 45–79 designed to examine onset and progression of knee OA, Riddle, Kong, and Fitzgerald (2011) found that depressive symptoms were an independent predictor of yearly change (over 2 years) in self-reported disability, walking distance, and chair stand performance in addition to pain. However, while statistical significance was obtained, the authors suggested that the findings were not clinically significant. Examining the prognostic impact of depressive symptoms on future pain and functioning, the authors found that depression was required to be chronic and persist for multiple years in order to produce a meaningful impact on future pain and disability.

On the other hand, another longitudinal study of community-dwelling individuals (n = 257) (Sharma et al., 2003) found that baseline factors associated with poor functional outcome (measured by the Western Ontario and McMaster osteoarthritis index [WOMAC]) at 3 years included higher Body Mass Index, greater knee pain intensity, increased laxity, and reduced aerobic exercise, as well as lower psychosocial functioning in terms of mental health, self-efficacy, and social support. The impact of psychological distress on functional outcomes appears to be latent, with pain intensity the only baseline factor to predict functioning at 18 months. In terms of chair-stand performance, there was no difference between those with poor and those with good WOMAC scores. Self-efficacy was the only psychosocial factor that contributed to both 3-year self-reported functional decline and objective chair-stand performance. Importantly, differences in self-efficacy between those who sustained high functioning over time compared to those that saw a decline or sustained low function were the largest of any predictor. This finding is supported by other longitudinal research (Rejeski, Miller, Foy, Messier, & Rapp, 2001).

Pain and Disease Activity

In chronic pain patients, poor psychological functioning is generally associated with more pain sites, pain intensity duration, and severity and interference (Bair, Robinson, Katon, & Kroenke, 2003; Bair, Wu, Damush, Sutherland, & Kroenke, 2008). In arthritis, most studies have examined the role of pain on psychological outcomes as opposed to the reverse. In an early clinical study of 400 RA patients attending a rheumatological clinic on average for 3 years, Hawley and Wolfe (1988) found that depression and anxiety were associated with number of outpatients visits, while depression (although highly correlated with anxiety) contributed to continued high levels of pain at follow-up. Meanwhile, in a longitudinal analysis of 238 patients with RA (aged 20–70), Odegard et al. (2007) found that anxiety alongside female gender, disease activity (defined as ESR), and physical function (measured by grip strength) independently explained the course of pain over the 10-year study period. While depression and anxiety were found to be interrelated longitudinally, depression (measured by the AIMS or General Health Questionnaire) did not contribute to the final model. These findings were consistent using two different measures of pain (VAS and AIMS).

In another study focused on early inflammatory arthritis, Looper et al. (2011) found that patients with a history of major depression had higher overall disease activity. Importantly, joint symptoms measured by the DAS28 showed significantly higher values according to depression history for both patient and physician assessment of the illness. Objective disease indicators such as tender and swollen joints and CRP levels were not related to depression history. Likewise, pain was not associated with depression history. This contrasts with an earlier study of 188 postmenopausal women with RA and OA (Zautra & Smith, 2001). In this study, Zautra and Smith found that increased pain sensitivity was associated with depressive symptoms. More specifically, weekly pain reports in RA patients were predicted by depressive symptoms, perceived stress, and an interaction between perceived stress and depression. For those with OA, weekly pain was predicted by independent associations of depression and perceived stress, with no interaction noted. The differences in findings between the two studies may have been related to how depression was classified (recurrent as opposed to history) and the population studied.

In a later study examining the effects of depression and anxiety on weekly pain in a mixed RA and OA sample, Smith and Zautra (2008) found that when examined separately, depression and anxiety had similar effects on the reporting of weekly pain, both current and next week (although the effects were nearly twice as large for anxiety). However, when examined in concert, depression was reduced to nonsignificance. This finding was supported by Harris et al. (2012) who examined the relative effects of self-reported diagnosed depression and anxiety in arthritis within a comprehensive model.

The impact of psychological factors on physical outcomes has less often been examined in an OA only population. Kim et al. (2011), in a cross-sectional study of 660 older Koreans with knee OA, found that coexisting depression was associated with knee pain. The strength of this relationship (after adjustment for confounders) was as strong as pathomorphologic damage. Particularly, the presence of depression was associated with a six-fold increase in reporting symptomatic knee OA. However, this influence was only noted in patients with minimal to moderate radiographic severity (measured by the Kellgren–Lawrence grading system). The presence of a depressive disorder was not associated with the risk of symptomatic knee OA in patients with severe OA (Kellgren–Lawrence grade 4). As a result, the authors argued that the findings suggested that depression contributes substantially to the discrepancy between symptoms and radiographic degenerative changes observed in knee OA.

The Pain–Disability–Depression Link: It's Complicated

The findings suggest that the influence of depression and anxiety on physical and psychological outcomes appears to be largely associated with subjective physical (in conjunction with psychosocial) factors as opposed to objective measures, with disease factors alone unable to reliably predict poor outcomes. The interrelation between these factors, however, appears much more complex. For instance, Crotty et al. (1994) suggested that the degree of pain and depression is a precursor to physical disability that may appear later in the disease course. Further, Covic et al. (2003), in their biopsychosocial assessment of 157 men and women with early RA, found, using path analysis, that the suggested biopsychosocial model accounted for a large proportion of the cross-sectional and longitudinal variance for pain (52–94 % and 29–43 %, respectively) and depression (37–71 % and 21–33 %, respectively). It was found that physical disability, along with helplessness and passive coping, contributed to the levels of pain and depression in RA. Importantly physical disability was the most significant predictor of pain. This is supported in other research (Hodkinson et al., 2012). Escalante and del Rincon (Covic et al., 1999), in particular, found that only one-third of the variance associated with physical disability in RA is explained by disease-related factors, including disease duration, joint symptoms, and objective functional limitations. Meanwhile, 20 % of the variance could be explained by psychosocial factors such as helplessness and self-efficacy. This is supported by other studies which have found that passive coping strategies, including those involving helplessness and catastrophizing, have been found to be associated with pain sensitivity (Evers et al., 2003; Naidoo & Pretorius, 2006), while active coping strategies and the development of self-efficacy have been found to have a positive impact on pain reduction (Savelkoul, de Witte, & Post, 2003).

Using factor analysis, Kojima et al. (2009) identified four principal components that represented the interrelationship between psychosocial factors and clinical factors in RA—disease activity, current symptoms, physical status, and psychosocial factors. Psychosocial factors, comprised of satisfaction with social support, number of available supporting individuals, anxiety, and depression were correlated with symptomatology and physical status, but not with disease activity. Likewise, all factors were associated with physical status and current symptoms (see Fig. 4.3). This study, however, was cross-sectional in nature and may not be generalizable, with participants being regular attendees at a university hospital rheumatology clinic.

Meanwhile, Hawker et al. (2011) examined the longitudinal relationship between pain and depressive symptoms in a community sample of older adults ($n=834$) with symptomatic hip and knee OA. Controlling for psychosocial and demographic factors and taking into account important disease outcomes; (fatigue and disability); a cyclical relationship was identified in which arthritis pain predicted subsequent functional disability, which, in turn, led to depression and worsening of arthritis pain and disability. This cyclical path model is illustrated in Fig. 4.4.

A variety of pathways have been suggested to explain the link between pain symptoms and depression. Although pain may contribute to depression through psychosocial and behavioral pathways such as passive coping, helplessness, low self-efficacy, and sleep disturbance (Covic et al., 2003; Dersh, Polatin, & Gatchel, 2002; Kundermann, Hemmeter-Spernal, Huber, Krieg, & Lautenbacher, 2008; Williams, Jacka, Pasco, Dodd, & Berk, 2006), depression is also responsible for neurotransmitter imbalance. Dysregulation of key modulating neurotransmitters such as serotonin, norepinephrine, and dopamine, coupled with alterations to shared central pain processing, has the ability to create ongoing pain sensitivity (Bair et al., 2003). Meanwhile, the effects of anxiety on pain have been linked to anxiety sensitivity (Schmidt & Cook, 1999). Using event-related functional MRI, Ploghaus et al. (2001) found that anxiety-induced pain sensitivity was associated with activation of the hippocampal network, particularly the entorhinal cortex of the hippocampal formation. Using the Gray–McNaughton theory of

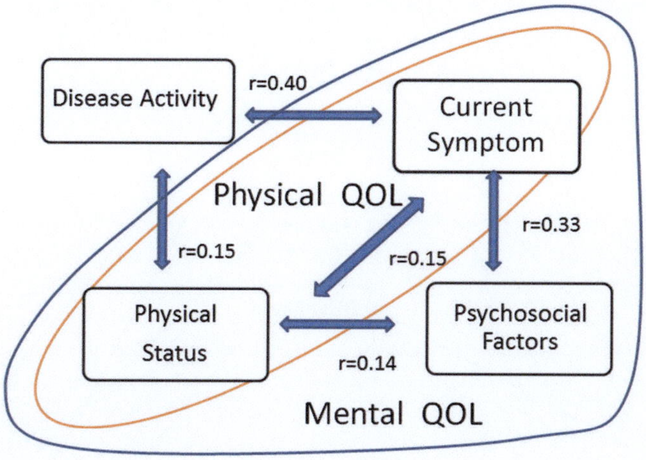

Fig. 4.3 Interrelationships between psychosocial factors, disease activity, current symptoms, and physical status. Based on the results of the factor analysis derived from the clinical and psychosocial variable data of 120 patients with RA. Reprinted from Journal of Psychosomatic Research, 67(5), Kojima M, Kojima T, Ishiguro, N, Oguchi, T, Oba, M, Tsuchiya, H, et al., Psychosocial factors, disease status, and quality of life in patients with rheumatoid arthritis, p. 429. Copyright (2009) with permission from Elsevier

anxiety (Gray & McNaughton, 2000), the authors posited that during the experience of anxiety, the hippocampal formation increases the response to aversive stimuli by behavioral priming responses to consider the worst possible outcome. This may result in a chronic cycle of pain and anxiety.

Are Psychological Disorders Risk Factors for the Onset of Arthritis?

While significant progress has been made regarding the understanding of particular aspects of arthritis, notably relating to disease progression (e.g., development of new treatment options, assessment of treatment efficacy), the pathogenesis of arthritis remains unclear. In the absence of a single genetic vulnerability, arthritis is viewed as a disease of multifactorial origin, with both genetic and environmental factors contributing to its occurrence and expression (Alamanos & Drosos, 2005; Felson, 1996; Silman & Pearson, 2002). Consequently, prevention strategies have focused on identifying factors which place an individual at heightened risk for disease development (Cooper et al., 2000; Felson, 1996). Box 4.1 provides an overview of the key nonmodifiable and modifiable factors associated with increased risk of developing OA and RA. Psychological factors, particularly depression, are now being considered as risk factors for diseases other than arthritis (Clarke & Currie, 2009). Within the arthritis literature, limited evidence exists regarding the role of depression and anxiety in disease onset.

In a ten-country cross-sectional study, Scott et al. (2011) found that early onset (i.e., diagnosed prior to age 21) mental health disorders were associated with increased risk of OA. All examined disorders were associated with increased reporting of OA. The highest Hazard Ratio was associated with posttraumatic stress disorder (1.91), followed by generalized anxiety disorder (1.69), and panic disorder (1.68). Major depression had the lowest hazard ratio of all the mental health disorders (1.52). This finding is supported longitudinally by Von Korff et al. (2009) who noted that the experience of mental health problems (depression and anxiety) prior to age 21 was associated with an increased risk of developing adult onset arthritis.

Further, in a 12-year prospective population-based study, Karkus and Patton (2011) indicated that depression was associated with a 1.5 increase in odds of reporting arthritis. This finding is

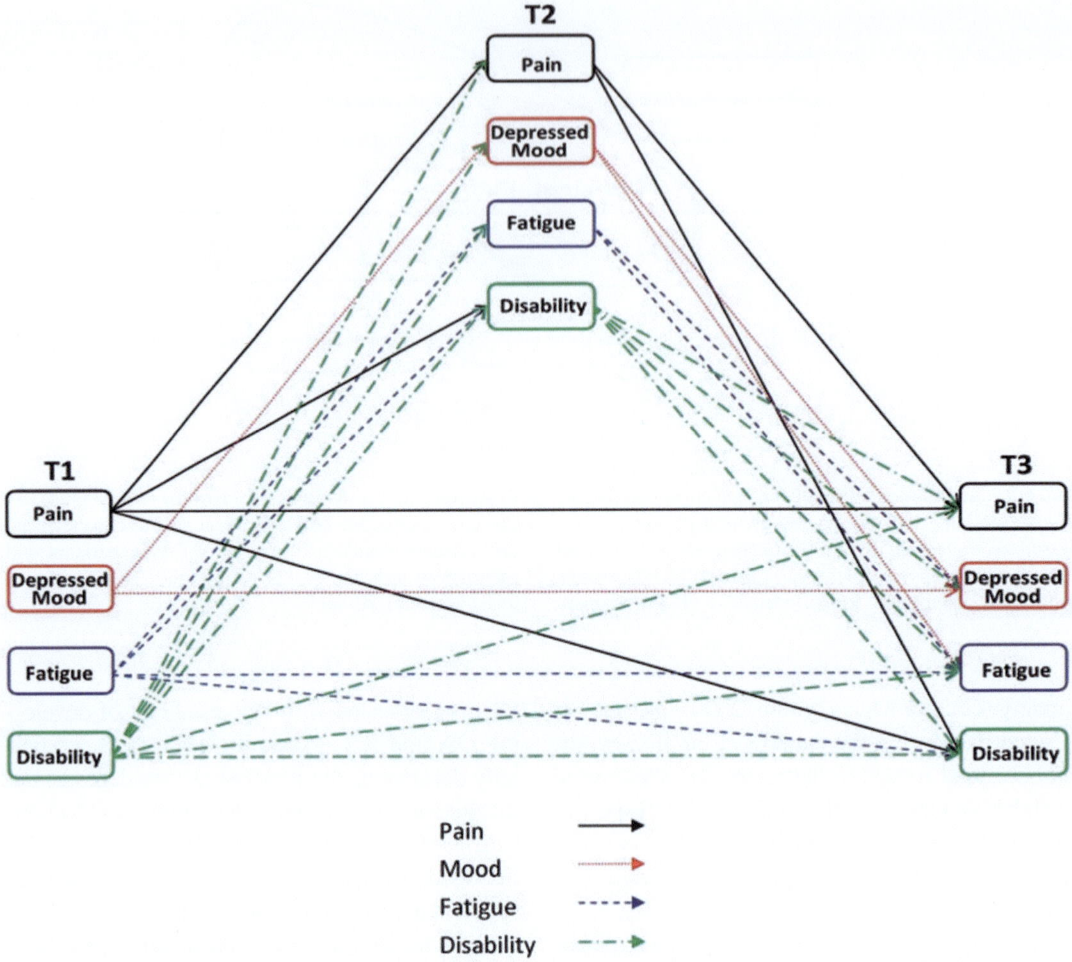

Fig. 4.4 Result for the final path model, adjusting for covariates. T1 = baseline; T2 = 1-year follow-up; T3 = 2-year follow-up. Reprinted from Arthritis Care and Research, 63(10), Hawker GA, Gignac MA, Badley E, Davis AM, French MR, Li Y, et al., A longitudinal study to explain the pain-depression link in older adults with osteoarthritis, p. 1387. Copyright (2011) with permission from American College of Rheumatology

supported by a 20-year prospective study which found five or more depressive symptoms associated with arthritis onset (Seavey, Kurata, & Cohen, 2003). In contrast, van't Land et al. (2010) aimed to untangle the direction of the relationship between arthritis and psychiatric disorders. In a 2-year prospective study of 90 municipalities in the Netherlands, it was found that having arthritis was a risk factor for the development of a mood disorder. When the temporal relationship between psychiatric disorders and arthritis onset was examined over a 3-year period, no significant association was detected following adjustment for confounders.

Lastly, one study has used sophisticated statistical techniques in order to examine the temporal relationship between psychological factors and arthritis onset. In a 9-year prospective (nationally representative) study that had the primary aim of examining perceived stress as a risk factor for arthritis onset in older Australian women, it was found that self-reported diagnosed depression conferred the same risk as low levels of chronic stress (Harris, Loxton, Sibbritt, & Byles, 2013). Following the adjustment for confounders, longitudinal analyses revealed a 1.4 (95 % CI 1.2, 1.5; $p < 0.001$) increase in odds of having arthritis. An analysis employing a time

Box 4.1: Established Nonmodifiable and Potentially Modifiable Risk Factors for Osteoarthritis (OA) and Rheumatoid Arthritis (RA)

Nonmodifiable	Potentially modifiable
• Age	• Overweight and obesity (OA only)
• Female gender	• Joint trauma (OA only)
• Family history	• Physical activity/ inactivity[a] (OA only)
• Female sex hormones—estrogen	• Joint overload (OA only)
• Congenital abnormalities (OA only)	• Socioeconomic status
• Bone density (OA only)	• Tobacco smoking (RA only)
• Ethnicity	

[a]Moderate physical activity has been found to be protective in OA development

lag was then conducted. This method examined whether the predictor (in this case depression) at time one was associated with arthritis diagnosis at time two, and so on. Using this approach, the risk for depression remained the same. A final sensitivity analysis was conducted excluding participants who reported no arthritis but experienced persistent joint pain. When this time-lag analysis was conducted, the odds of being diagnosed with arthritis rose slightly to 1.5 (95 % CI 1.1, 1.4; $p<0.001$).

Diagnosed anxiety was also examined in a similar fashion as depression. In the longitudinal model, the odds of having been diagnosed with arthritis was slightly elevated for those with anxiety (adjusted OR = 1.2, 95 % CI 1.1, 1.4; $p=0.001$). When the time-lag model was employed, however, the effect of anxiety on arthritis onset became nonsignificant. Coupled with the findings from van't Land et al. (2010), it suggests that anxiety is a consequence of arthritis and not a precursor, while a bidirectional relationship may exist with depression.

Mechanisms Implicated in the Depression–Arthritis Relationship

Depression has been posited to influence the onset of arthritis through multiple pathways. With stress hormones known to be elevated in depression (McEwen, 2003), the allostatic load model proposed by McEwen (1998a) (see Fig. 4.5) has generated increased attention in explaining the onset of disease within a biospychosocial framework. This model takes into account the physiological consequences (i.e., cumulative wear and tear) associated with elevated stress levels. Chronic stress (or alternatively chronic depression) has been suggested to affect homeostatic structures, set points, and processes that are designed to support physiological resilience via dysregulation of the HPA and sympathetic-adrenal-medullary (SAM) axes (Berntson & Cacioppo, 2000; McEwen, 1998a). The acute stress response involves the initiation of key allostatic systems, including central, autonomic, neuroendocrine, and immune systems as well as motor responses in response to real or perceived threats to homeostasis (Hawkley et al., 2005). Particularly, the SAM-axis releases catecholamines and the HPA axis secretes glucocorticoids that mobilize the 'fight or flight' response (Kudielka & Kirschbaum, 2005; Sapolsky, Romero, & Munck, 2000). This process is deemed adaptive and facilitates physiological resilience (Hawkley et al., 2005). Chronic activation of the SAM and HPA axes (as in depression) results in a stress-related hormonal cascade into surrounding interconnected systems. Chronic glucocorticoid release or blunting is hypothesized to instigate a negative feedback loop to the immune system (Marques-Deak, Cizza, & Sternberg, 2005). Coupled with amplification of pro-inflammatory cytokines, these maladaptive processes may result in lasting changes to these systems that are conducive to the onset of disease, such as those of an inflammatory nature (Eskandari, Webster, & Sternberg, 2003; McEwen, 1998b).

Less evidence exists for the role of psychological disorders in the onset of OA. It has been argued that elevated stress levels may also influence joint degeneration and pain pathways through

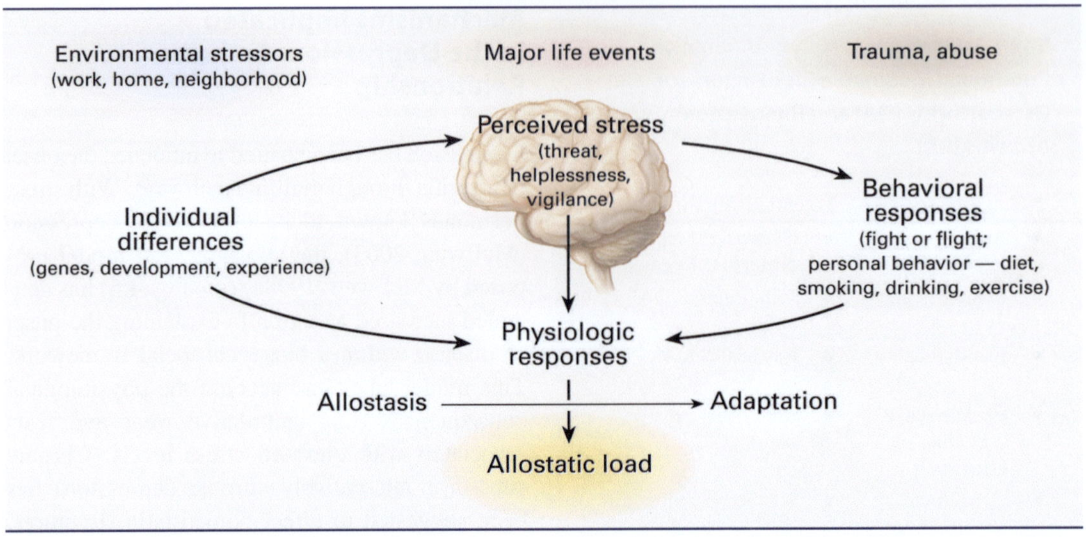

Fig. 4.5 The Stress Response and Development of Allostatic Load. The perception of stress is influenced by one's experiences, genetics, and behavior. When the brain perceives an experience as stressful, physiologic and behavioral responses are initiated, leading to allostasis and adaptation. Over time, allostatic load can accumulate, and the overexposure to mediators of neural, endocrine, and immune stress can have adverse effects on various organ systems, leading to disease. From The New England Journal of Medicine, McEwen BS, Protective and damaging effects of stress mediators, 338(3), p. 172. Copyright © (1998) Massachusetts Medical Society. Reprinted with permission from Massachusetts Medical Society

cellular aging or altered mood (Hawkley et al., 2005; Rome & Rome, 2000; Sibille et al., 2012). Chronic inflammatory stimulation (through increased tumor necrosis factor-α and interleukin-6 production) has been found to have direct effects on key disease-related features including cartilage breakdown and heightened pain sensitivity (Brenn, Richter, & Schaible, 2007; Dina, Green, & Levine, 2008). Likewise, it has been suggested that disease onset for arthritis, most notably OA, may occur through metabolic pathways as a result of adverse health behaviors such as obesity (Velasquez & Katz, 2010), or through psychosocial processes (e.g., poor coping), thus increasing allostatic load (McEwen & Stellar, 1993; Velasquez & Katz, 2010).

Chapter Highlights and Future Directions

The aim of this chapter was to provide an overview of psychological disorders in arthritis. More quality studies are needed (particularly around anxiety) in order to disentangle the relationship between psychological disorders, disease outcomes, and psychological adjustment. The findings to date, however, suggest that this process is extremely complex with a cyclical relationship noted between pain, physical function, and depression. This process is often complicated by psychosocial factors including passive coping, helplessness, and self-efficacy. Healthcare professionals who are at the coal face of chronic disease management are required to be more actively involved in the care of arthritis patients, monitoring not only symptoms but also routinely screening for psychosocial concerns (e.g., depression and anxiety). Psychosocial assessments of risk for poor emotional outcomes using standardized self-report measures with defined cut-off scores may be key to assisting with clinical referrals and supplementary treatment options (Boersma & Linton, 2005; Wolfe & Skevington, 2000). Simultaneous treatment of psychological disorders has been found to not only be effective in reducing psychological symptoms but also decreasing pain and improving functional status (Lin et al., 2003). Furthermore, while it appears that anxiety is a consequence of arthritis as opposed to a risk factor, further research is required that addresses the mechanisms associated with depression and the onset of arthritis. Such understanding may assist with improving current strategies in order to prevent or delay the onset of this preventable disease.

References

Achat, H., Kawachi, I., Spiro, A., III, DeMolles, D. A., & Sparrow, D. (2000). Optimism and depression as predictors of physical and mental health functioning: The Normative Aging Study. *Annals of Behavioral Medicine, 22*(2), 127–130.

Adams, R. J., Wilson, D. H., Taylor, A. W., Daly, A., Tursan d'Espaignet, E., Dal Grande, E., & Ruffin, R. E. (2004). Psychological factors and asthma quality of life: A population based study. *Thorax, 59*(11), 930–935.

Adler, B., Abraham, C. S., van Teijlinga, E., & Potter, M. (Eds.). (2009). *Psychology and sociology applied to medicine. An illustrated colour text* (3rd ed.). Sydney, New South Wales, Australia: Elsevier.

Alamanos, Y., & Drosos, A. A. (2005). Epidemiology of adult rheumatoid arthritis. *Autoimmunity Reviews, 4*(3), 130–136.

Allison, P. J., Guichard, C., & Gilain, L. (2000). A prospective investigation of dispositional optimism as a predictor of health-related quality of life in head and neck cancer patients. *Quality of Life Research, 9*(8), 951–960.

Andrianakos, A. A., Miyakis, S., Trontzas, P., Kaziolas, G., Christoyannis, F., Karamitsos, D., Karanikolas, G., & Dantis, P. (2005). The burden of the rheumatic diseases in the general adult population of Greece: The ESORDIG study. *Rheumatology (Oxford), 44*(7), 932–938.

Ang, D. C., Choi, H., Kroenke, K., & Wolfe, F. (2005). Comorbid depression is an independent risk factor for mortality in patients with rheumatoid arthritis. *The Journal of Rheumatology, 32*(6), 1013–1019.

Australian Institute of Health and Welfare. (2005). *Arthritis and musculoskeletal conditions in Australia, 2005*. Canberra, Australian Capital Territory: AIHW.

Australian Institute of Health and Welfare. (2006). *Chronic diseases and associated risk factors in Australia*. Canberra, Australian Capital Territory: AIHW.

Axford, J., Butt, A., Heron, C., Hammond, J., Morgan, J., Alavi, A., Bolton, J., & Bland, M. (2010). Prevalence of anxiety and depression in osteoarthritis: Use of the Hospital Anxiety and Depression Scale as a screening tool. *Clinical Rheumatology, 29*(11), 1277–1283.

Bair, M. J., Robinson, R. L., Katon, W., & Kroenke, K. (2003). Depression and pain comorbidity: A literature review. *Archives of Internal Medicine, 163*(20), 2433–2445.

Bair, M. J., Wu, J., Damush, T. M., Sutherland, J. M., & Kroenke, K. (2008). Association of depression and anxiety alone and in combination with chronic musculoskeletal pain in primary care patients. *Psychosomatic Medicine, 70*(8), 890–897.

Baird, C. L. (2000). Living with hurting and difficulty doing: Older women with osteoarthritis. *Clinical Excellence for Nurse Practitioners, 4*(4), 231–237.

Belza, B. L. (1995). Comparison of self-reported fatigue in rheumatoid arthritis and controls. *The Journal of Rheumatology, 22*(4), 639–643.

Berntson, G. G., & Cacioppo, J. T. (2000). From homeostasis to allodynamic regulation. In G. G. Berntson & J. T. Cacioppo (Eds.), *Handbook of psychophysiology* (2nd ed., pp. 459–481). Cambridge, England: Cambridge University Press.

Boersma, K., & Linton, S. J. (2005). Screening to identify patients at risk: Profiles of psychological risk factors for early intervention. *The Clinical Journal of Pain, 21*(1), 38–43.

Branch, V. K., Lipsky, K., Nieman, T., & Lipsky, P. E. (1999). Positive impact of an intervention by arthritis patient educators on knowledge and satisfaction of patients in a rheumatology practice. *Arthritis Care and Research, 12*(6), 370–375.

Brenn, D., Richter, F., & Schaible, H. G. (2007). Sensitization of unmyelinated sensory fibers of the joint nerve to mechanical stimuli by interleukin-6 in the rat: An inflammatory mechanism of joint pain. *Arthritis and Rheumatism, 56*(1), 351–359.

Brenner, G. F., Melamed, B. G., & Panush, R. S. (1994). Optimism and coping as determinants of psychosocial adaptation to rheumatoid arthritis. *Journal of Clinical Psychology in Medical Settings, 1*, 115–134.

Brown, G. K., Nicassio, P. M., & Wallston, K. A. (1989). Pain coping strategies and depression in rheumatoid arthritis. *Journal of Consulting and Clinical Psychology, 57*(5), 652–657.

Brown, G. K., Wallston, K. A., & Nicassio, P. M. (1989). Social support and depression in rheumatoid arthritis: A one-year prospective study. *Journal of Applied Social Psychology, 19*, 1164–1181.

Buckwalter, J. A., Saltzman, C., Brown, T. (2004). The impact of osteoarthritis: Implications for research. *Clinical Orthopaedics and Related Research*, (427 Suppl), S6–S15.

Carver, C. S., Pozo-Kaderman, C., Harris, S. D., Noriega, V., Scheier, M. F., Robinson, D. S., Ketcham, A. S., Moffat, F. L., Jr., & Clark, K. C. (1994). Optimism versus pessimism predicts the quality of women's adjustment to early stage breast cancer. *Cancer, 73*(4), 1213–1220.

Centers for Disease Control and Prevention. (2005). Racial/ethnic differences in the prevalence and impact of doctor-diagnosed arthritis—United States, 2002. *MMWR. Morbidity and Mortality Weekly Report, 54*(5), 119–123.

Clark, L. A., & Watson, D. (1991). Tripartite model of anxiety and depression: Psychometric evidence and taxonomic implications. *Journal of Abnormal Psychology, 100*(3), 316–336.

Clarke, D. M., & Currie, K. C. (2009). Depression, anxiety and their relationship with chronic diseases: A review

of the epidemiology, risk and treatment evidence. *The Medical Journal of Australia, 190*(7 Suppl), S54–S60.
Cooper, C., Snow, S., McAlindon, T. E., Kellingray, S., Stuart, B., Coggon, D., & Dieppe, P. A. (2000). Risk factors for the incidence and progression of radiographic knee osteoarthritis. *Arthritis and Rheumatism, 43*(5), 995–1000.
Courvoisier, D. S., Agoritsas, T., Glauser, J., Michaud, K., Wolfe, F., Cantoni, E., Perneger, T. V., & Finckh, A. (2012). Pain as an important predictor of psychosocial health in patients with rheumatoid arthritis. *Arthritis Care and Research, 64*(2), 190–196.
Covic, T., Adamson, B., & Hough, M. (2000). The impact of passive coping on rheumatoid arthritis pain. *Rheumatology (Oxford), 39*(9), 1027–1030.
Covic, T., Adamson, B., Spencer, D., & Howe, G. (2003). A biopsychosocial model of pain and depression in rheumatoid arthritis: A 12-month longitudinal study. *Rheumatology (Oxford), 42*(11), 1287–1294.
Covic, T., Tyson, G., Spencer, D., & Howe, G. (2006). Depression in rheumatoid arthritis patients: Demographic, clinical, and psychological predictors. *Journal of Psychosomatic Research, 60*(5), 469–476.
Crotty, M., McFarlane, A. C., Brooks, P. M., Hopper, J. L., Bieri, D., & Taylor, S. J. (1994). The psychosocial and clinical status of younger women with early rheumatoid arthritis: A longitudinal study with frequent measures. *British Journal of Rheumatology, 33*(8), 754–760.
Curtis, R., Groarke, A., Coughlan, R., & Gsel, A. (2004). The influence of disease severity, perceived stress, social support and coping in patients with chronic illness: A 1-year follow up. *Psychology, Health and Medicine, 9*, 456–475.
Curtis, R., Groarke, A., Coughlan, R., & Gsel, A. (2005). Psychological stress as a predictor of psychological adjustment and health status in patients with rheumatoid arthritis. *Patient Education and Counseling, 59*(2), 192–198.
Dager, T. N., Kjeken, I., Fjerstad, E., & Hauge, M. I. (2012). "It is about taking grips and not let myself be ravaged by my body": A qualitative study of outcomes from in-patient multidisciplinary rehabilitation for patients with chronic rheumatic diseases. *Disability and Rehabilitation, 34*(11), 910–916.
Dekkers, J. C., Geenen, R., Evers, A. W., Kraaimaat, F. W., Bijlsma, J. W., & Godaert, G. L. (2001). Biopsychosocial mediators and moderators of stress-health relationships in patients with recently diagnosed rheumatoid arthritis. *Arthritis and Rheumatism, 45*(4), 307–316.
Demange, V., Guillemin, F., Baumann, M., Suurmeijer, T. P., Moum, T., Doeglas, D., Briancon, S., & van den Heuvel, W. J. (2004). Are there more than cross-sectional relationships of social support and support networks with functional limitations and psychological distress in early rheumatoid arthritis? The European Research on Incapacitating Diseases and Social Support Longitudinal Study. *Arthritis and Rheumatism, 51*(5), 782–791.
Dersh, J., Polatin, P. B., & Gatchel, R. J. (2002). Chronic pain and psychopathology: Research findings and theoretical considerations. *Psychosomatic Medicine, 64*(5), 773–786.
Descartes, R. (1968). *Discourse on method and the meditations*. Harmondsworth, England: Penguin.
Dickens, C., McGowan, L., Clark-Carter, D., & Creed, F. (2002). Depression in rheumatoid arthritis: A systematic review of the literature with meta-analysis. *Psychosomatic Medicine, 64*(1), 52–60.
Dina, O. A., Green, P. G., & Levine, J. D. (2008). Role of interleukin-6 in chronic muscle hyperalgesic priming. *Neuroscience, 152*(2), 521–525.
Dunlop, D. D., Lyons, J. S., Manheim, L. M., Song, J., & Chang, R. W. (2004). Arthritis and heart disease as risk factors for major depression: The role of functional limitation. *Medical Care, 42*(6), 502–511.
Ehrlich, G. E. (2003). Osteoarthritis beginning with inflammation. Definitions and correlations. 1975. *Bulletin of the World Health Organization, 81*(9), 691–693.
El-Miedany, Y. M., & El-Rasheed, A. H. (2002). Is anxiety a more common disorder than depression in rheumatoid arthritis? *Joint, Bone, Spine, 69*(3), 300–306.
Engel, G. L. (1977). The need for a new medical model: A challenge for biomedicine. *Science, 196*(4286), 129–136.
Escalante, A., & del Rincon, I. (1999). How much disability in rheumatoid arthritis is explained by rheumatoid arthritis? Arthritis and Rheumatism, 42(8), 1712-1721..
Eskandari, F., Webster, J. I., & Sternberg, E. M. (2003). Neural immune pathways and their connection to inflammatory diseases. *Arthritis Research and Therapy, 5*(6), 251–265.
Ethgen, O., Vanparijs, P., Delhalle, S., Rosant, S., Bruyere, O., & Reginster, J. Y. (2004). Social support and health-related quality of life in hip and knee osteoarthritis. *Quality of Life Research, 13*(2), 321–330.
Evers, A. W., Kraaimaat, F. W., Geenen, R., & Bijlsma, J. W. (1997). Determinants of psychological distress and its course in the first year after diagnosis in rheumatoid arthritis patients. *Journal of Behavioral Medicine, 20*(5), 489–504.
Evers, A. W., Kraaimaat, F. W., Geenen, R., Jacobs, J. W., & Bijlsma, J. W. (2002). Longterm predictors of anxiety and depressed mood in early rheumatoid arthritis: A 3 and 5 year followup. *The Journal of Rheumatology, 29*(11), 2327–2336.
Evers, A. W., Kraaimaat, F. W., Geenen, R., Jacobs, J. W., & Bijlsma, J. W. (2003). Stress-vulnerability factors as long-term predictors of disease activity in early rheumatoid arthritis. *Journal of Psychosomatic Research, 55*(4), 293–302.
Felson, D. T. (1996). Does excess weight cause osteoarthritis, and if so, why? *Annals of the Rheumatic Diseases, 55*(9), 668–670.
Ferreira, V. M., & Sherman, A. M. (2007). The relationship of optimism, pain and social support to well-being in older adults with osteoarthritis. *Aging and Mental Health, 11*(1), 89–98.

Folkman, S., & Greer, S. (2000). Promoting psychological well-being in the face of serious illness: When theory, research and practice inform each other. *Psychooncology, 9*(1), 11–19.

Fournier, M., de Ridder, D., & Bensing, J. (2002). How optimism contributes to the adaptation of chronic illness: A prospective study into the enduring effects of optimism on adaptation moderated by the controllability of chronic illness. *Personality and Individual Differences, 33*, 1163–1183.

Franklin, A. L., & Harrell, T. H. (2013). Impact of fatigue on psychological outcomes in adults living with rheumatoid arthritis. *Nursing Research, 62*(3), 203–209.

Gignac, M. A., Cott, C., & Badley, E. M. (2000). Adaptation to chronic illness and disability and its relationship to perceptions of independence and dependence. *The Journals of Gerontology. Series B, Psychological Sciences and Social Sciences, 55*(6), 362–372.

Godha, D., Shi, L., & Mavronicolas, H. (2010). Association between tendency towards depression and severity of rheumatoid arthritis from a national representative sample: The medical expenditure panel survey. *Current Medical Research and Opinion, 26*(7), 1685–1690.

Gray, J. A., & McNaughton, N. (2000). *The neuropsychology of anxiety*. Oxford, England: Oxford University Press.

Gronning, K., Lomundal, B., Koksvik, H. S., & Steinsbekk, A. (2011). Coping with arthritis is experienced as a dynamic balancing process. A qualitative study. *Clinical Rheumatology, 30*(11), 1425–1432.

Gureje, O., Von Korff, M., Simon, G. E., & Gater, R. (1998). Persistent pain and well-being: A World Health Organization Study in Primary Care. *The Journal of the American Medical Association, 280*(2), 147–151.

Harris, M. L., Byles, J. E., Sibbritt, D., & Loxton, D. (2015). "Just get on with it": Qualitative insights of coming to terms with a deteriorating body for older women with osteoarthritis. *PLoS One, 10*(3), e0120507.

Harris, M. L., Loxton, D., Sibbritt, D. W., & Byles, J. E. (2012). The relative importance of psychosocial factors in arthritis: Findings from 10,509 Australian women. *Journal of Psychosomatic Research, 73*(4), 251–256.

Harris, M. L., Loxton, D., Sibbritt, D. W., & Byles, J. E. (2013). The influence of perceived stress on the onset of arthritis in women: Findings from the Australian Longitudinal Study on Women's Health. *Annals of Behavioral Medicine, 46*(1), 9–18.

Hawker, G. A., Gignac, M. A., Badley, E., Davis, A. M., French, M. R., Li, Y., Perruccio, A. V., Power, J. D., Sale, J., & Lou, W. (2011). A longitudinal study to explain the pain-depression link in older adults with osteoarthritis. *Arthritis Care and Research, 63*(10), 1382–1390.

Hawkley, L. C., Berntson, G. G., Engeland, C. G., Marucha, P. T., Masi, C. M., & Cacioppo, J. T. (2005). Stress, aging and resilience: Can accrued wear and tear be slowed? *Canadian Psychology, 46*(3), 115–125.

Hawley, D. J., & Wolfe, F. (1988). Anxiety and depression in patients with rheumatoid arthritis: A prospective study of 400 patients. *The Journal of Rheumatology, 15*(6), 932–941.

Hawley, D. J., & Wolfe, F. (1993). Depression is not more common in rheumatoid arthritis: A 10-year longitudinal study of 6,153 patients with rheumatic disease. *The Journal of Rheumatology, 20*(12), 2025–2031.

Hill, C. L., Gill, T., Taylor, A. W., Daly, A., Grande, E. D., & Adams, R. J. (2007). Psychological factors and quality of life in arthritis: A population-based study. *Clinical Rheumatology, 26*(7), 1049–1054.

Ho, R. C., Fu, E. H., Chua, A. N., Cheak, A. A., & Mak, A. (2011). Clinical and psychosocial factors associated with depression and anxiety in Singaporean patients with rheumatoid arthritis. *International Journal of Rheumatic Diseases, 14*(1), 37–47.

Hodkinson, B., Musenge, E., Ally, M., Meyer, P. W. A., Anderson, R., & Tikly, M. (2012). Functional disability and health-related quality of life in South Africans with early rheumatoid arthritis. *Scandinavian Journal of Rheumatology, 41*(5), 366–374.

Hyrich, K., Symmons, D., Watson, K., Silman, A., BSRBR Control Centre Consortium, & British Society for Rheumatology Biologics Register. (2006). Baseline comorbidity levels in biologic and standard DMARD treated patients with rheumatoid arthritis: Results from a national patient register. *Annals of the Rheumatic Diseases, 65*(7), 895–898.

Isik, A., Koca, S. S., Ozturk, A., & Mermi, O. (2007). Anxiety and depression in patients with rheumatoid arthritis. *Clinical Rheumatology, 26*(6), 872–878.

Jones, A., & Doherty, M. (1995). ABC of rheumatology. Osteoarthritis. *British Medical Journal, 310*(6977), 457–460.

Jung, C. (1972). *Collected works of CG Jung* (2nd ed.). Princeton, NJ: Princeton University Press.

Karakus, M. C., & Patton, L. C. (2011). Depression and the onset of chronic illness in older adults: A 12-year prospective study. *The Journal of Behavioral Health Services & Research, 38*(3), 373–382.

Katz, P. P., & Yelin, E. H. (1993). Prevalence and correlates of depressive symptoms among persons with rheumatoid arthritis. *The Journal of Rheumatology, 20*(5), 790–796.

Kean, W. F., Kean, R., & Buchanan, W. W. (2004). Osteoarthritis: Symptoms, signs and source of pain. *Inflammopharmacology, 12*(1), 3–31.

Kim, K. W., Han, J. W., Cho, H. J., Chang, C. B., Park, J. H., Lee, J. J., Lee, S. B., Seong, S. C., & Kim, T. K. (2011). Association between comorbid depression and osteoarthritis symptom severity in patients with knee osteoarthritis. *The Journal of Bone and Joint Surgery. American Volume, 93*(6), 556–563.

Kojima, M., Kojima, T., Ishiguro, N., Oguchi, T., Oba, M., Tsuchiya, H., Sugiura, F., Furukawa, T. A., Suzuki, S., & Tokudome, S. (2009). Psychosocial factors, disease status, and quality of life in patients with rheumatoid arthritis. *Journal of Psychosomatic Research, 67*(5), 425–431.

Kraaimaat, F. W., Van Dam-Baggen, R. M., & Bijlsma, J. W. (1995). Association of social support and the spouse's reaction with psychological distress in male and female patients with rheumatoid arthritis. *The Journal of Rheumatology, 22*(4), 644–648.

Kroenke, K., Wu, J., Bair, M. J., Krebs, E. E., Damush, T. M., & Tu, W. (2011). Reciprocal relationship between pain and depression: A 12-month longitudinal analysis in primary care. *The Journal of Pain, 12*(9), 964–973.

Kudielka, B. M., & Kirschbaum, C. (2005). Sex differences in HPA axis responses to stress: A review. *Biological Psychology, 69*(1), 113–132.

Kundermann, B., Hemmeter-Spernal, J., Huber, M. T., Krieg, J. C., & Lautenbacher, S. (2008). Effects of total sleep deprivation in major depression: Overnight improvement of mood is accompanied by increased pain sensitivity and augmented pain complaints. *Psychosomatic Medicine, 70*(1), 92–101.

Lazarus, R. S., & Folkman, S. (1987). Transactional theory and research on emotions and coping. *European Journal of Personality, 1*(3), 141–169.

Leserman, J., Jackson, E. D., Petitto, J. M., Golden, R. N., Silva, S. G., Perkins, D. O., Cai, J., Folds, J. D., & Evans, D. L. (1999). Progression to AIDS: The effects of stress, depressive symptoms, and social support. *Psychosomatic Medicine, 61*(3), 397–406.

Leskela, U., Rytsala, H., Komulainen, E., Melartin, T., Sokero, P., Lestela-Mielonen, P., & Isometsa, E. (2006). The influence of adversity and perceived social support on the outcome of major depressive disorder in subjects with different levels of depressive symptoms. *Psychological Medicine, 36*(6), 779–788.

Lin, E. H., Katon, W., Von Korff, M., Tang, L., Williams, J. W., Jr., Kroenke, K., Hunkeler, E., Harpole, L., Hegel, M., Arean, P., Hoffing, M., Della Penna, R., Langston, C., Unutzer, J., & Impact Investigators (2003). Effect of improving depression care on pain and functional outcomes among older adults with arthritis: A randomized controlled trial. *The Journal of the American Medical Association, 290*(18), 2428–2429.

Lok, E. Y. C., Mok, C. C., Cheng, C. W., Cheung, E. F. C. (2010). Prevalence and determinants of psychiatric disorders in patients with rheumatoid arthritis. *Psychosomatics, 51*(4), 338–338.e8.

Long, B. C., & Sangster, J. I. (1993). Dispositional optimism/pessimism and coping strategies: Predictors of psychosocial adjustment of rheumatoid and osteoarthritis patients. *Journal of Applied Social Psychology, 23*, 1069–1091.

Looper, K., Mustafa, S., Zelkowitz, P., Purden, M., Baron, M., & McGill Early Arthritis Research Group. (2011). History of depressive episodes as a risk factor for illness severity in early inflammatory arthritis. *Journal of Psychosomatic Research, 71*(1), 28–31.

Lutze, U., & Archenholtz, B. (2007). The impact of arthritis on daily life with the patient perspective in focus. *Scandinavian Journal of Caring Sciences, 21*(1), 64–70.

Margaretten, M., Yelin, E., Imboden, J., Graf, J., Barton, J., Katz, P., & Julian, L. (2009). Predictors of depression in a multiethnic cohort of patients with rheumatoid arthritis. *Arthritis and Rheumatism, 61*(11), 1586–1591.

Marks, R. (2013). Depressive symptoms among community-dwelling older adults with mild to moderate knee osteoarthritis: Extent, interrelationships, and predictors. *American Journal of Medicine Studies, 1*(3), 11–18.

Marks, R., & Allegrante, J. P. (2002). Comorbid disease profiles of adults with end-stage hip osteoarthritis. *Medical Science Monitor, 8*(4), CR305–CR309.

Marques-Deak, A., Cizza, G., & Sternberg, E. (2005). Brain-immune interactions and disease susceptibility. *Molecular Psychiatry, 10*(3), 239–250.

Masuda, A., Anderson, P. L., Wendell, J. W., Chou, Y.-Y., Price, M., & Feinstein, A. B. (2011). Psychological flexibility mediates the relations between self-concealment and negative psychological outcomes. *Personality and Individual Differences, 50*(2), 243–247.

McEwen, B. S. (1998a). Protective and damaging effects of stress mediators. *The New England Journal of Medicine, 338*(3), 171–179.

McEwen, B. S. (1998b). Stress, adaptation, and disease. Allostasis and allostatic load. *Annals of the New York Academy of Sciences, 840*, 33–44.

McEwen, B. S. (2003). Mood disorders and allostatic load. *Biological Psychiatry, 54*(3), 200–207.

McEwen, B. S., & Stellar, E. (1993). Stress and the individual. Mechanisms leading to disease. *Archives of Internal Medicine, 153*(18), 2093–2101.

McLaughlin, T. P., Khandker, R. K., Kruzikas, D. T., & Tummala, R. (2006). Overlap of anxiety and depression in a managed care population: Prevalence and association with resource utilization. *The Journal of Clinical Psychiatry, 67*(8), 1187–1193.

Melanson, P. M., & Downe-Wamboldt, B. (2003). Confronting life with rheumatoid arthritis. *Journal of Advanced Nursing, 42*(2), 125–133.

Mella, L. F., Bertolo, M. B., & Dalgalarrondo, P. (2010). Depressive symptoms in rheumatoid arthritis. *Revista Brasileira de Psiquiatria, 32*(3), 257–263.

Moussavi, S., Chatterji, S., Verdes, E., Tandon, A., Patel, V., & Ustun, B. (2007). Depression, chronic diseases, and decrements in health: Results from the World Health Surveys. *Lancet, 370*(9590), 851–858.

Murphy, S., Creed, F., & Jayson, M. I. (1988). Psychiatric disorder and illness behaviour in rheumatoid arthritis. *British Journal of Rheumatology, 27*(5), 357–363.

Murphy, L. B., Sacks, J. J., Brady, T. J., Hootman, J. M., & Chapman, D. P. (2012). Anxiety and depression among US adults with arthritis: Prevalence and correlates. *Arthritis Care and Research, 64*(7), 968–976.

Naidoo, P., & Pretorius, T. B. (2006). The moderating role of helplessness in rheumatoid arthritis, a chronic disease. *Social Behavior and Personality, 34*, 103–112.

Norton, S., Sacker, A., Young, A., & Done, J. (2011). Distinct psychological distress trajectories in rheumatoid arthritis: Findings from an inception cohort. *Journal of Psychosomatic Research, 71*(5), 290–295.

Odegard, S., Finset, A., Mowinckel, P., Kvien, T. K., & Uhlig, T. (2007). Pain and psychological health status over a 10-year period in patients with recent onset rheumatoid arthritis. *Annals of the Rheumatic Diseases, 66*(9), 1195–1201.

Olson, M. M., Trevino, D. B., Islam, J., & Denner, L. (2010). The biopsychosocial milieu of type 2 diabetes: An exploratory study of the impact of social relationships on a chronic inflammatory disease. *International Journal of Psychiatry in Medicine, 40*(3), 289–305.

Palkonyai, E., Kolarz, G., Kopp, M., Bogye, G., Temesvari, P., Palkonyay, L., Ratko, I., & Meszaros, E. (2007). Depressive symptoms in early rheumatoid arthritis: A comparative longitudinal study. *Clinical Rheumatology, 26*(5), 753–758.

Patten, S. B., Williams, J. V., & Wang, J. (2006). Mental disorders in a population sample with musculoskeletal disorders. *BMC Musculoskeletal Disorders, 7*, 37.

Pembroke, T. P., Rasul, F., Hart, C. L., Davey Smith, G., & Stansfeld, S. A. (2006). Psychological distress and chronic obstructive pulmonary disease in the Renfrew and Paisley (MIDSPAN) study. *Journal of Epidemiology and Community Health, 60*(9), 789–792.

Persson, L. O., Larsson, B. M., Nived, K., & Eberhardt, K. (2005). The development of emotional distress in 158 patients with recently diagnosed rheumatoid arthritis: A prospective 5-year follow-up study. *Scandinavian Journal of Rheumatology, 34*(3), 191–197.

Peters, T. J., Sanders, C., Dieppe, P., & Donovan, J. (2005). Factors associated with change in pain and disability over time: A community-based prospective observational study of hip and knee osteoarthritis. *The British Journal of General Practice, 55*(512), 205–211.

Ploghaus, A., Narain, C., Beckmann, C. F., Clare, S., Bantick, S., Wise, R., Matthews, P. M., Rawlins, J. N., & Tracey, I. (2001). Exacerbation of pain by anxiety is associated with activity in a hippocampal network. *The Journal of Neuroscience, 21*(24), 9896–9903.

Porcelli, P., Zaka, S., Centonze, S., & Sisto, G. (1994). Psychological distress and levels of disease activity in inflammatory bowel disease. *The Italian Journal of Gastroenterology, 26*(3), 111–115.

Ramjeet, J., Koutantji, M., Barrett, E. M., & Scott, D. G. (2005). Coping and psychological adjustment in recent-onset inflammatory polyarthritis: The role of gender and age. *Rheumatology (Oxford), 44*(9), 1166–1168.

Rasul, F., Stansfeld, S. A., Smith, G. D., Shlomo, Y. B., & Gallacher, J. (2007). Psychological distress, physical illness and risk of myocardial infarction in the Caerphilly study. *Psychological Medicine, 37*(9), 1305–1313.

Rejeski, W. J., Miller, M. E., Foy, C., Messier, S., & Rapp, S. (2001). Self-efficacy and the progression of functional limitations and self-reported disability in older adults with knee pain. *The Journals of Gerontology. Series B, Psychological Sciences and Social Sciences, 56*(5), S261–S265.

Riddle, D. L., Kong, X., & Fitzgerald, G. K. (2011). Psychological health impact on 2-year changes in pain and function in persons with knee pain: Data from the Osteoarthritis Initiative. *Osteoarthritis and Cartilage, 19*(9), 1095–1101.

Rome, H. P., Jr., & Rome, J. D. (2000). Limbically augmented pain syndrome (LAPS): Kindling, corticolimbic sensitization, and the convergence of affective and sensory symptoms in chronic pain disorders. *Pain Medicine, 1*(1), 7–23.

Rosemann, T., Laux, G., & Szecsenyi, J. (2007). Osteoarthritis: Quality of life, comorbidities, medication and health service utilization assessed in a large sample of primary care patients. *Journal of Orthopaedic Surgery and Research, 2*, 12.

Sapolsky, R. M., Romero, L. M., & Munck, A. U. (2000). How do glucocorticoids influence stress responses? Integrating permissive, suppressive, stimulatory, and preparative actions. *Endocrine Reviews, 21*(1), 55–89.

Sareen, J., Cox, B. J., Clara, I., & Asmundson, G. J. (2005). The relationship between anxiety disorders and physical disorders in the U.S. National Comorbidity Survey. *Depression and Anxiety, 21*(4), 193–202.

Savelkoul, M., de Witte, L., & Post, M. (2003). Stimulating active coping in patients with rheumatic diseases: A systematic review of controlled group intervention studies. *Patient Education and Counseling, 50*(2), 133–143.

Scheier, M. F., & Carver, C. S. (1985). Optimism, coping, and health: Assessment and implications of generalized outcome expectancies. *Health Psychology, 4*(3), 219–247.

Scheier, M. F., & Carver, C. S. (1987). Dispositional optimism and physical well-being: The influence of generalized outcome expectancies on health. *Journal of Personality, 55*(2), 169–210.

Scheier, M. F., Matthews, K. A., Owens, J. F., Magovern, G. J., Sr., Lefebvre, R. C., Abbott, R. A., & Carver, C. S. (1989). Dispositional optimism and recovery from coronary artery bypass surgery: The beneficial effects on physical and psychological well-being. *Journal of Personality and Social Psychology, 57*(6), 1024–1040.

Scheier, M. F., Weintraub, J. K., & Carver, C. S. (1986). Coping with stress: Divergent strategies of optimists and pessimists. *Journal of Personality and Social Psychology, 51*(6), 1257–1264.

Schmidt, N. B., & Cook, J. H. (1999). Effects of anxiety sensitivity on anxiety and pain during a cold pressor challenge in patients with panic disorder. *Behaviour Research and Therapy, 37*(4), 313–323.

Scott, K. M., Von Korff, M., Angermeyer, M. C., Benjet, C., Bruffaerts, R., de Girolamo, G., Haro, J. M., Lepine, J. P., Ormel, J., Posada-Villa, J., Tachimori, H., & Kessler, R. C. (2011). Association of childhood adversities and early-onset mental disorders with adult-onset chronic physical conditions. *Archives of General Psychiatry, 68*(8), 838–844.

Seavey, W. G., Kurata, J. H., & Cohen, R. D. (2003). Risk factors for incident self-reported arthritis in a 20 year followup of the Alameda County Study Cohort. *The Journal of Rheumatology, 30*(10), 2103–2111.

Sharma, L., Cahue, S., Song, J., Hayes, K., Pai, Y. C., & Dunlop, D. (2003). Physical functioning over three years in knee osteoarthritis: Role of psychosocial, local mechanical, and neuromuscular factors. *Arthritis and Rheumatism, 48*(12), 3359–3370.

Shaul, M. P. (1995). From early twinges to mastery: The process of adjustment in living with rheumatoid arthritis. *Arthritis Care and Research, 8*(4), 290–297.

Sherman, A. M. (2003). Social relations and depressive symptoms in older adults with knee osteoarthritis. *Social Science and Medicine, 56*(2), 247–257.

Shih, M., Hootman, J. M., Strine, T. W., Chapman, D. P., & Brady, T. J. (2006). Serious psychological distress in U.S. adults with arthritis. *Journal of General Internal Medicine, 21*(11), 1160–1166.

Sibille, K. T., Langaee, T., Burkley, B., Gong, Y., Glover, T. L., King, C., Riley, J. L., 3rd, Leeuwenburgh, C., Staud, R., Bradley, L. A., & Fillingim, R. B. (2012). Chronic pain, perceived stress, and cellular aging: An exploratory study. *Molecular Pain, 8*(1), 12.

Silman, A. J., & Pearson, J. E. (2002). Epidemiology and genetics of rheumatoid arthritis. *Arthritis Research, 4*(Suppl 3), S265–S272.

Sinclair, V. G., & Wallston, K. A. (2010). Psychological vulnerability predicts increases in depressive symptoms in individuals with rheumatoid arthritis. *Nursing Research, 59*(2), 140–146.

Smedstad, L. M., Moum, T., Vaglum, P., & Kvien, T. K. (1996). The impact of early rheumatoid arthritis on psychological distress. A comparison between 238 patients with RA and 116 matched controls. *Scandinavian Journal of Rheumatology, 25*(6), 377–382.

Smedstad, L. M., Vaglum, P., Moum, T., & Kvien, T. K. (1997). The relationship between psychological distress and traditional clinical variables: A 2 year prospective study of 216 patients with early rheumatoid arthritis. *British Journal of Rheumatology, 36*(12), 1304–1311.

Smith, B. W., & Zautra, A. J. (2008). The effects of anxiety and depression on weekly pain in women with arthritis. *Pain, 138*(2), 354–361.

Snow-Turek, A. L., Norris, M. P., & Tan, G. (1996). Active and passive coping strategies in chronic pain patients. *Pain, 64*(3), 455–462.

Soderlin, M. K., Hakala, M., & Nieminen, P. (2000). Anxiety and depression in a community-based rheumatoid arthritis population. *Scandinavian Journal of Rheumatology, 29*(3), 177–183.

Sokka, T., Kautiainen, H., Mottonen, T., & Hannonen, P. (1999). Work disability in rheumatoid arthritis 10 years after the diagnosis. *The Journal of Rheumatology, 26*(8), 1681–1685.

Stamm, T., Lovelock, L., Stew, G., Nell, V., Smolen, J., Jonsson, H., Sadlo, G., & Machold, K. (2008). I have mastered the challenge of living with a chronic disease: Life stories of people with rheumatoid arthritis. *Qualitative Health Research, 18*(5), 658–669.

Strine, T. W., Hootman, J. M., Okoro, C. A., Balluz, L., Moriarty, D. G., Owens, M., & Mokdad, A. (2004). Frequent mental distress status among adults with arthritis age 45 years and older, 2001. *Arthritis and Rheumatism, 51*(4), 533–537.

Theis, K. A., Helmick, C. G., & Hootman, J. M. (2007). Arthritis burden and impact are greater among U.S. women than men: Intervention opportunities. *Journal of Women's Health, 16*(4), 441–453.

Thomten, J., Soares, J. J., & Sundin, O. (2011). The influence of psychosocial factors on quality of life among women with pain: A prospective study in Sweden. *Quality of Life Research, 20*(8), 1215–1225.

Timonen, M., Viilo, K., Hakko, H., Sarkioja, T., Ylikulju, M., Meyer-Rochow, V. B., Vaisanen, E., & Rasanen, P. (2003). Suicides in persons suffering from rheumatoid arthritis. *Rheumatology (Oxford), 42*(2), 287–291.

Treharne, G. J., Lyons, A. C., Booth, D. A., & Kitas, G. D. (2007). Psychological well-being across 1 year with rheumatoid arthritis: Coping resources as buffers of perceived stress. *British Journal of Health Psychology, 12*(Pt 3), 323–345.

Treharne, G. J., Lyons, A. C., & Kitas, G. D. (2000). Suicidal ideation in patients with rheumatoid arthritis. Research may help identify patients at high risk. *British Medical Journal, 321*(7271), 1290.

Uhlig, T., Smedstad, L. M., Vaglum, P., Moum, T., Gerard, N., & Kvien, T. K. (2000). The course of rheumatoid arthritis and predictors of psychological, physical and radiographic outcome after 5 years of follow-up. *Rheumatology (Oxford), 39*(7), 732–741.

van der Heide, A., Jacobs, J. W., Haanen, H. C., & Bijlsma, J. W. (1995). Is it possible to predict the first year extent of pain and disability for patients with rheumatoid arthritis? *The Journal of Rheumatology, 22*(8), 1466–1470.

van Dijk, G. M., Dekker, J., Veenhof, C., & van den Ende, C. H. (2006). Course of functional status and pain in osteoarthritis of the hip or knee: A systematic review of the literature. *Arthritis and Rheumatism, 55*(5), 779–785.

van Lankveld, W., Naring, G., van't Pad Bosch, P., & van de Putte, L. (2000). The negative effect of decreasing the level of activity in coping with pain in rheumatoid arthritis: An increase in psychological distress and disease impact. *Journal of Behavioral Medicine, 23*(4), 377–391.

van't Land, H., Verdurmen, J., Ten Have, M., van Dorsselaer, S., Beekman, A., & de Graaf, R. (2010). The association between arthritis and psychiatric disorders: Results from a longitudinal population-based study. *Journal of Psychosomatic Research, 68*(2), 187–193.

Velasquez, M. T., & Katz, J. D. (2010). Osteoarthritis: Another component of metabolic syndrome? *Metabolic Syndrome and Related Disorders, 8*(4), 295–305.

Von Korff, M., Alonso, J., Ormel, J., Angermeyer, M., Bruffaerts, R., Fleiz, C., de Girolamo, G., Kessler, R. C., Kovess-Masfety, V., Posada-Villa, J., Scott, K. M., & Uda, H. (2009). Childhood psychosocial stressors and adult onset arthritis: Broad spectrum risk factors and allostatic load. *Pain, 143*(1–2), 76–83.

Vriezekolk, J. E., van Lankveld, W. G., Geenen, R., & van den Ende, C. H. (2011). Longitudinal association between coping and psychological distress in rheumatoid arthritis: A systematic review. *Annals of the Rheumatic Diseases, 70*(7), 1243–1250.

Watson, M., Homewood, J., Haviland, J., & Bliss, J. M. (2005). Influence of psychological response on breast cancer survival: 10-year follow-up of a population-based cohort. *European Journal of Cancer, 41*(12), 1710–1714.

WHO Scientific Group. (2003). *The burden of musculoskeletal conditions at the start of the new millennium: Report of a WHO Scientific Group* (WHO Technical Report Series 919). Geneva, Switzerland: World Health Organization.

Williams, L. J., Jacka, F. N., Pasco, J. A., Dodd, S., & Berk, M. (2006). Depression and pain: An overview. *Acta Neuropsychiatrica, 18*(2), 79–87.

Wilson, A., Yu, H. T., Goodnough, L. T., & Nissenson, A. R. (2004). Prevalence and outcomes of anemia in rheumatoid arthritis: A systematic review of the literature. *The American Journal of Medicine, 116*(Suppl 7A), 50S–57S.

Wittchen, H. U., Kessler, R. C., Pfister, H., & Lieb, M. (2000). Why do people with anxiety disorders become depressed? A prospective-longitudinal community study. *Acta Psychiatrica Scandinavica - Supplement, 406*, 14–23.

Wolfe, F., & Cathey, M. A. (1991). The assessment and prediction of functional disability in rheumatoid arthritis. *The Journal of Rheumatology, 18*(9), 1298–1306.

Wolfe, F., & Hawley, D. J. (1998). The longterm outcomes of rheumatoid arthritis: Work disability: A prospective 18 year study of 823 patients. *The Journal of Rheumatology, 25*(11), 2108–2117.

Wolfe, F., Hawley, D. J., & Wilson, K. (1996). The prevalence and meaning of fatigue in rheumatic disease. *The Journal of Rheumatology, 23*(8), 1407–1417.

Wolfe, F., & Michaud, K. (2006). Anemia and renal function in patients with rheumatoid arthritis. *The Journal of Rheumatology, 33*(8), 1516–1522.

Wolfe, F., & Michaud, K. (2009). Predicting depression in rheumatoid arthritis: The signal importance of pain extent and fatigue, and comorbidity. *Arthritis and Rheumatism, 61*(5), 667–673.

Wolfe, F., & Skevington, S. M. (2000). Measuring the epidemiology of distress: The rheumatology distress index. *The Journal of Rheumatology, 27*(8), 2000–2009.

World Health Organization. (1948). *Preamble to the constitution of the World Health Organization as adopted by the International Health Conference, New York, 19–22 June, 1946; signed on 22 July 1946 by the representatives of 61 States (official records of the World Health Organization, no. 2, p. 100) and entered into force on 7 April 1948.*

World Health Organization. (2002). *The world health report 2002: Reducing risks, promoting healthy life.* Geneva, Switzerland: WHO.

Zautra, A. J., & Smith, B. W. (2001). Depression and reactivity to stress in older women with rheumatoid arthritis and osteoarthritis. *Psychosomatic Medicine, 63*(4), 687–696.

Zochling, J., Stucki, G., Grill, E., & Braun, J. (2007). A comparative study of patient-reported functional outcomes in acute rheumatoid arthritis. *The Journal of Rheumatology, 34*(1), 64–69.

Stress in Arthritis

5

Dhwani J. Kothari, Mary C. Davis,
and Kirti Thummala

Arthritic conditions are characterized by chronic pain that contributes to functional impairments in physical, and often mental, health. In fact, arthritis is the most common cause of disability in the United States, affecting over 52 million adults; the number of individuals affected is expected to reach 67 million by the year 2030 (Centers for Disease Control and Prevention, 2013). Adjustment to arthritis and its sequelae varies considerably among individuals, however, fueling efforts to identify factors that can be modified to promote better adaptation. Such factors can then be integrated into interventions aimed at enhancing functional health and quality of life among patients. These efforts are especially important from a public health perspective, given the increasing prevalence of arthritis conditions.

The chronic pain that characterizes arthritis is influenced by a dynamic interplay of biological, psychological, and social factors that may be amenable to interventions. An enormous body of research has focused on the central role of stress as a key influence on adjustment to arthritis, although the relations among stress, pain, and disability are not straightforward. Rather, the deleterious impact of stress varies across individuals and within individuals depending on context. The diathesis-stress model provides one framework that is useful for understanding these complex associations. According to this approach, a predisposing vulnerability (e.g., diathesis) and a precipitating environmental agent (e.g., stress) interact to exacerbate disease or disability via physiological as well as psychosocial mechanisms.

The current chapter examines the mechanisms that underlie the relation between stress and adjustment in arthritis. In particular, the biopsychosocial effects of stress are reviewed for three debilitating arthritic pain conditions: osteoarthritis (OA), rheumatoid arthritis (RA), and systemic lupus erythematosus (SLE). First, an overview of each condition is provided, describing its specific symptoms, prevalence, and risk factors. Next, the diathesis-stress process that links stress with health is discussed, including emotional, cognitive, and behavioral factors that moderate the relations between stress and outcomes in OA, RA, and SLE. Third, empirically supported treatments and promising treatments that target stress management in arthritis are reviewed. Finally, future directions for research and practice are briefly highlighted.

D.J. Kothari, MA (✉) • M.C. Davis, PhD
K. Thummala, MA
Department of Psychology, Arizona State University, PO Box 871104, Tempe, AZ, 85287-1104, USA
e-mail: Dhwani.Kothari@asu.edu; Mary.Davis@asu.edu; Kirti.Thummala@asu.edu

P.M. Nicassio (ed.), *Psychosocial Factors in Arthritis*, DOI 10.1007/978-3-319-22858-7_5

Overview of Arthritic Conditions

Osteoarthritis (OA)

OA is a joint disease that involves the degradation of joints, leading to cartilage destruction, bone erosions and regrowth, inflammation of the synovial tissue surrounding the affected joint, and other metabolic effects (Hinton, Moody, Davis, & Thomas, 2002). As cartilage begins to deteriorate, bone-on-bone contact restricts movement and triggers pain in the affected joint area. The effects of OA are limited to one or more impaired joints, with knees, hips, hands, and spine being the most frequently affected joints and wrists, shoulders, and elbows being the least frequently affected joints (Lawrence et al., 2008). Depression is a frequent comorbid condition, with approximately 19 % of OA patients in a primary care setting reporting moderately severe levels of depression (Rosemann et al., 2007), a rate that is substantially higher than the rate of approximately 9 % in unselected primary care patients of similar age (Backenstrass et al., 2006).

OA is the most prevalent arthritic condition, affecting an estimated 27 million adults in the United States (Lawrence et al., 2008). The risk of developing OA significantly increases with age, especially in those 65 years and older (Felson et al., 2000). Among those with OA, older adults report greater physical disability whereas younger individuals experience greater psychological disability and pain (Weinberger, Tierney, Booher, & Hiner, 1990). Before the age of 50, the incidence of OA in most joints is greater in men than women; however, after the age of 50, women show a greater incidence of OA in the knees, feet, and hands than men (as cited in Felson et al., 2000). Additional risk factors of OA include obesity, joint injury, muscle weakness, genetic predisposition, and the presence of additional arthritic conditions.

Rheumatoid Arthritis (RA)

RA is a systemic autoimmune disease characterized by attacks on the synovial tissue lining the joints by the body's own immune cells. As a result, the affected joint area becomes inflamed, causing tenderness, pain, stiffness, and fatigue (Harris, 1993). The most commonly affected joints are the proximal interphalangeal, metacarpophalangeal, and the wrists. More severe forms of RA involve widespread joint inflammation. RA is also associated with increased risk of psychopathology; more than 40 % of RA patients experience clinical levels of depression, anxiety, or both (Bruce, 2008; Covic et al., 2012).

The estimated prevalence of RA in the United States is 1.6 million individuals, which includes both juvenile and adult diagnoses (Helmick et al., 2008). Of note, juvenile forms of arthritis apply to individuals who are under the age of 16. Similar to OA, RA becomes more prevalent with increasing age. Individuals who develop RA at a younger age (e.g., 60 or younger) experience more severe disease activity (Harris, 1993) and greater psychological disability (e.g., depression; Wright et al., 1998), relative to those who have a later onset. Further, the risk of developing RA increases 2–4 times if first-degree relatives have been diagnosed (Silman & Pearson, 2002). In fact, studies demonstrate that two-thirds of RA risk may be heritable (Oliver & Silman, 2006). Current research evidence suggests that genetic predisposition alone is not sufficient for producing RA, however, and points to interactions between genes and environment as determining factors in the condition's onset (e.g., Mahdi et al., 2009).

Systemic Lupus Erythematosus (SLE)

Like RA, SLE is an autoimmune disease. However, in SLE, the body's immune system may target not only the joints but also the skin, blood vessels, and organs. Symptoms of pain and fatigue vary from person to person and over time, but a prominent feature of SLE is the development of nonerosive arthritis, with wrists, hands, fingers, and knees being the most frequently affected joints (Hochberg, 1997). The cause of SLE is unknown and its symptoms can range from mild to extreme, depending on the tissues that are attacked by the body's immune system. For instance, affected individuals may develop skin rashes, cardiovascular conditions (e.g., stroke), gastrointestinal or renal diseases, or neuropsychiatric conditions (Smith & Gordon, 2010). Significant levels of psychological distress are also common among individuals with SLE, with up to 40 % qualifying for a psychological diagnosis (Segui et al., 2000). In fact, the rate of psychiatric disorders is higher in SLE than in other autoimmune conditions, including RA (Sundquist, Li, Hemminki, & Sundquist, 2008). Moreover, levels of distress have been associated with disease activity in SLE (Dobkin et al., 1998). Over time, however, both physical and psychological functioning among patients with SLE can improve (Dobkin et al., 2001).

The prevalence of SLE is lower than that of OA and RA, affecting an estimated 161,000–322,000 adults in the United States (Helmick et al., 2008). Although women are more often diagnosed with SLE than are men, men experience higher rates of morbidity than women. For example, men with SLE more frequently manifest hypertension and renal dysfunction than do women. The risk for developing SLE also varies by ethnicity; African-Americans and African-Caribbeans demonstrate an increased incidence of SLE compared to Caucasians (Hopkinson, Doherty, & Powell, 1994), a pattern that has been attributed to genetic as well as socioeconomic differences (e.g., Hopkinson, Jenkinson, Muir, Doherty, & Powell, 2000). Although the average age at onset for SLE is in the early 30s, it often develops earlier in African-Americans than in Caucasians (Petri, 2002).

Stress and Adaptation in Arthritis

Within the framework of the diathesis-stress model, stressors in life are seen as circumstances that are challenging to all individuals, but harmful only to individuals who have diatheses or vulnerabilities (Banks & Kerns, 1996). Although stress has been defined in a variety of ways, for the purposes of this chapter, it is defined in terms of responses to a provocation; that is, stress is reflected in the physiological, emotional, cognitive, and/or behavioral responses to a situation that is appraised as threatening or beyond one's ability to manage (Lazarus & Folkman, 1984). It is worth noting that for arthritis patients, the stressful situation is often the fluctuating, intense, or unpredictable pain and other symptoms that characterize their condition. One crucial dimension of stressful events is their magnitude (Miller & Smith, 1997). Minor events are those short-lasting circumstances that occur routinely in everyday life (e.g., work deadlines, conflict, hassles, minor pain flare), whereas major life events are circumstances that initiate significant disruptions in life (e.g., divorce, bereavement). How individuals appraise challenging circumstances is fundamental to determining the degree of perceived stress they experience, which sets in motion the cascade of responses they employ to cope with this perceived stress. In this section, we discuss the somatic, physiological, psychological, and social aspects of the stress response in OA, RA, and SLE.

Somatic Responses

A substantial body of work links the experience of minor life stresses with worsening of physical and psychological symptoms in arthritis patients. Among individuals with OA, for example, increases in daily life stressors are linked with greater pain, fatigue, and disability (Parrish, Zautra, & Davis, 2008; Weinberger et al., 1990). Psychological stress also contributes to disease activity and poorer outcomes in RA patients over time. In a comprehensive review of 27 independent studies involving over 3,000 patients, the stress of minor life events lasting hours to days was associated with increased disease activity among adult RA patients (Herrmann, Schölmerich, & Straub, 2000). For instance, minor daily stressors experienced by RA patients on one day were linked to their disease activity several days later (Zautra et al., 1997; Zautra et al., 1998). Moreover, elevations in daily stress have been related to increased next-day fatigue (Parrish et al., 2008) and to more bony erosions and a poorer outcome 5 years later in RA (Feigenbaum, Masi, & Kaplan, 1979). A similar pattern is evident among individuals with SLE (Adams, Dammers, Saia, Brantley, & Gaydos, 1994; Affleck, Tennen, Urrows, & Higgins, 1994; Pawlak et al., 2003). For example, among SLE patients who were followed daily over a 6-month period, experiencing worsened stress on one day was associated with worsened same-day and next-day clinical symptoms (Peralta-Ramírez, Jiménez-Alonso, Godoy-García, & Pérez-García, 2004). Although research comparing patient groups is fairly limited, some evidence suggests that SLE patients may be more vulnerable than are RA patients to the effects of everyday stress, with stronger links between daily stress and physical and psychological status in SLE versus RA patients (Wekking, Vingerhoets, van Dam, Nossent, & Swaak, 1991). RA patients, in turn, may be more vulnerable than OA patients; RA patients show more substantial increases in disease activity as well as depression and poor coping than do OA patients associated with elevations in daily stress (Zautra, Burleson, Matt, Roth, & Burrows, 1994).

Although the experience of minor life stress appears to heighten disease activity and disability, the evidence linking major life stress to health in arthritis patients is mixed. Some evidence suggests that exposure to major life stressors may dampen disease activity and symptoms. For example, a case study of a female RA patient followed weekly over 12 weeks revealed that her disease went into temporary remission during a week when she reported two unexpected family deaths (Potter & Zautra, 1997). In contrast, her minor stressors were related to symptom increases. These findings are consistent with data linking bereavement with immunosuppression in healthy individuals (Schleifer, Keller, Camerino, Thornton, & Stein, 1983). However, other data regarding major life stress and disease activity suggest that recent exposure to major events has no relation to current disease activity in RA or SLE (Chou & Hwang, 2002; Haller, Holzner, Mur, & Günther, 1997; Wallace & Metzger, 1994), and there is no evidence to suggest worsening in functional health over the long term (Da Costa et al., 1999).

Physiological Responses

The link between stress and health outcomes among arthritis patients may be due at least in part to stress-induced physiological responses. Experiencing stress sets in motion physiological changes, particularly in the nervous and endocrine systems that have evolved to promote survival and restore homeostasis. Two axes of the physiological stress response have been extensively studied: the sympathetic-adrenal medullary (SAM) axis, and the hypothalamic-pituitary-adrenocortical (HPA) axis.

The SAM axis is responsible for instigating the "fight or flight" response via activation of the sympathetic nerves that directly innervate not only the heart, blood vessels, immune organs, and other tissues, but also the adrenal medulla. When stress stimulates the SAM axis, the ensuing effects are immediate. Heart rate and blood pressure increase, and the adrenal medulla releases epinephrine and norepinephrine into the blood stream (Cannon, 1932), thereby propagating physiological arousal. Beyond producing cardiovascular arousal, acute activation of the SAM axis can influence the immune system via the anti-inflammatory effects of norepinephrine that is released not only into the bloodstream but also at sympathetic nerve terminals in the joints and other tissues (Elenkov, Wilder, Chrousos, & Vizi, 2000).

Whereas the SAM axis has both nervous system and endocrine components, the HPA axis is mainly an endocrine system, in which hormones released from glands travel through the bloodstream to target organs. Stimulation of the HPA axis begins when stress initiates the release of corticotropin-releasing hormone (CRH) from the hypothalamus, a gland within the central nervous system. CRH then travels to the anterior pituitary where it stimulates the release of adrenal corticotrophic hormone (ACTH), which in turn, travels to the adrenal cortex where it triggers release of cortisol. Because it involves a cascade of hormones, the HPA axis is slower acting than the SAM axis; elevations in circulating levels of cortisol are evident approximately 20–30 min after the onset of stress. In healthy individuals, cortisol acts to dampen inflammation. Thus, by enhancing cortisol secretion, stress can serve an anti-inflammatory purpose and act to reestablish homeostasis. However, the impact of stress on cortisol varies depending on the nature of the stress experience. Short-term acute stressors that are characterized by uncontrollable social threat and long-term stressors that involve major life events are the types of stressors that most consistently elicit increases in cortisol (Dickerson & Kemeny, 2004).

The SAM and HPA axes respond in a coordinated fashion to influence immune functioning; thus, dysregulation in one or both systems can have profound implications for chronic inflammatory conditions like RA and SLE. Indeed, existing evidence points to dysregulation of these stress response axes in RA and perhaps SLE. Data gleaned from RA and SLE patients suggests that sympathetic tone is elevated in both conditions (Glück et al., 2000; Härle et al., 2006). Although increased SAM activity in healthy individuals is associated with anti-inflammatory effects, it may be ineffective in dampening inflammation or even fuel inflammation in patients with RA. For example, increased sympathetic activation fuels a pro-inflammatory immune profile in animal models of inflammatory arthritis, whereas blocking SAM activation attenuates inflammation and symptoms in RA patients (Bellinger et al., 2008). The absence of the usual anti-inflammatory effects of the SAM system in patients with autoimmune pain disorders may be at least in part because their immune cell receptors are relatively insensitive to SAM stimulation (Bellinger et al., 2008), and/or they experience a dramatic loss of sympathetic nerve fibers in inflamed tissue (Straub & Kalden, 2009).

Not only do RA and SLE patients show diminished benefits from SAM activation, but also they show decreased responsiveness of the HPA axis to provocation (Geenen, Van Middendorp, & Bijlsma, 2006; Härle et al., 2006; Straub, Dhabhar, Bijlsma, & Cutolo, 2005). In the face of short-term stressors, for example, individuals with RA fail to mount a significant HPA axis response, yielding an inadequate level of circulating cortisol in relation to the level of systemic inflammation (Capellino & Straub, 2008; Dekkers et al., 2001). Moreover, receptors on the surface of immune cells in RA patients show a diminished responsiveness to the anti-inflammatory effects of cortisol (Miller, Jüsten, Schölmerich, & Straub, 2000; Pawlak et al., 1999; Straub et al., 2005), particularly under conditions of minor daily stress (Davis et al., 2008). Taken together, the disturbances of the SAM and HPA axes in these pain conditions appear to create a pro-inflammatory physiological state that facilitates stress-induced aggravation of disease activity (Straub et al., 2005).

Physiological stress response systems are crucial components of the diathesis-stress model; individuals with a preexisting vulnerability at any point in the stress process may be unable to appropriately terminate a stress response and restore homeostasis. Although physiological and psychological responses to stress are determined to a significant extent by the magnitude and duration of stress, the extent of those responses hinges on the effectiveness of efforts to address the demands of the stressors. Thus, being able to manage emotional, cognitive, and behavioral responses to stress are key to sustaining psychological and functional health in patients with arthritis (e.g., Penninx et al., 1997).

Psychosocial Factors That Impact Adjustment to Stress

Emotional Responses

The influence of stressors on somatic and physiological responses, and ultimately quality of life in arthritic conditions may depend on the ability to effectively manage emotional stress responses. The dynamic model of affect (DMA) offers a lens through which to view emotional responses to stress in chronic pain (Davis, Zautra, & Smith, 2004), positing that the complexity of emotional processing depends on the stressfulness of the context. According to the DMA, circumstances characterized by low stress allow complex processing of emotional and other information.

During times of relative calm, negative and positive affect are experienced on separate dimensions and are relatively independent, and appropriate cognitive resources can be allocated to judge both positive and negative aspects of the environment and subsequently develop an adaptive response. In the face of stress, including the stress of pain, individuals experience more rudimentary emotional processing that is characterized by elevated negative affect and dampened positive affect (Zautra, Reich, Davis, Potter, & Nicolson, 2000). Thus, negative and positive affects are experienced as "black or white," on a single dimension without complexity or subtlety. Likewise, attention narrows and information processing becomes quick, simple, and readily focused on the negative and demanding aspects of the environment. Such focused affective and cognitive processing is reflexive and is an appropriate response to situations that pose an imminent threat and require an immediate response. In that context, narrowed processing results in a limited ability to fully evaluate and employ the most adaptive response available (Hart, Wade, & Martelli, 2003).

The DMA framework is especially relevant for understanding emotional regulation among pain populations with arthritis. The chronic stress engendered by pain is capable of producing both simplified cognitive processing (Reich, Zautra, & Potter, 2001) and affective dysregulation that is characterized by a heightened level of negative affect and a diminished ability to sustain positive affect (e.g., depression; Romano & Turner, 1985). This affective disturbance is associated with poorer adaptation, reflected in greater pain and fatigue and reports of more frequent stressful experiences among patients (Sale, Gignac, & Hawker, 2008). Perhaps the most significant consequence of the emotion dysregulation experienced by many pain patients is the decline in positive affect, because it impairs the ability to recover from stress (Davis, Thummala, & Zautra, 2014). Numerous studies have documented the benefits of positive affect for limiting the negative impact of stressors and preserving functional health (Finan & Garland, 2015). For example, among women with OA or RA, those who were able to sustain their positive affect during weeks of high stress due to conflict and pain were protected from stress-related elevations in negative affect (Strand et al., 2006; Zautra, Johnson, & Davis, 2005). Boosts in positive affect may also help patients speed their recovery. For example, among depressed OA patients who discussed a stressful interpersonal event, those who subsequently viewed a video to boost positive mood showed decreases in pain relative to those who watched a neutral video (Davis et al., 2014).

It is worth noting that very little work examining affective regulation in response to pain and stress has been conducted in patients with SLE. As noted above, stress is an even more prominent component of daily life in individuals with SLE relative to those with RA (Wekking et al., 1991). In fact, SLE patients primarily perceive their physical health in terms of daily stressors (Dobkin et al., 1998). As a result, individuals with SLE experience higher levels of depressive symptoms and greater psychological distress overall than do individuals with RA (Kozora, Ellison, Waxmonsky, Wamboldt, & Patterson, 2005), which is especially prevalent among SLE patients with more active disease states who experience greater pain, helplessness, and physical disability (Seawell & Danoff-Burg, 2004). Thus, due to ongoing daily stressors, pain, and other disabling aspects of SLE, affective disturbances tend to become ingrained as part of the illness experience. The extent to which positive affect can offset the deleterious effects of stress among SLE remains to be determined, although there is no reason to expect that the pattern of findings evident for OA and RA patients will not hold for SLE patients as well.

One means for overcoming the emotional simplification associated with stress is maintaining or boosting positive mood, which acts as a source of resilience (i.e., Strand et al., 2006; Zautra et al., 2005). A second, less developed line of work points to another potential avenue to promote adaptive emotional regulation during stressful events: the development of mood clarity (Salovey & Mayer, 1989). Mood clarity refers to the ability to be able to distinguish between different emotions, an individual difference that should be relevant to sustaining affective differentiation during times of stress. In healthy subjects, higher levels of mood clarity are related to lower levels of depression, social anxiety, and cortisol secretion during stressful days (Salovey, Stroud, Woolery, & Epel, 2002), and among older adults to an attenuated relation between pain and subsequent depression (Kennedy et al., 2010). In pain patients, higher levels of mood clarity are linked with more distinct experiences of negative and positive affect, reflecting greater affective differentiation (Study 1; Zautra, Smith, Affleck, & Tennen, 2001). Thus, the accruing evidence points to the adaptive value of sustaining affective differentiation in general, and positive affect during times of stress in particular, for individuals managing chronic pain.

Cognitive Responses

According to the Lazarus and Folkman (1984) model of stress and coping, cognitive-affective appraisals, or people's evaluation of their pain, its meaning and significance, and the resources they have available to cope with it are all important determinants of adaptation to the stress of chronic pain. Pain-related beliefs and appraisals have often been found to be more important determinants of outcomes in arthritic conditions. One such cognitive appraisal, pain self-efficacy, characterized by positive expectancies about one's ability to successfully cope with pain, has been proven to be one of the most potent predictors of improved outcomes and successful adaptation in arthritis patients (for a review, see Marks, Allegrante, & Lorig, 2005). On the other hand, excessive negative expectancies of future pain experiences, termed pain catastrophizing, have been proven to be an equally consistent and powerful predictor of poor adaptation among individuals with chronic pain (for a review, see Sullivan et al., 2001).

Self-efficacy has been established as an important construct that is predictive of positive emotional, physical, and functional outcomes for pain patients. Arthritis self-efficacy, in particular, is defined as an individual's belief in his or her ability to successfully manage arthritic pain and other stressors generated by arthritis (Bandura, 1997). Studies in arthritis patients have shown that individuals vary in their self-efficacy for managing pain, with some feeling confident in their ability to cope with pain and its related stress, and others feeling less able to effectively manage the condition (Lorig, Chastain, Ung, Shoor, & Holman, 1989). Within OA patients, pain self-efficacy has been shown to account for a significant proportion of variance in physical health outcomes, with patients with higher self-efficacy reporting lower pain (Pells et al., 2008). Further, an inverse relationship between emotional distress and self-efficacy has often been demonstrated in RA patients; higher self-efficacy expectations consistently predict lower levels of stress, anxiety, and depression (Arnstein, Caudill, Mandle, Norris, & Beasley, 1999; Lowe et al., 2008; O'Leary, Shoor, Lorig, & Holman, 1988). Although the role of self-efficacy has not been extensively studied in SLE patients, many studies with chronic pain populations have demonstrated that individuals with greater self-efficacy experience less interference from pain in their daily physical functioning (Arnstein, 2000; da Cunha Menezes Costa, Maher, McAuley, Hancock, & Smeets, 2011).

Because pain self-efficacy is consistently linked to most of the markers of better adaptation to stress, several researchers have suggested inclusion of pain self-efficacy as a target in interventions for arthritis patients (American College of Rheumatology Subcommittee on Rheumatoid Arthritis, 2002; Marks et al., 2005; McKnight, Afram, Kashdan, Kasle, & Zautra, 2010). In fact, treatment-outcome studies in OA, RA, and SLE patients have shown that an increase in self-efficacy is not only related to improvements in psychological and functional variables such as reduced helplessness, anxiety, depression, and fatigue, and pain perception, but that it is also important to long-term maintenance of treatment gains (Chui, Lau, & Yau, 2004; Lorig, Mazonson, & Holman, 1993; Karlson et al., 2004; Keefe, Caldwell, et al., 1996; Keefe, Kashikar-Zuck, et al., 1996; for reviews, see Marks, 2001 and Seawell & Danoff-Burg, 2004).

While appraisals such as a self-efficacy are considered positive strengths, maladaptive cognitive responses such as catastrophizing are also powerful predictors of adaptation to stress and other outcomes for arthritis patients. Pain-related catastrophizing is the tendency to magnify the perception of pain or make exaggerated predictions about its damaging consequences (Rosenstiel & Keefe, 1983; Sullivan, Bishop, & Pivik, 1995). A propensity to catastrophize about pain has been associated with several negative outcomes, including higher levels of negative affect, increased risk of depression, and greater anxiety and overall emotional distress (Keefe et al., 1991; Moldovan, Onac, Vantu, Szentagotai, & Onac, 2009). In fact, within OA patients, pain catastrophizing has been shown to account for a significant proportion of variance in pain, both psychological and physical disability, and gait speed (Somers et al., 2009). Functional disability has also been consistently predicted by pain catastrophizing in RA patients (e.g., Keefe, Brown, Wallston, & Caldwell, 1989; Parker et al., 1989). This association between pain catastrophizing and increased disability may be due in part to high pain catastrophizers focusing more attention and coping efforts on potential or actual pain signals. A similar link between pain catastrophizing and functional outcomes likely exists in SLE patients, although this relation has not been examined to date.

Results of treatment studies demonstrate the importance of catastrophizing and self-efficacy appraisals in mediating and sustaining improvements in pain outcomes, but in the opposite directions. Pain catastrophizing is associated with increased disability and poor adaptation, whereas pain self-efficacy predicts a more resilient response. Thus, while both constructs are beliefs about one's ability to cope with chronic pain, they tend to be inversely related (Asghari & Nicholas, 2001; Keefe et al., 1997; McKnight et al., 2010). Pain catastrophizing, in fact, may interfere with the development of self-efficacy because individuals dwell on their pain or the threat of pain, and interpret it as being out of their control. This sense of helplessness about one's ability to deal with pain leads to further maladaptive cognitive processes, such as a hypervigilance to pain or the anticipation of pain onset. When attention is narrowed to this threat, opportunities for adaptive self-regulation become limited because switching to other adaptive behaviors or cognitions requires significant cognitive resources. However, some findings that suggest that well-timed, pain-relevant social support may provide a means of interrupting the cycle linking catastrophizing with poor functioning. In a daily diary study of individuals with RA, higher satisfaction with spousal pain-related support was protective against the detrimental effects of pain catastrophizing on subsequent increases in negative affect and pain (Holtzman & DeLongis, 2007).

More recently, the capacity to accept pain and other stressors has come to the fore as a potentially important cognitive coping response linked to better functional health among those in pain. Acceptance of pain is defined as the capacity to respond to pain without attempting to control or avoid it, and to remain willing to stay engaged in life despite pain (McCracken, 1998). The body of evidence, which to date is based primarily on general samples of chronic pain patients, points to the benefits of pain acceptance in promoting positive adaptation to pain and other stressors (McCracken & Zhao-O'Brien, 2010). Pain acceptance shows cross-sectional associations with reports of lower pain intensity, pain-related distress and avoidance, depression, and disability (McCracken & Eccleston, 2006), and explains more variance in outcomes than more traditional coping strategies (McCracken & Eccleston, 2006). It is also linked with the capacity to limit increases in negative affect associated with acute pain flares in daily life (Kratz, Davis, & Zautra, 2007) and has been prospectively linked to decreased future pain and better functional health (McCracken & Eccleston, 2005). Some evidence suggests that the benefits of pain acceptance may be mediated via lessened attention to pain, greater engagement in daily activities, and higher efficacy to perform day-to-day activities (Viane, Crombez, Eccleston, Devulder, & De Corte, 2004).

Behavioral Responses

Behavioral responses to pain and other stressors are influenced by two independent motivational systems: the avoidance system and the approach system (e.g., Davidson, 1992; Elliot & Thrash, 2002; Gray, 1994). Specifically, the avoidance system of motivation is activated by self-protective biases, aimed at escaping from an undesired state that is perceived to be threatening. In contrast, the approach system of motivation promotes behaviors and associated cognitions and emotions that are aimed at achieving a desired end state. Together, the motivational systems function to promote self-regulation and adaptation to positive and negative circumstances.

The fear-avoidance model of pain (Vlaeyen & Linton, 2000) posits that although avoidance may be adaptive in the acute pain stage by preventing further injury, for chronic pain sufferers, fear of pain and associated stressors may lead to consistent avoidance of important daily activities. Thus, the heightened attention to pain, difficulty disengaging from the threat of pain, and worry may fuel avoidance behaviors that have a deleterious effect on physical and emotional functioning over the long term. In addition to employing strategies to escape or avoid pain, pain patients may adopt another maladaptive pain management approach: withdrawal from engagement in valued activities. When preoccupied with the fear of pain, chronic pain sufferers refrain from initiating desirable activities or persisting in meeting meaningful goals. They may also withdraw socially from friends and family, thereby cutting off beneficial social support.

Among chronic pain patients, the motivational influences of behaviors often become geared primarily toward preventing or alleviating the ongoing stress of pain. Many pain patients become fearful of pain or (re)injury, which triggers conditioned responses to escape pain. Not only is this avoidance related to functional disability and affective disturbances (Leeuw et al., 2007; Vlaeyen & Linton, 2000), but also a hypervigilance to pain (Crombez, Van Damme, & Eccleston, 2005). As a result of attempting to avoid pain, patients experience less enjoyment in life and have fewer distractions from their pain (as cited in Keefe, Caldwell et al., 1996; Keefe, Kashikar-Zuck et al., 1996).

Perhaps the most oft-cited behavior pain patients avoid to prevent exacerbation of pain is exercise and related physical activity (e.g., Holla et al., 2015). Paradoxically, numerous research studies have documented the benefits of such activity for the management of arthritis and other pain conditions. For instance, in both OA and RA patients, exercise interventions have been shown to improve physical fitness and increase the perceived ability to perform activities of daily living (Suomi & Collier, 2003). Further, in RA patients, physical activity provides greater meaningfulness in life (Loeppenthin et al., 2014). Similar benefits of exercise have also been documented in SLE patients (for a review, see Ayán & Martín, 2007). Although SLE patients are less likely to engage in physical activity when stressed (Mancuso, Perna, Sargent, & Salmon, 2010), research findings suggest that physical activity can have a positive influence on disease activity (i.e., through a reduced risk of developing atherosclerosis; Volkmann et al., 2010).

Avoidance-oriented behaviors are also related to poor sleep quality. Most pain patients, including those with OA, RA, and SLE, experience impairments in sleep (e.g., Chandrasekhara, Jayachandran, Rajasekhar, Thomas, & Narsimulu, 2009; Sariyildiz et al., 2014; Taylor-Gjevre, Gjevre, Nair, Skomro, & Lim, 2011). Of importance, sleep disturbance significantly exacerbates pain in a range of chronic pain conditions (for a review, see Finan, Goodin, & Smith, 2013). In fact, improving sleep in OA and RA patients, for instance, has been shown to decrease pain (Vitiello, Rybarczyk, Von Korff, & Stepanski, 2009). This evidence may suggest that sleep impairment contributes to avoidance of activities in arthritis patients through heightened levels of pain. After being exposed to additional stress, the harmful relations among poor sleep, pain, and avoidance of activities may become further exacerbated.

While avoidance-oriented coping strategies decrease engagement in activities, approach-oriented strategies improve activity engagement. Patients who engage in approach-oriented behaviors despite experiencing pain accrue a host of positive outcomes, including an increased tolerance of pain (e.g., Zelman, Howland, Nichols, & Cleeland, 1991) and overall better functioning (McCracken & Eccleston, 2005). A key factor that motivates this engagement in activities is positive social support. In fact, McCracken (2005) demonstrated an association between the quality of social support and chronic pain patients' engagement in activities. Specifically, patients who received less negative responses from their significant others were more likely to engage in activities and accept pain. Further, receiving or perceiving positive social support has been associated with better health outcomes in OA, RA, and SLE patients (e.g., Jump et al., 2005; Radojevic, Nicassio, & Weisman, 1993; Sherman, 2003). Researchers have increasingly argued that sustaining engagement in desirable activities and pursuit of meaningful goals is at least as important as minimizing avoidance behaviors in determining resilient outcomes (Culos-Reed & Brawley, 2003; Fish, Hogan, Morrison, Stewart, & McGuire, 2013; Kranz, Bollinger, & Nilges, 2010; Sturgeon & Zautra, 2013).

Psychosocial Treatments for Arthritis

The impact of OA, RA, and SLE on individuals' health and quality of life very much depends on their capacity to manage life's inevitable stressors, including the stress of chronic pain. Not surprisingly, psychosocial interventions have been developed to bolster that capacity in order to alleviate physical and psychological symptoms and promote well-being. In fact, empirical evidence highlights the utility of psychosocial approaches to treatment. A recent meta-analysis of 27 randomized clinical trials showed that psychosocial interventions significantly impact pain intensity, and psychological and physical functioning in arthritis patients (Dixon, Keefe, Scipio, Perri, & Abernethy, 2007). In particular, cognitive-behavioral therapy (CBT) has emerged as one of the most common forms of psychosocial treatment. From a CBT perspective, it is an individual's belief regarding physical symptoms and physical limitations, and the coping responses that stem from those beliefs that promote better or worse adaptation to the chronic pain condition. To address faulty cognitions and maladaptive coping, CBT typically employs multiple components, including biofeedback, relaxation exercises, education, mastery, modeling, and cognitive reappraisal, with the goal of improving targeted aspects of health status such as pain tolerance, mobility, self-management, and self-efficacy. In fact, CBT has emerged as the "gold standard" treatment for chronic pain and yields improvements in pain, depression, disease activity, and health care utilization in individuals with arthritis (for a review, see Nicassio & Greenberg, 2001). Of note, the utility of CBT has been thoroughly tested in OA and RA patients, but fewer data are available regarding its efficacy in SLE patients. Nevertheless, the limited evidence suggests that CBT is likely to improve physical and psychological functioning among those with SLE (e.g., Greco, Rudy, & Manzi, 2004; Navarrete-Navarrete et al., 2010).

Rather than focusing primarily on altering pain- and stress-related coping through CBT, an alternative approach focuses solely on increasing physical activity to treat the symptoms and disability that accompany OA, RA, and SLE. Empirical evidence points to significant health benefits of exercise programs across chronic pain conditions. Overall, exercise produces moderate improvements in pain and disability among those with OA (for a review, see Roddy, Zhang, & Doherty, 2005). For example, individuals with knee OA who were randomly assigned to either aerobic exercise or strength training showed more improvement in physical function and perceived health status than did those in an education condition; the effects of the interventions were mediated in part by improvements in pain and self-efficacy (Rejesky, Martin, Ettinger, & Morgan, 1998). Available evidence also suggests that aerobic and strength training exercise helps to improve symptoms and functional health in patients with RA (Metsios et al., 2008) and SLE (for a review, see Ayán & Martín, 2007). Thus, the armamentarium of treatment options for musculoskeletal conditions now routinely includes exercise as a key component of care (Westby, 2001).

Despite the effectiveness of available psychosocial and behavioral treatments, many patients continue to experience significant physical and emotional symptoms associated with their pain condition. More recently, a growing body of work has pointed to the potential value of approaches that focus on acceptance of pain and other aversive experiences to enhance the capacity of pain patients to manage the physical, emotional, and social demands of their illness (Kabat-Zinn, Lipworth, & Burney, 1985). Rather than encouraging control of pain and dysfunctional thoughts, which ironically may serve to intensify those experiences (Wegner, 1997), an approach grounded in acceptance targets enhanced awareness and acceptance of current aversive experiences (Ma & Teasdale, 2004). The acceptance of all current experiences allows for awareness of, and attention, to the positive features that may also be present in the moment. Some treatments go further and explicitly include an emphasis on meaningful values and/or engagement in rewarding activity to bolster social connectedness and positive affect (Hayes, Luoma, Bond, Masuda, & Lillis, 2006; Zautra et al., 2008). The available evidence shows that an acceptance-based approach leads to improvements in functional health among OA patients (Morone, Greco, & Weiner, 2008), and for RA patients who are especially vulnerable to emotion dysregulation and disability (e.g., McCracken, Vowles, & Eccleston, 2005; Vowles & McCracken, 2008). For example, in RA patients with a history of recurrent depression, mindful-acceptance treatment yielded greater improvements in pain, fatigue, positive and negative affect, and inflammation at posttreatment and 6-month follow-up compared to CBT and an education control (Zautra et al., 2008). Thus, the capacity to attend to both positive and negative experiences in an intentional way and to build greater social connectedness may be valuable in promoting better functional health in at least some subgroups of arthritis patients.

Future Directions

Despite continuing advances in medical approaches to the treatment of OA, RA, and SLE, stress continues to play an important role in the functional health and well-being among individuals coping with these conditions. Far fewer data are available regarding the role of psychosocial factors in SLE, but the evidence that has accrued suggests that prevailing models apply to that condition as well. Our efforts to understand and ameliorate the negative effects of stress on adaptation to arthritis have yielded significant benefits to patients. Going forward, a systematic focus on effectively tapping into broader social resources, including spouses, families, and communities may be fruitful. For example, capitalizing on existing social systems (i.e., family, peers, and health care providers) to address barriers to build stress management skills and increase compliance with other treatment recommendations may prove beneficial (Keefe, Caldwell et al., 1996; Keefe, Kashikar-Zuck et al., 1996). The rapid rise of social media and technological advancements increase the feasibility of such an approach. A second advancement would be a more thorough integration of a resilience perspective into our models of adaptation and treatment of chronic pain. As we have noted here, positive affect, social support, and engagement in life can coexist with stress and pain, and are essential to living a full life despite pain. And that, after all, is the primary goal of our care.

References

Adams, S. G., Jr., Dammers, P. M., Saia, T. L., Brantley, P. J., & Gaydos, G. R. (1994). Stress, depression, and anxiety predict average symptom severity and daily symptom fluctuation in systemic lupus erythematosus. *Journal of Behavioral Medicine, 17*(5), 459–477.

Affleck, G., Tennen, H., Urrows, S., & Higgins, P. (1994). Person and contextual features of daily stress reactivity: Individual differences in relations of undesirable daily events with mood disturbance and chronic pain intensity. *Journal of Personality and Social Psychology, 66*(2), 329–340.

American College of Rheumatology Subcommittee on Rheumatoid Arthritis. (2002). Guidelines for the management of arthritis: 2002 update. *Arthritis and Rheumatism, 46*(2), 328–346.

Arnstein, P. (2000). The mediation of disability by self efficacy in different samples of chronic pain patients. *Disability and Rehabilitation, 22*(17), 794–801.

Arnstein, P., Caudill, M., Mandle, C. L., Norris, A., & Beasley, R. (1999). Self efficacy as a mediator of the relationship between pain intensity, disability and depression in chronic pain patients. *Pain, 80*(3), 483–491.

Asghari, A., & Nicholas, M. K. (2001). Pain self-efficacy beliefs and pain behavior. A prospective study. *Pain, 94*(1), 85–100.

Ayán, C., & Martín, V. (2007). Systemic lupus erythematosus and exercise. *Lupus, 16*(1), 5–9.

Backenstrass, M., Frank, A., Joest, K., Hingmann, S., Mundt, C., & Kronmüller, K. T. (2006). A comparative study of nonspecific depressive symptoms and minor depression regarding functional impairment and associated characteristics in primary care. *Comprehensive Psychiatry, 47*(1), 35–41.

Bandura, A. (1997). *Self-efficacy: The exercise of self-control*. Gordonsville, VA: WH Freeman.

Banks, S. M., & Kerns, R. D. (1996). Explaining high rates of depression in chronic pain: A diathesis-stress framework. *Psychological Bulletin, 119*(1), 95–110.

Bellinger, D. L., Millar, B. A., Perez, S., Carter, J., Wood, C., ThyagaRajan, S., … Lorton, D. (2008). Sympathetic modulation of immunity: Relevance to disease. *Cellular Immunology, 252*(1), 27–56.

Bruce, T. O. (2008). Comorbid depression in rheumatoid arthritis: Pathophysiology and clinical implications. *Current Psychiatry Reports, 10*(3), 258–264.

Cannon, W. B. (1932). *The wisdom of the body*. New York, NY: W. W. Norton.

Capellino, S., & Straub, R. H. (2008). Neuroendocrine immune pathways in chronic arthritis. *Best Practice & Research. Clinical Rheumatology, 22*(2), 285–297.

Centers for Disease Control and Prevention. (2013). Prevalence of doctor-diagnosed arthritis and arthritis-attributable activity limitation—United States, 2010-2012. *Morbidity and Mortality Weekly Report, 62*(44), 869–873.

Chandrasekhara, P. K. S., Jayachandran, N. V., Rajasekhar, L., Thomas, J., & Narsimulu, G. (2009). The prevalence and associations of sleep disturbances in patients with systemic lupus erythematosus. *Modern Rheumatology, 19*(4), 407–415.

Chou, C. T., & Hwang, C. M. (2002). Changes in the clinical and laboratory features of lupus patients after the big earthquake in Taiwan. *Lupus, 11*(2), 109–113.

Chui, D. Y. Y., Lau, J. S. K., & Yau, I. T. Y. (2004). An outcome evaluation study of the rheumatoid arthritis self-management programme in Hong Kong. *Psychology, Health & Medicine, 9*(3), 286–292.

Covic, T., Cumming, S. R., Pallant, J. F., Manolios, N., Emery, P., Conaghan, P. G., & Tennant, A. (2012). Depression and anxiety in patients with rheumatoid arthritis: Prevalence rates based on a comparison of the Depression, Anxiety and Stress Scale (DASS) and the Hospital, Anxiety and Depression Scale (HADS). *BMC Psychiatry, 12*, 1–6.

Crombez, G., Van Damme, S., & Eccleston, C. (2005). Hypervigilance to pain: An experimental and clinical analysis. *Pain, 116*(1–2), 4–7.

Culos-Reed, S. N., & Brawley, L. R. (2003). Self-efficacy predicts physical activity in individuals with fibromyalgia. *Journal of Applied Biobehavioral Research, 8*(1), 27–41.

Da Costa, D., Dobkin, P. L., Pinard, L., Fortin, P. R., Danoff, D. S., Esdaile, J. M., & Clarke, A. E. (1999). The role of stress in functional disability among women with systemic lupus erythematosus: A prospective study. *Arthritis Care & Research, 12*(2), 112–119.

da Cunha Menezes Costa, L., Maher, C. G., McAuley, J. H., Hancock, M., & Smeets, R. J. (2011). Self-efficacy is more important than fear of movement in mediating the relationship between pain and disability in chronic low back pain. *European Journal of Pain, 15*(2), 213–219.

Davidson, R. J. (1992). Emotion and affective style: Hemispheric substrates. *Psychological Science, 3*(1), 39–43.

Davis, M. C., Thummala, K., & Zautra, A. J. (2014). Stress-related clinical pain and mood in women with chronic pain: Moderating effects of depression and positive mood induction. *Annals of Behavioral Medicine, 48*(1), 61–70.

Davis, M. C., Zautra, A. J., & Smith, B. (2004). Chronic pain, stress, and the dynamics of affective differentiation. *Journal of Personality, 72*(6), 1133–1159.

Davis, M. C., Zautra, A. J., Younger, J., Motivala, S. J., Attrep, J., & Irwin, M. R. (2008). Chronic stress and regulation of cellular markers of inflammation in rheumatoid arthritis: Implications for fatigue. *Brain, Behavior, and Immunity, 22*, 24–32.

Dekkers, J. C., Geenen, R. I. N. I. E., Godaert, G. L., Glaudemans, K. A., Lafeber, F. P., van Doornen, L. J., & Bijlsma, J. W. (2001). Experimentally challenged reactivity of the hypothalamic pituitary adrenal axis in patients with recently diagnosed rheumatoid arthritis. *The Journal of Rheumatology, 28*(7), 1496–1504.

Dickerson, S. S., & Kemeny, M. E. (2004). Acute stressors and cortisol responses: A theoretical integration and synthesis of laboratory research. *Psychological Bulletin, 130*(3), 355–391.

Dixon, K. E., Keefe, F. J., Scipio, C. D., Perri, L. M., & Abernethy, A. P. (2007). Psychological interventions for arthritis pain management in adults: A meta-analysis. *Health Psychology, 26*(3), 241–250.

Dobkin, P. L., Da Costa, D., Fortin, P. R., Edworthy, S., Barr, S., Esdaile, J. M., … Clarke, A. E. (2001). Living with lupus: A prospective pan-Canadian study. *The Journal of Rheumatology, 28*(11), 2442–2448.

Dobkin, P. L., Fortin, P. R., Joseph, L., Esdaile, J. M., Danoff, D. S., & Clarke, A. E. (1998). Psychosocial contributors to mental and physical health in patients with systemic lupus erythematosus. *Arthritis and Rheumatism, 11*(1), 23–31.

Elenkov, I. J., Wilder, R. L., Chrousos, G. P., & Vizi, E. S. (2000). The sympathetic nerve—An integrative interface between two supersystems: The brain and the immune system. *Pharmacological Reviews, 52*(4), 595–638.

Elliot, A. J., & Thrash, T. M. (2002). Approach-avoidance motivation in personality: Approach and avoidance temperaments and goals. *Journal of Personality and Social Psychology, 82*, 804–818.

Feigenbaum, S. L., Masi, A. T., & Kaplan, S. B. (1979). Prognosis in rheumatoid arthritis: A longitudinal study of newly diagnosed younger adult patients. *The American Journal of Medicine, 66*(3), 377–384.

Felson, D. T., Lawrence, R. C., Dieppe, P. A., Hirsch, R., Helmick, C. G., Jordan, J. M., … Fries, J. F. (2000). Osteoarthritis: New insights. Part 1: The disease and its risk factors. *Annals of Internal Medicine, 133*(8), 635–646.

Finan, P. H., & Garland, E. L. (2015). The role of positive affect in pain and its treatment. *Clinical Journal of Pain, 31*, 177–187.

Finan, P. H., Goodin, B. R., & Smith, M. T. (2013). The association of sleep and pain: An update and a path forward. *The Journal of Pain, 14*(12), 1539–1552.

Fish, R. A., Hogan, M. J., Morrison, T. G., Stewart, I., & McGuire, B. E. (2013). Willing and able: A closer look at pain willingness and activity engagement on the Chronic Pain Acceptance Questionnaire (CPAQ-8). *The Journal of Pain, 14*(3), 233–245.

Geenen, R., Van Middendorp, H., & Bijlsma, J. W. (2006). The impact of stressors on health status and hypothalamic-pituitary-adrenal axis and autonomic nervous system responsiveness in rheumatoid arthritis. *Annals of the New York Academy of Sciences, 1069*(1), 77–97.

Glück, T., Oertel, M., Reber, T., Zietz, B., Schölmerich, J., & Straub, R. H. (2000). Altered function of the hypothalamic stress axes in patients with moderately active systemic lupus erythematosus. I. The hypothalamus-autonomic nervous system axis. *The Journal of Rheumatology, 27*(4), 903–910.

Gray, J. A. (1994). Three fundamental emotion systems. In P. Ekman & R. J. Davidson (Eds.), *The nature of emotion* (pp. 243–247). New York, NY: Oxford University Press.

Greco, C. M., Rudy, T. E., & Manzi, S. (2004). Effects of a stress-reduction program on psychological function, pain, and physical function of systemic lupus erythematosus patients: A randomized controlled trial. *Arthritis Care & Research, 51*(4), 625–634.

Haller, C., Holzner, B., Mur, E., & Günther, V. (1997). The impact of life events on patients with rheumatoid arthritis: A psychological myth? *Clinical and Experimental Rheumatology, 15*(2), 175–179.

Härle, P., Straub, R. H., Wiest, R., Mayer, A., Schölmerich, J., Atzeni, F., … Sarzi-Puttini, P. (2006). Increase of sympathetic outflow measured by neuropeptide Y and decrease of the hypothalamic-pituitary-adrenal axis tone in patients with systemic lupus erythematosus and rheumatoid arthritis: Another example of uncoupling of response systems. *Annals of the Rheumatic Diseases, 65*(1), 51–56.

Harris, E. D. (1993). Clinical features of rheumatoid arthritis. In W. N. Kelley, E. D. Harris, S. Ruddy, & C. B. Sledge (Eds.), *Textbook of rheumatology* (4th ed., pp. 874–911). Philadelphia, PA: Saunders.

Hart, R. P., Wade, J. B., & Martelli, M. F. (2003). Cognitive impairment in patients with chronic pain: The significance of stress. *Current Pain and Headache Reports, 7*(2), 116–126.

Hayes, S. C., Luoma, J. B., Bond, F. W., Masuda, A., & Lillis, J. (2006). Acceptance and commitment therapy: Model, processes and outcomes. *Behaviour Research and Therapy, 44*(1), 1–25.

Helmick, C. G., Felson, D. T., Lawrence, R. C., Gabriel, S., Hirsch, R., Kwoh, C. K., … Stone, J. H. (2008). Estimates of the prevalence of arthritis and other rheumatic conditions in the United States: Part I. *Arthritis and Rheumatism, 58*(1), 15–25.

Herrmann, M., Schölmerich, J., & Straub, R. H. (2000). Stress and rheumatic diseases. *Rheumatic Disease Clinics of North America, 26*(4), 737–763.

Hinton, R., Moody, R. L., Davis, A. W., & Thomas, S. F. (2002). Osteoarthritis: Diagnosis and therapeutic considerations. *American Family Physician, 65*(5), 841–848.

Hochberg, M. C. (1997). Updating the American College of Rheumatology revised criteria for the classification of systemic lupus erythematosus. *Arthritis and Rheumatism, 40*(9), 1725.

Holla, J. F., Leeden, M., Knol, D. L., Roorda, L. D., Hilberdink, W. K., Lems, W. F., … Dekker, J. (2015). Predictors and outcome of pain-related avoidance of activities in persons with early symptomatic knee osteoarthritis: A 5-year follow-up study. *Arthritis Care & Research, 67*(1), 48–57.

Holtzman, S., & DeLongis, A. (2007). One day at a time: The impact of daily satisfaction with spouse responses on pain, negative affect and catastrophizing among individuals with rheumatoid arthritis. *Pain, 131*(1–2), 202–213.

Hopkinson, N. D., Doherty, M., & Powell, R. J. (1994). Clinical features and race-specific incidence/prevalence rates of systemic lupus erythematosus in a geographically complete cohort of patients. *Annals of the Rheumatic Diseases, 53*(10), 675–680.

Hopkinson, N. D., Jenkinson, C., Muir, K. R., Doherty, M., & Powell, R. J. (2000). Racial group, socioeconomic status, and the development of persistent proteinuria in systemic lupus erythematosus. *Annals of the Rheumatic Diseases, 59*(2), 116–119.

Jump, R. L., Robinson, M. E., Armstrong, A. E., Barnes, E. V., Kilbourn, K. M., & Richards, H. B. (2005). Fatigue in systemic lupus erythematosus: Contributions of disease activity, pain, depression, and perceived social support. *The Journal of Rheumatology, 32*(9), 1699–1705.

Kabat-Zinn, J., Lipworth, L., & Burney, R. (1985). The clinical use of mindfulness meditation for the self-regulation of chronic pain. *Journal of Behavioral Medicine, 8*(2), 163–190.

Karlson, E. W., Liang, M. H., Eaton, H., Huang, J., Fitzgerald, L., Rogers, M. P., & Daltroy, L. H. (2004). A randomized clinical trial of a psychoeducational intervention to improve outcomes in systemic lupus erythematosus. *Arthritis and Rheumatism, 50*(6), 1832–1841.

Keefe, F., Brown, G., Wallston, K., & Caldwell, D. (1989). Coping with rheumatoid-arthritis pain: Catastrophizing as a maladaptive strategy. *Pain, 37*(1), 51–56.

Keefe, F. J., Caldwell, D. S., Baucom, D., Salley, A., Robinson, E., Timmons, K., … Helms, M. (1996). Spouse-assisted coping skills training in the management of osteoarthritic knee pain. *Arthritis Care & Research, 9*(4), 279–291.

Keefe, F. J., Caldwell, D. S., Martinez, S., Nunley, J., Beckham, J., & Williams, D. A. (1991). Analyzing pain in rheumatoid arthritis patients. Pain coping strategies in patients who have had knee replacement surgery. *Pain, 46*(2), 153–160.

Keefe, F. J., Kashikar-Zuck, S., Opiteck, J., Hage, E., Dalrymple, L., & Blumenthal, J. A. (1996). Pain in arthritis and musculoskeletal disorders: The role of coping skills training and exercise interventions. *Journal of Orthopaedic & Sports Physical Therapy, 24*(4), 279–290.

Keefe, F. J., Kashikar-Zuck, S., Robinson, E., Salley, A., Beaupre, P., Caldwell, D., Haythornthwaite, J. (1997). Pain coping strategies that predict patients' and spouses' ratings of patients' self-efficacy. *Pain, 73*(2), 191–199.

Kennedy, L. A., Cohen, T. R., Panter, A. T., Devellis, B. M., Yamanis, T. J., Jordan, J. M., & Devellis, R. F. (2010). Buffering against the emotional impact of pain: Mood clarity reduces depressive symptoms in older adults. *Journal of Social and Clinical Psychology, 29*(9), 975–987.

Kozora, E., Ellison, M. C., Waxmonsky, J. A., Wamboldt, F. S., & Patterson, T. L. (2005). Major life stress, coping styles, and social support in relation to psychological distress in patients with systemic lupus erythematosus. *Lupus, 14*(5), 363–372.

Kranz, D., Bollinger, A., & Nilges, P. (2010). Chronic pain acceptance and affective well-being: A coping perspective. *European Journal of Pain, 14*(10), 1021–1025.

Kratz, A. L., Davis, M. C., & Zautra, A. J. (2007). Pain acceptance moderates the relation between pain and negative affect in female osteoarthritis and fibromyalgia patients. *Annals of Behavioral Medicine, 33*(3), 291–301.

Lawrence, R. C., Felson, D. T., Helmick, C. G., Arnold, L. M., Choi, H., Deyo, R. A., … Wolfe, F. (2008). Estimates of the prevalence of arthritis and other rheumatic conditions in the United States: Part II. *Arthritis and Research, 58*(1), 26–35.

Lazarus, R. S., & Folkman, S. (1984). *Stress, appraisal, and coping*. New York, NY: Springer.

Leeuw, M., Goossens, M. E. J. B., Linton, S. J., Crombez, G., Boersma, K., & Vlaeyen, J. W. S. (2007). The fear-avoidance model of musculoskeletal pain: Current state of scientific evidence. *Journal of Behavioral Medicine, 30*(1), 77–94.

Loeppenthin, K., Esbensen, B. A., Ostergaard, M., Jennum, P., Thomsen, T., & Midtgaard, J. (2014). Physical activity maintenance in patients with rheumatoid arthritis: A qualitative study. *Clinical Rehabilitation, 28*(3), 289–299.

Lorig, K., Chastain, R. L., Ung, E., Shoor, S., & Holman, H. R. (1989). Development and evaluation of a scale to measure perceived self-efficacy in people with arthritis. *Arthritis and Rheumatism, 32*(1), 37–44.

Lorig, K. R., Mazonson, P. D., & Holman, H. R. (1993). Evidence suggesting that health education for self-management in patients with chronic arthritis has sustained health benefits while reducing health care costs. *Arthritis and Rheumatism, 36*(4), 439–446.

Lowe, R., Cockshott, Z., Greenwood, R., Kirwan, J. R., Almeida, C., Richards, P., & Hewlett, S. (2008). Self-efficacy as an appraisal that moderates the coping-emotion relationship: Associations among people with rheumatoid arthritis. *Psychology & Health, 23*(2), 155–174.

Ma, S. H., & Teasdale, J. D. (2004). Mindfulness-based cognitive therapy for depression: Replication and exploration of differential relapse prevention effects. *Journal of Consulting and Clinical Psychology, 72*(1), 31–40.

Mahdi, H., Fisher, B. A., Källberg, H., Plant, D., Malmström, V., Rönnelid, J., … Lundberg, K. (2009). Specific interaction between genotype, smoking and autoimmunity to citrullinated α-enolase in the etiology of rheumatoid arthritis. *Nature Genetics, 41*(12), 1319–1324.

Mancuso, C. A., Perna, M., Sargent, A. B., & Salmon, J. E. (2010). Perceptions and measurements of physical activity in patients with systemic lupus erythematosus. *Lupus, 20*(3), 231–242.

Marks, R. (2001). Efficacy theory and its utility in arthritis rehabilitation: Review and recommendations. *Disability and Rehabilitation, 23*(7), 271–280.

Marks, R., Allegrante, J. P., & Lorig, K. (2005). A review and synthesis of research evidence for self-efficacy-enhancing interventions for reducing chronic disability: Implications for health education practice (Part I). *Health Promotion Practice, 6*(1), 37–43.

McCracken, L. M. (1998). Learning to live with pain: Acceptance of pain predicts adjustment in persons with chronic pain. *Pain, 74*, 21–27.

McCracken, L. M. (2005). Social context and acceptance of chronic pain: The role of solicitous and punishing responses. *Pain, 113*(1), 155–159.

McCracken, L. M., & Eccleston, C. (2005). A prospective study of acceptance of pain and patient functioning with chronic pain. *Pain, 118*(1), 164–169.

McCracken, L. M., & Eccleston, C. (2006). A comparison of the relative utility of coping and acceptance-based measures in a sample of chronic pain sufferers. *European Journal of Pain, 10*(1), 23–29.

McCracken, L. M., Vowles, K. E., & Eccleston, C. (2005). Acceptance-based treatment for persons with complex, long standing chronic pain: A preliminary analysis of treatment outcome in comparison to a waiting phase. *Behaviour Research and Therapy, 43*(10), 1335–1346.

McCracken, L. M., & Zhao-O'Brien, J. (2010). General psychological acceptance and chronic pain: There is more to accept than the pain itself. *European Journal of Pain, 14*(2), 170–175.

McKnight, P. E., Afram, A., Kashdan, T. B., Kasle, S., & Zautra, A. (2010). Coping self-efficacy as a mediator between catastrophizing and physical functioning: Treatment target selection in an osteoarthritis sample. *Journal of Behavioral Medicine, 33*(3), 239–249.

Metsios, G. S., Stavropoulos-Kalinoglou, A., Veldhuijzen van Zanten, J. J. C. S., Treharne, G. J., Panoulas, V. F., Douglas, K. M. J., … Kitas, G. D. (2008). Rheumatoid arthritis, cardiovascular disease and physical exercise: A systematic review. *Rheumatology, 47*(3), 239–248.

Miller, L. E., Jüsten, H., Schölmerich, J., & Straub, R. H. (2000). The loss of sympathetic nerve fibers in the synovial tissue of patients with rheumatoid arthritis is accompanied by increased norepinephrine release from synovial macrophages. *The FASEB Journal, 14*(13), 2097–2107.

Miller, L. H., & Smith, A. D. (1997). *The stress solution*. Washington, DC: American Psychological Association.

Moldovan, A. R., Onac, I. A., Vantu, M., Szentagotai, A., & Onac, I. (2009). Emotional distress, pain catastrophizing and expectancies in patients with low back pain. *Journal of Cognitive and Behavioral Psychotherapies, 9*(1), 83–93.

Morone, N. E., Greco, C. M., & Weiner, D. K. (2008). Mindfulness meditation for the treatment of chronic low back pain in older adults: A randomized controlled pilot study. *Pain, 134*(3), 310–319.

Navarrete-Navarrete, N., Peralta-Ramírez, M. I., Sabio, J. M., Martínez-Egea, I., Santos-Ruiz, A., & Jiménez-Alonso, J. (2010). Quality-of-life predictor factors in patients with SLE and their modification after cognitive behavioural therapy. *Lupus, 19*(14), 1632–1639.

Nicassio, P. M., & Greenberg, M. A. (2001). The effectiveness of cognitive-behavioral and psychoeducational interventions in the management of arthritis. In M. H. Weisman, M. Weinblatt, & J. Louie (Eds.), *Treatment of rheumatic diseases* (2nd ed., pp. 147–161). Orlando, FL: William Saunders.

O'Leary, A., Shoor, S., Lorig, K., & Holman, H. R. (1988). A cognitive-behavioral treatment for rheumatoid arthritis. *Health Psychology, 7*(6), 527–544.

Oliver, J. E., & Silman, A. J. (2006). Risk factors for the development of rheumatoid arthritis. *Scandinavian Journal of Rheumatology, 35*(3), 169–174.

Parker, J., Smarr, K., Buescher, K., Phillips, L., Frank, R., Beck, N., … Walker, S. (1989). Pain control and rational thinking. Implications for rheumatoid-arthritis. *Arthritis and Rheumatism, 32*(8), 984–990.

Parrish, B. P., Zautra, A. J., & Davis, M. C. (2008). The role of positive and negative interpersonal events on daily fatigue in women with fibromyalgia, rheumatoid arthritis, and osteoarthritis. *Health Psychology, 27*(6), 694–702.

Pawlak, C. R., Jacobs, R., Mikeska, E., Ochsmann, S., Lombardi, M. S., Kavelaars, A., … Schedlowski, M. (1999). Patients with systemic lupus erythematosus differ from healthy controls in their immunological response to acute psychological stress. *Brain, Behavior, and Immunity, 13*(4), 287–302.

Pawlak, C. R., Witte, T., Heiken, H., Hundt, M., Schubert, J., Wiese, B, … Schedlowski, M. (2003). Flares in patients with systemic lupus erythematosus are associated with daily psychological stress. *Psychotherapy and Psychosomatics, 72*(3), 159–165.

Pells, J. J., Shelby, R. A., Keefe, F. J., Dixon, K. E., Blumenthal, J. A., LaCaille, L., … Kraus, V. B. (2008). Arthritis self-efficacy and self-efficacy for resisting eating: Relationships to pain, disability, and eating behavior in overweight and obese individuals with osteoarthritic knee pain. *Pain, 136*(3), 340–347.

Penninx, B. W., Van Tilburg, T., Deeg, D. J., Kriegsman, D. M., Boeke, A. J. P., & Van Eijk, J. (1997). Direct and buffer effects of social support and personal coping resources in individuals with arthritis. *Social Science & Medicine, 44*(3), 393–402.

Peralta-Ramírez, M. I., Jiménez-Alonso, J., Godoy-García, J. F., & Pérez-García, M. (2004). The effects of daily stress and stressful life events on the clinical symptomatology of patients with lupus erythematosus. *Psychosomatic Medicine, 66*(5), 788–794.

Petri, M. (2002). Epidemiology of systemic lupus erythematosus. *Best Practice & Research. Clinical Rheumatology, 16*(5), 847–858.

Potter, P. T., & Zautra, A. J. (1997). Stressful life events' effects on rheumatoid arthritis disease activity. *Journal of Consulting and Clinical Psychology, 65*(2), 319–323.

Radojevic, V., Nicassio, P. M., & Weisman, M. H. (1993). Behavioral intervention with and without family support for rheumatoid arthritis. *Behavior Therapy, 23*(1), 13–30.

Reich, J. W., Zautra, A. J., & Potter, P. T. (2001). Cognitive structure and the independence of positive and negative affect. *Journal of Social and Clinical Psychology, 20*(1), 99–115.

Rejesky, W. J., Martin, K., Ettinger, W. H., & Morgan, T. (1998). Treating disability in knee osteoarthritis with exercise therapy: A central role for self-efficacy and pain. *Arthritis and Rheumatism, 11*(2), 94–101.

Roddy, E., Zhang, W., & Doherty, M. (2005). Aerobic walking or strengthening exercise for osteoarthritis of the knee? A systematic review. *Annals of the Rheumatic Diseases, 64*(4), 544–548.

Romano, J. M., & Turner, J. A. (1985). Chronic pain and depression: Does the evidence support a relationship? *Psychological Bulletin, 97*(1), 18–34.

Rosemann, T., Backenstrass, M., Joest, K., Rosemann, A., Szecsenyi, J., & Laux, G. (2007). Predictors of depression in a sample of 1,021 primary care patients with osteoarthritis. *Arthritis Care & Research, 57*(3), 415–422.

Rosenstiel, A. K., & Keefe, F. J. (1983). The use of coping strategies in chronic low back pain patients: Relationship to patient characteristics and current adjustment. *Pain, 17*(1), 33–44.

Sale, J. E., Gignac, M., & Hawker, G. (2008). The relationship between disease symptoms, life events, coping and treatment, and depression among older adults with osteoarthritis. *The Journal of Rheumatology, 35*(2), 335–342.

Salovey, P., & Mayer, J. D. (1989). Emotional intelligence. *Imagination, Cognition and Personality, 9*(3), 185–211.

Salovey, P., Stroud, L. R., Woolery, A., & Epel, E. S. (2002). Perceived emotional intelligence, stress reactivity, and symptom reports: Further explorations using the trait meta-mood scale. *Psychology and Health, 17*(5), 611–627.

Sariyildiz, M. A., Batmaz, I., Bozkurt, M., Bez, Y., Cetincakmak, M. G., Yazmalar, L., … Celepkolu, T. (2014). Sleep quality in rheumatoid arthritis: Relationship between the disease severity, depression, functional status and the quality of life. *Journal of Clinical Medicine Research, 6*(1), 44–52.

Schleifer, S. J., Keller, S. E., Camerino, M., Thornton, J. C., & Stein, M. (1983). Suppression of lymphocyte stimulation following bereavement. *The Journal of the American Medical Association, 250*(3), 374–377.

Seawell, A. H., & Danoff-Burg, S. (2004). Psychosocial research on systemic lupus erythematosus: A literature review. *Lupus, 13*(12), 891–899.

Segui, J., Ramos-Casals, M., Garcia-Carrasco, M., De Flores, T., Cervera, R., Valdeés, M., … Ingelmo, M. (2000). Psychiatric and psychosocial disorders in patients with systemic lupus erythematosus: A longitudinal study of active and inactive stages of the disease. *Lupus, 9*(8), 584–588.

Sherman, A. M. (2003). Social relations and depressive symptoms in older adults with knee osteoarthritis. *Social Science & Medicine, 56*(2), 247–257.

Silman, A. J., & Pearson, J. E. (2002). Epidemiology and genetics of rheumatoid arthritis. *Arthritis Research, 4*(Suppl 3), S265–S272.

Smith, P. P., & Gordon, C. (2010). Systemic lupus erythematosus: Clinical presentations. *Autoimmunity Reviews, 10*(1), 43–45.

Somers, T. J., Keefe, F. J., Pells, J. J., Dixon, K. E., Waters, S. J., Riordan, P. A., … Rice, J. R. (2009). Pain catastrophizing and pain-related fear in osteoarthritis patients: Relationships to pain and disability. *Journal of Pain and Symptom Management, 37*(5), 863–872.

Strand, E. B., Zautra, A. J., Thoresen, M., Ødegård, S., Uhlig, T., & Finset, A. (2006). Positive affect as a factor of resilience in the pain-negative affect relationship in patients with rheumatoid arthritis. *Journal of Psychosomatic Research, 60*(5), 477–484.

Straub, R. H., Dhabhar, F. S., Bijlsma, J. W., & Cutolo, M. (2005). How psychological stress via hormones and nerve fibers may exacerbate rheumatoid arthritis. *Arthritis and Rheumatism, 52*(1), 16–26.

Straub, R. H., & Kalden, J. R. (2009). Stress of different types increases the proinflammatory load in rheumatoid arthritis. *Arthritis Research and Therapy, 11*(3), 114.

Sturgeon, J. A., & Zautra, A. J. (2013). Psychological resilience, pain catastrophizing, and positive emotions: Perspectives on comprehensive modeling of individual pain adaptation. *Current Pain and Headache Reports, 17*(3), 1–9.

Sullivan, M. J. L., Bishop, S. R., & Pivik, J. (1995). The Pain Catastrophizing Scale: Development and validation. *Psychological Assessment, 7*(4), 524–532.

Sullivan, M. J. L., Thorn, B., Haythornthwaite, J. A., Keefe, F., Martin, M., Bradley, L. A., & Lefebvre, J. C. (2001). Theoretical perspectives on the relation between catastrophizing and pain. *The Clinical Journal of Pain, 17*(1), 52–64.

Sundquist, K., Li, X., Hemminki, K., & Sundquist, J. (2008). Subsequent risk of hospitalization for neuropsychiatric disorders in patients with rheumatic diseases: A nationwide study from Sweden. *Archives of General Psychiatry, 65*(5), 501–507.

Suomi, R., & Collier, D. (2003). Effects of arthritis exercise programs on functional fitness and perceived activities of daily living measures in older adults with arthritis. *Archives of Physical Medicine and Rehabilitation, 84*(11), 1589–1594.

Taylor-Gjevre, R. M., Gjevre, J. A., Nair, B., Skomro, R., & Lim, H. J. (2011). Components of sleep quality and sleep fragmentation in rheumatoid arthritis and osteoarthritis. *Musculoskeletal Care, 9*(3), 152–159.

Viane, I., Crombez, G., Eccleston, C., Devulder, J., & De Corte, W. (2004). Acceptance of the unpleasant reality of chronic pain: Effects upon attention to pain and engagement with daily activities. *Pain, 112*(3), 282–288.

Vitiello, M. V., Rybarczyk, B., Von Korff, M., & Stepanski, E. J. (2009). Cognitive behavioral therapy for insomnia improves sleep and decreases pain in older adults with co-morbid insomnia and osteoarthritis. *Journal of Clinical Sleep Medicine, 5*(4), 355–362.

Vlaeyen, J. W. S., & Linton, S. J. (2000). Fear-avoidance and its consequences in chronic musculoskeletal pain: A state of the art. *Pain, 85*(3), 317–332.

Volkmann, E. R., Grossman, J. M., Sahakian, L. J., Skaggs, B. J., FitzGerald, J., Ragavendra, N., … McMahon, M. (2010). Low physical activity is associated with proinflammatory high-density lipoprotein and increased subclinical atherosclerosis in women with systemic lupus erythematosus. *Arthritis Care & Research, 62*(2), 258–265.

Vowles, K. E., & McCracken, L. M. (2008). Acceptance and values-based action in chronic pain: A study of treatment effectiveness and process. *Journal of Consulting and Clinical Psychology, 76*(3), 397–407.

Wallace, D. J., & Metzger, A. L. (1994). Can an earthquake cause flares of rheumatoid arthritis or lupus nephritis? *Arthritis and Rheumatism, 37*(12), 1826–1828.

Wegner, D. M. (1997). When the antidote is the poison: Ironic mental control processes. *Psychological Science, 8*(3), 148–150.

Weinberger, M., Tierney, W. M., Booher, P., & Hiner, S. L. (1990). Social support, stress, and functional status in patients with osteoarthritis. *Social Science & Medicine, 30*(4), 503–508.

Wekking, E. M., Vingerhoets, A. J. J. M., van Dam, A. P., Nossent, J. C., & Swaak, A. J. J. G. (1991). Daily stressors and systemic lupus erythematosus: A longitudinal analysis—First findings. *Psychotherapy and Psychosomatics, 55*(2–4), 108–113.

Westby, D. M. (2001). A health professional's guide to exercise prescription for people with arthritis: A review of aerobic fitness activities. *Arthritis Care & Research, 45*(6), 501–511.

Wright, G. E., Parker, J. C., Smarr, K. L., Johnson, J. C., Hewett, J. E., & Walker, S. E. (1998). Age, depressive symptoms, and rheumatoid arthritis. *Arthritis and Rheumatism, 41*(2), 298–305.

Zautra, A. J., Burleson, M. H., Matt, K. S., Roth, S., & Burrows, L. (1994). Interpersonal stress, depression, and disease activity in rheumatoid arthritis and osteoarthritis patients. *Health Psychology, 13*(2), 139–148.

Zautra, A. J., Davis, M. C., Reich, J. W., Nicassario, P., Tennen, H., Finan, P., … Irwin, M. R. (2008). Comparison of cognitive behavioral and mindfulness meditation interventions on adaptation to rheumatoid arthritis for patients with and without history of recurrent depression. *Journal of Consulting and Clinical Psychology, 76*(3), 408–421.

Zautra, A. J., Hoffman, J. M., Matt, K. S., Yocum, D., Potter, P. T., Castro, W. L., & Roth, S. (1998). An examination of individual differences in the relationship between interpersonal stress and disease activity among women with rheumatoid arthritis. *Arthritis & Rheumatism, 11*(4), 271–279.

Zautra, A. J., Hoffman, J., Potter, P., Matt, K. S., Yocum, D., & Castro, L. (1997). Examination of changes in interpersonal stress as a factor in disease exacerbations among women with rheumatoid arthritis. *Annals of Behavioral Medicine, 19*(3), 279–286.

Zautra, A. J., Johnson, L. M., & Davis, M. C. (2005). Positive affect as a source of resilience for women in chronic pain. *Journal of Consulting and Clinical Psychology, 73*(2), 212–220.

Zautra, A. J., Reich, J. W., Davis, M. C., Potter, P. T., & Nicolson, N. A. (2000). The role of stressful events in the relationship between positive and negative affects: Evidence from field and experimental studies. *Journal of Personality, 68*(5), 927–951.

Zautra, A., Smith, B., Affleck, G., & Tennen, H. (2001). Examinations of chronic pain and affect relationships: Applications of a dynamic model of affect. *Journal of Consulting and Clinical Psychology, 69*(5), 786.

Zelman, D. C., Howland, E. W., Nichols, S. N., & Cleeland, C. S. (1991). The effects of induced mood on laboratory pain. *Pain, 46*(1), 105–111.

Socioeconomic Disparities in Arthritis

6

Antoine R. Baldassari and Leigh F. Callahan

Introduction

There is little debate that health status varies by socioeconomic status (SES); notwithstanding challenges in precisely defining and measuring SES, the observation that socioeconomically disadvantaged people shoulder a greater disease burden and have broadly worse health than those in higher socioeconomic strata is nearly ubiquitous across fields of health. Although the documentation of health disparities long predates modern research, the issue rose to political prominence throughout the second half of the twentieth century and was propelled to the forefront of public policy following the 1980 publication of the Black report, a landmark presentation of health inequities in the United Kingdom (Townsend & Davidson, 1992). Today, the reduction in health disparities features prominently among the goals of public administrations. In the United States, the Department of Health and Human Services lists social determinants of health as important targets of its 10-year goal set, Healthy People 2020 (US Department of Health and Human Services and Office of Disease Prevention and Health Promotion, 2012). This chapter first introduces some of the challenges involved in health disparities research. We will then present the current evidence for socioeconomic patterns of disease onset and health outcomes in arthritis and discuss the suspected mechanisms involved.

A.R. Baldassari (✉)
Thurston Arthritis Research Center, School of Medicine, University of North Carolina at Chapel Hill, 3300 Thurston Building, CB # 7280, Chapel Hill, NC, 27599-7330, USA
e-mail: baldassa@email.unc.edu

L.F. Callahan, PhD
Thurston Arthritis Research Center, School of Medicine, University of North Carolina at Chapel Hill, 3300 Thurston Building, CB # 7280, Chapel Hill, NC, 27599-7330, USA

Department of Medicine and Social Medicine, University of North Carolina at Chapel Hill, Chapel Hill, NC, USA
e-mail: leigh_callahan@med.unc.edu

Challenges in Health Disparities Research

The consistent identification of health disparities across fields of health belies the challenges involved in the measurement and use of socioeconomic data. The enthusiasm gap between the use of SES in health research and the development and adoption of unified methods has led to great heterogeneity in health disparities research (Oakes & Rossi, 2003). This is notable even within relatively narrow inquiries such as in the efforts to assess socioeconomic patterns of self-reported health outcomes among people with rheumatoid arthritis (RA), so far conducted disparately using

P.M. Nicassio (ed.), *Psychosocial Factors in Arthritis*, DOI 10.1007/978-3-319-22858-7_6

education, income, employment status, area-level measures, composite instruments, homeownership, and housing data (Ghawi et al., 2015). We bring attention to four key methodological considerations: (1) the need to measure SES using multiple indicators, (2) the likelihood of effect-measure modification between communities and demographic groups, (3) graded and nonlinear patterns of health inequities, and (4) upcoming models of life-course SES.

SES is commonly measured with a single instrument (often, income, education, or area-level variables); however, while socioeconomic indicators covary to a degree, they can operationalize very different aspects of the relationship between SES and health. Illustratively, studies jointly evaluating multiple SES dimensions as predictors of health often find patterns of inequities to differ between SES measures. For instance, we found RA disease severity to primarily vary by homeownership status and income and less so by occupation and education in a cohort of African Americans with RA (Baldassari et al., 2014).

Additional complexity arises from variations in the meaning of SES indicators across populations, including by age group, gender, race/ethnicity (Williams et al., 2010), and between countries. For instance, education may not yield the same SES gains among African Americans in the United States as it does among Whites due to complex structural factors including employment discrimination; low-SES may also tie into gender-associated health determinants, such as physically demanding occupations for men and single parenthood for women; further, limited financial resources may differentially affect access to health services depending on universal care availability.

Health inequities are typically hypothesized to occur either past a certain threshold triggering poorer health, or along a graded pattern of increasingly worse health with decreasing SES; whereas empirical evidence supports the latter case in many instances (Adler et al., 1994), studies of health disparities still often limit themselves to the detection of threshold effects by their use of dichotomized SES indicators. To again take RA research as an example, most studies of the association between education and physical health among people with RA only compare two categories of education, whereas the minority of those allowing for multiple levels of education suggest a gradient effect.

Studies of socioeconomic health disparities have increasingly emphasized the importance of socioeconomic disadvantage throughout the life-course as a lasting determinant of health (Ben-Shlomo & Kuh, 2002). The manner in which to evaluate the childhood SES and health relationship remains a subject of debate and ultimately depends on an investigator's research question. Typically, three classes of analytic models are distinguished (Ben-Shlomo & Kuh, 2002): those involving additive effects of SES at different life stages on health (accumulation model), models placing special importance on SES during vulnerable life stages (critical phase model), and those hypothesizing that changes in SES drive health disparities (social mobility model). While accumulation models are primarily used in chronic disease disparities research, methods today allow investigators to concurrently evaluate all three approaches in nested models (Mishra et al., 2009).

The Unequal Distribution of Arthritis

The literature on health disparities in arthritis goes back several decades and presents overwhelming evidence that low-SES individuals not only develop a broad range of rheumatic diseases at a higher rate, but also experience worse disease progression and more adverse outcomes than their higher-SES counterparts. Arthritis is composed of a wide range of etiologically distinct disorders, and we focus this section on archetypical forms of the disease: osteoarthritis and rheumatoid arthritis. As a word of caution, self-reported arthritis and OA are sufficiently common that odds ratios used to quantify their associations with SES in logistic regressions substantially overestimate risk ratios and may not be conflated with them.

Osteoarthritis

Osteoarthritis (OA) is characterized by the progressive degradation of articular cartilage and represents a sizable majority of all arthritis cases. OA is a main cause of disability worldwide, with disease of the knees and hips jointly accounting for more activity limitation than any other disorder. Women shoulder two thirds of all OA cases and disease risk increases progressively with age, reaching an estimated one in three adults over the age of 65 in the United States (Lawrence et al., 2008).

Much of the early work on social determinants of OA was motivated by the hypothesis that occupational joint strain could increase susceptibility to OA, and the data accumulated over the past half-century, reviewed by McWilliams and colleagues for knee OA (McWilliams et al., 2011), provide strong empirical support for associations between various occupational features and the onset of OA. Tasks mobilizing load-bearing joints, such as repeated knee-bending, lifting/carrying, or kneeling, have intuitive mechanistic ties to OA pathogenesis; however, occupational differences in OA risk, particularly when described by job title or by blue—or white—collar status, also hint at socioeconomic patterns of OA susceptibility that extend beyond the workplace.

For the purpose of this overview, we will distinguish between studies of health disparities assessed in radiographically diagnosed OA and those using self-reported instruments.

Radiographically Assessed OA

We present an overview of health disparities in radiographically diagnosed arthritis in Table 6.1. Investigations predominantly originate from two cohort studies in the United States: the first part of the National Health and Nutrition Examination Survey (Anderson & Felson, 1988; Hannan et al., 1992; Tepper & Hochberg, 1993) and the Johnston County Osteoarthritis project (Callahan et al., 2010; Callahan, Cleveland, et al., 2011; Cleveland et al., 2013). Data from those cohorts provide overlapping evidence for differences in OA risk by income, education, and occupational class, both for hip OA and knee OA, and Johnston County data further suggest a relationship between area-level SES and OA risk.

Self-Reported Arthritis

Ascertainment of arthritis can be challenging in large-scale studies, and self-reported case definitions are often used to facilitate the evaluation of disease burden. Case definitions used in most studies involve participant reports of any prior receipt of an arthritis or rheumatic disease diagnosis from a health professional; self-reported chronic arthritis symptoms have also been used, rarely as a stand-alone criterion and typically together with a self-reported doctor diagnosis. There is evidence that self-reported case definitions for arthritis have satisfactory sensitivity for population surveillance purposes, but suffer from low specificity, particularly among individuals less than 65 years old (Bombard, Powell, Martin, Helmick, & Wilson, 2005). Nevertheless, there is no evidence that instrument validity for self-reported arthritis definitions varies by SES, as could systematically bias estimates of the SES and self-reported arthritis association. To the extent that most self-reported arthritis involves OA of the hips, knees, or hands, the evidence for its differential prevalence by SES complements that presented in our section on radiographic OA.

We summarize some of the work on socioeconomic differences in the risk of self-reported arthritis in Table 6.2. These studies span decades, geographic regions, and demographic groups, yet almost unanimously find meaningful differences in the risk of self-reported arthritis by a number of socioeconomic characteristics, including education, income, neighborhood disadvantage, or occupational class. There is equivocal evidence for effect-measure modification by race/ethnicity. Cunningham and colleagues notably found gradient patterns of increased self-reported arthritis susceptibility with lower SES, but only among non-indigenous participants in a sample of Australian participants (Cunningham, 2011); in comparison, data from a cohort study in rural North Carolina (USA) did not suggest significantly different patterns of inequities between Whites and African Americans (Callahan et al., 2008).

Table 6.1 Overview of socioeconomic disparities in radiographically diagnosed OA (r-kOA), including symptomatic OA (s-kOA)

Study	Reference	Data (country)	Size	Adjusted for	SES variables	Results
Leigh 1991	Leigh and Fries (1991a)	NHANES-I, QES73, SDW78, NHIS86 (USA)				
Hannan 1992	Hannan et al. (1992)	NHANES-I (USA)	6880	Income, BMI, smoking, knee injury	Education: HS, <HS	Greater risk among <HS than ≥HS
					Income	
Wang 2000	Peter Wang et al. (2000)	NPHS (Canada)	39,240	Education, BMI	Income	Greater prevalence in group with low income based on family size (e.g., <$15,000 for one- or two-person family) vs. not-low income participants
					Education	
Busija 2007	Busija et al. (2007)	VPHS (Australia)	7500	BMI		
Callahan 2008	Callahan et al. (2008)	NC-FM-RN (NC, USA)	7306			
Cañizares 2008	Cañizares et al. (2008)	Community health survey (Canada)	127,513			
Grotle (2008)	Grotle et al. (2008)	Community survey (Norway)	3266			
Cunningham 2011	Cunningham (2011)	NATSIHS (Australia)	18,340			
Brennan 2012	Brennan and Turrell (2012)	HABITAT (Australia)	10,757		Education	
					Income	
					Area SES	
Baldassari 2013	Baldassari et al. (2013a)	NC-FM-RN (NC, USA)		Age, sex, race	Count of low education, non-homeowner-ship and low SES occupation	
					Count of low maternal: education, non-parental homeownership and low-SES paternal occupation	

Anderson 1988	Anderson and Felson (1988)	NHANES-I (USA)	5193		Income: (continuous scale)	*KNEE OA*
						Decreased risk with \$5000/year income increments, similarly for both men and women (OR = 0.8). Not significant in fully adjusted models
					Education: <8 years, 9–12 years, >12 years	Decreased risk per increase in education category. OR = 0.7 for men, OR = 0.8 for women. Not significantin fully adjusted models
Hannan 1992	Hannan et al. (1992)	NHANES-I (USA)	6880	Age, race, sex, smoking	Education	*KNEE OA*
						Greater prevalence with fewer years of education,for r-kOA (lowest vs. highest OR = 1.5) and s-kOA (lowest vs. highest OR = 1.3). Explained by BMI for r-kOA but not s-kOA
Tepper 1993	Tepper and Hochberg (1993)	NHANES-I (USA)	2358	Age, race, sex, marital status, other SES variable	Education	*HIP OA*
						Greater prevalence in <12 years of schooling vs. ≥12 years, slightly short of significance at $\alpha = 0.05$ (OR = 1.64). Possibly stronger association among men
					Income	No significant associations, imprecise estimates show possible U-shaped relation between higher family income and hip OA
Andrianakos 2006	Andrianakos et al. (2006)	Population-based study (Greece)	8740	Age, gender,	Education: ≤12 years, >12 years	*KNEE, HIP, AND HAND OA*
						Greater risk of knee OA for ≤12 years vs. >12 years (OR = 2.8) but not for hand or hip OA
					Occupation: non-manual, others	Lower risk for hand OA for non-manual occupations vs. others (OR = 0.6), but not hip OA or knee OA

(continued)

Table 6.1 (continued)

Study	Reference	Data (country)	Size	Adjusted for	SES variables	Results
Callahan 2008	Callahan, Cleveland, et al., (2011)	Johnston County OA project (USA)	3552	Age, gender, race, BMI, physical activity	Education: <12 years, ≥12 years	*KNEE OA*
						Greater risk in <12 years of schooling vs. ≥12 years for unilateral (OR = 2.1) and bilateral r-kOA, and symptomatic unilateral (OR = 2.2) and bilateral r-kOA
					Occupation: managerial, others	Greater risk for non-managerial vs. managerial, for r-kOA (OR = 1.4) and s-kOA (OR = 1.5). Explained by other SES variables
					Area poverty: high, medium, low	Greater risk in medium and high poverty vs. low poverty. OR for High vs. low poverty = 1.9 (r-kOA) and 1.4 (s-kOA)
Callahan 2010	Callahan et al. (2010)	Johnston County OA project (USA)	2627	Age, race/ethnicity, stratified by gender	Education: <12 years, ≥12 years	*KNEE OA*
						Greater prevalence for <12 years vs. ≥12 years, for r-kOA (women only: OR = 1.6) and s-kOA (Men: OR = 1.55, Women: OR = 1.9). Unexplained by BMI, smoking, alcohol use, previous knee injury, hormone replacement therapy
Cleveland 2013	Cleveland et al. (2013)	Johnston County OA project (USA)	3087	Age, gender, race, BMI, smoking, prior hip injury, workplace physical demands	Education: <12 years, ≥12 years	*HIP OA*
						Greater risk in <12 years of schooling vs. ≥12 years for unilateral (OR = 1.4) and bilateral s-hOA (OR = 2.0), and for bilateral s-hOA (OR = 1.3)
					Occupation: managerial, others	Greater risk for non-managerial vs. managerial, for r-hOA (OR = 1.4) and s-hOA (OR = 1.5). Explained by other SES variables
					Area poverty: high, medium, low	Greater risk in medium and high poverty vs. low poverty. Unilateral/bilateral High vs. low OR = 1.3/2.0 (r-kOA) and 1.6/NS (s-kOA)
Rodriguez-Amado 2014	Rodriguez-Amado et al. (2014)	Population-based study (Mexico)	17,566			*ANY OA*

NHANES National Health and Nutrition Examination Survey

Table 6.2 Overview of socioeconomic disparities in self-reported doctor-diagnosed arthritis prevalence

Study	Reference	Data (country)	Size	Adjusted for	SES variables	Results
Hannan 1992	Hannan et al. (1992)	Population health survey: NHANES-I (USA)	6880	Age, gender, race, smoking	Education: 0–8 years, 9–11 years, 12 years, ≥13 years	Increasing risk with lower educational category. Lowest vs. highest OR = 1.51. Unchanged by further adjustments for BMI and knee injury
Wang 2000	Peter Wang et al. (2000)	Population health survey: NPHS (Canada)	39,240	Age, gender, ethnic group, other SES variables	Education: <secondary, ≥secondary	No difference by low education status
					Income: low for, family size, not low	Greater risk in low income group than not-low group (OR = 1.14)
					Occupation: unskilled, semiskilled, professional	No meaningful difference in risk by occupation
Busija 2007	Busija et al. (2007)	Population health survey: VPHS (Australia)	7500	Age, gender, BMI, area of residence, other SES variables	Education: primary, secondary, tertiary	No meaningful independent associations
					Income: <$A 20 K, 20–40 K, 40–60 K, >60 K	Increasing risk with decreasing income; vs. highest category, ORs = 0.8, 0.6 and 0.5 respectively
					Occupation: professional, others	No meaningful independent associations
Callahan 2008	Callahan et al. (2008)	Primary-care patients: NC-FM-RN (NC, USA)	7306	Age, gender, BMI, stratified by race.	Education: <12 years, 12 years, ≥12 years	Greater risk in <12 years vs. >12 years; OR = 1.55 for Whites and 1.92 for African Americans
					Area poverty: low %, medium %, high %	No independent main effects, but meaningful interaction of greatest poverty with highest education category: OR = 1.55 for Whites, 2.06 for African Americans
Cañizares 2008	Cañizares et al. (2008)	Community health survey (Canada)	127,513	Age, gender, race, smoking, physical activity, immigration status,, area characteristic, other SES variables	Education: <secondary, secondary, >secondary	No meaningful independent association
					Income: <$A 20 K, 20–40 K, 40–60 K, ≥60 K	Increasing risk in decreasing income categories; vs. ≥60 K, OR = 1.49, 1.26, and 1.13, respectively
					Area poverty: % low-SES	Greater risk with increasing % of low-income families (OR = 1.3 for 10 % increase), but not with increasing % of low-education families
Grotle 2008	Grotle et al. (2008)	Community survey (Norway)	3266	Age, gender	Education: ≤9 years, 9–12 years, >12 years	*Uses self-reported osteoarthritis rather than any arthritis*
						Evenly greater self-reported OA risk for lower two education categories vs. >12 years, for any OA (OR ≈ 2.1), hip OA (OR ≈ 2.8), knee OA (OR ≈ 2.3), and hand OA (OR ≈ 1.5)

(continued)

Table 6.2 (continued)

Study	Reference	Data (country)	Size	Adjusted for	SES variables	Results
Cunningham 2011	Cunningham (2011)	Population health survey NATSIHS (Australia)	18,340	Age, gender, stratified by indigenous status	Education: <12 years, ≥12 years, or no degree, certificate, diploma, university	*Associations only found among non-indigenous participants, except for greater risk for lowest* vs. *highest income quartile among indigenous* (*OR* = *1.6*)
						Lower risk for ≥12 years than less than years (OR = 0.6)
						Decreasing risk with higher categories of education than no degree. University vs. no degree OR = 0.5
					Income: quintiles	Increasing risk with lower income quintiles than Q3-5. Q1 vs. Q3-5 OR = 2.1
					Area poverty: quintiles	Increasing risk with lower area poverty. Q1 (poorest) vs. Q5 (richest) OR = 1.7
					Housing tenure	No meaningful association
Brennan 2012	Brennan and Turrell (2012)	Population-based cross-sectional study: HABITAT (Australia)	10,757		Education: Secondary, Certificate, Diploma, Bachelor	Greater disease in categories lower than highest education, similar in all three lower categories (OR ≈ 1.3)
					Income: <$A 26 K, 26–42 K, 42–73 K, 73–130 K, >130 K	Progressively higher risk with decreasing income category: respectively, OR = 1.96, 1.75, 1.51, 1.28
					Occupation: blue collar, white collar, professional	No meaningful independent association with work status among the employed
					Area poverty: quintiles	Greater risk among people in quintile 2 or 3 (OR ≈ 1.2) and quintile 1 (lowest SES, OR = 1.42) vs. quintile 5 (highest SES)
Baldassari 2013	Baldassari, Cleveland, and Callahan (2013b)	Primary-care patients: NC-FM-RN (NC, USA)	1276	Age, sex, race	Current SES: Count of low education, non-homeowner-ship and low SES occupation	Increasing risk of self-reported arthritis with increasing count of low-SES factors. Not explained by childhood SES or BMI: lowest vs. highest OR = 2.08 in fully adjusted models
					Count of low maternal: education, non-parental homeownership and low-SES paternal occupation	Increasing risk with higher count of childhood low-SES factors. Lowest vs. highest SES difference remained significant after adjusting for current SES and BMI (OR = 1.39)

NHANES-I National Health and Nutrition Examination Survey, *QES* Quality of Employment Survey, *SDW* Survey of Disability and Work, *NHIS* National Health Interview Survey, NPHS National Population Health Survey, VPHS Victorian Population Health Survey, *NC-FM-RN* North-Carolina Family-Medicine Research Network, *NATSIHS* National Aboriginal and Torres Strait Islander Health Survey, *HABITAT* How Areas in Brisbane Influence Health and Activity study

Rheumatoid Arthritis

With a prevalence between 0.5 and 1 %, rheumatoid arthritis (RA) is the most common autoimmune disorder; women represent two thirds of all cases (Gabriel, 2001) and the disease typically occurs between the age of 50 and 75. Current genetic heritability estimates for RA do not exceed 50 % (Frisell et al., 2013), leaving ample room for modifiable determinants which, with the exception of smoking (Silman, Newman, & Macgregor, 1996), remain largely unknown.

We provide an overview of studies on socioeconomic differences in RA risk in Table 6.3. While early studies found no clear associations of socioeconomic status with RA development (Bankhead et al., 1996; Uhlig et al., 1999), more recent work consistently suggests that people with low SES are at an increased susceptibility for RA. Intriguing data further indicate that socioeconomic disadvantage chiefly increases susceptibility to seropositive disease (Bengtsson et al., 2005; Pedersen et al., 2006), as characterized by rheumatoid factors, supporting the increasingly adopted notion that seropositive and seronegative RA constitute etiologically distinct phenotypes.

Other Arthritis

While health disparities in the rheumatic diseases have been primarily studied within OA, RA, and self-reported arthritis, they likely extend to other arthritis subtypes. For instance, studies in the United Kingdom and New Zealand found patterns of greater gout prevalence with, respectively, lower income (Hayward et al., 2013) and greater area deprivation (Taylor et al., 2004); in contrast, gout was found to be more prevalent among white-collar than blue-collar workers in a sample of Black South-Africans from a Johannesburg hospital (Tikly et al., 1998). Further, modest socioeconomic patterns of lupus erythematous prevalence (but not lupus nephritis) were discerned at the county level in a study of American Medicaid claims data (Feldman et al., 2013).

SES and Health Outcomes in Arthritis

General Patterns in Arthritis

As observed in the general population, patterns of worse health with lower SES are consistently found among individuals with arthritis, as reviewed by our group in OA (Luong et al., 2012). These health disparities are apparent across self-reported instruments monitoring physical health and function in the rheumatic diseases; notably, participant scores on the Health Assessment Questionnaire, the physical component summary of the Short-Form Health Survey, and the Western Ontario and McMaster Universities Osteoarthritis Index are typically found to vary by SES among people with arthritis, including by education, income, and area deprivation (Brekke et al., 1999; ERAS Study Group, 2000; Harrison et al., 2005; Jacobi et al., 2003; Knight et al., 2011; Marra et al., 2004; McEntegart et al., 1997; Vliet Vlieland et al., 1994). The extent of those differences varies between studies, but appears important beyond mere statistical significance: in our published analyses of primary-care patients with self-reported arthritis, differences in HAQ and SF-12 physical scores between the lowest (<$15,000) and highest household income groups (>$45,000) exceeded the minimally important clinical differences used for these instruments (Callahan, Martin, et al., 2011).

Patterns in Osteoarthritis: Joint Replacement Outcomes and SES

Total joint arthroplasty (TJA) is an increasingly common surgical treatment for severe joint pain and loss of function from chronic musculoskeletal disorders, primarily OA of the hips or knees. Socioeconomic status has been shown to predict the effectiveness of, and recovery from, TJA at 6 (Agabiti et al., 2007; Jenkins et al., 2009) and 12 (Clement et al., 2011) months, leading Clement and colleagues to warn against the confounding potential of socioeconomic factors in comparative evaluations of total hip arthroplasty providers (Clement et al., 2011).

Table 6.3 Overview of studies of socioeconomic disparities in rheumatoid arthritis risk

Study	Reference	Data (country)	Size	Adjusted for	SES variables	Results
Bankhead 1996	Bankhead et al. (1996)	Population-based register NOAR (USA)	687	Stratified by gender	Five census-level variables	No strong correlation between SES variables and arthritis incidence (r_s between 0 and 0.3)
Uhlig 1999	Uhlig, Hagen, and Kvien (1999)	County RA register (Norway)	361 cases, 5851 controls	Age, gender, smoking	Education	Not associated with RA risk
Olsson 2001	Olsson, Skogh, and Wingren (2001)	Single hospital records (Denmark)	281 cases, 507 controls	Age, smoking, high-risk occupation	Education	Lower incidence for secondary/upper secondary and university vs. compulsory school only (RR $\approx$ 0.5). Similar disparities among men and women
Jaakola and Gissler 2004	Jaakkola and Gissler (2005)	1987 national birth cohort, (Finland)	56,632	Age (birth cohort), gender, birth order, maternal age, marital status, current SES index	Maternal occupation	Increased risk of inflammatory polyarthropathies (incl. RA) (OR = 2.11) and juvenile RA (OR = 2.12) for blue-collar vs. upper white-collar maternal occupation. Imprecise estimates; not statistically significant
Bengtsson 2005	Bengtsson et al. (2005)	Population-based case-control study EIRA (Sweden)	930 cases, 1126 controls	Age, residential area, smoking	Education	Greater incidence of RA among participants in both educational categories below university degree (RR $\approx$ 1.7), similarly among men and women. Associations stronger for RF-positive RA than for RF-negative RA
					Occupation	Higher RA incidence among women in the manual occupational class vs. non-manual (RR $\approx$ 1.3). Associations stronger for RF-positive RA than for RF-negative RA
Pedersen 2006	Pedersen et al. (2006)	Nationwide hospital records over 5 years (Denmark)	515 cases, 769 controls	Gender, year of birth, year of diagnosis, place of residence	Education	Lower risk with greater education in graded pattern (linear trend $p < 0.001$, highest vs. lowest education RR $\approx$ 0.4). Only observed for RF-positive RA
					Current affluence	Lower risk in middle and most affluent thirds vs. least affluent thirds (OR 0.9 and 0.66), not significant at $\alpha = 0.05$
					Affluence during childhood	Lower risk in middle and most affluent thirds vs. least affluent thirds (OR 0.90 and 0.66), not significant at $\alpha = 0.05$

Schneider 2006	Schneider, Schmitt, and Richter (2006)	National Health survey (Germany)	6491	Age, sex	Occupation	Top-level office workers, and white-collar vs. manual OR = 0.27 and 0.54. Unexplained by lifestyle factors and other sociodemographic variables
					Education	Highest category and high school vs. no high school OR = 0.5 and 0.72
					Social status	Upper class and middle class vs. Lower class OR = 0.54 and 0.86
Bergstrom 2011	Bergström et al. (2011)	Citywide Preventative screening program (Sweden)	290 cases, 1006 controls	Crude analyses	Occupation	Greater incidence of RA among blue-collar workers than among white collar (OR = 1.54), similar for men and women. Unexplained by current smoking or chronic obstructive pulmonary disease
Parks 2013	Parks et al. (2013)	NIEHS Sister Study (USA)	50,884	Age, gender, race	Education	Greater RA risk at lower education levels: vs. graduate/professional degree, OR = 1.5 for high-school only, OR = 1.7 for less than high-school
					Income	Greater RA risk among low income/poor vs. well-off/middle income (OR = 1.3)
					Early-life SES markers	Gradient pattern of more RA with additional factors of low early-life SES (OR = 3.0 for four factors vs. 0)
Ghawi 2015	Ghawi et al. (2015)	Population-based study (USA)	604 cases, 564 controls	Age, gender, date of RA incidence	Education	Greater risk of RA for all three categories of education lower than graduate school (OR = 1.92 for < high school)
					Housing quality index	Greater RA risk in middle two quartiles of housing quality index vs. quartile of highest SES (Q2 vs. Q1 OR = 1.42; Q3 vs. Q1 OR = 1.37). No RA risk difference between lowest and highest quartiles

NOAR Norfolk arthritis registry, *EIRA* Epidemiological Investigation of Rheumatoid Arthritis, *NIEHS* National Institute of Environmental Health Sciences

Patterns in Rheumatoid Arthritis: Disease Severity, Inflammation, and SES

In addition to socioeconomic disparities in self-reported physical (Allaire et al., 2009; Barton et al., 2011; Berkanovic et al., 1996; Callahan, Martin, et al., 2011; ERAS Study Group, 2000; Harrison et al., 2005; Jacobi et al., 2003; Leigh & Fries, 1991b; Linde et al., 2009; Marra et al., 2004; Massardo et al., 2012; McEntegart et al., 1997; Vliet Vlieland et al., 1994) and mental health (Brekke et al., 1999; Callahan, Martin, et al., 2011; Harrison et al., 2005; Jacobi et al., 2003), studies of RA patients have found robust associations of SES (primarily education and income) with scores on the commonly used Disease Activity Score (Harrison et al., 2005; Jacobi et al., 2003) and with tender and painful joint counts (Brekke et al., 1999; Callahan & Pincus, 1988; ERAS Study Group, 2000; Harrison et al., 2005; Vliet Vlieland et al., 1994). Socioeconomic patterns in RA mortality, which remains increased compared to the general population (Dadoun et al., 2013), have also been discerned according to area deprivation in the UK (Maiden et al., 1999).

In contrast, data remain inconsistent with socioeconomic disparities in joint erosion scores on the Sharp/van der Heijde scale (ERAS Study Group, 2000; Harrison et al., 2005; Massardo et al., 2012; Vliet Vlieland et al., 1994) or in acute-phase inflammation as measured by erythrocyte sedimentation rate or serum C-reactive protein concentration (Callahan & Pincus, 1988; ERAS Study Group, 2000; Marra et al., 2004; Massardo et al., 2012; McEntegart et al., 1997). Consistent with the notion that differential susceptibility to RA by SES may primarily involve seropositive disease (see above) (Bengtsson et al., 2005; Pedersen et al., 2006), there is some evidence that low-SES individuals with RA are more likely to be positive for rheumatoid factor autoantibodies and anti-citrullinated protein antibodies (Bengtsson et al., 2005; Mackie et al., 2012; Pedersen et al., 2006), although results have been occasionally mixed: Mackie and colleagues, for instance, found that English participants from socioeconomically deprived communities were at an elevated risk for RF but not ACPA (Mackie et al., 2012).

While research on health inequities in RA has predominantly focused on populations of European descent, comparable patterns were found among African Americans from the Southeastern United States, in the Consortium for the Evaluation of African Americans with Rheumatoid Arthritis (CLEAR) (Baldassari et al., 2014).

It is as yet unclear whether health disparities in RA persist or subside with increasing disease duration. So far, a Dutch study found the health status of RA patients to equalize across SES groups following disease presentation (Harrison et al., 2005), whereas a British study found disparities to remain at 3 years (ERAS Study Group, 2000), and our aforementioned work on CLEAR participants found wider disparities among people with established RA than those with early disease (≤2 years) (Baldassari et al., 2014). One possible explanation for these different results lies in the differing abilities of healthcare systems to equitably deliver effective RA therapies, although this remains speculative absent of more conclusive data.

Patterns in Other Arthritis

Outside OA and RA, socioeconomic determinants of health in arthritis have predominantly been investigated in lupus, where these are convincingly associated with disease activity and mortality (Alarcon et al., 2004; Bertoli et al., 2008; Karlson et al., 1995; Pons-Estel et al., 2010). Various aspects of lupus morbidity are likewise observed to follow socioeconomic patterns, with severe renal disease having a well-studied relationship with SES in lupus (Alarcón et al., 2006; Petri et al., 1991).

Life-Course SES and Arthritis

Studies of health disparities in the rheumatic diseases have sparingly evaluated the independent contribution of socioeconomic factors in early life. The literature on early SES and self-reported arthritis so far includes the findings that low parental income and low-status paternal occupation are, respectively, associated with a higher risk of self-reported arthritis among middle-aged and elderly individuals (Blackwell, Hayward, & Crimmins, 2001; Ziol-Guest et al., 2012). While the relationship between childhood SES and the onset of RA has been comparatively more researched, its independence from later socioeconomic characteristics remains uncertain (Carlens et al., 2009; Jaakkola & Gissler, 2005; Parks et al., 2013; Pedersen et al., 2006); notably, Parks and colleagues reported that a low SES during childhood was associated with a greater risk for RA among women from a US national cohort, provided that SES remained low across the life-course (Parks et al., 2013).

Our recent work on participants in a North Carolina primary care cohort found that low childhood SES aggregated across dimensions was meaningfully associated with self-reported arthritis independently of current socioeconomic circumstances, with further analyses pointing to excess body mass as a primary mechanism for the association (Baldassari, Cleveland, & Callahan, 2013b). Within that same primary-care cohort (Baldassari, Cleveland, & Callahan, 2013a), childhood SES was associated with participant scores on the HAQ index of disability and the physical component summary of the SF-12, independently of current SES; in contrast, associations with mental health outcomes did not remain after adjustment for current status. While these associations of childhood SES with physical health outcomes among people with arthritis have yet to be corroborated in other studies, they are consistent with the mounting evidence in other chronic diseases that health status takes its root in early life, as predominantly exemplified to date in studies of cardiovascular diseases (Galobardes, Smith, & Lynch, 2006).

Pathways to Disparities

Arthritis encompasses diverse, etiologically complex disorders, and a vast range of mechanisms plausibly underlie the socioeconomic patterns in its distribution and severity (Fig. 6.1).

Lifestyle factors prominently feature as mechanisms of health disparities in the social epidemiology literature, and they may be especially germane in arthritis. In particular, the importance of excess body mass in both OA (probably including non-weight bearing joints (Yusuf et al., 2010)) and RA susceptibility, combined with the clear socioeconomic patterns in obesity and overweightness, makes it plausibly central to SES differences in arthritis incidence and outcomes.

Other lifestyle factors have less homogeneous affiliations with the rheumatic diseases, although they obviously remain important in the health status of patients. For instance, cigarette smoking does not independently increase the risk of OA and may even have a small protective effect (Felson & Zhang, 2015); conversely, smoking is a major preventable risk factor for seropositive RA, as it strongly interacts with a family of human leukocyte antigen (HLA) alleles promoting the self-recognition of post-translationally modified proteins found in the inflamed lungs (Klareskog & Catrina, 2015).

The powerful, genetically moderated relationship between cigarette smoking and RA is currently suspected to involve lung inflammation rather than nicotine compounds, and case-control studies have found a greater RA risk among workers occupationally exposed to irritating dusts (Olsson et al., 2004; Stolt et al., 2005). These data open the door to a possible role for atmospheric lung irritants in RA pathogenesis (Farhat et al., 2011) and, to the extent that exposure to air quality is unevenly distributed across socioeconomic strata, exposure to inflammatory air pollutants could constitute a link from SES to RA risk. This notwithstanding, the literature on air pollution and RA is in its infancy and the data remain inconclusive (Hart et al., 2013; Hart, Laden, Puett, Costenbader, & Karlson, 2009).

The access to, utilization, and effectiveness of healthcare services, particularly specialist care, vary broadly by SES, even among societies with universal care (Dixon et al., 2007; Veugelers & Yip, 2003). These patterns are a plausible factor driving health outcomes disparities in arthritis, especially considering the high costs of some key treatments. Notably, socioeconomic patterns in

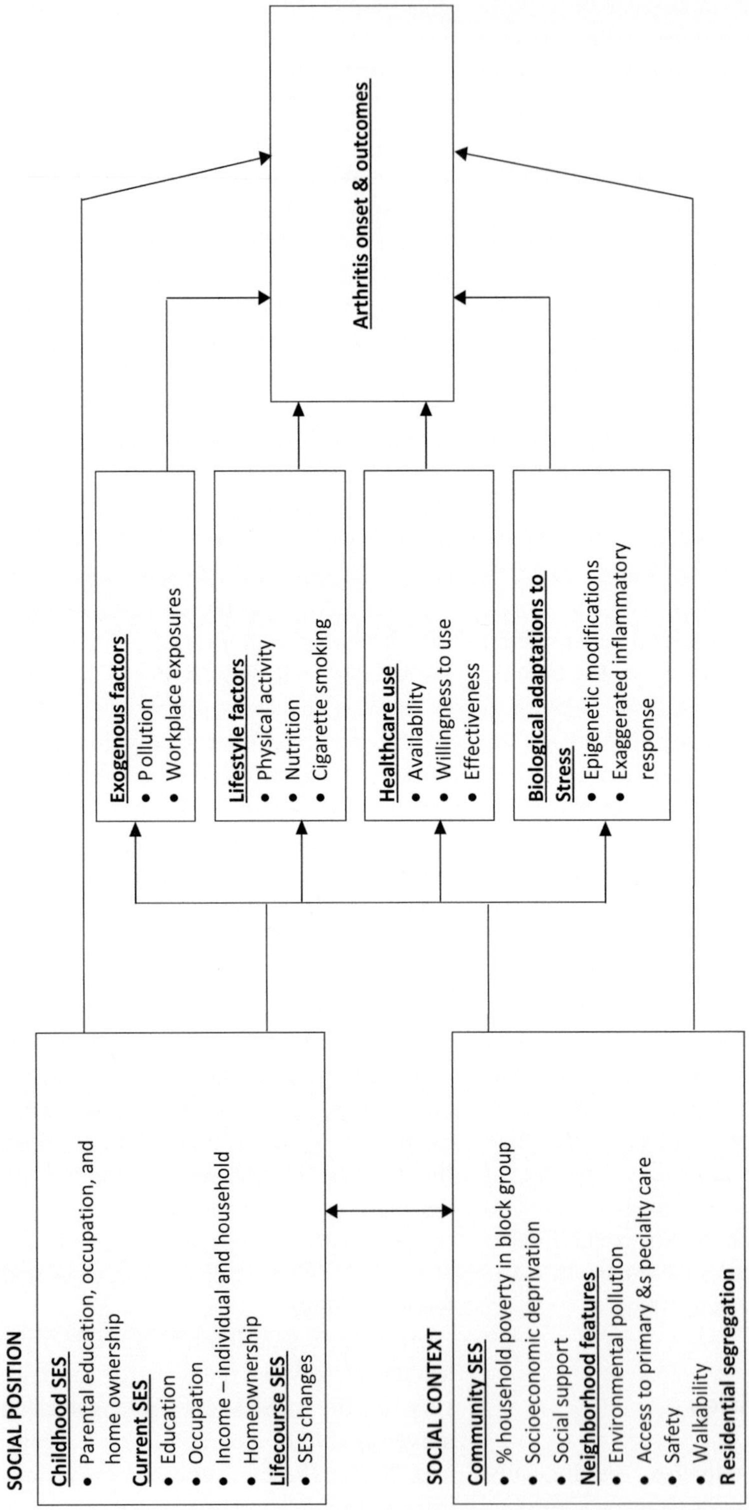

Fig. 6.1 Theoretical framework linking socioeconomic status to arthritis onset and outcomes

the utilization of TJR among OA patients are well-established (Dixon, Shaw, Ebrahim, & Dieppe, 2004) and may stem from not only financial strain, but also from socioeconomic differences in treatment preference, health literacy, and effective communication with healthcare providers. In RA, time-to-diagnosis, a critical component of disease management, is delayed among low SES individuals (Molina, Del Rincon, Restrepo, Battafarano, & Escalante, 2015) and the utilization of biologic medications likewise follows socioeconomic patterns likely contributing to inequities in disease activity (Schmajuk et al., 2011).

Psychosocial factors likely constitute a chief mechanism underlying health disparities. There is strong evidence for socioeconomic patterns in exposure to stress and in key characteristics modulating the stress response such as coping skills and threat perception (Matthews, Gallo, & Taylor, 2010). The importance of psychosocial factors is apparent in arthritis: notably, the experience of grave childhood adversity has robust, independent associations with arthritis susceptibility (Fuller-Thomson, Stefanyk, & Brennenstuhl, 2009; Springer, Sheridan, Kuo, & Carnes, 2007; Walker et al., 1997). While the precise biological systems linking psychosocial states to arthritis pathogenesis remain unclear, recent findings have shown that biological adaptations to chronic stress may lastingly dysregulate the inflammatory response (Azad et al., 2012; Carroll, Cohen, & Marsland, 2011). It is possible that such dysregulation may constitute a potential pathway for the onset of arthritis, and more research is needed to address this important question.

References

Adler, N. E., Boyce, T., Chesney, M. A., Cohen, S., Folkman, S., Kahn, R. L., & Syme, S. L. (1994). Socioeconomic status and health: The challenge of the gradient. *American Psychologist, 49*(1), 15.

Agabiti, N., Picciotto, S., Cesaroni, G., Bisanti, L., Forastiere, F., Onorati, R., … Spadea, T. (2007). The influence of socioeconomic status on utilization and outcomes of elective total hip replacement: A multicity population-based longitudinal study. *International Journal for Quality in Health Care, 19*(1), 37–44.

Alarcón, G. S., Bastian, H. M., Beasley, T. M., Roseman, J. M., Tan, F. K., Fessler, B. J., … Group, L. S. (2006). Systemic lupus erythematosus in a multi-ethnic cohort (LUMINA): Contributions of admixture and socioeconomic status to renal involvement. *Lupus, 15*(1), 26–31. doi:10.1191/0961203306lu2260oa.

Alarcon, G. S., McGwin, G., Jr., Sanchez, M. L., Bastian, H. M., Fessler, B. J., Friedman, A. W., … Reveille, J. D. (2004). Systemic lupus erythematosus in three ethnic groups. XIV. Poverty, wealth, and their influence on disease activity. *Arthritis and Rheumatism, 51*(1), 73–77. doi:10.1002/art.20085.

Allaire, S., Wolfe, F., Niu, J., LaValley, M. P., Zhang, B., & Reisine, S. (2009). Current risk factors for work disability associated with rheumatoid arthritis: Recent data from a US national cohort. *Arthritis and Rheumatism, 61*(3), 321–328. doi:10.1002/art.24281.

Anderson, J. J., & Felson, D. T. (1988). Factors associated with osteoarthritis of the knee in the first national health and nutrition examination survey (HANES I): Evidence for an association with overweight, race, and physical demands of work. *American Journal of Epidemiology, 128*(1), 179–189.

Andrianakos, A. A., Kontelis, L. K., Karamitsos, D. G., Aslanidis, S. I., Georgountzos, A. I., Kaziolas, G. O., … Group, E. S. (2006). Prevalence of symptomatic knee, hand, and hip osteoarthritis in Greece. The ESORDIG study. *The Journal of Rheumatology, 33*(12), 2507–2513.

Azad, M. B., Lissitsyn, Y., Miller, G. E., Becker, A. B., HayGlass, K. T., & Kozyrskyj, A. L. (2012). Influence of socioeconomic status trajectories on innate immune responsiveness in children. *PLoS One, 7*(6), e38669. doi:10.1371/journal.pone.0038669.

Baldassari, A. R., Cleveland, R. J., & Callahan, L. F. (2013a). Independent associations of childhood and current socioeconomic status with risk of self-reported doctor-diagnosed arthritis in a family-medicine cohort of North-Carolinians. *BMC Musculoskeletal Disorders, 14*(1), 327.

Baldassari, A. R., Cleveland, R. J., & Callahan, L. F. (2013b). Independent influences of current and childhood socioeconomic status on health outcomes in a North Carolina family practice sample of arthritis patients. *Arthritis Care & Research, 65*(8), 1334–1342.

Baldassari, A. R., Cleveland, R. J., Jonas, B. L., Conn, D. L., Moreland, L. W., Bridges, S. L., & Callahan, L. F. (2014). Socioeconomic disparities in the health of African Americans with rheumatoid arthritis from the Southeastern United States. *Arthritis Care & Research, 66*(12), 1808–1817.

Bankhead, C., Silman, A., Barrett, B., Scott, D., & Symmons, D. (1996). Incidence of rheumatoid arthritis is not related to indicators of socioeconomic deprivation. *The Journal of Rheumatology, 23*(12), 2039–2042.

Barton, J. L., Trupin, L., Schillinger, D., Gansky, S. A., Tonner, C., Margaretten, M., … Yelin, E. (2011). Racial and ethnic disparities in disease activity and function among persons with rheumatoid arthritis from university-affiliated clinics. *Arthritis Care &*

Research (Hoboken), 63(9), 1238–1246. doi:10.1002/acr.20525.

Bengtsson, C., Nordmark, B., Klareskog, L., Lundberg, I., & Alfredsson, L. (2005). Socioeconomic status and the risk of developing rheumatoid arthritis: Results from the Swedish EIRA study. *Annals of the Rheumatic Diseases, 64*(11), 1588–1594. doi:10.1136/ard.2004.031666.

Ben-Shlomo, Y., & Kuh, D. (2002). A life course approach to chronic disease epidemiology: Conceptual models, empirical challenges and interdisciplinary perspectives. *International Journal of Epidemiology, 31*(2), 285–293.

Bergström, U., Jacobsson, L. T., Nilsson, J.-Å., Berglund, G., & Turesson, C. (2011). Pulmonary dysfunction, smoking, socioeconomic status and the risk of developing rheumatoid arthritis. *Rheumatology, 50*(11), 2005–2013.

Berkanovic, E., Oster, P., Wong, W. K., Bulpitt, K., Clements, P., Sterz, M., & Paulus, H. (1996). The relationship between socioeconomic status and recently diagnosed rheumatoid arthritis. *Arthritis Care & Research, 9*(6), 257–262.

Bertoli, A. M., Vilá, L. M., Reveille, J. D., Alarcón, G. S., & LUMINA Study Group. (2008). Systemic lupus erythaematosus in a multiethnic US cohort (LUMINA) LIII: Disease expression and outcome in acute onset lupus. *Annals of the Rheumatic Diseases, 67*(4), 500–504. doi:10.1136/ard.2007.076059.

Blackwell, D. L., Hayward, M. D., & Crimmins, E. M. (2001). Does childhood health affect chronic morbidity in later life? *Social Science and Medicine, 52*(8), 1269–1284.

Bombard, J. M., Powell, K. E., Martin, L. M., Helmick, C. G., & Wilson, W. H. (2005). Validity and reliability of self-reported arthritis: Georgia senior centers, 2000–2001. *American Journal of Preventive Medicine, 28*(3), 251–258.

Brekke, M., Hjortdahl, P., Thelle, D. S., & Kvien, T. K. (1999). Disease activity and severity in patients with rheumatoid arthritis: Relations to socioeconomic inequality. *Social Science and Medicine, 48*(12), 1743–1750.

Brennan, S., & Turrell, G. (2012). Neighborhood disadvantage, individual-level socioeconomic position, and self-reported chronic arthritis: A cross-sectional multilevel study. *Arthritis Care & Research, 64*(5), 721–728.

Busija, L., Hollingsworth, B., Buchbinder, R., & Osborne, R. H. (2007). Role of age, sex, and obesity in the higher prevalence of arthritis among lower socioeconomic groups: A population-based survey. *Arthritis Care & Research, 57*(4), 553–561.

Callahan, L. F., Cleveland, R. J., Shreffler, J., Schwartz, T. A., Schoster, B., Randolph, R., … Jordan, J. M. (2011). Associations of educational attainment, occupation and community poverty with knee osteoarthritis in the Johnston County (North Carolina) osteoarthritis project. *Arthritis Research and Therapy, 13*(5), R169.

Callahan, L. F., Martin, K. R., Shreffler, J., Kumar, D., Schoster, B., Kaufman, J. S., & Schwartz, T. A. (2011). Independent and combined influence of homeownership, occupation, education, income, and community poverty on physical health in persons with arthritis. *Arthritis Care & Research, 63*(5), 643–653. doi:10.1002/acr.20428.

Callahan, L. F., & Pincus, T. (1988). Formal education level as a significant marker of clinical status in rheumatoid arthritis. *Arthritis and Rheumatism, 31*(11), 1346–1357.

Callahan, L. F., Shreffler, J., Mielenz, T., Schoster, B., Kaufman, J. S., Xiao, C., … Sloane, P. D. (2008). Arthritis in the family practice setting: Associations with education and community poverty. *Arthritis Care & Research, 59*(7), 1002–1008. doi:10.1002/art.23834.

Callahan, L. F., Shreffler, J., Siaton, B. C., Helmick, C. G., Schoster, B., Schwartz, T. A., … Jordan J. M. (2010). Limited educational attainment and radiographic and symptomatic knee osteoarthritis: A cross-sectional analysis using data from the Johnston County (North Carolina) Osteoarthritis Project. *Arthritis Research and Therapy, 12*(2), R46.

Cañizares, M., Power, J. D., Perruccio, A. V., & Badley, E. M. (2008). Association of regional racial/cultural context and socioeconomic status with arthritis in the population: A multilevel analysis. *Arthritis Care & Research, 59*(3), 399–407. doi:10.1002/art.23316.

Carlens, C., Jacobsson, L., Brandt, L., Cnattingius, S., Stephansson, O., & Askling, J. (2009). Perinatal characteristics, early life infections and later risk of rheumatoid arthritis and juvenile idiopathic arthritis. *Annals of the Rheumatic Diseases, 68*(7), 1159–1164. doi:10.1136/ard.2008.089342.

Carroll, J. E., Cohen, S., & Marsland, A. L. (2011). Early childhood socioeconomic status is associated with circulating interleukin-6 among mid-life adults. *Brain, Behavior, and Immunity, 25*(7), 1468–1474. doi:10.1016/j.bbi.2011.05.016.

Clement, N. D., Muzammil, A., MacDonald, D., Howie, C. R., & Biant, L. C. (2011). Socioeconomic status affects the early outcome of total hip replacement. *Journal of Bone and Joint Surgery (British Volume), 93-B*(4), 464–469. doi:10.1302/0301-620x.93b4.25717.

Cleveland, R. J., Schwartz, T. A., Prizer, L. P., Randolph, R., Schoster, B., Renner, J. B., … Callahan, L. F. (2013). Associations of educational attainment, occupation, and community poverty with hip osteoarthritis. *Arthritis Care & Research, 65*(6), 954–961. doi:10.1002/acr.21920.

Cunningham, J. (2011). Socioeconomic disparities in self-reported arthritis for Indigenous and non-Indigenous Australians aged 18–64. *International Journal of Public Health, 56*(3), 295–304.

Dadoun, S., Zeboulon-Ktorza, N., Combescure, C., Elhai, M., Rozenberg, S., Gossec, L., & Fautrel, B. (2013). Mortality in rheumatoid arthritis over the last fifty years: Systematic review and meta-analysis. *Joint, Bone, Spine, 80*(1), 29–33. doi:10.1016/j.jbspin.2012.02.005.

Dixon, A., Le Grand, J., Henderson, J., Murray, R., & Poteliakhoff, E. (2007). Is the British National Health Service equitable? The evidence on socioeconomic differences in utilization. *Journal of Health Services Research & Policy, 12*(2), 104–109. doi:10.1258/135581907780279549.

Dixon, T., Shaw, M., Ebrahim, S., & Dieppe, P. (2004). Trends in hip and knee joint replacement: Socioeconomic inequalities and projections of need. *Annals of the Rheumatic Diseases, 63*(7), 825–830.

ERAS Study Group. (2000). Socioeconomic deprivation and rheumatoid disease: What lessons for the health service? Early Rheumatoid Arthritis Study. *Annals of the Rheumatic Diseases, 59*(10), 794–799.

Farhat, S. C. L., Silva, C. A., Orione, M. A. M., Campos, L. M. A., Sallum, A. M. E., & Braga, A. L. F. (2011). Air pollution in autoimmune rheumatic diseases: A review. *Autoimmunity Reviews, 11*(1), 14–21. doi:10.1016/j.autrev.2011.06.008.

Feldman, C. H., Hiraki, L. T., Liu, J., Fischer, M. A., Solomon, D. H., Alarcón, G. S., … Costenbader, K. H. (2013). Epidemiology and sociodemographics of systemic lupus erythematosus and lupus nephritis among US adults with Medicaid coverage, 2000–2004. *Arthritis and Rheumatism, 65*(3), 753–763. doi:10.1002/art.37795.

Felson, D. T., & Zhang, Y. (2015). Smoking and osteoarthritis: A review of the evidence and its implications. *Osteoarthritis and Cartilage, 23*(3), 331–333. doi:10.1016/j.joca.2014.11.022.

Frisell, T., Holmqvist, M., Källberg, H., Klareskog, L., Alfredsson, L., & Askling, J. (2013). Familial risks and heritability of rheumatoid arthritis: Role of rheumatoid factor/anti-citrullinated protein antibody status, number and type of affected relatives, sex, and age. *Arthritis and Rheumatism, 65*(11), 2773–2782. doi:10.1002/art.38097.

Fuller-Thomson, E., Stefanyk, M., & Brennenstuhl, S. (2009). The robust association between childhood physical abuse and osteoarthritis in adulthood: Findings from a representative community sample. *Arthritis and Rheumatism, 61*(11), 1554–1562. doi:10.1002/art.24871.

Gabriel, S. E. (2001). The epidemiology of rheumatoid arthritis. *Rheumatic Disease Clinics of North America, 27*(2), 269–281.

Galobardes, B., Smith, G. D., & Lynch, J. W. (2006). Systematic review of the influence of childhood socioeconomic circumstances on risk for cardiovascular disease in adulthood. *Annals of Epidemiology, 16*(2), 91–104.

Ghawi, H., Crowson, C. S., Rand-Weaver, J., Krusemark, E., Gabriel, S. E., & Juhn, Y. J. (2015). A novel measure of socioeconomic status using individual housing data to assess the association of SES with rheumatoid arthritis and its mortality: A population-based case-control study. *BMJ Open, 5*(4), e006469. doi:10.1136/bmjopen-2014-006469.

Grotle, M., Hagen, K. B., Natvig, B., Dahl, F. A., & Kvien, T. K. (2008). Prevalence and burden of osteoarthritis: Results from a population survey in Norway. *The Journal of Rheumatology, 35*(4), 677–684.

Hannan, M. T., Anderson, J. J., Pincus, T., & Felson, D. T. (1992). Educational attainment and osteoarthritis: Differential associations with radiographic changes and symptom reporting. *Journal of Clinical Epidemiology, 45*(2), 139–147. doi:10.1016/0895-4356(92)90006-9.

Harrison, M. J., Tricker, K. J., Davies, L., Hassell, A., Dawes, P., Scott, D. L., … Symmons, D. P. (2005). The relationship between social deprivation, disease outcome measures, and response to treatment in patients with stable, long-standing rheumatoid arthritis. *The Journal of Rheumatology, 32*(12), 2330–2336.

Hart, J. E., Källberg, H., Laden, F., Costenbader, K. H., Yanosky, J. D., Klareskog, L., … Karlson, E. W. (2013). Ambient air pollution exposures and risk of rheumatoid arthritis. *Arthritis Care & Research (Hoboken), 65*(7), 1190–1196. doi:10.1002/acr.21975.

Hart, J. E., Laden, F., Puett, R. C., Costenbader, K. H., & Karlson, E. W. (2009). Exposure to traffic pollution and increased risk of rheumatoid arthritis. *Environmental Health Perspectives, 117*(7), 1065–1069.

Hayward, R. A., Rathod, T., Roddy, E., Muller, S., Hider, S. L., & Mallen, C. D. (2013). The association of gout with socioeconomic status in primary care: A cross-sectional observational study. *Rheumatology, 52*(11), 2004–2008. doi:10.1093/rheumatology/ket262.

Jaakkola, J. J., & Gissler, M. (2005). Maternal smoking in pregnancy as a determinant of rheumatoid arthritis and other inflammatory polyarthropathies during the first 7 years of life. *International Journal of Epidemiology, 34*(3), 664–671. doi:10.1093/ije/dyi006.

Jacobi, C. E., Mol, G. D., Boshuizen, H. C., Rupp, I., Dinant, H. J., & Van Den Bos, G. A. (2003). Impact of socioeconomic status on the course of rheumatoid arthritis and on related use of health care services. *Arthritis and Rheumatism, 49*(4), 567–573. doi:10.1002/art.11200.

Jenkins, P., Perry, P., Ng, C. Y., & Ballantyne, J. (2009). Deprivation influences the functional outcome from total hip arthroplasty. *The Surgeon, 7*(6), 351–356.

Karlson, E. W., Daltroy, L. H., Lew, R. A., Wright, E. A., Partridge, A. J., Roberts, W. N., … Liang, M. H. (1995). The independence and stability of socioeconomic predictors of morbidity in systemic lupus erythematosus. *Arthritis and Rheumatism, 38*(2), 267–273. doi:10.1002/art.1780380217.

Klareskog, L., & Catrina, A. I. (2015). Autoimmunity: Lungs and citrullination. *Nature Reviews. Rheumatology, 11*(5), 261–262.

Knight, J. B., Callahan, L. F., Luong, M.-L. N., Shreffler, J., Schoster, B., Renner, J. B., & Jordan, J. M. (2011). The association of disability and pain with individual and community socioeconomic status in people with hip osteoarthritis. *The Open Rheumatology Journal, 5*, 51–58. doi:10.2174/1874312901105010051.

Lawrence, R. C., Felson, D. T., Helmick, C. G., Arnold, L. M., Choi, H., Deyo, R. A., … Hunder, G. G. (2008). Estimates of the prevalence of arthritis and other rheumatic conditions in the United States: Part II. *Arthritis and Rheumatism, 58*(1), 26–35.

Leigh, J. P., & Fries, J. F. (1991a). Occupation, income, and education as independent covariates of arthritis in four national probability samples. *Arthritis and Rheumatism, 34*(8), 984–995.

Leigh, J. P., & Fries, J. F. (1991b). Education level and rheumatoid arthritis: Evidence from five data centers. *The Journal of Rheumatology, 18*(1), 24–34.

Linde, L., Sorensen, J., Ostergaard, M., Horslev-Petersen, K., Rasmussen, C., Jensen, D. V., & Hetland, M. L. (2009). What factors influence the health status of patients with rheumatoid arthritis measured by the SF-12v2 Health Survey and the Health Assessment Questionnaire? *The Journal of Rheumatology, 36*(10), 2183–2189. doi:10.3899/jrheum.090134.

Luong, M.-L. N., Cleveland, R. J., Nyrop, K. A., & Callahan, L. F. (2012). Social determinants and osteoarthritis outcomes. *Aging Health, 8*(4), 413–437. doi:10.2217/ahe.12.43.

Mackie, S. L., Taylor, J. C., Twigg, S., Martin, S. G., Steer, S., Worthington, J., … Morgan, A. W. (2012). Relationship between area-level socio-economic deprivation and autoantibody status in patients with rheumatoid arthritis: Multicentre cross-sectional study. *Annals of the Rheumatic Diseases, 71*(10), 1640–1645. doi:10.1136/annrheumdis-2011-201003.

Maiden, N., Capell, H., Madhok, R., Hampson, R., & Thomson, E. (1999). Does social disadvantage contribute to the excess mortality in rheumatoid arthritis patients? *Annals of the Rheumatic Diseases, 58*(9), 525–529.

Marra, C. A., Lynd, L. D., Esdaile, J. M., Kopec, J., & Anis, A. H. (2004). The impact of low family income on self-reported health outcomes in patients with rheumatoid arthritis within a publicly funded health-care environment. *Rheumatology (Oxford), 43*(11), 1390–1397. doi:10.1093/rheumatology/keh334.

Massardo, L., Pons-Estel, B. A., Wojdyla, D., Cardiel, M. H., Galarza-Maldonado, C. M., Sacnun, M. P., … Furst, D. E. (2012). Early rheumatoid arthritis in Latin America: Low socioeconomic status related to high disease activity at baseline. *Arthritis Care & Research (Hoboken), 64*(8), 1135–1143. doi:10.1002/acr.21680.

Matthews, K. A., Gallo, L. C., & Taylor, S. E. (2010). Are psychosocial factors mediators of socioeconomic status and health connections? *Annals of the New York Academy of Sciences, 1186*(1), 146–173. doi:10.1111/j.1749-6632.2009.05332.x.

McEntegart, A., Morrison, E., Capell, H. A., Duncan, M. R., Porter, D., Madhok, R., & Thomson, E. A. (1997). Effect of social deprivation on disease severity and outcome in patients with rheumatoid arthritis. *Annals of the Rheumatic Diseases, 56*(7), 410–413.

McWilliams, D. F., Leeb, B. F., Muthuri, S. G., Doherty, M., & Zhang, W. (2011). Occupational risk factors for osteoarthritis of the knee: A meta-analysis. *Osteoarthritis and Cartilage, 19*(7), 829–839. doi:10.1016/j.joca.2011.02.016.

Mishra, G., Nitsch, D., Black, S., De Stavola, B., Kuh, D., & Hardy, R. (2009). A structured approach to modelling the effects of binary exposure variables over the life course. *International Journal of Epidemiology, 38*(2), 528–537. doi:10.1093/ije/dyn229.

Molina, E., Del Rincon, I., Restrepo, J. F., Battafarano, D. F., & Escalante, A. (2015). Association of socioeconomic status with treatment delays, disease activity, joint damage and disability in rheumatoid arthritis. *Arthritis Care & Research (Hoboken), 67*(7), 940–946. doi:10.1002/acr.22542.

Oakes, J. M., & Rossi, P. H. (2003). The measurement of SES in health research: Current practice and steps toward a new approach. *Social Science & Medicine, 56*(4), 769–784.

Olsson, Å. R., Skogh, T., Axelson, O., & Wingren, G. (2004). Occupations and exposures in the work environment as determinants for rheumatoid arthritis. *Occupational and Environmental Medicine, 61*(3), 233–238. doi:10.1136/oem.2003.007971.

Olsson, Å. R., Skogh, T., & Wingren, G. (2001). Comorbidity and lifestyle, reproductive factors, and environmental exposures associated with rheumatoid arthritis. *Annals of the Rheumatic Diseases, 60*(10), 934–939.

Parks, C. G., D'Aloisio, A. A., DeRoo, L. A., Huiber, K., Rider, L. G., Miller, F. W., & Sandler, D. P. (2013). Childhood socioeconomic factors and perinatal characteristics influence development of rheumatoid arthritis in adulthood. *Annals of the Rheumatic Diseases, 72*(3), 350–356. doi:10.1136/annrheumdis-2011-201083.

Pedersen, M., Jacobsen, S., Klarlund, M., & Frisch, M. (2006). Socioeconomic status and risk of rheumatoid arthritis: A Danish case-control study. *The Journal of Rheumatology, 33*(6), 1069–1074.

Peter Wang, P., Elsbett-Koeppen, R., Geng, G.-Y., & Badley, E. M. (2000). Arthritis Prevalence and Place of Birth: Findings from the 1994 Canadian National Population Health Survey. *American Journal of Epidemiology, 152*(5), 442–445. doi:10.1093/aje/152.5.442.

Petri, M., Perez-Gutthann, S., Longenecker, J. C., & Hochberg, M. (1991). Morbidity of systemic lupus erythematosus: Role of race and socioeconomic status. *The American Journal of Medicine, 91*(4), 345–353. doi:10.1016/0002-9343(91)90151-M.

Pons-Estel, G. J., Alarcón, G. S., Scofield, L., Reinlib, L., & Cooper, G. S. (2010). Understanding the epidemiology and progression of systemic lupus erythematosus. *Seminars in Arthritis and Rheumatism, 39*(4), 257–268. doi:10.1016/j.semarthrit.2008.10.007.

Rodriguez-Amado, J., Moreno-Montoya, J., Alvarez-Nemegyei, J., Goycochea-Robles, M., Sanin, L., Burgos-Vargas, R., … Pelaez-Ballestas, I. (2014). The Social Gap Index and the prevalence of osteoarthritis in the community: A cross-sectional multilevel study in Mexico. *Clinical Rheumatology*, 1–8. doi:10.1007/s10067-014-2776-y.

Schmajuk, G., Trivedi, A. N., Solomon, D. H., Yelin, E., Trupin, L., Chakravarty, E. F., & Yazdany, J. (2011). Receipt of disease-modifying antirheumatic drugs among patients with rheumatoid arthritis in medicare managed care plans. *JAMA, 305*(5), 480–486. doi:10.1001/jama.2011.67.

Schneider, S., Schmitt, G., & Richter, W. (2006). Prevalence and correlates of inflammatory arthritis in Germany: Data from the First National Health Survey. *Rheumatology International, 27*(1), 29–38. doi:10.1007/s00296-006-0153-0.

Silman, A. J., Newman, J., & Macgregor, A. J. (1996). Cigarette smoking increases the risk of rheumatoid arthritis: Results from a nationwide study of disease-discordant twins. *Arthritis and Rheumatism, 39*(5), 732–735.

Springer, K. W., Sheridan, J., Kuo, D., & Carnes, M. (2007). Long-term physical and mental health consequences of childhood physical abuse: Results from a large population-based sample of men and women. *Child Abuse and Neglect, 31*(5), 517–530. doi:10.1016/j.chiabu.2007.01.003.

Stolt, P., Källberg, H., Lundberg, I., Sjögren, B., Klareskog, L., & Alfredsson, L. (2005). Silica exposure is associated with increased risk of developing rheumatoid arthritis: Results from the Swedish EIRA study. *Annals of the Rheumatic Diseases, 64*(4), 582–586. doi:10.1136/ard.2004.022053.

Taylor, W., Smeets, L., Hall, J., & McPherson, K. (2004). The burden of rheumatic disorders in general practice: Consultation rates for rheumatic disease and the relationship to age, ethnicity, and small-area deprivation. *New Zealand Medical Journal, 117*(1203), U1098.

Tepper, S., & Hochberg, M. C. (1993). Factors associated with hip osteoarthritis: Data from the First National Health and Nutrition Examination Survey (NHANES-I). *American Journal of Epidemiology, 137*(10), 1081–1088.

Tikly, M., Bellingan, A., Lincoln, D., & Russell, A. (1998). Risk factors for gout: A hospital-based study in urban black South Africans. *Revue du Rhumatisme (English Ed.), 65*(4), 225–231.

Townsend, P., & Davidson, N. (1992). *Inequalities in health: The Black report*. Harmondsworth, UK: Penguin.

Uhlig, T., Hagen, K., & Kvien, T. (1999). Current tobacco smoking, formal education, and the risk of rheumatoid arthritis. *The Journal of Rheumatology, 26*(1), 47–54.

US Department of Health and Human Services and Office of Disease Prevention and Health Promotion. (2012). *Healthy people 2020*. Washington, DC: US Department of Health and Human Services and Office of Disease Prevention and Health Promotion.

Veugelers, P. J., & Yip, A. M. (2003). Socioeconomic disparities in health care use: Does universal coverage reduce inequalities in health? *Journal of Epidemiology and Community Health, 57*(6), 424–428. doi:10.1136/jech.57.6.424.

Vliet Vlieland, T. P., Buitenhuis, N. A., van Zeben, D., Vandenbroucke, J. P., Breedveld, F. C., & Hazes, J. M. (1994). Sociodemographic factors and the outcome of rheumatoid arthritis in young women. *Annals of the Rheumatic Diseases, 53*(12), 803–806.

Walker, E. A., Keegan, D., Gardner, G., Sullivan, M., Bernstein, D., & Katon, W. J. (1997). Psychosocial factors in fibromyalgia compared with rheumatoid arthritis: II. Sexual, physical, and emotional abuse and neglect. *Psychosomatic Medicine, 59*(6), 572–577.

Williams, D. R., Mohammed, S. A., Leavell, J., & Collins, C. (2010). Race, socioeconomic status, and health: Complexities, ongoing challenges, and research opportunities. *Annals of the New York Academy of Sciences, 1186*(1), 69–101.

Yusuf, E., Nelissen, R., Ioan-Facsinay, A., Stojanovic-Susulic, V., DeGroot, J., van Osch, G., … Kloppenburg, M. (2010). Association between weight or Body Mass Index and hand osteoarthritis: A systematic review. *Annals of the Rheumatic Diseases, 69*(4), 761–765. doi:10.1136/ard.2008.106930.

Ziol-Guest, K. M., Duncan, G. J., Kalil, A., & Boyce, W. T. (2012). Early childhood poverty, immune-mediated disease processes, and adult productivity. *Proceedings of the National Academy of Sciences of the United States of America, 109*(Suppl 2), 17289–17293. doi:10.1073/pnas.1203167109.

The Heart of Clinical Relationships: Doctor–Patient Communication in Rheumatology

7

M. Cameron Hay

Introduction

What makes for the best clinical relationships in rheumatology? In reflecting on an appointment, one patient praised his rheumatologist saying, "Her patients might get well just by talking to her!" Although hyperbole, this highlights the key importance of communication as the heart of a solid clinical relationship.

There is no magic formula for excellent communications during clinical interactions, but research has identified the ingredients that make excellent doctor–patient communications possible. The foundation of clinical communication in rheumatology is clinical competence, and thus our discussion starts there, with the recognition that clinical competence must be balanced by communicative competence. Communicative competence necessitates the ability to anticipate expectations, frame interactions appropriately, listen empathically, and provide the needed care, all within the external constraints of a clinical appointment time-slot.

M.C. Hay, PhD (✉)
Department of Anthropology, Miami University, Oxford, Ohio, USA

Center for Culture and Health, Semel Institute for Neuroscience and Human Behavior, UCLA, Los Angeles, California, USA
e-mail: hayrolmc@miamioh.edu

Throughout this chapter, illustrative examples are drawn from original anthropological data collected in two rheumatology clinics in a major American medical center. The IRB-approved study included interviews and audio-recordings of doctor–patient interactions for 8 rheumatologists and 121 of their patients at every appointment over a 20-month period. In this chapter, comments and dialogue illustrate dynamics affecting doctor–patient communications in rheumatology.

In comparison to other medical fields, doctor–patient communication in rheumatology has not received much attention (Suarez-Almazor, 2004), despite the fact that communication may be particularly critical in caring for patients with the chronic, debilitating, incurable diseases common to rheumatology. The excellent available work on doctor-patient communication in rheumatology (e.g. Daltroy, 1993; Suarez-Almazor, 2004), is augmented by work from other scholarly perspectives including sociology (e.g., Heritage & Maynard, 2006a, 2006b; Waitzkin, 1993), psychology/psychiatry (e.g., Hahn et al., 1993; Halpern, 2001; Mishler, 1984; Moore et al., 2004), public health (e.g., Hall, Roter, Milburn & Daltroy, 1996; Roter, 1977), and law (e.g., Katz, 1984). To this scholarly conversation, anthropologists contribute a holistic perspective, linking the micro-level analysis of individual concerns and clinical dialogues with macro-level social-cultural processes (e.g., Good, 1994, 1995; Kleinman, 1995; Rouse, 2009, 2010). In this

P.M. Nicassio (ed.), *Psychosocial Factors in Arthritis*, DOI 10.1007/978-3-319-22858-7_7

chapter, doctor–patient communication is examined incorporating both patients' and rheumatologists' perspectives.

The Two Legs of Competence

There are over 150 rheumatic conditions, many of which are complex, autoimmune disorders difficult to diagnosis and even more difficult to manage. It is unsurprising then that clinical competence is central to training in rheumatology to ensure the consistent application of the highest standards of care (Rudd & Bosch, 1966; Woolf, 2002). Rheumatic disorders are often systemic and many are rare, thus a physician in general practice may not have ever seen a case of systemic sclerosis, for example, and thus not pick up on the clues that would include it as a differential. When a patient comes to a rheumatologist, it is usually after a circuitous road with many physicians guessing at different diagnoses and trying different treatments along the way (e.g., Salt & Peden, 2011). Patients in our study commonly had seen multiple physicians before finally getting a diagnosis that made sense and led to a treatment that worked. As one patient said, "I can't do anything other than doing nothing 'cause I don't have the stamina. It could be lupus, rheumatoid arthritis, it could be muscular, fibromyalgia. It could be, it could be laziness. I want some kind of diagnosis. I want answers." Another reported: "I'd had 5–6 hospitalizations …before coming here. They couldn't figure out what was wrong with me. I had a whole team of specialists…. I was bleeding from everywhere, and no one knew what was wrong. I was close to death, and that's when I came here, and I've been coming back ever since." The clinical competence that enables rheumatologists to provide answers to contain diverse and frightening symptoms with a diagnosis is an essential component of patient care.

However, treating patients with clinical competence alone is like trying to stand on one leg. One may be able to do it for a while, but it is difficult to stay balanced for long and nearly impossible to move forward gracefully especially over any distance. Because almost all rheumatological conditions are chronic, a rheumatologist–patient relationship is one that must be sustainable over the long haul. Rheumatologists need a second leg to stand on, and that second leg is communicative competence. Indeed, the American College of Rheumatology curriculum includes interpersonal skills and communication among its recommended core competencies, although the extent to which programs provide dedicated time and training in these skills varies substantially and indeed may not be explicitly addressed at all (Patwardhan, Henrickson, Laskosz, Duyenhong, & Spencer, 2014).

Communicative competence is a concept originally developed by linguistic anthropologist, Dell Hymes (2001), to argue against Chomsky's (1965) notion that mastery of a language could be achieved with grammatical and lexical accuracy. Hymes (2001) contended that communication depends on awareness of the social-cultural context, semiotic assumptions, and potential interpretations of speech. In other words, the goal of language is not linguistic mastery per se, but communicative competence with its ability to convey meaning successfully in interactions. To become medical professionals, providers spend years mastering the Latin lexicon of medicine and learning how to communicate as a professional to other professionals: to summarize cases and write soap notes with all of the medically relevant information and omitting "extraneous" details such as the consequences of disease on patient's lives (Good & Delvecchio Good, 1993; Konner, 1987). "Soap" is an acronym standing for the key elements of a case description needed for patient charts: subjective findings (patient-reported complaints), objective (physical and laboratory findings), assessment (differential diagnosis), and plan (treatment strategy). Physicians sometimes recorded soap notes orally during clinical interactions, and in them we can see clearly Mishler's "voice of medicine" (1984):

> Patient is a 41-year-old woman with joint pain of approximately 4 months duration. Patient had the onset of pain in her right hip region …The pain became more severe and she had difficulty walking, subsequently the pain progressed to involve the left hip on the medial aspect of the thigh, and uh, subsequently with swelling of the knees, hands,

elbows, ankles, tops of the feet, temporal-mandibular joint, and uh, cervical spine… She was started on Prednisone …. This has been of partial but not complete benefit to her. Uh, the uh, over the last three weeks the patient has been unable to work. ….

The oral soap notes continued with the numerical findings from her bloodwork, a review of her "systems" (e.g., "chest was clear to percussion auscultation"), findings from the rheumatologic examination (e.g., "tenderness of several of the MCP's"), an assessment that she has markers of early rheumatoid arthritis, and concludes with a recommendation that "Laboratory profile needs to be filed on a regular basis to see if there's conversion of her laboratory tests to positive." In other words, the physician is so clinically competent that he correctly recognizes the disease prior to laboratory confirmation.

This soap note hardly hints at the impact her condition has had on her lifeworld, other than to note her "difficulty walking" and being "unable to work." The transcript of the entire doctor–patient interaction, however, is filled with the patient's tears, her husband's concerns that she is "very depressed," her worries about being on disability, and her helplessness at being "in bed for days" overwhelmed by pain. None of this enters the medicalized case summary. The physician shows his awareness of how poorly she is doing when at one point he comments to the husband, "She's really not doing well." While it is clear that the physician understands how ill the patient is and how much pain she is in, the language of medicine requires that he mask it. While the patient and her husband were present when the physician dictated the note, they make no comment on it. Soap notes miss what is salient for patients: the disease's impact on their everyday lives. Physicians, to be communicatively competent, must go beyond what Mishler (1984) called the "voice of medicine"—the detached, technical, objectifying lexicon of medicine—and incorporate, at least with patients, the "voice of the lifeworld"—the everyday ways of speaking that highlight the problems and personal and emotional concerns that the patient feels are inextricably tied to illness.

The concept of the lifeworld (German, *Lebenswelt*) originated in philosophy with Husserl (1970) to denote the experience of actively engaging with others in the world. Schutz (1973) and Habermas (1984) augmented the understanding of lifeworld to include subjective experience of engaging in the shifting of meaningful activities and relationships of everyday life within the constraints of material circumstances. Mishler used the concept of lifeworld to highlight how patients frame disease in terms of their everyday lives (1984). While Mishler's focus was on the communicative gap between the voice of medicine and the voice of the lifeworld, more recent work has highlighted how engagement with the lifeworld is necessarily through embodiment or the medium of one's body—its senses and capabilities (Csordas, 1990; Desjarlais & Jason Throop, 2011; Jackson, 2012). Thus, the ways patients embody a disease fundamentally shape their daily experiences to engage meaningfully with their dynamic lifeworlds. For a patient, talking about their lifeworld is an effort to draw physicians into the experiences that matter most to them.

It is difficult to master the kind of communicative competence that enables a physician to smoothly code-switch from the professional medical language and ways of speaking (e.g., summarizing and treating a "case") to a way of speaking that engages with the patient-at-hand's embodied experience within his or her lifeworld. While some patients expect physicians to fully engage with their lifeworld concerns, others strive to themselves code-switch into the language of medicine, seeing it as their responsibility.

For example, consider the interaction below, taken from the patient's third appointment, after the patient had started treatment and heard the diagnosis name multiple times at previous appointments. In those previous appointments, the physician had never explained the disease, nor had the patient ever asked. The transcription below is written for readability, highlighting only a few markers of speech: pauses such as "(…5)" indicates a 5-s pause, often marking hesitation and concern to frame speech in a socially acceptable way, laughter such as "(h)," and brackets indicating overlapping speech. Below is an excerpt from the patient's interaction with his physician that begins with the physician's answer to the patient's question about the blood tests:

Dr: Yeah. Oh the tests that we did were negative.
Pt: Negative for (h) what things were we looking (h) [for…?
Dr: [Looking] for signs of significant inflammation. Looking for um (…1) uh any potential for another kind of arthritis, for Rheumatoid Arthritis, for instance on top of it. And it's negative. So that's good.
Pt: And so as you said it was sero negatives (…3)?
Dr: Spinal arthropathy.
Pt: Spinal arthropathy. Uh that, I want to go ahead and understand what that is. It is related to the psoriasis and the skin condition?
Dr: Yeah.
Pt: I guess I don't know much about psoriasis so I always thought psoriasis was just a skin condition, but it is can be related to the [blood] (…1) and…?
Dr: [It can be]
Dr: It can be related to arthritis. About 15 % of people with psoriasis also have arthritis with it.
Pt: Mmhmm.
Dr: In other words, a bulk of people don't.
Pt: Mmm.
Dr: When I was in medical school I was taught that psoriasis was a condition of healthy people.
Pt: Oh. (h) Okay.
Dr: So often that's all they had.
Pt: Mmhmm.
Dr: But we now know that there can be arthritis. And the arthritis can be significant. So we like to keep tabs on it and make sure it doesn't start eating up joints.
Pt: Mmhmm.
Dr: Because we now have very effective therapies for it.

Note that it has taken three visits for the patient to feel comfortable enough to ask what his diagnosis means and the reason for the tests he had already taken. The physician had not thought to translate the medical terms and tests for the patient. By using laughter to soften his questioning, the patient is indicating that he realizes he is straying into delicate waters and does so hesitantly (Haakana, 2001), using laughter to mark that the patient is striving not to create a breach in the relationship (Jefferson, 2004). This careful framing on the part of the patient does not successfully communicate to the physician how intent the patient is in gaining an informed understanding of his condition. The patient then drops the laughter frame, seeking to understand if spinal arthopathy is related to psoriasis and skin conditions. Rather than elaborating, the physician just says "Yeah." The patient tries again, framing his statement with blanks that the physician needs to fill in by ending the "and" with the rising intonation of a question. The physician fills in with statistics. The patient encourages further information with his "mmhmm"'s and "oh" continuers, indicating that he is listening intently. But the physician does not go into the details of the disease, simply confirming that psoriasis can be connected with arthritis and can start "eating up joints," which sounds ominous until the physician transitions to the topic of treatment with "very effective therapies." In essence, the physician suggests that the simplistic understanding offered is all the information the patient needs. The physician maintains control of expert information, overly simplifying for the patient what the physician thinks the patient needs to know. Is this communicative competence?

A pub-med search for communicative competence primarily brings up literature on how to teach communicative competence to those who lack fundamental skills in talking, hearing, and appropriately interacting in a social scenario: normal infants, children, and adults on the autism spectrum, or people with auditory challenges (Happé, 1993; Ochs & Schieffelin, 2008; Teachman & Gibson, 2014). There are some writings on communicative competence for healthcare providers, primarily on testing for communicative competence in medical schools (e.g., Gillotti, Thompson, & McNeilis, 2002) or on the challenges of communicating to patients with different cultural assumptions about health and illness (e.g., Gregg & Saha, 2007). But largely communicative competence is something healthcare providers are assumed to master over time and the accumulation of experience in the clinic; the problem, of course, is that the mastery of communication in the clinic involves mastery of social nuances, as subtle as the clinical nuances of rheumatoid arthritis and as easy to miss.

Why Is Doctor–Patient Communication Difficult?

"One of the essential qualities of the clinician is interest in humanity, for the secret of the care of the patient is in caring for the patient" (Peabody, 1927).

The conclusion of the Peabody address to medical students in 1927 is an oft-quoted reminder of the importance of the clinical relationship between doctors and patients. What is curious is that nearly a century after Peabody's revelation of the secret of the care of the patient, and despite countless studies and programs to improve clinical communications, doctor–patient relationships still can be challenging. There are three primary reasons for continuing difficulties in clinical relationships: (1) there is so much at stake for patients in the communications, (2) there are many external constraints on the communications, and (3) there is variation in expectations for patient and physician roles; in other words, in the twenty-first century there are shifting expectations for clinical appointments and what constitutes a good patient or a good physician within those appointments. In reverse order, each is outlined below.

The Changing Expectations of Patients and Physicians

The challenges of clinical relationships are magnified when curing is not an option, especially as the role expectations of American medicine were largely codified with acute or curable diseases in mind. Expectations are one's thoughts about what should occur during an appointment or interaction (Bell, Kravitz, Thom, & Krupat, 2002). According to Talcott Parsons who first outlined the expected roles of physicians and patients (Parsons, 1951), the physician as the expert in medical knowledge is expected to diagnose and treat disease, maintaining clinical distance from the patient. The patient's role is to give the physician information to facilitate diagnosis and to follow the physician's instructions so that he or she may quickly return to normal levels of productive life (Hay, 2006). In the heady decades of medical discoveries and breakthroughs—from methotrexate to Salk's polio vaccine to lung transplants—there was an expectation that medical knowledge could solve any problem (Fanu & Le, 1999), which itself reinforced Parsonian roles. The idea of the expert physician who wields the miracles of medicine on behalf of the compliant patient still seeps into clinical interactions; it is "part of the mythic world of the patient as well as the physician" (Kirmayer, 2000, p. 170).

While rheumatologists with the best technologies at their disposal have made enormous strides in lengthening life-spans, stabilizing disease, and improving quality of life, much of rheumatology consists of palliative care. The diseases tend to be chronic, painful, debilitating, and life-limiting so that even if patients follow physicians' instructions precisely, disease will continue to haunt them and their futures. The lack of a cure challenges classic expectations of physician and patient roles, leaving rheumatologists and their patients to negotiate a relationship that maximizes patient well-being and quality of life over the long term.

There is also a second problem with the classic roles as outlined by Parsons: they have been undermined by a convergence of processes encouraging distrust. These processes include increased availability of medical information combined with the consumerism of neoliberal economic policies and the empowerment movement of advocacy groups. Increasingly towards the end of the twentieth century, patients were deemed responsible for gathering information and making their own health decisions (Giddens, 1991). This is a dramatic shift away from the

Parsonian model in which the patient's only job was to follow the physician's directives.

Consumer advertising encouraged this neoliberal responsibility of the patient, while also reframing patient-consumers as responsible for providing information to the physician. In the United States, legal constraints on direct-to-consumer pharmaceutical advertising were relaxed so that by 1985 pharmaceutical companies could market their products directly to consumers in print ads using small print on risks associated with a medication (Ventola, 2011). In 1997 and again in 2004, the Federal Drug Administration further relaxed requirements, enabling pharmaceutical companies to market their drugs on broadcast television with minimal information on risks (Ventola, 2011). The advertisements, illustrating happy people living pain-free lives, regularly conclude that the consumer should "talk to your doctor to see if (*brand name*) is right for you." In so doing, pharmaceutical advertisements simultaneously undermined the image of the physician-as-expert and made the patient responsible for gathering information to ensure that they received the "right" prescription (Dumit, 2012).

Advocacy groups likewise gained momentum during the 1980s and 1990s and increasingly emphasized that patients must advocate for their own right to health. That advocacy was primarily directed at health insurers, funding agencies, and after the passing of the Americans with Disabilities Act in 1990, at employers (Heath, Rapp, & Taussig, 2007), but such activism required that patients argue on their own behalf, becoming empowered through knowledge acquisition. "Knowledge is power" was, by the early and mid-2000s, a common phrase on disease advocacy sites and patient-support media sites.

Over the same period that pharmaceutical companies exponentially increased their direct-to-consumer advertising framing patients as the ones who had to educate their physicians about medications, and advocacy groups framed patients as being responsible for "arming" themselves with knowledge, medical information became widely available online. In 1991, the world wide web was made publicly available, and by 1998, approximately 48 % of American households owned a computer and 26 % had access to the internet (National Science Board, 2000). That number too grew exponentially, so that by 2005, 66 % of American adults were using the internet (Fox & Rainie, 2014) and by 2006, 64 % were using the internet to search for health information (Fox, 2006). As early as 1999, Hardey could describe a world in which "the Internet forms the site of a new struggle over expertise in health that will transform the relationship between health professions and their clients" (1999, p. 820). Today the internet has become a key resource for patients, and it is increasingly used to self-diagnose, check, or even replace information from a physician (Fox & Duggan, 2013), but patients are not necessarily discussing that information with their physicians (Diaz et al., 2002; Hay et al., 2008).

The collusion of these three broader societal trends—direct-to-consumer pharmaceutical marketing, patient advocacy, and the availability of online health information—together reframed patients as responsible for educating themselves and their physicians about medications, advocating for themselves, and being the experts in their own healthcare. If one looks solely at these social trends, one could conclude that the physicians' role has become one of gatekeeper to diagnostic tests and prescriptions listening to the demands of the patient-consumer, and the patient must now be the expert, responsible for their own well-being. In fact, what has happened is that role expectations are unpredictable, making doctor–patient communications particularly challenging.

In rheumatology, a handful of studies on expectations suggest that patients' expectations are often unmet. In one study of patients who had established relationships with their physicians, one third of patients reported unmet expectations for their appointments (Rao, Weinberger, Anderson, & Kroenke, 2004). In another study of over 1000 patients, nearly 1/3 reported unmet health needs which were associated with poor health outcomes (Kjeken et al., 2006).

Given this, it is unsurprising that recommendations for rheumatologists include eliciting patient expectations at the outset of an appointment (Main, Buchbinder, Porcheret, & Foster, 2010). In our research, participating rheumatologists always began appointments with some version of the question, "What would you like to accomplish here today?", thereby soliciting patients' explicit wants or concerns, but role expectations are often unconscious notions of how an interaction should proceed and what responsibilities belong to whom. In the exit interviews, even though their explicit expectations had been solicited, it was not uncommon for patients to voice disappointment. Those disappointments often had less to do with explicit care or information received (cf. Rao et al., 2004), than with role expectations and concerns about trustworthiness. Patients want trusting relationships (e.g., Berrios-Rivera et al., 2006; Salt & Peden, 2011), but to demonstrate trust, caregivers must meet often unconscious expectations.

Based on our research on clinical interactions, some patients want a somewhat Parsonian doctor, an expert to make the decisions on their behalf, and the provider that welcomes patients as active decision-makers will have patients leave frustrated saying, "Who am I to decide? He's the expert!" (Notice that even those that want a Parsonian-style doctor still reserve the very twenty-first century right to grumble about the physician). Other patients judge the quality of care based on health outcomes: one patient noted "I really need to wait and see if this medication works before I can say for sure"—in other words, her evaluation of the physician's care would be based on her health outcome using a consumer logic. Most patients have expectations that fall somewhere along the continuum between these two extremes. Some are willing to take on a Parsonian patient role, but yearn for a non-Parsonian physician; as one patient put it, "You know, we have to be respectful of the doctor, because they are the doctors, but they aren't necessarily respectful of their patients." Some do not necessarily want to be partners, but they do want to be told all the relevant information, as one patient said, "He was just so condescending, very distant, as if I didn't know anything about it. Doctors have to have more humanity when talking to patients. Don't be dominant. The patient shouldn't be made to feel subservient." Other patients seem completely complacent in clinical interactions, accepting prescriptions and recommendations without question, only to double check online everything the physician says: "Well he wants me to go on something new. It's still experimental, and he said they don't know whether it'll help or not, but we're going to try it. I'm going to read up on it online before I start it though." Healthcare providers in the twenty-first century have to be equally ready for patients who want them to be the experts or to include patients as partners in decision-making, and for every possible role in between (e.g., Street, Gordon, Ward, Krupat, & Kravitz, 2005). Patient's expectations are wide-ranging, yet they are critical to meet because they have potential clinical consequences (Kravitz, 2001).

At this point, care providers might be tempted to throw up their hands in despair, and it is worth remembering that patients often feel the same way. The unpredictability of role expectations has made clinical interactions challenging, particularly given the structural constraints of clinical appointments.

Structural Constraints on Clinical Interactions

Clinical communication is typically seen as dyadic, between physician and patient. What is rarely taken into account are the external pressures on consultations that shape the contours of doctor–patient communications.

From the patient's point of view, seeing a physician means overcoming a series of barriers. First, one must find a provider who accepts one's insurance or Medicare, which may mean multiple inquiries, longer wait-times for appointments, and greater travel distance (e.g., Gillis et al., 2007; Hagglund, Clark, Hilton & Hewett, 2005). Second, one must make an appointment, and wait times for appointments in rheumatology can be significant ranging from 43 to 105 days (Hurst et al., 2000). While modifications in scheduling can lead to much quicker appointments (Newman, Harrington, Olenginski, & Perruquet, 2004), delays are often caused by the acute current shortage of rheumatologists (Badley & Davis, 2012; Deal et al., 2007). Studies have found that only between 25 and 34 % of patients were able to see a rheumatologist within 3 months of symptom onset (Deluarier, Bernatsky, Baron, Légaré, & Feldman, 2012; Jamal, Alibhai, Badley, & Bombardier, 2011), even though delays in treatment are known to have adverse affects on disease activity and function (e.g., Schneider & Krüger, 2013). Third, one must get to the appointment, which can be a significant concern in large urban centers, where the distance to the clinic and concerns about traffic may be significantly linked with the patient's wish to continue care (Agrawal et al., 2012). Fourth, for those patients who arrive late or become agitated in the waiting room, receptionists are often perceived as gatekeepers that a patient must get past to see the physician (Strathmann & Hay, 2008). Because clinics may overbook appointments to increase provider productivity (Laganga & Lawrence, 2007), these may lead to longer waiting room time and increased frustration for patients. Overall then, from the patient's point of view, while clinics should facilitate access to a physician, in fact, there are so many barriers that clinics may be perceived as thwarting access.

Once with the physician, patients find that their time is often constricted with appointment time slots dictated by clinic administrators. Short appointments are associated with a number of indicators of poor doctor–patient communication. For example, patients are five times more likely to report unmet expectations if their appointment was 10 min long or less (Rao et al., 2004; Ward, 2004). In rheumatology, initial appointment time slots may be more generous, with 40–60 min initial visit appointments. In our study, there were also occasions when appointments stretched to 2 h, if the physician deemed it necessary to give the patient needed care. When this happened, physicians felt the pressure of the bulging number of patients kept waiting for their appointments. According to a study of 422 general practitioners and internists (Linzer et al., 2009), over 50 % reported time pressure during consultations, over 48 % reported a chaotic work pace, and 26.5 % reported burnout. In a survey among rheumatologists, high stress levels with associated emotional exhaustion and high patient loads were both associated with low work satisfaction (McNearney, Hunnicutt, Maganti, & Rice, 2008). Rheumatologists spend disproportionate amounts of time in clinic and attending to the paperwork in comparison with other medical specialties (Foley, 2005), which was anecdotally noted in our study as well. One physician sighed that he used to see 36 patients a day in clinic, but now could barely handle 12–14 because of the increased paperwork. From the physicians' point of view, then, seeing a patient means working within the time-pressure and other administrative constraints of the clinic.

Constraints on clinical appointments directly affect communication. When a physician doesn't pay attention, interrupts, or initiates abrupt topic changes (e.g., Ainsworth-Vaughn, 1998; Waitzkin, 1993; West, 1993,1984), it undermines the patient's sense that his or her concerns are important. It was not uncommon for a physician to have to review the patient's files while gathering the patient's history: "Go ahead and tell me what happened. While I look at it your files, you tell me your version." Frequently, a few moments later the physician would have to interrupt the narrative, to ask the patient to repeat something: "I'm sorry…um—I was reading when you just said the last—What did you say there?" While it is easy to point a finger at physicians, in fact, relatively brief appointments are the real culprit. Brief appointments handicap a physician's ability to listen to patients' narratives—there simply isn't time. Thus, it isn't surprising that even though between 17 and 40 % of patients with arthritis have some kind of mood problem, brief appointments mean that depression is much less likely to be identified or treated (Nicassio, 2008). These external constraints on clinical communication negatively impact patient well-being.

Patient Vulnerability

The final challenge to smooth clinical communication is that patients have so much at stake. For patients, the significance of clinical appointments is heavy with patients' hopes for answers and treatments. The insidiousness of rheumatological disorders like lupus or fibromyalgia or dermatomyositis, as for other chronic diseases, is that through pain and disability they undermine a person's identity or core sense of self (cf. Charmaz, 1993; Murphy, 1987). Indeed, wait times for appointments can be particularly frustrating because they can be perceived as delays in treatment that then further delay the hope of "being able to be more myself" (Hay, 2010, p. 266).

For patients, illness is not simply a disease confined to their bodies, it spills over, staining everything it touches. In addition to pain and disability, rheumatological conditions undermine people's ability to be productive. In societies like the US in which productivity is associated with value, not being able to be productive may exacerbate suffering (Hay, 2010). This increase in suffering through lack of productivity is evident as one patient opened her appointment with an uncontrolled rush of words denoting the ways her identity had been discombobulated by disease "My thing is—is that if *anything* will help—improve my—(0.1) my uh my—just my life quality-um:m I'm 38. I'm very active. I don't want to be sittin' around" (emphasis in original). Rheumatic conditions often cause worlds to unravel. It is unsurprising that helplessness is common in rheumatological disorders and has been associated with less physical functionality, more depression and mood disorders, and more pain in rheumatoid arthritis, fibromyalgia, osteoarthritis, and lupus (e.g., Nicassio, Schuman, Radojevic & Weisman, 1999; Nicassio, Wallston, Callahan, & Pincus, 1985; Tayer, Nicassio, Radojevic, & Krall, 1996). Depression is likewise common in rheumatic disorders like rheumatoid arthritis (17–39 %, Matcham, Rayner, Steer, & Hotopf, 2013; Withers, Moran, Nicassio, Weisman, & Karpouzas, 2014), lupus (30 %, Huang, Magder, & Petri, 2014), and scleroderma (10–23 %, Jewett, Razykov, Hudson, Baron, & Thombs, 2012). Even those who are not depressed are likely to experience distress with scleroderma (Newton, Thombs, & Groleau, 2012) and rheumatoid arthritis (Treharne, Kitas, Lyons, & Booth, 2005). Catastrophizing (ruminating about one's condition) is common in rheumatic disorders and associated with helplessness, depression, sleeplessness, and pain (Edwards, Cahalan, Mensing, Smith, & Haythornthwaite, 2011).

All of these negatively affect a patient's lifeworld, and for these reasons, patients often seek empathy during their consultations (e.g., Halpern, 2007; Stamer, Schmacke, & Richter, 2013). But while patients often seek physician understanding and empathy, rheumatologists have a job to do and may need to stay on task as this excerpt demonstrates:

Pt: I was dancing professionally, … and couldn't make it through rehearsal and class and getting so that I was vomiting all the time. Had lots of blood tests and they figured a connective disease something was going on—

Dr: Where was that at?

Pt: That was in S__ and eventually after about a year I was diagnosed with lupus. Ummm, [the physician] tried to control it with prednisone and plaquinil, and get the prednisone high enough so that I could keep dancing. But it just—

Dr: How high of a dose?

Pt: On the prednisone? I don't think it ever got really, really high. …And that didn't bring the energy level up. So I quit dancing and started teaching umm, and …kind of muddled through.…I had also at a point in there lost my health insurance because I couldn't afford it, so I was off all meds at that point. So my boyfriend in P__ was able to put me on his medical insurance and I moved there, got rid of the dance studio, went to work at a desk job and I've had a history of really severe migraines which got worse at the desk job. I started … missing so much work that I lost my job there.

Dr: And when was this?

In this excerpt, the patient tells of how lupus has thoroughly undermined her lifeworld—professionally, financially, socially, geographically, and physically. The physician stays on the course of the medical interview, often interrupting her to do so. Each of the patient's speech turns are, according to Suchman, Markakis, Beckman, and Frankel (1997), potential empathic opportunities in which the patient voices suffering. Physicians have reason to be concerned that offering empathy may take precious time, but often a statement like "You've had a really hard time" followed up with a statement like "Let's do this first, and then I can see what we can do to help out with [fill in problem here]" simultaneously offers patients the empathy they need and helps keep them on track to do the clinical work of the appointment.

Literature suggests that just listening may be sufficient to calm a patient's concerns in doctor–patient interactions (Jagosh, Donald Boudreau, Steinert, Macdonald, & Ingram, 2011). Active listening has been associated in doctor–patient communication with eye-contact (Ruusuvuori, 2001) and improved understanding of patient history and the nuances of the complaint (Lang, Floyd, & Beine, 2000). Patients, particularly those whose condition is largely invisible (Hay, 2010), also need the reassurance that they have been believed and their suffering is affirmed as real. In the example below, the rheumatologist asked "does that hurt" as he pressed on her body during the exam. She mentioned a number of times that although it did not hurt during the exam, it did hurt in the mornings:

Dr: Mmhmm. How about here?
Pt: No. But in the morning, yes. Mornings, everything is swollen.
Dr: I understand, but we're not talking about morning right now. I understand. I believe you. Don't worry.

Patients are in vulnerable positions. They need someone who understands the disease and will find ways to help them regain pieces of their lives and their sense of self. As one patient put it: "You can't afford to insult them…. If you aren't careful, aren't respectful, they won't give you what you need." The vulnerability of patients makes them cautious. On the one hand, their suffering compels them to give voice to their lifeworlds. On the other hand, they worry about irritating the physician, concerned that if they do so, the physician may not give them the best possible care—a concern that reflects the extent of patient vulnerability, not the professionalism or clinical competence of physicians (Hay et al., 2008).

Movements within medicine recently have highlighted cultural competency training to better enable engagement with patients' perspectives, particularly when patients have cultural backgrounds that differ from those of the provider. It is abundantly clear that the cultural backgrounds of patients and their providers influence clinical interactions and health outcomes (Kleinman & Benson, 2006) and yet it is equally clear that cultural assumptions are not static nor do they necessarily map onto skin color, regional origins, or linguistic background. Cultural competency has gained popularity as a tool for making healthcare accessible and communicating with diverse patient groups (Kirmayer, 2012), thereby theoretically addressing health disparities (Smedley, Stith, & Nelson, 2003). Locally developed and implemented cultural competence training programs have proven successful (Kirmayer, 2013); however, the majority of studies of cultural competence training have shown no significant impact on provider behaviors or patient outcomes (Beach et al., 2005; Thom, Tirado, Woon, & McBride, 2006). Cultural competence training may even be detrimental if available "cultural profiles" reinforce stereotypes which are then used to orient providers' communicative strategies (Weisner & Hay, 2015).

Arthur Kleinman, a leading physician-scholar, has devoted much of his career to examining healthcare providers in different contexts and exploring how they can best meet the most salient concerns of their patients. To better help physicians understand the perspectives of patients, Kleinman developed eight questions that would reveal what Kleinman calls patient explanatory models, the foundational assumptions with which one makes sense of disease (Kleinman, 1988). The questions are: What do you call this problem? What do you believe is the cause of this problem? What course do you expect it to take/how serious is it? What do you think this problem does inside your body? How does it affect your body and your mind? What do you most fear about this condition? What do you most fear about the treatment? (Kleinman, 1988; Kleinman & Benson, 2006, p. 1674). While not every question may be necessary with every patient, this intentional focus on the patient and the patient's concerns is the essence of what constitutes a patient-centered interview (Platt et al., 2001). Patient-centeredness ultimately involves seeking to understand and acknowledge the patient's concerns regarding his or her condition and its effects on his or her lifeworld.

A patient-centered approach is not a patient-led approach; patients need to be able to rely on the physician to give them the best possible evidence-based clinical care, but that care must take into account his or her lifeworld realities.

How Much Does Communication Matter?

As long as the physician prescribes methotrexate, does it really matter how little the physician interrupts the patient or how often the physician provides empathy? Evidence suggests that, yes, communication does matter.

Good communication with patients is associated with better adherence and better health outcomes (e.g., Arbuthnott & Sharpe, 2009). Current adherence rates in rheumatic disorders can be low ranging from 30 to 80 % (Harrold & Andrade, 2009), but rheumatology patients are more likely to adhere to a treatment regime if there is a good physician–patient relationship (Pasma et al., 2014). In a 3-year study on quality of contact, healthcare providers showed that a higher quality relationship was associated with more consistent adherence to medications over time (Viller et al., 1999). Another study found that if patients are satisfied with their consultations and believe that their medications are necessary, they report higher adherence (Treharne, Lyons, & Kitas, 2004). Multiple studies have linked trust in the provider with higher levels of adherence (e.g., Martin et al., 2008), and a trusting, cooperative relationship is built by and facilitates communication. As a leading rheumatologist noted "…the most important goal in arthritis patient education may be to develop a cooperative relationship between physician and patient so that the patient adheres to a mutually-agreed-upon regimen, and so that the physician's search for the best regimen is guided by accurate feedback from the patient" (Daltroy, 1993, p. 221).

Good communication that incorporates the patient's lifeworld makes clinical sense in rheumatic diseases, many of which are systemic. Systemic disease, particularly systemic autoimmune disease in which psychosocial stress is associated with flares, means that clinically the whole body needs to be taken into account; it is but a short step to additionally take the person's lifeworld into account communicatively. Doing so may lead to more refined treatments, as Daltroy suggests, and communicates that a relationship that is not *about* disease but *between* persons. As one patient puts it, in reflecting after her appointment, "The doctor must be professional, yes, but don't treat the patient like an object, we're people." Communicative competence is a pathway to improve patient trust, belief in medications, communication, adherence, and ultimately health outcomes.

Communication in Rheumatology: Future Possibilities for Improvement

Communicative competence is, like clinical competence, an ongoing practice, one that needs constant attention and improvement. Just as a clinically competent rheumatologist keeps track of the emergent evidence-based literature, modifying clinical practice in keeping with locally acquired experiential knowledge as a clinician, so too communicatively competent physician moves fluidly between "the stance of expert and the stance of learner" (Browning, 2002, p. 25), listening for the particular perspectives of the patient and assuming that just as the EBM literature changes on a daily basis, so too do the nuances of a patient's lifeworld.

Jerome Groopman has noted that while hospitals have a process for learning from the clinical errors, called the Morbidity and Mortality—M & M—conference, "there was no similar conference about language. No analysis of errors in judgment or technique about what we say to patients and their families" (2003, p. 51). Groopman implies that physicians would benefit from the learning experience like an M&M-type session that focuses on language and communication. Such an event could be called a C&S conference, for Communication and Suffering, and might go a long way to enabling clinicians to thoughtfully improve their communication.

Given how much is at stake for patients, we need a better way of understanding how patient experience impacts clinical communications and patient health outcomes. Specifically, we know that rheumatology patients often have high levels of distress—helplessness, perceived stress, mood, maladaptive coping skills as measured by standardized instruments (e.g., Nicassio et al., 2011), but how or whether that distress surfaces in clinical interactions is yet unknown. Similarly, do all patients need empathy, or do some at some points need empathy more than others? We know that patients may see multiple physicians and experience sometimes years of failed treatments before being correctly diagnosed with a rheumatological disorder; are there specific communicative markers common to appointments that lead to a failed diagnosis or treatment? Likewise are there specific communication markers that are associated with higher adherence and patient well-being? Also, given that doctor–patient relationships tend to be long-term in rheumatology, how does the quality of communication shift over time and affect patient health outcomes?

Finally, the emphasis in doctor–patient communication research to date has focused on the impact of communication on patients and their health outcomes. It is worth considering the impact of communication on physicians and their well-being as well. Recall the voiced frustration of the doctor who can only see 12 patients a day because of high administrative paperwork. The rheumatologists I know and have worked with delight in talking with their patients and figuring out the puzzle of their conditions. When rheumatologists leave consultations irritated, it may be a result of mismatched expectations. For example, while rheumatologists were extremely patient and professional with patients whose health was seriously failing (see also Hall et al., 1996), they could become irritated when, given the short prescribed appointment lengths, patients wanted more appointment time than was physically warranted, wanting the physician to consider a pharmaceutical that the patient had seen advertised or to look over a stack of materials printed from the Internet. The burden of poor communication thus may weigh not only on patients, but also on rheumatologists and their well-being.

The tools physicians use to ease suffering only begin with mastery of the biomedical literature, technology, pharmaceuticals, and skills of clinical competence. As has been argued here, these clinical skills must be matched by strong interpersonal and communicative skills—these are the second leg of competence.

Acknowledgments The author is grateful to Perry Nicassio, participating rheumatologists and patients, the Department of Anthropology at Miami University, and the UCLA Center for Culture and Health. Material in this chapter is based upon work supported by the National Science Foundation under Grant No. 0137921.

References

Agrawal, H., Hay, M. C., Volkmann, E. R., Maranian, P., Khanna, D., & Furst, D. E. (2012). Satisfaction and access to clinical care in a rheumatology clinic at a large urban medical center. *Journal of Clinical Rheumatology, 18*(4), 209–211. doi:10.1097/RHU.0b013e318259aa1b.

Ainsworth-Vaughn, N. (1998). *Claiming power in doctor-patient talk* (p. 224). Oxford, UK: Oxford University Press.

Arbuthnott, A., & Sharpe, D. (2009). The effect of physician-patient collaboration on patient adherence in non-psychiatric medicine. *Patient Education and Counseling, 77*(1), 60–67. doi:10.1016/j.pec.2009.03.022.

Badley, E. M., & Davis, A. M. (2012). Meeting the challenge of the ageing of the population: Issues in access to specialist care for arthritis. *Best Practice and Research. Clinical Rheumatology, 26*(5), 599–609. doi:10.1016/j.berh.2012.09.002.

Beach, M. C., Price, E. G., Gary, T. L., Robinson, K. A., Gozu, A., Palacio, A., … Cooper, L. A. (2005). Cultural competency: A systematic review of health care provider educational interventions. *Medical Care, 43*(4), 356–373.

Bell, R. A., Kravitz, R. L., Thom, D., & Krupat, E. (2002). Unmet expectations for care and the patient-physician relationship. *Journal of General Internal Medicine, 17*, 817–824.

Berrios-Rivera, J. P., Jr., Street, R. L., Popa-Lisseanu, M. G. G., Kallen, M. A., Richardson, M. N., Janssen, N. M., … Suarez-Almazor, M. E. (2006). Trust in physicians and elements of the medical interaction in patients with rheumatoid arthritis and systemic lupus erythematosus. *Arthritis Care & Research, 55*(3), 385–393.

Browning, D. (2002). "To Show Our Humanness–Relational and Communicative Competence in Pediatric Pallative Care." *Bioethics Forum, 18*(3/4), 23–28.

Charmaz, K. C. (1993). *Good days, bad days: The self in chronic illness and time*. New Brunswick, NJ: Rutgers University Press. Retrieved from http://books.google.com/books?id=8CYzSaI4oUQC&pg=PP5&dq=on+the+experience+of+time&sig=LSqYyrf3_or2IfGufMO24JG3m1A#PPP5,M1

Chomsky, N. (1965). *The aspects of the theory of syntax*. Cambridge, MA: MIT Press.

Csordas, T. (1990). Embodiment as a paradigm for anthropology. *Ethos, 18*(1), 5–47.

Daltroy, L. H. (1993). Doctor-patient communication in rheumatological disorders. *Baillière's Clinical Rheumatology, 7*(2), 221–239. doi:10.1016/S0950-3579(05)80087-1.

Deal, C. L., Hooker, R., Harrington, T., Birnbaum, N., Hogan, P., Bouchery, E., … Barr, W. (2007). The United States rheumatology workforce: Supply and demand, 2005–2025. *Arthritis and Rheumatism, 56*(3), 722–729. doi:10.1002/art.22437.

Deluarier, A., Bernatsky, S., Baron, M., Légaré, J., & Feldman, D. (2012). Wait times for rheumatology consultation: Is rheumatoid arthritis prioritized? *Journal of Clinical Rheumatology, 18*(7), 341–344. doi:10.1097/RHU.0b013e31826d6408.

Desjarlais, R., & Jason Throop, C. (2011). Phenomenological approaches in anthropology. *Annual Review of Anthropology, 40*(1), 87–102. doi:10.1146/annurev-anthro-092010-153345.

Diaz, J. A., Griffith, R. A., Ng, J. J., Reinert, S. E., Friedmann, P. D., & Moulton, A. W. (2002). Patients' use of the internet for medical information. *Journal of General Internal Medicine, 17*(3), 180–185.

Dumit, J. (2012). *Drugs for life: How pharmaceutical companies define our health* (p. 262). Durham, NC: Duke University Press.

Edwards, R. R., Cahalan, C., Mensing, G., Smith, M., & Haythornthwaite, J. A. (2011). Pain, catastrophizing, and depression in the rheumatic diseases. *Nature Reviews. Rheumatology, 7*, 216–224. doi:10.1038/nrrheum.2011.66.

Fanu, M. D., & Le, J. (1999). *The rise and fall of modern medicine* (p. 426). New York, NY: Carroll and Graf.

Foley, K. (2005). Vital signs: Rheumatologists worked nearly 47 clinical hours per week in 2003. *Rheumatology News, 4*(2), 1.

Fox, S. (2006). *Online health search 2006*. Washington, DC: Pew Internet and American Life Project.

Fox, S., & Duggan, M. (2013). Health online 2013. *Health,* 1–55. Retrieved from http://www.pewinternet.org/~/media//Files/Reports/PIP_HealthOnline.pdf

Fox, S., & Rainie, L. (2014). The Web at 25 in the U.S. *The Pew Research Center*, 1–41. Retrieved from http://www.pewinternet.org/2014/02/25/the-web-at-25-in-the-u-s

Giddens, A. (1991). *Modernity and self-identity: Self and society in the late modern age* (p. 264). Stanford, CA: Stanford University Press.

Gillis, J. Z., Yazdany, J., Trupin, L., Julian, L., Panopalis, P., Criswell, L. A, … Yelin, E. (2007). Medicaid and access to care among persons with systemic lupus erythematosus. *Arthritis and Rheumatism, 57*(4), 601–607. doi:10.1002/art.22671.

Gillotti, C., Thompson, T., & McNeilis, K. (2002). Communicative competence in the delivery of bad news. *Social Science and Medicine, 54*(7), 1011–1023.

Good, B. J. (1994). *Medicine, rationality, and experience: An anthropological perspective. Lewis Henry Morgan lecture series*. Cambridge, MA: Cambridge University Press.

Good, M. J. D. (1995). *American medicine: The quest for competence*. Berkeley: University of California Press.

Good, B., & Delvecchio Good, M.-J. (1993). "Learning medicine": The constructing of medical knowledge at Harvard Medical School. In S. Lindenbaum & M. Lock (Eds.), *Knowledge, power, and practice* (pp. 81–107). Berkeley: University of California.

Gregg, J., & Saha, S. (2007). Communicative competence: A framework for understanding language barriers in health care. *Journal of General Internal Medicine, 22*(Suppl 2), 368–370. doi:10.1007/s11606-007-0364-4.

Groopman, J. (2003). *Anatomy of hope: How people prevail in the face of illness*. New York, NY: Random House.

Haakana, M. (2001). Laughter as a patient's resource: Dealing with delicate aspects of medical interaction. *Text—Interdisciplinary Journal for the Study of Discourse, 21*, 187–219.

Habermas, J. (1984). *The theory of communicative action* (Lifeworld and system, Vol. 2). Boston, MA: Beacon Press.

Hagglund, K. J., Clark, M. J., Hilton, S. A., & Hewett, J. E. (2005). Access to healthcare services among persons with osteoarthritis and rheumatoid arthritis. *American Journal of Physical Medicine and Rehabilitation, 84*(9), 702–711.

Hahn, S. R., Kroenke, K., Spitzer, R. L., Brody, D., Williams, J. B. W., Linzer, M., & Verloin, F. (1993). The difficult patient: Prevalence, psychopathology, and functional impairment. *Journal of Clinical Epidemiology, 6*, 647–657.

Hall, J., Roter, D. L., Milburn, M., & Daltroy, L. H. (1996). Patients' health as a predictor of physician and patient behavior in medical visits: A synthesis of four studies. *Medical Care, 34*(12), 1205–1218.

Halpern, J. (2001). *From detached concern to empathy: Humanizing medical practice*. Oxford, UK: Oxford University Press.

Halpern, J. (2007). Empathy and patient-physician conflicts. *Journal General Internal Medicine, 22*, 696–701. doi:10.1007/sl.

Happé, F. G. E. (1993). Communicative competence and theory of mind in autism: A test of relevance theory. *Cognition, 48*, 101–119.

Hardey, M. (1999). Doctor in the house: The Internet as a source of lay health knowledge and the challenge to expertise. *Sociology of Health & Illness, 21*(6), 820–835. doi:10.1111/1467-9566.00185.

Harrold, L. R., & Andrade, S. E. (2009). Medication adherence of patients with selected rheumatic conditions: a systematic review of the literature. *Seminars in Arthritis and Rheumatism, 38*(5), 396–402.

Hay, M. C. (2006). Sick role. In *Encyclopedia of disability*. Thousand Oaks, CA: Sage.

Hay, M. C. (2010). Suffering in a productive world. *American Ethnologist, 37*(2), 259–274. doi:10.1111/j.1548-1425.2010.01254.x.

Hay, M. C., Cadigan, R. J., Khanna, D., Strathmann, C., Lieber, E. L. I., Altman, R. O. Y., … Furst, D. E. (2008). Prepared patients: Internet information seeking by new rheumatology patients. *Arthritis Care and Research, 59*(4), 575–582. doi:10.1002/art.23533.

Heath, D., Rapp, R., & Taussig, K.-S. (2007). Genetic citizenship. In D. Nugent & J. Vincent (Eds.), *A companion to the anthropology of politics* (pp. 152–167). Oxford, UK: Blackwell. doi:10.1002/9780470693681.ch10.

Heritage, J., & Maynard, D. W. (2006a). Introduction: Analyzing Interaction between doctors and patients in primary care encounters. In J. Heritage & D. W. Maynard (Eds.), *Communication in medical care* (Vol. 20). Cambridge, MA: Cambridge University Press.

Heritage, J., & Maynard, D. W. (2006b). Problems and prospects in the study of physician-patient interaction: 30 years of research. *Annual Review of Sociology, 32*(1), 351–374. doi:10.1146/annurev.soc.32.082905.093959.

Huang, X., Magder, L. S., & Petri, M. (2014). Predictors of survival in systemic lupus erythematosus. *Journal of Rheumatology, 41*(9), 1823–1833. doi:10.1097/01.md.0000224709.70133.f7.

Hurst, N. P., Lambert, C. M., Forbes, J., Lochhead, A., Major, K., & Lock, P. (2000). Does waiting matter? A randomized controlled trial of new non-urgent rheumatology out-patient referrals. *Rheumatology (Oxford, England), 39*, 369–376.

Husserl, E. (1970). *The crisis of European sciences and transcendental phenomenology*. Evanston, IL: Northwestern University Press.

Hymes, D. (2001). On communicative competence. In *Linguistic anthropology* (pp. 53–73). Malden, MA: Blackwell.

Jackson, M. (2012). *Lifeworlds: Essays in existential anthropology*. Chicago, IL: University of Chicago Press.

Jagosh, J., Donald Boudreau, J., Steinert, Y., Macdonald, M. E., & Ingram, L. (2011). The importance of physician listening from the patients' perspective: Enhancing diagnosis, healing, and the doctor-patient relationship. *Patient Education and Counseling, 85*(3), 369–374. doi:10.1016/j.pec.2011.01.028.

Jamal, S., Alibhai, S. M. H., Badley, E. M., & Bombardier, C. (2011). Time to treatment for new patients with rheumatoid arthritis in a major metropolitan city. *The Journal of Rheumatology, 38*(7), 1282–1288. doi:10.3899/jrheum.101315.

Jefferson, G. (2004). A note on laughter in "male–female" interaction. *Discourse Studies, 6*(1), 117–133. doi:10.1177/1461445604039445.

Jewett, L. R., Razykov, I., Hudson, M., Baron, M., & Thombs, B. D. (2012). Prevalence of current, 12-month and lifetime major depressive disorder among patients with systemic sclerosis. *Rheumatology, 52*, 669–675. doi:10.1093/rheumatology/kes347.

Katz, J. (1984). *The silent world of doctor and patient* (p. 263). New York, NY: Free Press.

Kirmayer, L. J. (2000). Broken narratives: Clinical encounters and the poetics of illness experience. In C. Mattingly & L. C. Garro (Eds.), *Narrative and the cultural construction of illness and healing* (pp. 153–180). Berkeley: University of California Press.

Kirmayer, L. J. (2012). Rethinking cultural competence. *Transcultural Psychiatry, 49*(2), 149–164. doi:10.1177/1363461512444673.

Kirmayer, L. J. (2013). Embracing uncertainty as a path to competence: Cultural safety, empathy, and alterity in clinical training. *Culture, Medicine and Psychiatry, 37*(2), 365–372. doi:10.1007/s11013-013-9314-2.

Kjeken, I., Dagfinrud, H., Mowinckel, P., Uhlig, T., Kvien, T. K., & Finset, A. (2006). Rheumatology care: Involvement in medical decisions, received information, satisfaction with care, and unmet health care needs in patients with rheumatoid arthritis and ankylosing spondylitis. *Arthritis Care and Research, 55*(3), 394–401. doi:10.1002/art.21985.

Kleinman, A. (1988). *The illness narratives: Suffering, healing, and the human condition*. New York, NY: Basic Books.

Kleinman, A. (1995). *Writing at the margin: Discourse between anthropology and medicine*. Berkeley: University of California Press.

Kleinman, A., & Benson, P. (2006). Anthropology in the clinic: The problem of cultural competency and how to fix it. *PLoS Medicine, 3*(10), e294. doi:10.1371/journal.pmed.0030294.

Konner, M. (1987). *Becoming a doctor: A journey of initiation in medical school*. New York, NY: Penguin.

Kravitz, R. L. (2001). The physician–patient relationship measuring patients' expectations and requests. *Annals of Internal Medicine, 134*, 881–888.

Laganga, L. R., & Lawrence, S. R. (2007). Clinic overbooking to improve patient access and increase provider productivity. *Decision Sciences, 38*(2), 251–276. doi:10.1111/j.1540-5915.2007.00158.x.

Lang, F., Floyd, M. R., & Beine, K. L. (2000). Clues to patients' explanations and concerns about their illnesses. A call for active listening. *Archives of Family Medicine, 9*, 222–227. doi:10.1001/archfami.9.3.222.

Linzer, M., Manwell, L. B., Williams, E. S., Bobula, J. A., Brown, R. L., Varkey, A. B., … Schwartz, M. D. (2009). Improving patient care annals of internal medicine working conditions in primary care:

Physician reactions and care quality. *Annals of Internal Medicine, 151*(1), 28–36.
Main, C. J., Buchbinder, R., Porcheret, M., & Foster, N. (2010). Addressing patient beliefs and expectations in the consultation. *Best Practice & Research. Clinical Rheumatology, 24*(2), 219–225. doi:10.1016/j.berh.2009.12.013.
Martin, R. W., Head, A. J., René, J., Swartz, T. J., Fiechtner, J. J., McIntosh, B. A., & Holmes-Rovner, M. (2008). Patient decision-making related to anti-rheumatic drugs in rheumatoid arthritis: The importance of patient trust of physician. *Journal of Rheumatology, 35*, 618–624.
Matcham, F., Rayner, L., Steer, S., & Hotopf, M. (2013). The prevalence of depression in rheumatoid arthritis: A systematic review and meta-analysis. *Rheumatology (Oxford, England), 52*, 2136–2148. doi:10.1093/rheumatology/ket169.
McNearney, T. A., Hunnicutt, S. E., Maganti, R., & Rice, J. (2008). What factors relate to job satisfaction among rheumatologists. *Journal of Clinical Rheumatology, 14*(3),133–137.doi:10.1097/RHU.0b013e318177274d.
Mishler, E. G. (1984). *The discourse of medicine: Dialectics of medical interviews*. Norwood, NJ: Ablex.
Moore, P. J., Sickel, A. E., Malat, J., Williams, D., Jackson, J., & Adler, N. E. (2004). Psychosocial factors in medical and psychological treatment avoidance: The role of the doctor-patient relationship. *Journal of Health Psychology, 9*, 421–433. doi:10.1177/1359105304042351.
Murphy, R. F. (1987). The damaged self. In *The body silent*. New York, NY: Norton.
National Science Board. (2000). Science and engineering indicators—2000 (Vol. 1). Arlington, VA: National Science Board. Retrieved from http://www.nsf.gov/statistics/seind00/
Newman, E. D., Harrington, T. M., Olenginski, T. P., & Perruquet, J. L. (2004). "The rheumatologist can see you now": Successful implementation of an advanced access model in a rheumatology practice. *Arthritis Care and Research, 51*(2), 253–257. doi:10.1002/art.20239.
Newton, E. G., Thombs, B. D., & Groleau, D. (2012). The experience of emotional distress among women with scleroderma. *Qualitative Health Research, 22*(9), 1195–1206. doi:10.1177/1049732312449207.
Nicassio, P. M. (2008). The problem of detecting and managing depression in the rheumatology clinic. *Arthritis Care and Research, 59*(2), 155–158. doi:10.1002/art.23348.
Nicassio, P. M., Kay, M. a, Custodio, M. K., Irwin, M. R., Olmstead, R., & Weisman, M. H. (2011). An evaluation of a biopsychosocial framework for health-related quality of life and disability in rheumatoid arthritis. *Journal of Psychosomatic Research, 71*(2), 79–85.
Nicassio, P. M., Schuman, C., Radojevic, V., & Weisnman, M. H. (1999). Helplessness as a Mediator of Health Status in Fibromyalgia. *Cognitive Therapy and Research, 23*(2), 181–196.
Nicassio, P., Wallston, K. A., Callahan, L. F., & Pincus, T. (1985). The measurement of helplessness in rheumatoid arthritist: The development of the arthritis helplessness index. *The Journal of Rheumatology, 12*, 462–467.
Ochs, E., & Schieffelin, B. (2008). Language socialization: An historical overview. In N. Hornberger (Ed.), *Encyclopedia of language and education SE-193* (pp. 2580–2594). New York, NY: Springer. doi:10.1007/978-0-387-30424-3_193.
Parsons, T. (1951). Illness and the role of the physician: A sociological perspective. *American Journal of Orthopsychiatry, 21*, 452–460.
Pasma, A., van't Spijker, A., Luime, J. J., Walter, M. J. M., Busschbach, J. J. V., & Hazes, J. M. W. (2014). Facilitators and barriers to adherence in the initiation phase of disease-modifying antirheumatic drug (DMARD) use in patients with arthritis who recently started their first DMARD treatment. *The Journal of Rheumatology, 42*(3), 379–385. doi:10.3899/jrheum.140693.
Patwardhan, A., Henrickson, M., Laskosz, L., Duyenhong, S., & Spencer, C. H. (2014). Current pediatric rheumatology fellowship training in the United States: What fellows actually do. *Pediatric Rheumatology Online Journal, 12*(1), 8. doi:10.1186/1546-0096-12-8.
Peabody, F. W. (1927). The care of the patient. *JAMA, 88*(12), 877–882.
Platt, F. W., Gaspar, D. L., Coulehan, J. L., Fox, L., Adler, A. J., Weston, W. W., … Stewart, M. (2001). "Tell me about yourself": The patient-centered interview. *Annals of Internal Medicine, 134*(11), 1079–1085.
Rao, J. K., Weinberger, M., Anderson, L. A., & Kroenke, K. (2004). Predicting reports of unmet expectations among rheumatology patients. *Arthritis and Rheumatism, 51*(2), 215–221. doi:10.1002/art.20246.
Roter, D. L. (1977). Patient participation in the patient-provider interaction: The effects of patient question asking on the quality of interaction, satisfaction and compliance. *Health Education & Behavior, 5*(4), 281–315. doi:10.1177/109019817700500402.
Rouse, C. M. (2009). *Uncertain suffering: Racial health care disparities and sickle cell disease* (p. 314). Berkeley: University of California Press. doi:10.1093/jhmas/jrq007.
Rouse, C. (2010). Patient and practitioner noncompliance: Rationing, therapeutic uncertainty, and the missing conversation. *Anthropology & Medicine, 17*(2), 187–200. doi:10.1080/13648470.2010.493602.
Rudd, E., & Bosch, S. J. (1966). Education and training of rheumatologists. *Arthritis & Rheumatism, 9*(6), 830–833.
Ruusuvuori, J. (2001). Looking means listening: Coordinating displays of engagement in doctor–patient interaction. *Social Science & Medicine, 52*(7), 1093–1108. doi:10.1016/S0277-9536(00)00227-6.
Salt, E., & Peden, A. (2011). The complexity of the treatment: The decision-making process among women with rheumatoid arthritis. *Qualitative Health Research, 21*(2), 214–222. doi:10.1177/1049732310381086.
Schneider, M., & Krüger, K. (2013). Rheumatoid arthritis—Early diagnosis and disease management. *Deutsches Ärzteblatt International, 110*(27–28), 477–484. doi:10.3238/arztebl.2013.0477.

Schutz, A. (1973). *Structures of the life-world* (Vol. 1, p. 335). Evanston, IL: Northwestern University Press.
Smedley, B. D., Stith, A. Y., & Nelson, A. R. (2003). Unequal treatment: What healthcare providers need to know about racial and ethnic disparities in healthcare. In G. E. Henderson, S. E. Estroff, L. R. Churchill, N. M. P. King, J. Oberlander, & R. P. Strauss (Eds.), *The social medicine reader: Social and cultural contributions to health, difference, and inequality* (pp. 123–132). Durham, NC: Duke University Press.
Stamer, M., Schmacke, N., & Richter, P. (2013). Noncompliance: A never-ending story. Understanding the perspective of patients with rheumatoid arthritis. *Forum: Qualitative Social Research, 14*(3), Art. 7.
Strathmann, C., & Hay, M. C. (2008). I'm paying your salary here!: Social inequality, consumerism, and the politics of space in medical clinics. *Human Organization, 67*(1), 49–60.
Street, R. L., Gordon, H. S., Ward, M. M., Krupat, E., & Kravitz, R. L. (2005). Patient participation in medical consultations: Why some patients are more involved than others. *Medical Care, 43*(10), 960–969. doi:10.1097/01.mlr.0000178172.40344.70.
Suarez-Almazor, M. E. (2004). Patient-physician communication. *Current Opinion in Rheumatology, 58*(152), 357–361. doi:10.1097/00002281-200403000-00003.
Suchman, A. L., Markakis, K., Beckman, H. B., & Frankel, R. (1997). A model of empathic communication in the medical interview. *JAMA 277*, 678–682. doi:10.1001/jama.277.8.678.
Tayer, W. G., Nicassio, P. M., Radojevic, V., & Krall, T. (1996). Pain and helplessness as correlates of depression in systemic lupus erythematosus. *British Journal of Health Psychology, 1*, 253–262.
Teachman, G., & Gibson, B. E. (2014). "Communicative competence" in the field of augmentative and alternative communication: A review and critique. *International Journal of Language & Communication Disorders/ Royal College of Speech & Language Therapists, 49*(1), 1–14. doi:10.1111/1460-6984.12055.
Thom, D. H., Tirado, M. D., Woon, T. L., & McBride, M. R. (2006). Development and evaluation of a cultural competency training curriculum. *BMC Medical Education, 6*, 38. doi:10.1186/1472-6920-6-38.
Treharne, G. J., Kitas, G. D., Lyons, A. C., & Booth, D. A. (2005). Well-being in rheumatoid arthritis: The effects of disease duration and psychosocial factors. *Journal of Health Psychology, 10*, 457–474. doi:10.1177/1359105305051416.
Treharne, G., Lyons, A., & Kitas, G. (2004). Medication adherence in rheumatoid arthritis: Effects of psychosocial factors. *Psychology, Health & Medicine, 9*(3), 337–349. doi:10.1080/13548500410001721909.
Ventola, C. (2011). Direct-to-consumer pharmaceutical advertising: Therapeutic or toxic? *Pharmacy and Therapeutics, 36*(10), 669–684. Retrieved from http://www.pubmedcentral.nih.gov/articlerender.fcgi?artid=3278148&tool=pmcentrez&rendertype=abstracthttp://www.ncbi.nlm.nih.gov/pmc/articles/PMC3278148/pdf/ptj3610669.pdfhttp://www.ncbi.nlm.nih.gov/pmc/articles/PMC3278148/?tool=pmcentrez
Viller, F., Guillemin, F., Briançon, S., Moum, T., Suurmeijer, T., & van den Heuvel, W. (1999). Compliance to drug treatment of patients with rheumatoid arthritis: A 3 year longitudinal study. *The Journal of Rheumatology, 26*(10), 2114–2122. Retrieved from http://europepmc.org/abstract/MED/10529126
Waitzkin, H. (1993). *The politics of medical encounters: How patients and doctors deal with social problems* (p. 327). New Haven, CT: Yale University Press.
Ward, M. M. (2004). Rheumatology care, patient expectations, and the limits of time. *Arthritis and Rheumatism, 51*(3), 307–308. doi:10.1002/art.20417.
Weisner, T. S., & Hay, M. C. (2015). Practice to research: Integrating evidence-based practices with culture and context. *Transcultural Psychiatry, 52*(2), 222–243.
West, C. (1984). Medical misfires: Mishearings, misgivings, and misunderstandings in physician-patient dialogues. *Discourse Processes, 7*(2), 107–134. doi:10.1080/01638538409544586.
West, C. (1993). Reconceptualizing gender in physician-patient relationships. *Social Science and Medicine, 36*(1), 57–66. doi:10.1016/0277-9536(93)90305-N.
Withers, M., Moran, R., Nicassio, P., Weisman, M. H., & Karpouzas, G. A. (2014). Perspectives of vulnerable US hispanics with rheumatoid arthritis on depression: Awareness, barriers to disclosure and treatment options. *Arthritis Care & Research, 67*(4), 484–492. doi:10.1002/acr.22462.
Woolf, A. D. (2002). Specialist training in rheumatology in Europe. *Rheumatology, 41*, 1062–1066.

Resilience to Chronic Arthritis Pain Is Not About Stopping Pain That Will Not Stop: Development of a Dynamic Model of Effective Pain Adaptation

8

John A. Sturgeon and Alex J. Zautra

Chronic pain poses a challenge to all aspects of self-regulation. In this chapter, we examine the key problems that people face and offer some tentative solutions to guide the refinement of existing interventions and the design of new programs to boost resilient responding in this population. Individuals with chronic pain face changes to their physical states, which are frequently accompanied by significant behavioral changes and alterations to their states of mind. There is a wealth of information that suggests that pain adversely affects all aspects of functioning, including more frequent and disruptive maladaptive thoughts about pain (Sturgeon & Zautra, 2013b), increased prevalence of depression and anxiety (Pincus, Griffith, Pearce, & Isenberg, 1996), decreased positive emotions and positive social engagement (Sturgeon, Zautra, & Arewasikporn, 2014), proliferation of clinically significant fatigue (Wolfe, Hawley, & Wilson, 1996), sleep disturbance (Nicassio & Wallston, 1992), and increased rates of disability (Wolfe & Hawley, 1998). Historically, these accounts have been largely one-dimensional: They have focused on how the presence of pain predicts poorer overall functioning for most people, though not for everyone.

This focus on the deleterious consequences of chronic pain is understandable, given the problem-focused nature of traditional medical and psychological research. Indeed, attention on the negative consequences of chronic pain has yielded much clinically useful insight. However, adoption of a perspective that gives predominant weight only to the negative consequences of pain leads to a single-minded goal of eliminating pain altogether, a prospect that is frequently unattainable. As Blalock et al. have shown, a mindset bound by precepts concerning the prevention of harm cannot find ways forward to find and value the positive (Blalock et al., 2015). A new approach is needed to widen the scope of these inquiries to characterize the ways and means of positive adaptation. Of late, there has been a proliferation of studies devoted to factors that facilitate effective adaptation to chronic pain, commonly referred to as pain resilience (Karoly & Ruehlman, 2006; Ramirez-Maestre, Esteve, & Lopez, 2012; Strand et al., 2006; Sturgeon & Zautra, 2010, 2013a; Zautra, Johnson, & Davis, 2005). It is these studies that provide the basis for our review and provide the foundation for our call for new initiatives to address the problem of pain in the lives of arthritis patients.

J.A. Sturgeon, PhD (✉)
Department of Anesthesia, Perioperative, and Pain Medicine, Stanford University, 1070 Arastradero Road, Suite 200, Palo Alto, CA, 94304, USA
e-mail: jasturge@gmail.com

A.J. Zautra, PhD
Department of Psychology, Arizona State University, Tempe, AZ, USA

P.M. Nicassio (ed.), *Psychosocial Factors in Arthritis*, DOI 10.1007/978-3-319-22858-7_8

Resilience in Chronic Pain

There are many ways to define resilience to pain. It is reasonable to define pain resilience according to the prevention of the development or progression of chronic pain. Indeed, recent studies have suggested that one possible way of examining resilience is through studying the lack of coherence between objective radiographic findings of a disease like osteoarthritis and clinical complaints of pain (Finan et al., 2013). In many cases, however, the development of pain, a symptom that accompanies arthritis, is both unavoidable and incurable. We advocate for a more generic model of resilience that does not focus on the pain itself, but rather on the ways in which the person responds adaptively to the stressful aspects of the pain experience. Three characteristic dimensions of resilient adaptation appear worthy of study: (1) recovery, (2) sustainability, and (3) psychological growth (Zautra & Reich, 2011). Recovery refers to how quickly and completely a person returns to baseline levels of emotional and physical functioning after a painful flare-up of her/his condition. If the person in pain has been able to maintain meaningful positive engagements in spite of the presence of pain, he or she receives high marks on sustainability, regardless of how well they have recovered emotionally. Inquiries regarding growth ask whether the person has learned new skills, developed new strengths, and/or gained in knowledge as a consequence of the pain experience (Sturgeon & Zautra, 2010). In previous studies (Sturgeon & Zautra, 2010, 2013a), we have pointed out that resilience to pain must account for both static contributors to pain resilience such as personality and social status, referred to as *resilience resources*, and dynamic factors that may be activated to aid in effective adaptation to pain factors such as positive social engagements and the positive emotions that accompany those engagements, referred to as *resilience mechanisms* (see Fig. 8.1, adapted from a model originally published in Sturgeon & Zautra, 2010). Further, the social context of pain adaptation highlighted by other studies (Sturgeon, Zautra & Arewasikporn, 2014; Yeung, Arewasikporn, & Zautra, 2012) also needs to be considered when investigating resilience. Chronic pain poses a number of challenges to social relationships, and how the person and the people he or she cares about respond can both enhance and/or hinder pain adaptation.

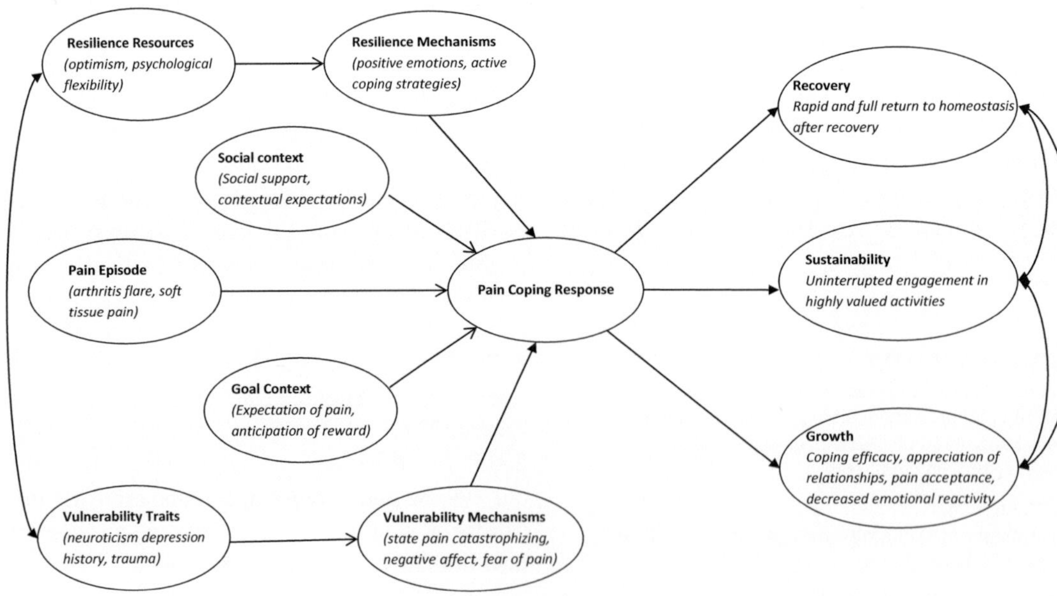

Fig. 8.1 Conceptual path model for resilience in chronic pain (adapted from Sturgeon & Zautra, 2010)

Although it remains a relatively new topic of inquiry in chronic pain, measures of resilience have already demonstrated utility as a predictor of health, coping, and quality of life in chronic pain. Resilience has been connected to a variety of positive outcomes in chronic pain, including increased feelings of vitality (Salathé et al., 2013) and physical function (Torma, Houck, Wagnild, Messecar, & Jones, 2013), decreased ratings of symptom burden (McAllister et al., 2013), and lower rates of disability and mortality (Elliott, Burton, & Hannaford, 2014).

Although the aforementioned model of resilience in chronic pain can help to organize the multitude of factors that predict positive functioning in chronic pain, some aspects of this model would benefit from further development. For example, paying greater attention to the phenomenological experience of pain, understanding the nature of pain adaptation from the perspective of the sufferer and giving weight to both person-centered and contextual factors in adaptation, may enhance our understanding of chronic pain (Karoly & Ruehlman, 2006; Masi, White, & Pilcher, 2002). Though experimental and observational studies serve an important purpose in identifying and clarifying processes related to positive pain adaptation, the clinical and empirical utility of such models may be limited if they do not meaningfully reflect the experience of pain by the sufferer. This perspective can help to highlight important new areas of inquiry that have remained dormant in existing models. For example, there is a large body of literature that has emphasized the context of pain coping. Though the social context of pain experience has rightfully garnered increased attention in recent years, there is also an expanding body of literature that examines the roles of goal orientation (Ceulemans, Karsdorp, & Vlaeyen, 2013a, 2013b; Coffey, Gallagher, Desmond, & Ryall, 2014) and reward processing in pain (Becker, Gandhi, & Schweinhardt, 2012; Leknes & Tracey, 2008) that may underlie chronic pain processing and adaptation. In many cases, individual goals and the perception of reward involve and interact with interpersonal processes to promote resilience to pain, thereby shaping the experience of the pain sufferer and direct their coping efforts accordingly. Examining contextual goals and reward processing in chronic pain can help to explain many of the subtleties that are inherent in explaining resilient responses to pain from a motivational standpoint, which has remained a relatively understudied area of pain adaptation (Crombez, Eccleston, Van Damme, Vlaeyen, & Karoly, 2012).

Additionally, chronic pain may place a higher demand on an individual's self-regulatory processes (Solberg Nes, Carlson, Crofford, de Leeuw, & Segerstrom, 2010). The role of self-regulation is key to understanding how individuals with chronic pain are able to override tendencies to avoid pain and to continue to function meaningfully. However, these resources are not boundless, and the process of depletion and recovery of self-regulatory resources may help to explain the trajectories of adaptation inherent within chronic pain. We will pay particular attention to the construct of fatigue, which may reflect a state of depleted self-regulatory resources and may also serve as a significant barrier to functioning in chronic pain.

In sum, this chapter will examine multiple factors that contribute to resilience to pain by identifying specific contributors to sustainability, recovery, and growth. We will also examine the importance of the timeframe of pain adaptation and the very human contexts, both within the person in terms of idiosyncratic goals and motivations and the social relationships that support or interfere with adaptive responses to episodic pain.

Characterizing Sustainability Processes

Defined in terms of chronic pain resilience, *sustainability* refers to continued positive engagement: the persistence in valued activities in the presence of pain (Sturgeon & Zautra, 2010). Traditionally, studies have examined pain tolerance, which may function as a marker of sustainability. Pain tolerance has been acknowledged as an important factor in resilience in past studies

(Karoly & Ruehlman, 2006; Zautra et al., 2005), and there is a logical connection between pain tolerance and sustainability in the face of pain. Individuals who cannot tolerate their pain are, by definition, unlikely to function effectively in its presence. Experimental studies have identified a variety of factors that can modify pain tolerance, including cognitive strategies (Fernandez & Turk, 1989), and a number of variables that predict individual differences in pain tolerance, including gender (Riley, Robinson, Wise, Myers, & Fillingim, 1998), genetic dispositions (Compton, Geschwind, & Alarcon, 2003), emotional temperament (de Wied & Verbaten, 2001), and medication use (Skarke, Darimont, Schmidt, Geisslinger, & Lotsch, 2003). Pain tolerance also shows some utility as a clinical construct, as it has been found to predict treatment response following multidisciplinary interventions for chronic pain (Edwards, Doleys, Lowery, & Fillingim, 2003).

Though useful, pain tolerance has too limited a range to encapsulate resilient responding. Tolerance of induced pain in an experimental setting may not generalize to living with chronic pain (Sturgeon & Zautra, 2013a). Furthermore, indiscriminant persistence when in pain is not inherently adaptive. Put simply, resilience to pain is neither necessary nor likely in cases where the ultimate outcome is of little importance to the pain sufferer; the goals of the individual uniquely identify his or her resilience agenda. Pursuit of valued goals can serve to enhance positive emotions and buffer against negative emotions in the context of dealing with a painful medical condition (Coffey et al., 2014). Similarly, optimism and hope, which reflect an ability to identify one's goals and to identify the ways to reach these valued goals, are important predictors of positive functioning despite pain (Hood, Pulvers, Carrillo, Merchant, & Thomas, 2012; Wright et al., 2011). Higher levels of optimism have been found to be protective against pain, emotional distress, and catastrophic thinking (Bruce et al., 2014; Hanssen, Peters, Vlaeyen, Meevissen, & Vancleef, 2013) and reduce the deleterious effects of pain on higher-order cognitive functioning (Boselie, Vancleef, Smeets, & Peters, 2014). Indeed, optimism has also been shown to sustain behavioral efforts in a painful task (Solberg Nes, Carlson, Crofford, de Leeuw, & Segerstrom, 2011).

Recently, research has taken steps to clarify the role of goal orientation in sustainability processes using experimental paradigms. The Mood-As-Inputmodel posits that individuals use information gleaned from their emotional states to determine whether to persist or discontinue engagement in an indefinite task (Ceulemans et al., 2013b). Hedonic goals, such as an innate and immediate desire to continue performing a task, can enhance persistence in that task (Ceulemans et al., 2013b), as does the interpretation of a painful task as a challenge (Jackson, Wang, & Fan, 2014) or in terms of achievement (Karsdorp, Ranson, Nijst, & Vlaeyen, 2013). Further, individuals will also persist in a painful task for longer periods if they are acting according to a sense of personal responsibility (Ceulemans et al., 2013a); this finding may suggest that the presence of eudaimonic goals, which are less concrete and oriented towards outcomes that are abstract or occur in the longer term than hedonic goals, may also enhance persistence. Interestingly, negative emotions may also provide an initial impetus for persistence despite pain, as persistence in a painful task was found to be higher for individuals with higher induced levels of negative emotion (Ceulemans et al., 2013a). However, the motivating effects of negative emotion come at a cost to adaptation; more intense negative emotional states in these experiments were also predictive of higher levels of reported pain later in the procedure (Karsdorp & Vlaeyen, 2011). These studies suggest that cognitive interpretation, goal orientation, and emotional states may modify the willingness of an individual to function under painful conditions, and these effects may be relatively independent forces (Ceulemans et al., 2013a). Although these studies provide valuable support for the importance of goals in sustainability, we do not yet know whether these effects can be generalized outside of an experimental setting and whether they persist over time. Similarly, most of the evidence for the Mood-As-Input model has been gleaned from healthy individuals. Though promising, the importance of goal orientation in resilience to chronic pain awaits further study with clinical populations.

Another valuable model of sustainability can be borrowed from a recently proposed model of stress resilience (Smith, Epstein, Ortiz, Christopher, & Tooley, 2013). Smith and colleagues propose a temporal model of resilience, in which individuals undergo a sequential process of confronting a stressful event, identifying a desired outcome, and mobilizing coping efforts. This model of resilience is valuable, both because it incorporates time as an important factor in resilience and also implicates different variables in the promotion of resilience at each stage. The authors posit that mindful awareness and clarity of mood enhance the ability of an individual to initially confront a stressful event, optimism and a purpose in life help to identify a desired future event, and active coping strategies and social support help the individual to mobilize coping efforts. This model of resilience can be reasonably applied to the experience of pain as well: as individuals experience a new pain or a flare in their existing pain, they may be able to employ similar strategies in orienting to pain, identifying a desired goal, and mobilizing coping efforts for pain in a more coherent way. In terms of resilient responses to chronic pain, however, this model may require expansion across a longer span of time, as the experience of stressful experiences of pain may not be discrete events and may not resolve completely. Many individuals with recurrent pain do not experience an end to the experience of their pain and, thus, may not be able to adequately recover from the exposure to the stressful event in the same way as they might from an acute stressor.

A related system underlying sustained functioning in the face of pain is the perception and pursuit of reward. A recent review of the overlap of pain and reward systems in the brain suggests that chronic pain has implications for both the hedonic and motivational aspects of reward processing (Becker et al., 2012). Becker et al. discuss the "Motivation-Decision Model" of pain and reward, which explores the immediate and often unconscious prioritization of competing impulses of pain-related escape and reward pursuit. As an acute pain signal acts as a potent signal to stop or avoid a painful stimulus, the value of a reward stimulus must exceed the impulse to escape a painful stimulus if the organism is to employ a non-avoidant behavioral response. This model provides an intuitive and important concept in explaining the phenomenon of persistence through painful experiences in humans; in order for an individual to persist in a task that is causing him or her pain, the individual must be able to perceive or call to mind an impending or likely reward that is more salient than the experience of pain.

The Motivation-Decision Model also holds value in conceptualizing chronic pain, as it provides a perspective on how patterns of behavior develop in chronic pain as a function of operant learning (Leknes & Tracey, 2010). By understanding how maladaptive behavioral patterns develop in chronic pain, we can better define the meaning of sustainability from the perspective of the pain sufferer. It has been posited that pain relief may function as a salient reward. There is evidence to support this claim; reward and pain relief demonstrate similar patterns of activation in the orbitofrontal cortex and nucleus accumbens (Becker et al., 2012). Considered from an operant learning perspective, pain relief appears to function as a reward through negative reinforcement, or increasing the likelihood of a behavior by removing an aversive or noxious stimulus, while increases in pain serve as a punishment, which introduce a noxious stimulus like pain. This perspective can help to explain the initial development of unhealthy or maladaptive behavioral patterns after the onset of pain, such as behavioral avoidance: if each time an individual engages in physical movement, they also experience an increased level of pain, a natural consequence of this pattern would be an increase in learned avoidant responses. This pattern would be further reinforced by the relief experienced by individuals when they are not performing those activities that cause increases in their pain. Such responses may be adaptive in the case of acute pain, as individuals could be expected to experience activation in their reward processing circuits when they are able to successfully escape danger, thereby reinforcing behavior that will promote safety in the future.

However, the implications of reinforcing avoidant behaviors become more sinister in the case of chronic pain. As the pattern of pain experience becomes chronic, expectancy of increased pain may develop, making more salient those occasions when pain is absent or at a lower level. This pattern may thus reinforce learned responses to pain that are adaptive in the short term (i.e., through avoidance of or relief from pain), but are problematic in the long term; there is ample evidence that behavioral avoidance enhances the risk of longer-term disability in individuals suffering from a chronic musculoskeletal pain condition (Vlaeyen & Linton, 2000).

The difficulty of sustainability in the face of recurrent pain, then, becomes apparent: resilient responses to chronic pain necessitate identification of important goals whose value exceeds the value of short-term relief from pain. As individuals continue to make decisions about whether to persist in or avoid an activity that exacerbates their pain but may yield another reward, the feedback from these decisions, such as temporary relief from pain or achieving their desired goal, will then reinforce the decision that is made. This process of chosen behavior and reinforcement will then inform future decisions about whether to approach or avoid opportunities when they arise. When individuals are faced with an opportunity to pursue a meaningful goal, but also maintain an expectation that goal pursuit will be accompanied by increased pain, their decision to persist or discontinue their pursuit will be contingent on the rewards they received from previous attempts at goal pursuit or avoidance (see Fig. 8.2). From an operant perspective, those individuals who prove to be resilient to their pain are those who pursue opportunities and are sufficiently reinforced by reaching them. As a result, they become willing to tolerate pain in order to reach a greater reward in the future.

Though it is often said that chronic pain is pain that has lost its utility as a biological signal (as it no longer signals continuing damage or dangerous physical changes in the body), it retains some value as a harbinger of future symptoms in the framework of coping with pain in the long term. More specifically, those individuals who disregard their level of pain and attempt to significantly increase their level of activity despite their pain typically demonstrate poorer overall functioning across time (McCracken & Samuel, 2007). Yet, those individuals who

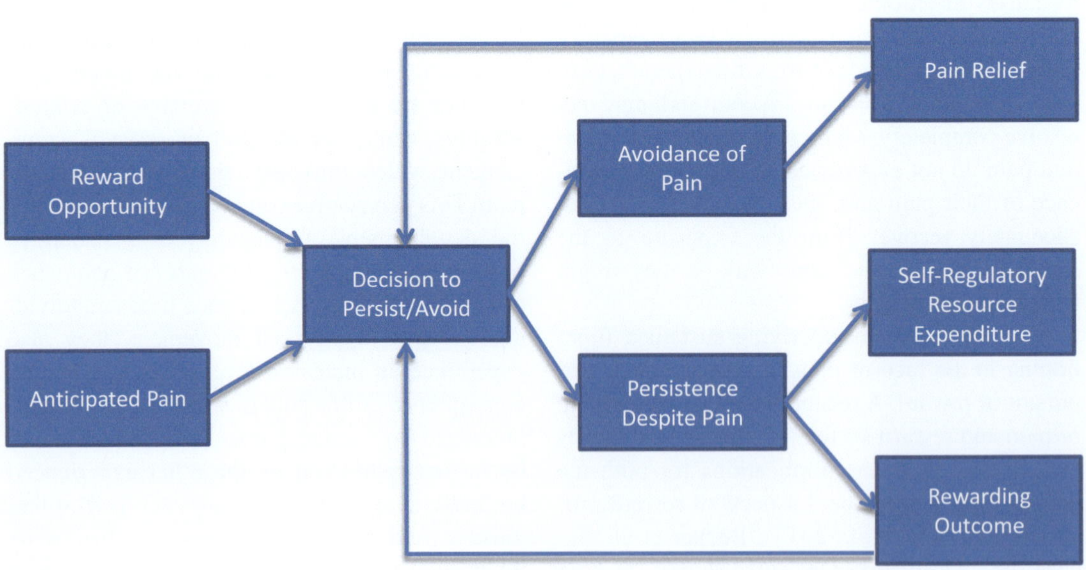

Fig. 8.2 Process of sustainability in chronic pain

attempt to avoid physical activity because of their pain may experience increased pain through deconditioning if they attempt to disregard their pain completely. These patterns of pain coping would suggest that there may be an optimal level of physical activity in which in individual can engage that balances the immediate costs of physical exertion with the long-term benefits of activity (Karsdorp & Vlaeyen, 2011). This concept has been used as a basis for developing behavioral pacing strategies, which are a hallmark intervention of cognitive-behavioral therapy for pain (Keefe, 1996). Curiously, however, even pain-coping styles that center on attempts to pace oneself may predispose an individual to poorer overall functioning (McCracken & Samuel, 2007). Instead, effective sustainability despite pain appears to be dependent on multiple coinciding psychological factors, including a low level of behavioral avoidance, in conjunction with high levels of both physical activity and acceptance of pain (McCracken & Samuel, 2007). In short, the process of sustainability in chronic pain must: (1) engage reward processes oriented towards approach-type or active behaviors; (2) be sensitive enough to immediate, activity-related changes in pain, allowing the individual to persist in these goals across time without the occurrence of significant worsening of pain itself; and (3) maintain a low level of emotional distress related to the experience of pain itself.

Fatigue and Recovery Mechanisms in Chronic Pain

An underappreciated aspect of resilience in chronic pain is the capacity to recover from the deleterious consequences of pain. The costs of sustained functioning despite the presence of significant pain may demand a greater capacity for self-regulatory resources than in healthy individuals, which may manifest in reports of greater fatigue (Solberg Nes et al., 2010). We suggest that fatigue, which is a complex construct comprised of behavioral, cognitive, and emotional components (Nes, Ehlers, Whipple, & Vincent, 2013), should also be understood as a failure of recovery processes in chronic pain. Fatigue has been reported as a significant barrier to functioning and quality of life in osteoarthritis (Murphy, Smith, Clauw, & Alexander, 2008) and rheumatoid arthritis (Pollard, Choy, Gonzalez, Khoshaba, & Scott, 2006), as well as several other chronic pain conditions (Burke, Elliott, & Fleissner, 1999; Feuerstein, Carter, & Papciak, 1987; Kop et al., 2005). Fatigue is also significantly related to anxiety (Roy-Byrne et al., 2002) and shows a reciprocal relationship with depression, such that individuals with complaints of fatigue appear to be at increased risk of developing a future major depressive episode (Addington, Gallo, Ford, & Eaton, 2001), and individuals with depression are more likely to report significant fatigue in the future (Skapinakis, Lewis, & Mavreas, 2004).

Although it is logical to expect fatigue to present a challenge to overall functioning, its role in daily life for an individual with a chronic pain condition is not always appreciated. For example, individuals with chronic pain may be informed by their medical providers about the positive effects of physical exercise for their health, even with recurrent pain. Consequently, many individuals with pain may seek to follow this advice and incorporate greater levels of physical activity into their daily lives and may ultimately experience long-term benefit. Experientially, however, incorporating higher levels of physical activity for an individual with chronic pain may be more difficult than for an individual without chronic pain for several reasons. First, individuals with chronic pain are faced with the task of overcoming a natural impulse to avoid activity and further pain if their symptoms flare up in response to physical activity; this impulse, while frequently adaptive in response to acute pain, may also contribute to longer-term deconditioning and later worsening the experience of pain (Asmundson, Norton, & Norton, 1999). Further, the process of re-introducing physical activity itself into a routine devoid of exercise may initially require significant regulatory effort, as individuals with chronic pain may face increased levels of physical deconditioning if they have fallen into a pattern of behavioral avoidance that frequently accompanies chronic pain conditions (Vlaeyen & Linton, 2000). Additionally, the experience of pain itself may deplete the availability of these self-regulatory resources; individuals with some chronic pain disorders, such as fibromyalgia and temporomandibular joint disorder, demonstrate chronically elevated levels of self-regulatory fatigue, which appear to be partially explained by the intensity of their pain (Solberg Nes et al., 2010). Thus, as a natural consequence of returning to a higher level of physical activity, individuals with chronic pain may experience immediate or prolonged states of regulatory depletion, which may manifest as fatigue (Hagger, Wood, Stiff, & Chatzisarantis, 2010; Segerstrom & Nes, 2007; Solberg Nes et al., 2010; Sturgeon, Yeung, & Zautra, 2014).

As noted previously, some individuals may be prone to maladaptive attempts to excessively increase their levels of physical activity without regard for their level of deconditioning or the severity of their physical symptoms, thereby exacerbating these symptoms (McCracken & Samuel, 2007). In this instance, individuals may appear to be demonstrating some aspects of resilience through *sustainability*, in that they continue to function despite their pain for a period of time. However, they may be simultaneously demonstrating failures in *recovery*, as their attempts may prove unsuccessful in the long term because of the unsustainable intensity of activity and disregard for future symptoms, which may make continued functioning progressively more difficult. The role of recovery is particularly important in this case, as resilience cannot continue indefinitely; even the positive effects of optimism on persistence in a painful task can be compromised by those individuals dealing with greater depletion of their self-regulatory resources (Solberg Nes et al., 2011).

Although individuals with chronic pain may be susceptible to greater depletion of their self-regulatory resources, there are several factors that have been implicated in effective recovery from pain. One important factor for recovery is positive emotion. Positive emotion has been implicated in resilience in a multitude of ways. Broadly, positive emotions aid in recovery from cardiovascular disease (Fredrickson & Levenson, 1998), emotional (DeWall et al., 2011; Tugade & Fredrickson, 2004), and cognitive (Boselie et al., 2014) recovery from stress and also appear to have beneficial effects for the immune system (Pressman & Black, 2012). Positive emotional states also appear to enhance cognition, as happier individuals are better able to think broadly and flexibly than they might under conditions of greater emotional distress (Fredrickson, 2001). Similarly, bolstered positive emotional states appear to underlie some of the cognitive benefits of optimism (Boselie et al., 2014). Individuals with chronic pain who are better able to sustain their positive emotions report less intense pain clinically and under experimental conditions (Finan, Quartana, & Smith, 2013) and appear to be less susceptible to catastrophizing about their pain (Hood et al., 2012) and to behavioral avoidance due to fear of their pain (Meulders, Meulders, & Vlaeyen, 2014). Individuals with an induced positive mood are also able to persist for longer periods under painful conditions (Karsdorp et al., 2013). Positive emotional states also appear to be a mechanism of resilience against problematic and habitual opioid medication misuse in individuals with chronic pain (Garland et al., 2014). Importantly for the purposes of resilience, there exists some evidence for the restorative effect of positive emotions for self-regulatory resources. A mutually influential relationship between positive states like enjoyment and levels of fatigue emerges in daily diary models, suggesting that increased levels of enjoyment may predict lower levels of later fatigue (Yeung, Aiken, MacKinnon, & Davis, 2014). Positive emotions thus appear to be a salient recovery factor in chronic pain.

Another key mechanism of recovery in chronic pain is sleep. Sleep quality, like resilience, is a multidimensional construct with effects in the behavioral, cognitive, affective, and physiological domains, and individual differences in sleep processes have been implicated in resilient coping. Sleep also plays a vital role in the development of memories and insight formation (Ellenbogen, 2005) and may be involved in the repair of damaged cells and neurons (Savage & West, 2007). Sleep quality has been associated with a variety of additional benefits, including lower fatigue (Bliwise, 1992) and lower psychological distress (Shaver & Paulsen, 1993). Good-quality sleep has also been implicated in enhanced physical (Haack & Mullington, 2005) and psychological recovery (Hamilton et al., 2008). Conversely, individuals with chronic pain who report more problematic sleep are more likely to experience significant pain (Finan, Goodin, & Smith, 2013), fatigue (Fishbain, Hall, Risser, & Gonzales, 2009), and poorer physical functioning (McCracken & Iverson, 2001). Greater sleep disruption also appears to be associated with greater complaints of both pain intensity and unpleasantness (Morin, Gibson, & Wade, 1998); this relationship may be informative with regard to the ways in which sleep enhances resilient responses to pain, as the ability to modulate attention towards and away from pain appears to be dependent to some degree on the quality of sleep (Affleck, Urrows, Tennen, Higgins, & Abeles, 1996, Edwards et al., 2003). Notably, sleep quality has also been implicated in the maintenance of positive emotional states in chronic pain (Hamilton, Catley, & Karlson, 2007), further strengthening the theoretical connection between both sleep and positive emotions and recovery processes in chronic pain. It is also instructive that cognitive-behavioral treatments focused specifically on sleep or pain demonstrate effects on both domains (Smith & Haythornthwaite, 2004), which indicates that there may be commonalities in the underlying etiologies of both processes.

Social Contributors to Pain Resilience

Although a great deal of research has traditionally been focused on intra-individual processes that contribute to resilient coping, the social world also plays a complex role in adaptation to chronic pain. In general, resilient individuals appear to effectively utilize social resources to recover from stress (Friborg et al., 2006) and can enhance resilience against a stressor by seeking out appropriate social support (Connor & Davidson, 2003). In individuals with chronic pain, a primary source of sustainable positive emotion is through continued positive social interactions (Smith & Zautra, 2008). Similarly, the presence of support from a loved one can buffer against the effects of stress and pain on the HPA axis (Hostinar, Sullivan, & Gunnar, 2014), preserves physical and psychological functioning during times of increased pain (Taylor, Davis, & Zautra, 2013), and predicts decreased pain and central nervous system activity during a pain induction procedure (Montoya, Larbig, Braun, Preissl, & Birbaumer, 2004).

However, individuals with chronic pain may also face unique challenges to their social worlds. Individuals with chronic pain may lose their ability to view their relationships with the appropriate degree of flexibility when experiencing increased pain (Davis, Zautra, & Smith, 2004), may be more likely to become irritable or angry and experience social conflict (Feldman, Downey, & Schaffer-Neitz, 1999), and show a greater tendency to decrease their levels of positive social engagement in the face of significant pain (Sturgeon, Zautra & Arewasikporn, 2014). It has been suggested that some individuals may also adopt a stoic attitude towards their pain, choosing not to seek out appropriate support from their social environment, even if it is available, thereby compromising the beneficial effects of a responsive social network (Moore, Grime, Campbell, & Richardson, 2013). When one's relationships are damaged, an important source of positive emotion is threatened; in these cases, recovery processes become increasingly important. Recent evidence suggests that a capacity to forgive and to repair damaged social relationships may enhance resilience in chronic pain (Toussaint et al., 2014).

Further, although social relations are fundamental to resilience in pain, a social network that is too large or that enhances dependency rather than rewarding competence may undermine the person's self-efficacy, leading to poorer long-term pain coping (Franks, Cronan, & Oliver, 2004). Similarly, social goals that are focused on receiving validation from others rather than contributing to the well-being of others may lessen, rather than boost, sustainability (Hamilton, Karoly, & Zautra, 2005). Social resilience in chronic pain thus may be best defined as an ability to maintain engagement in, and appreciation for, valued social relationships, even during painful moments, and to repair meaningful interpersonal relationships when they are damaged. Given the many challenges faced by those dealing with recurrent pain, social support can be an important contributor to successful adaptation, but only within the context of relationships that preserve an individual's motivation to take an active and meaningful part in shaping one's life course trajectory.

Growth and New Learning in Response to Chronic Pain

One implicit assumption in our model of resilience is that an individual experiences many opportunities to be resilient to chronic pain that can be measured across time. An individual may find a way to cope effectively with pain immediately, such that it does not meaningfully disrupt his or her immediate emotional, cognitive, or behavioral states. In those cases where pain does lead to poorer functioning, however, individuals may show resilience to pain by effectively bouncing back and returning to their baseline or homeostatic set points. Finally, those individuals who strive and fail, but ultimately bounce back from their pain-related challenges may acquire important new information about how to cope with pain in an effective way, catalyzing long-term growth.

These patterns of pain-coping responses may thus evolve across time; the occurrence of learning, which may spur alternative strategies for coping with pain, expectations about the experience of pain itself, and belief in one's own ability to cope, is dependent on the coping attempts that have occurred previously. Responses to pain and subsequent coping efforts also have a profound long-term impact; there is evidence that emotional reactivity to stressors can affect health status over a period of time as long as 10 years (Piazza, Charles, Sliwinski, Mogle, & Almeida, 2013). Consequently, it is necessary to expand models of pain resilience to incorporate time as an important contributing factor (Keefe & Wren, 2013); resilience to pain is "learned" through previous painful experiences, and only by acknowledging time as a factor can we understand how the phenomenon of resilience to pain may evolve within individuals as they progress from acute pain to chronic pain, and how they make adjustments to chronic pain itself. Some studies have begun to incorporate time in models of pain resilience by examining trajectories of intensity of specific pain complaints (Collins, Katz, Dervan, & Losina, 2014), which can serve as important characterizations of physical recovery from pain itself, while others have tracked the concomitant changes in pain and mood across time, reflecting psychological recovery from pain (Zhu, Galatzer-Levy, & Bonanno, 2014). We highlight the importance of long-term growth as a valuable temporal indicator of adaptation to chronic pain.

Missing in all models of adjustment, and in some models of resilience, is an appreciation for the capacity of the person with chronic pain to learn, not just to cope successfully, but to further their existing goals and develop new pursuits. Resilient *growth* in chronic pain occurs through adaptive efforts that are modified according to feedback to the individual and the environment. In early stages of chronic pain, individuals may naturally gravitate to different strategies when they believe their pain to be acute, rather than chronic. However, over time, many individuals discover that these strategies (e.g., behavioral avoidance) are maladaptive and may contribute to longer-standing problems. Further, some individuals may habituate to their pain naturally through the course of their daily lives, as recent findings suggest greater levels of resilience in older individuals with chronic physical ailments than in younger individuals (Terrill et al., 2014). Growth and new learning occurs through experience and, often, through failed attempts to adapt. Indeed, individuals who self-identify as resilient have reported drawing from coping with previous challenges and losses (Gattuso, 2003). Exposure to pain and stress is also important in fostering growth, as it provides an opportunity to learn and respond effectively to pain.

It is well-established that early life exposure to stressors can alter developmental trajectories; there is a robust literature suggesting that exposure to severe traumatic stressors or chronically elevated levels of stress exposure can manifest in poorer overall development and functioning later in life (Rutten et al., 2013). However, an optimal level of stress exposure may exist; put in another way, lack of exposure to stress during earlier developmental stages is unlikely to yield optimal levels of resilience in later developmental stages. A recent study by Seery et al. (2013) has demonstrated this phenomenon. These authors reported that moderate life stress exposure throughout adulthood has been found to predict greater levels of resilience to stress and pain, whereas resilience to these factors was lower in those with no significant life stress or very high levels of life stress. More specifically, individuals who reported moderate levels of life stress during their adult years demonstrated lower levels of situational catastrophizing, pain intensity, and pain unpleasantness to a cold pressor task, were able to tolerate cold pressor pain for longer periods, and also exhibited decreased physiological reactivity to a social stress paradigm in which they were asked to complete a nonverbal intelligence test (Seery, Leo, Lupien, Kondrak, & Almonte, 2013). In short, individuals who faced *significant but not overwhelming* stress as adults were better able to handle situational challenges like social stress and pain more effectively. Interestingly, individuals with chronic pain have shown decreased levels of emotional stress in response to future stressors after suffering the loss of a spouse, suggesting that resilience may develop even after particularly poignant losses and the ongoing experience of pain (Wade, Hart, Wade, Bajaj, & Price, 2013).

The inoculating effects of stress are also theorized to be present in childhood: early life exposure to periodic, but not necessarily prolonged, challenges like life stressors may contribute to resilience, while severe or prolonged stress exposure may sensitize the hypothalamic-pituitary-adrenal axis and may contribute to longer-term vulnerability to psychiatric disorders (Rutten et al., 2013). This phenomenon has been theorized to fit a quadratic or inverse-U function, such that too much or too little exposure to stress in childhood may contribute to greater vulnerability to poor stress response, while there is an optimal and moderate level of stress exposure (Parker & Maestripieri, 2011). Further, the process of resilient development appears to be modified by epigenetic factors, which may help to explain the large degree of variability of responses among individuals who are exposed to similar levels of challenge during their development (Rutten et al., 2013).

A similar parallel has been drawn to the benefits of a common and frequent physical challenge: physical exercise. Physical exercise presents a notable challenge to physiological adaptation (McEwen, 2003) and has been implicated as a promoting factor in resilience in earlier development (Strohle, 2009) and in resilient responses to stress in adults (Deuster & Silverman, 2013). Further, maintenance of physical exercise earlier in life is predictive of greater behavioral engagement in older age, despite the presence of chronic pain (Moore, Richardson, Sim, Bernard, & Jordan, 2014). However, physical activity in some forms may pose problems to individuals with chronic pain or fatigue, manifesting in increased inflammatory responses (McEwen, 2003). This evidence suggests that the effects of exercise, like stress, are not uniform across individuals in all forms and must be interpreted in the proper context.

Pain acceptance is another salient example of how the timeframe of pain adaptation plays a meaningful role in our understanding of resilience. Pain acceptance is defined as a process by which individuals acknowledge that they have pain, stop maladaptive attempts to prevent or cure their pain, and learn to live meaningful lives despite the presence of their pain (McCracken, 1998). Acceptance of pain may also reflect a greater degree of psychological flexibility, conferring an increased ability to maintain focus on values and goals during times of increased pain and distress, and helping individuals to act or adjust their behavior in ways that are most consistent with their values (Eccleston, Crombez, Aldrich, & Stannard, 2001). Acceptance of pain has proven to be a powerful predictor of better functioning in individuals with chronic pain, as individuals who accept their pain will show lower levels of emotional distress in response to pain and continue to maintain engagement in valued activities despite the presence of pain (McCracken, 2010). More recent studies of pain acceptance have tied this construct more directly to resilience, suggesting that acceptance of pain can buffer against negative consequences of pain on mood and functional impairment (Ramírez-Maestre & Esteve, 2014; Ramirez-Maestre, Esteve, & Lopez-Martinez, 2014) and may be a more salient factor in determining the severity of pain-related disability than negative cognitive factors such as pain catastrophizing (Mun, Okun, & Karoly, 2014).

However, pain acceptance may be a slow process, and the slowness of this process may be adaptive. In cases of acute pain, individuals may be better suited if they do not accept new pain sensations until they have run a normal course of medical evaluation and treatment, and it becomes clear that the pain does not signal a dangerous new problem, such as a new injury or illness. Indeed, the ability to detect and avoid danger is likely the primary evolutionary utility of pain itself, which manifests in specific behavioral responses to a new pain (Leknes & Bastian, 2014). Even in cases of pain that have not resolved over a period of a few months, individuals may naturally persist in seeking a cure to their pain and, in some cases, may find one. Once it becomes clear that pain will not resolve completely, acceptance becomes an especially important step. Individuals who maintain a rigid belief in a cure for their pain despite mounting evidence that no cure exists are likely to worsen their own emotional distress. It is only when their focus turns to returning to function in a meaningful way that their emotional distress will decrease, even if pain persists.

Though the differential effects of pain acceptance across time have not been well-studied to date, one recent study illustrates that this factor may be important. In a study of individuals with fibromyalgia and temporomandibular joint disorder, researchers found that, unsurprisingly, pain acceptance predicted better functioning and lower levels of self-regulatory fatigue (Eisenlohr-Moul, Burris, & Evans, 2013). Notably, however, the relationship between pain acceptance and fatigue was dependent on how long individuals had been experiencing their pain. Pain acceptance served as a stronger protective factor against fatigue in individuals who had been experiencing their pain for longer periods of time. Though this finding is somewhat unique at present, it serves to demonstrate the complex process of habituation and adaptation to chronic pain that is likely present in individuals dealing with pain.

The previous example also highlights the shifting nature of goals within chronic pain. While it may be valuable in the early stages of a painful episode to focus solely on pain relief, this strategy may prove unsatisfying in the long term, particularly in cases where the pain is poorly controlled, even with effective medical interventions. As individuals habituate and adapt to their pain (or fail to do so) across time, their identified needs may change. This topic has been discussed to some extent with regard to "stages of change." Individuals with pain may not yet recognize the need for more active engagement in their own pain management, or may recognize this need but be unaware about to engage, before they reach a stage of physical and psychological readiness to enact change in their lives by actively changing their attempts to cope with pain (Kerns, Rosenberg, Jamison, Caudill, & Haythornthwaite, 1997). Individual differences in one's "stage of change" may dictate the most appropriate degree of treatment that they receive; those individuals who have not yet reached the stage of recognizing the importance of taking an active approach to managing their pain may benefit more from an insight-focused or value-focused psychotherapeutic approach, allowing them to identify an impetus for behavior change (Kerns et al., 1997). Once a greater level of insight and motivation is reached, these individuals are able to more effectively seek and implement new strategies for changing their relationship with pain, as in cognitive-behavioral therapy. This process may develop naturally in some individuals, whereas other individuals may require more intensive intervention to reach later stages. It is in this way that we see that resilience to pain and, more specifically, resilient growth informed by chronic pain, may develop over time, not just to aid adaptation, but to deepen the meaning of a "good" life for someone in pain.

Conclusion

In order to more appropriately describe the full range of consequences of chronic pain, it becomes important to understand the experience of pain from the standpoint of the pain sufferer, while integrating the findings provided by previous research studies. Although we have traditionally viewed chronic pain as a strictly negative influence that involves only the physical and psychological states of the pain sufferer, this focus can be narrow and may underrepresent those individuals who continue to function meaningfully despite their pain. Our understanding of pain adaptation and resilience can be further improved by examining how the surrounding social environment and the goals and motivations of the person can change how and why they may choose to persist in pain. Adapting to a chronic pain condition requires constant effort to overcome a natural response to avoid pain; resilience occurs only when the individual is able to see past the immediate urge to avoid pain and pursue something more meaningful. Our understanding of resilience can be further enriched by incorporating a model in which each attempt at coping with pain informs future attempts: by characterizing how persistence and recovery from pain are intertwined, we can better explain the unique challenges of chronic, rather than episodic, pain, and how pain may lead to other problems that interfere with meaningful function, such as fatigue. In the longer term, individuals with long-lasting pain conditions may develop alternative and more effective ways of interpreting and coping with their pain that ultimately enhance well-being and functioning. In sum, expansion of the complexity of future clinical and empirical models will yield more useful insight into the wide-ranging consequences of and adaptation to chronic pain.

References

Addington, A., Gallo, J., Ford, D., & Eaton, W. (2001). Epidemiology of unexplained fatigue and major depression in the community: The Baltimore ECA follow-up, 1981–1994. *Psychological Medicine, 31*, 1037–1044.

Affleck, G., Urrows, S., Tennen, H., Higgins, P., & Abeles, M. (1996). Sequential daily relations of sleep, pain intensity, and attention to pain among women with fibromyalgia. *Pain, 68*, 363–368. doi:10.1016/S0304-3959(96)03226-5.

Asmundson, G. J., Norton, P. J., & Norton, G. R. (1999). Beyond pain: The role of fear and avoidance in chronicity. *Clinical Psychology Review, 19*, 97–119.

Becker, S., Gandhi, W., & Schweinhardt, P. (2012). Cerebral interactions of pain and reward and their relevance for chronic pain. *Neuroscience Letters, 520*, 182–187. doi:10.1016/j.neulet.2012.03.013.

Blalock, D., McKnight, P. E., Kashdan, T. B., Franz, S. C., Kasle, S., & Zautra, A. J. (2015). Predicting treatment course and outcome using a promotion and prevention framework in a community sample of arthritis sufferers. Manuscript in preparation.

Bliwise, N. G. (1992). Factors related to sleep quality in healthy elderly women. *Psychology and Aging, 7*, 83–88.

Boselie, J. J., Vancleef, L. M., Smeets, T., & Peters, M. L. (2014). Increasing optimism abolishes pain-induced impairments in executive task performance. *Pain, 155*, 334–340. doi:10.1016/j.pain.2013.10.014

Bruce, J., Thornton, A. J., Powell, R., Johnston, M., Wells, M., Heys, S. D., … for the Recovery Study Group. (2014). Psychological, surgical, and sociodemographic predictors of pain outcomes after breast cancer surgery: A population-based cohort study. *Pain, 155*, 232–243. doi:10.1016/j.pain.2013.09.028.

Burke, P., Elliott, M., & Fleissner, R. (1999). Irritable bowel syndrome and recurrent abdominal pain: A comparative review. *Psychosomatics, 40*, 277–285.

Ceulemans, K., Karsdorp, P. A., & Vlaeyen, J. W. (2013a). Effects of responsibility and mood on painful task persistence. *Journal of Behavior Therapy and Experimental Psychiatry, 44*, 186–193. doi:10.1016/j.jbtep.2012.10.005.

Ceulemans, K., Karsdorp, P. A., & Vlaeyen, J. W. (2013b). Mood, stop-rules and task persistence: No mood-as-input effects in the context of pain. *Journal of Behavior Therapy and Experimental Psychiatry, 44*, 463–468. doi:10.1016/j.jbtep.2013.06.002.

Coffey, L., Gallagher, P., Desmond, D., & Ryall, N. (2014). Goal pursuit, goal adjustment, and affective well-being following lower limb amputation. *British*

Journal of Health Psychology, 19, 409–424. doi:10.1111/bjhp.12051.

Collins, J. E., Katz, J. N., Dervan, E. E., & Losina, E. (2014). Trajectories and risk profiles of pain in persons with radiographic, symptomatic knee osteoarthritis: Data from the osteoarthritis initiative. *Osteoarthritis and Cartilage, 22*, 622–630. doi:10.1016/j.joca.2014.03.009.

Compton, P., Geschwind, D. H., & Alarcon, M. (2003). Association between human μ-opioid receptor gene polymorphism, pain tolerance, and opioid addiction. *American Journal of Medical Genetics Part B: Neuropsychiatric Genetics, 121*, 76–82.

Connor, K. M., & Davidson, J. R. (2003). Development of a new resilience scale: The Connor-Davidson Resilience Scale (CD-RISC). *Depression and Anxiety, 18*, 76–82. doi:10.1002/da.10113.

Crombez, G., Eccleston, C., Van Damme, S., Vlaeyen, J. W., & Karoly, P. (2012). Fear-avoidance model of chronic pain: The next generation. *The Clinical Journal of Pain, 28*, 475–483.

Davis, M. C., Zautra, A. J., & Smith, B. W. (2004). Chronic pain, stress, and the dynamics of affective differentiation. *Journal of Personality, 72*, 1133–1159. doi:10.1111/j.1467-6494.2004.00293.x.

de Wied, M., & Verbaten, M. N. (2001). Affective pictures processing, attention, and pain tolerance. *Pain, 90*, 163–172.

Deuster, P. A., & Silverman, M. N. (2013). Physical fitness: A pathway to health and resilience. *U.S. Army Medical Department Journal*, 24–35.

DeWall, C. N., Twenge, J. M., Koole, S. L., Baumeister, R. F., Marquez, A., & Reid, M. W. (2011). Automatic emotion regulation after social exclusion: Tuning to positivity. *Emotion, 11*, 623–636. doi:10.1037/a0023534.

Eccleston, C., Crombez, G., Aldrich, S., & Stannard, C. (2001). Worry and chronic pain patients: A description and analysis of individual differences. *European Journal of Pain, 5*, 309–318. doi:10.1053/eujp.2001.0252.

Edwards, R. R., Doleys, D. M., Lowery, D., & Fillingim, R. B. (2003). Pain tolerance as a predictor of outcome following multidisciplinary treatment for chronic pain: Differential effects as a function of sex. *Pain, 106*, 419–426. doi:10.1016/j.pain.2003.004.

Eisenlohr-Moul, T. A., Burris, J. L., & Evans, D. R. (2013). Pain acceptance, psychological functioning, and self-regulatory fatigue in temporomandibular disorder. *Health Psychology, 32*, 1236–1239. doi:10.1037/a0030150.

Ellenbogen, J. M. (2005). Cognitive benefits of sleep and their loss due to sleep deprivation. *Neurology, 64*, E25–E27.

Elliott, A. M., Burton, C. D., & Hannaford, P. C. (2014). Resilience does matter: Evidence from a 10-year cohort record linkage study. *BMJ Open, 4*, e003917. doi:10.1136/bmjopen-2013-003917.

Feldman, S. I., Downey, G., & Schaffer-Neitz, R. (1999). Pain, negative mood, and perceived support in chronic pain patients: A daily diary study of people with reflex sympathetic dystrophy syndrome. *Journal of Consulting and Clinical Psychology, 67*, 776–785.

Fernandez, E., & Turk, D. C. (1989). The utility of cognitive coping strategies for altering pain perception: A meta-analysis. *Pain, 38*, 123–135.

Feuerstein, M., Carter, R. L., & Papciak, A. S. (1987). A prospective analysis of stress and fatigue in recurrent low back pain. *Pain, 31*, 333–344.

Finan, P. H., Buenaver, L. F., Bounds, S. C., Hussain, S., Park, R. J., Haque, U. J., … Smith, M. T. (2013). Discordance between pain and radiographic severity in knee osteoarthritis findings from quantitative sensory testing of central sensitization. *Arthritis and Rheumatism, 65*, 363–372. doi:10.1002/Art.34646.

Finan, P. H., Goodin, B. R., & Smith, M. T. (2013). The association of sleep and pain: An update and a path forward. *The Journal of Pain, 14*, 1539–1552. doi:10.1016/j.jpain.2013.08.007.

Finan, P. H., Quartana, P. J., & Smith, M. T. (2013). Positive and negative affect dimensions in chronic knee osteoarthritis: Effects on clinical and laboratory pain. *Psychosomatic Medicine, 75*, 463–470. doi:10.1097/PSY.0b013e31828ef1d6.

Fishbain, D. A., Hall, J. A., Risser, R. C., & Gonzales, J. S. (2009). Does pain cause the perception of fatigue in patients with chronic pain? Findings from studies for management of diabetic peripheral neuropathic pain with duloxetine. *Pain Practice, 9*, 354–362.

Franks, H. M., Cronan, T. A., & Oliver, K. (2004). Social support in women with fibromyalgia: Is quality more important than quantity? *Journal of Community Psychology, 32*, 425–438.

Fredrickson, B. L. (2001). The role of positive emotions in positive psychology. The broaden-and-build theory of positive emotions. *The American Psychologist, 56*, 218–226.

Fredrickson, B. L., & Levenson, R. W. (1998). Positive emotions speed recovery from the cardiovascular sequelae of negative emotions. *Cognition and Emotion, 12*, 191–220. doi:10.1080/026999398379718.

Friborg, O., Hjemdal, O., Rosenvinge, J. H., Martinussen, M., Aslaksen, P. M., & Flaten, M. A. (2006). Resilience as a moderator of pain and stress. *Journal of Psychosomatic Research, 61*, 213–219. doi:10.1016/j.jpsychores.2005.12.007.

Garland, E. L., Manusov, E. G., Froeliger, B., Kelly, A., Williams, J. M., & Howard, M. O. (2014). Mindfulness-oriented recovery enhancement for chronic pain and prescription opioid misuse: Results from an early-stage randomized controlled trial. *Journal of Consulting and Clinical Psychology, 82*, 448–459. doi:10.1037/a0035798.

Gattuso, S. (2003). Becoming a wise old woman: Resilience and wellness in later life. *Health Sociology Review, 12*, 171–177.

Haack, M., & Mullington, J. M. (2005). Sustained sleep restriction reduces emotional and physical well-being. *Pain, 119*, 56–64. doi:10.1016/j.pain.2005.09.011.

Hagger, M. S., Wood, C., Stiff, C., & Chatzisarantis, N. L. (2010). Ego depletion and the strength model of self-control: A meta-analysis. *Psychological Bulletin, 136*, 495–525. doi:10.1037/a0019486.

Hamilton, N. A., Affleck, G., Tennen, H., Karlson, C., Luxton, D., Preacher, K. J., & Templin, J. L. (2008). Fibromyalgia: The role of sleep in affect and in negative event reactivity and recovery. *Health Psychology, 27*, 490–497. doi:10.1037/0278-6133.27.4.490.

Hamilton, N. A., Catley, D., & Karlson, C. (2007). Sleep and the affective response to stress and pain. *Health Psychology, 26*, 288–295. doi:10.1037/0278-6133.26.3.288.

Hamilton, N. A., Karoly, P., & Zautra, A. J. (2005). Health goal cognition and adjustment in women with fibromyalgia. *Journal of Behavioral Medicine, 28*, 455–466. doi:10.1007/s10865-005-9013-8.

Hanssen, M. M., Peters, M. L., Vlaeyen, J. W., Meevissen, Y. M., & Vancleef, L. M. (2013). Optimism lowers pain: Evidence of the causal status and underlying mechanisms. *Pain, 154*, 53–58. doi:10.1016/j.pain.2012.08.006.

Hood, A., Pulvers, K., Carrillo, J., Merchant, G., & Thomas, M. (2012). Positive traits linked to less pain through lower pain catastrophizing. *Personality and Individual Differences, 52*, 401–405. doi:10.1016/j.paid.2011.10.040.

Hostinar, C. E., Sullivan, R. M., & Gunnar, M. R. (2014). Psychobiological mechanisms underlying the social buffering of the hypothalamic-pituitary-adrenocortical axis: A review of animal models and human studies across development. *Psychological Bulletin, 140*, 256–282. doi:10.1037/a0032671.

Jackson, T., Wang, Y., & Fan, H. Y. (2014). Associations between pain appraisals and pain outcomes: Meta-analyses of laboratory pain and chronic pain literatures. *The Journal of Pain, 15*, 586–601. doi:10.1016/j.jpain.2014.01.499.

Karoly, P., & Ruehlman, L. S. (2006). Psychological "resilience" and its correlates in chronic pain: Findings from a national community sample. *Pain, 123*, 90–97. doi:10.1016/j.pain.2006.02.014.

Karsdorp, P. A., Ranson, S., Nijst, S., & Vlaeyen, J. W. (2013). Goals, mood and performance duration on cognitive tasks during experimentally induced mechanical pressure pain. *Journal of Behavior Therapy and Experimental Psychiatry, 44*, 240–247. doi:10.1016/j.jbtep.2012.07.009.

Karsdorp, P. A., & Vlaeyen, J. W. S. (2011). Goals matter: Both achievement and pain-avoidance goals are associated with pain severity and disability in patients with low back and upper extremity pain. *Pain, 152*, 1382–1390. doi:10.1016/j.pain.2011.02.018.

Keefe, F. J. (1996). Cognitive behavioral therapy for managing pain. *The Clinical Psychologist, 49*, 4–5.

Keefe, F. J., & Wren, A. A. (2013). Optimism and pain: A positive move forward. *Pain, 154*, 7–8. doi:10.1016/j.pain.2012.10.005.

Kerns, R. D., Rosenberg, R., Jamison, R. N., Caudill, M. A., & Haythornthwaite, J. (1997). Readiness to adopt a self-management approach to chronic pain: The Pain Stages of Change Questionnaire (PSOCQ). *Pain, 72*, 227–234.

Kop, W. J., Lyden, A., Berlin, A. A., Ambrose, K., Olsen, C., Gracely, R. H., … Clauw, D. J. (2005). Ambulatory monitoring of physical activity and symptoms in fibromyalgia and chronic fatigue syndrome. *Arthritis & Rheumatism, 52*, 296–303.

Leknes, S., & Bastian, B. (2014). The benefits of pain. *Review of Philosophy and Psychology, 5*, 57–70.

Leknes, S., & Tracey, I. (2008). A common neurobiology for pain and pleasure. *Nature Reviews. Neuroscience, 9*, 314–320. doi:10.1038/nrn2333.

Leknes, S., & Tracey, I. (2010). Pain and pleasure: Masters of mankind. In *Pleasures of the brain* (pp. 320–335).

Masi, A. T., White, K. P., & Pilcher, J. J. (2002). Person-centered approach to care, teaching, and research in fibromyalgia syndrome: Justification from biopsychosocial perspectives in populations. *Seminars in Arthritis and Rheumatism, 32*(2), 71–93.

McAllister, S. J., Vincent, A., Hassett, A. L., Whipple, M. O., Oh, T. H., Benzo, R. P., & Toussaint, L. L. (2013). Psychological resilience, affective mechanisms and symptom burden in a tertiary-care sample of patients with fibromyalgia. *Stress and Health*. doi:10.1002/smi.2555.

McCracken, L. M. (1998). Learning to live with the pain: Acceptance of pain predicts adjustment in persons with chronic pain. *Pain, 74*, 21–27.

McCracken, L. M. (2010). Toward understanding acceptance and psychological flexibility in chronic pain. *Pain, 149*, 420–421. doi:10.1016/j.pain.2010.02.036.

McCracken, L., & Iverson, G. (2001). Disrupted sleep patterns and daily functioning in patients with chronic pain. *Pain Research & Management, 7*, 75–79.

McCracken, L. M., & Samuel, V. M. (2007). The role of avoidance, pacing, and other activity patterns in chronic pain. *Pain, 130*, 119–125. doi:10.1016/j.pain.2006.11.016.

McEwen, B. S. (2003). Interacting mediators of allostasis and allostatic load: Towards an understanding of resilience in aging. *Metabolism, Clinical and Experimental, 52*, 10–16.

Meulders, A., Meulders, M., & Vlaeyen, J. W. (2014). Positive affect protects against deficient safety learning during extinction of fear of movement-related pain in healthy individuals scoring relatively high on trait anxiety. *The Journal of Pain, 15*, 632–644. doi:10.1016/j.jpain.2014.02.009.

Montoya, P., Larbig, W., Braun, C., Preissl, H., & Birbaumer, N. (2004). Influence of social support and emotional context on pain processing and magnetic brain responses in fibromyalgia. *Arthritis and Rheumatism, 50*, 4035–4044. doi:10.1002/art.20660.

Moore, A., Grime, J., Campbell, P., & Richardson, J. (2013). Troubling stoicism: Sociocultural influences and applications to health and illness behaviour. *Health (London, England), 17*, 159–173. doi:10.1177/1363459312451179.

Moore, A. J., Richardson, J. C., Sim, J., Bernard, M., & Jordan, K. P. (2014). Older people's perceptions of

remaining physically active and living with chronic pain. *Qualitative Health Research, 24*, 761–772. doi:10.1177/1049732314529663.
Morin, C. M., Gibson, D., & Wade, J. (1998). Self-reported sleep and mood disturbance in chronic pain patients. *The Clinical Journal of Pain, 14*, 311–314.
Mun, C. J., Okun, M. A., & Karoly, P. (2014). Trait mindfulness and catastrophizing as mediators of the association between pain severity and pain-related impairment. *Personality and Individual Differences, 66*, 68–73. doi:10.1016/j.paid.2014.03.016.
Murphy, S. L., Smith, D. M., Clauw, D. J., & Alexander, N. B. (2008). The impact of momentary pain and fatigue on physical activity in women with osteoarthritis. *Arthritis Care & Research, 59*, 849–856.
Nes, L. S., Ehlers, S. L., Whipple, M. O., & Vincent, A. (2013). Self-regulatory fatigue in chronic multisymptom illnesses: Scale development, fatigue, and self-control. *Journal of Pain Research, 6*, 181–188. doi:10.2147/JPR.S40014.
Nicassio, P. M., & Wallston, K. A. (1992). Longitudinal relationships among pain, sleep problems, and depression in rheumatoid-arthritis. *Journal of Abnormal Psychology, 101*, 514–520. doi:10.1037//0021-843x.101.3.514.
Parker, K. J., & Maestripieri, D. (2011). Identifying key features of early stressful experiences that produce stress vulnerability and resilience in primates. *Neuroscience and Biobehavioral Reviews, 35*, 1466–1483. doi:10.1016/j.neubiorev.2010.09.003.
Piazza, J. R., Charles, S. T., Sliwinski, M. J., Mogle, J., & Almeida, D. M. (2013). Affective reactivity to daily stressors and long-term risk of reporting a chronic physical health condition. *Annals of Behavioral Medicine, 45*, 110–120. doi:10.1007/s12160-012-9423-0.
Pincus, T., Griffith, J., Pearce, S., & Isenberg, D. (1996). Prevalence of self-reported depression in patients with rheumatoid arthritis. *British Journal of Rheumatology, 35*, 879–883.
Pollard, L., Choy, E., Gonzalez, J., Khoshaba, B., & Scott, D. (2006). Fatigue in rheumatoid arthritis reflects pain, not disease activity. *Rheumatology (Oxford), 45*, 885–889.
Pressman, S. D., & Black, L. L. (2012). Positive emotions and immunity. In *The Oxford handbook of psychoneuroimmunology* (pp. 92–104). New York, NY: Oxford University Press.
Ramírez-Maestre, C., & Esteve, R. (2014). The role of sex/gender in the experience of pain: Resilience, fear, and acceptance as central variables in the adjustment of men and women with chronic pain. *The Journal of Pain, 15*, 608–618.e1.
Ramirez-Maestre, C., Esteve, R., & Lopez, A. E. (2012). The path to capacity: Resilience and spinal chronic pain. *Spine, 37*, E251–E258. doi:10.1097/BRS.0b013e31822e93ab.
Ramirez-Maestre, C., Esteve, R., & Lopez-Martinez, A. (2014). Fear-avoidance, pain acceptance and adjustment to chronic pain: A cross-sectional study on a sample of 686 patients with chronic spinal pain. *Annals of Behavioral Medicine, 48*, 402–410. doi:10.1007/s12160-014-9619-6.
Riley, J. L., III, Robinson, M. E., Wise, E. A., Myers, C. D., & Fillingim, R. B. (1998). Sex differences in the perception of noxious experimental stimuli: A meta-analysis. *Pain, 74*, 181–187.
Roy-Byrne, P., Afari, N., Ashton, S., Fischer, M., Goldberg, J., & Buchwald, D. (2002). Chronic fatigue and anxiety/depression: A twin study. *The British Journal of Psychiatry, 180*, 29–34.
Rutten, B. P., Hammels, C., Geschwind, N., Menne-Lothmann, C., Pishva, E., Schruers, K., … Wichers, M. (2013). Resilience in mental health: Linking psychological and neurobiological perspectives. *Acta Psychiatrica Scandinavica, 128*, 3–20. doi:10.1111/acps.12095.
Salathé, C. R., Melloh, M., Kälin, W., Semmer, N., Roth, M., Müller, U., & Elfering, A. (2013). Comparison of pain-resilient working individuals to population-based case controls with/without momentary low back pain. *European Journal of Pain, 17*, 1411–1421.
Savage, V. M., & West, G. B. (2007). A quantitative, theoretical framework for understanding mammalian sleep. *Proceedings of the National Academy of Sciences of the United States of America, 104*, 1051–1056. doi:10.1073/pnas.0610080104.
Seebach, C. L., Kirkhart, M., Lating, J. M., Wegener, S. T., Song, Y., Riley, L. H., 3rd, & Archer, K. R. (2012). Examining the role of positive and negative affect in recovery from spine surgery. *Pain, 153*, 518–525. doi:10.1016/j.pain.2011.10.012.
Seery, M. D., Leo, R. J., Lupien, S. P., Kondrak, C. L., & Almonte, J. L. (2013). An upside to adversity? Moderate cumulative lifetime adversity is associated with resilient responses in the face of controlled stressors. *Psychological Science, 0956797612469210*.
Segerstrom, S. C., & Nes, L. S. (2007). Heart rate variability reflects self-regulatory strength, effort, and fatigue. *Psychological Science, 18*, 275–281. doi:10.1111/j.1467-9280.2007.01888.x.
Shaver, J. L., & Paulsen, V. M. (1993). Sleep, psychological distress, and somatic symptoms in perimenopausal women. *Family Practice Research Journal, 13*, 373–384.
Skapinakis, P., Lewis, G., & Mavreas, V. (2004). Temporal relations between unexplained fatigue and depression: Longitudinal data from an international study in primary care. *Psychosomatic Medicine, 66*, 330–335.
Skarke, C., Darimont, J., Schmidt, H., Geisslinger, G., & Lotsch, J. (2003). Analgesic effects of morphine and morphine-6-glucuronide in a transcutaneous electrical pain model in healthy volunteers. *Clinical Pharmacology and Therapeutics, 73*, 107–121. doi:10.1067/mcp.2003.5.
Smith, B. W., Epstein, E. M., Ortiz, J. A., Christopher, P. J., & Tooley, E. M. (2013). The foundations of resilience: What are the critical resources for bouncing back from stress? In *Resilience in children, adolescents, and adults* (pp. 167–187). New York, NY: Springer.
Smith, M. T., & Haythornthwaite, J. A. (2004). How do sleep disturbance and chronic pain inter-relate?

Insights from the longitudinal and cognitive-behavioral clinical trials literature. *Sleep Medicine Reviews, 8*, 119–132. doi:10.1016/S1087-0792(03)00044-3.

Smith, B. W., & Zautra, A. J. (2008). Vulnerability and resilience in women with arthritis: Test of a two-factor model. *Journal of Consulting and Clinical Psychology, 76*, 799–810. doi:10.1037/0022-006X.76.5.799.

Solberg Nes, L., Carlson, C. R., Crofford, L. J., de Leeuw, R., & Segerstrom, S. C. (2010). Self-regulatory deficits in fibromyalgia and temporomandibular disorders. *Pain, 151*, 37–44. doi:10.1016/j.pain.2010.05.009.

Solberg Nes, L., Carlson, C. R., Crofford, L. J., de Leeuw, R., & Segerstrom, S. C. (2011). Individual differences and self-regulatory fatigue: Optimism, conscientiousness, and self-consciousness. *Personality and Individual Differences, 50*, 475–480.

Strand, E. B., Zautra, A. J., Thoresen, M., Ødegård, S., Uhlig, T., & Finset, A. (2006). Positive affect as a factor of resilience in the pain—negative affect relationship in patients with rheumatoid arthritis. *Journal of Psychosomatic Research, 60*, 477–484.

Strohle, A. (2009). Physical activity, exercise, depression and anxiety disorders. *Journal of Neural Transmission, 116*, 777–784. doi:10.1007/s00702-008-0092-x.

Sturgeon, J. A., Yeung, E. W., & Zautra, A. J. (2014). Respiratory sinus arrhythmia: A marker of resilience to pain induction. *International Journal of Behavioral Medicine, 21*(6), 961–965. doi:10.1007/s12529-014-9386-6.

Sturgeon, J. A., & Zautra, A. J. (2010). Resilience: A new paradigm for adaptation to chronic pain. *Current Pain and Headache Reports, 14*, 105–112. doi:10.1007/s11916-010-0095-9.

Sturgeon, J. A., & Zautra, A. J. (2013a). Psychological resilience, pain catastrophizing, and positive emotions: Perspectives on comprehensive modeling of individual pain adaptation. *Current Pain and Headache Reports, 17*, 317. doi:10.1007/s11916-012-0317-4.

Sturgeon, J. A., & Zautra, A. J. (2013b). State and trait pain catastrophizing and emotional health in rheumatoid arthritis. *Annals of Behavioral Medicine, 45*, 69–77. doi:10.1007/s12160-012-9408-z.

Sturgeon, J. A., Zautra, A. J., & Arewasikporn, A. (2014). A multilevel structural equation modeling analysis of vulnerabilities and resilience resources influencing affective adaptation to chronic pain. *Pain, 155*, 292–298. doi:10.1016/j.pain.2013.10.007.

Taylor, S. S., Davis, M. C., & Zautra, A. J. (2013). Relationship status and quality moderate daily pain-related changes in physical disability, affect, and cognitions in women with chronic pain. *Pain, 154*, 147–153. doi:10.1016/j.pain.2012.10.004.

Terrill, A. L., Molton, I. R., Ehde, D. M., Amtmann, D., Bombardier, C. H., Smith, A. E., & Jensen, M. P. (2014). Resilience, age, and perceived symptoms in persons with long-term physical disabilities. *Journal of Health Psychology*. doi:10.1177/1359105314532973.

Torma, L. M., Houck, G. M., Wagnild, G. M., Messecar, D., & Jones, K. D. (2013). Growing old with fibromyalgia: Factors that predict physical function. *Nursing Research, 62*, 16–24. doi:10.1097/NNR.0b013e318273b853.

Toussaint, L. L., Vincent, A., Whipple, M. O., McAllister, S. J., Finnie, D. M., Hathaway, J. C., … Douglas, K. S. V. (2014). Forgiveness education in fibromyalgia: A qualitative inquiry. *Pain Studies and Treatment, 2*, 11–16.

Tugade, M. M., & Fredrickson, B. L. (2004). Resilient individuals use positive emotions to bounce back from negative emotional experiences. *Journal of Personality and Social Psychology, 86*, 320–333. doi:10.1037/0022-3514.86.2.320.

Vlaeyen, J. W., & Linton, S. J. (2000). Fear-avoidance and its consequences in chronic musculoskeletal pain: A state of the art. *Pain, 85*, 317–332.

Wade, J. B., Hart, R. P., Wade, J. H., Bajaj, J. S., & Price, D. D. (2013). The relationship between marital status and psychological resilience in chronic pain. *Pain Research and Treatment, 2013*.

Wolfe, F., & Hawley, D. J. (1998). The longterm outcomes of rheumatoid arthritis: Work disability: A prospective 18 year study of 823 patients. *The Journal of Rheumatology, 25*, 2108–2117.

Wolfe, F., Hawley, D. J., & Wilson, K. (1996). The prevalence and meaning of fatigue in rheumatic disease. *The Journal of Rheumatology, 23*, 1407–1417.

Wright, M. A., Wren, A. A., Somers, T. J., Goetz, M. C., Fras, A. M., Huh, B. K., … Keefe, F. J. (2011). Pain acceptance, hope, and optimism: Relationships to pain and adjustment in patients with chronic musculoskeletal pain. *The Journal of Pain, 12*, 1155–1162. doi:10.1016/j.jpain.2011.06.002.

Yeung, E. W., Aiken, L. S., MacKinnon, D. P., & Davis, M. C. (2014). The role of social enjoyment in daily fatigue among women with fibromyalgia. *Multivariate Behavioral Research, 49*, 301–301. doi:10.1080/00273171.2014.912930.

Yeung, E. W., Arewasikporn, A., & Zautra, A. J. (2012). Resilience and Chronic Pain. *Journal of Social and Clinical Psychology, 31*, 593–617.

Zautra, A. J., Johnson, L. M., & Davis, M. C. (2005). Positive affect as a source of resilience for women in chronic pain. *Journal of Consulting and Clinical Psychology, 73*, 212–220. doi:10.1037/0022-006X.73.2.212.

Zautra, A. J., & Reich, J. (2011). Resilience: The meanings, methods, and measures of a fundamental characteristic of human adaptation. In *The Oxford handbook on stress, health, and coping* (pp. 173–185).

Zhu, Z., Galatzer-Levy, I. R., & Bonanno, G. A. (2014). Heterogeneous depression responses to chronic pain onset among middle-aged adults: A prospective study. *Psychiatry Research, 217*, 60–66. doi:10.1016/j.psychres.2014.03.004.

Sleep Disturbance in Rheumatic Disease

9

Faith S. Luyster

Prevalence of Sleep Disturbances in Patients with Arthritis

Disturbed sleep is a serious concern for patients with arthritis (Kirwan et al., 2003). Sleep quality is an important aspect of the overall profile of sleep in patients with arthritis as it provides a global subjective measure of sleep that can, in some cases, contrast with objective assessments (Edinger et al., 2000; Hirsch et al., 1994; Mahowald, Mahowald, Bundlie, & Ytterberg, 1989). Sleep quality is typically evaluated by questionnaires, such as the Pittsburgh Sleep Quality Index (Buysse, Reynolds, Monk, Berman, & Kupfer, 1989) (PSQI), and defined as a composite score of sleep quantity, time needed to fall asleep (i.e., sleep latency), percentage of time asleep while in bed (i.e., sleep efficacy), sleep disturbances, and general satisfaction with sleep. Patients with arthritis have poor sleep quality (mean PSQI global scores: 7.0–8.4) (Luyster, Chasens, Wasko, & Dunbar-Jacob, 2011; Sariyildiz et al., 2014; Taylor-Gjevre, Gjevre, Nair, Skomro, & Lim, 2011; Westhovens, Van der Elst, Matthys, Tran, & Gilloteau, 2014), with 61–67 % identified as poor sleepers according to the suggested cutoff point for the PSQI global score (Buysse et al., 1989) (scores >5) (Luyster et al., 2011; Sariyildiz et al., 2014; Taylor-Gjevre et al., 2011). Poor sleep quality and sleep disturbances have been reported in 56–81.5 % of patients with systemic lupus erythematosus (SLE) (Chandrasekhara, Jayachandran, Rajasekhar, Thomas, & Narsimulu, 2009; Costa et al., 2005; Greenwood, Lederman, & Lindner, 2008; Tench, McCurdie, White, & D'Cruz, 2000). As compared to age- and sex-matched healthy controls, patients with rheumatoid arthritis had significantly worse sleep quality, longer sleep latency, lower sleep efficiency, more sleep disturbances, and a higher PSQI global score (Sariyildiz et al., 2014). Patients with SLE also have been found to have increased sleep latency, decreased total sleep time, increased number of arousals and awake time during the night, decreased sleep efficiency, and poorer sleep quality as compared to healthy controls and the general population (Chandrasekhara et al., 2009; Costa et al., 2005; Greenwood et al., 2008; Gudbjornsson & Hetta, 2001; Mckinley, Ouellette, & Winkel, 1995; Valencia-Flores et al., 1999; Vina, Green, Trivedi, Kwoh, & Utset, 2013). Insomnia is a common sleep disorder defined by difficulty initiating and maintaining sleep, early morning awakenings, or nonrestorative sleep associated with daytime impairments such as daytime sleepiness or decreased concentration (Buysse, Ancoli-Israel, Edinger, Lichstein, & Morin, 2006). Whether self-reported or based on diagnostic criteria, the

F.S. Luyster, PhD (✉)
School of Nursing, University of Pittsburgh, 3500 Victoria Street, Room 415, Pittsburgh, PA 15261, USA
e-mail: luysterfs@upmc.edu

P.M. Nicassio (ed.), *Psychosocial Factors in Arthritis*, DOI 10.1007/978-3-319-22858-7_9

prevalence of insomnia is significantly higher among patients with arthritis compared to those without arthritis (23–27 % and 16–20 %, respectively) (Budhiraja, Roth, Hudgel, Budhiraja, & Drake, 2011; Louie, Tektonidou, Caban-Martinez, & Ward, 2011). Population-based studies suggest that patients with arthritis are 1.5–2 times more likely than those without arthritis to have insomnia even after accounting for sociodemographic characteristics and other comorbid conditions (Budhiraja et al., 2011; Louie et al., 2011).

Objective Measurement of Sleep in Patients with Arthritis

Sleep can be measured objectively with polysomnography (PSG) or actigraphy. Polysomnography is a sleep study conducted in a sleep laboratory or a patient's home that uses EEG and other physiology-related measures to evaluate sleep and diagnose sleep disorders. Actigraphy utilizes a wrist actigraph to study sleep–wake patterns and circadian rhythms by assessing movement. Unlike polysomnography, actigraphy cannot provide information about sleep stages. Actigraphs are worn in the patient's home for extended periods of time, thus providing an objective measure of sleep that may more closely approximate habitual sleep patterns. Sleep architecture (i.e., total sleep time, rapid eye movement (REM) sleep latency, and percentage of time in non-REM (NREM) and REM sleep) in patients with arthritis is usually normal and similar to healthy controls (Drewes et al., 1998; Hirsch et al., 1994; Leigh, Hindmarch, Bird, & Wright, 1988; Mahowald et al., 1989; Moldofsky, Lue, & Smythe, 1983). Several studies have found an increase in alpha-EEG during most sleep cycles, which has been proposed to reflect internal arousal activity which may disturb sleep (Drewes, Svendsen, Nielsen, Taagholt, & Bjerregård, 1994). Sleep fragmentation may account for the subjective reports of poor sleep among patients with arthritis. Studies using PSG or actigraphy have shown frequent arousals and awakenings within both rheumatoid arthritis (RA) and osteoarthritis (OA) patients, with number of arousals per hour ranging from 9 to 52.5 (Drewes, Svendsen, et al., 1998; Lavie et al., 1992; Mahowald et al., 1989; Moldofsky, 1989) and number of awakenings per hour ranging from 3.4 to 19 (Crosby, 1988; Drewes, Svendsen, et al., 1998; Hirsch et al., 1994; Leigh et al., 1988; Mahowald et al., 1989). Findings for other sleep parameters including sleep latency, sleep efficacy, and wake time after sleep onset (WASO) from PSG and actigraphy studies are conflicting. Patients with RA have been shown to have longer sleep latencies, lower sleep efficiencies, and greater WASO than healthy controls (Crosby, 1988; Hirsch et al., 1994; Lavie et al., 1992); however, no differences in these sleep parameters have been found between both RA and OA patients and controls (Drewes, Svendsen, et al., 1998; Leigh et al., 1988; Louie et al., 2011). Limited studies using PSG in patients with SLE found a high percentage of alpha intrusions into NREM sleep, increased stage 1 sleep, decreased slow wave sleep (NREM stages 3–4), decreased sleep efficiency, and increased number of arousals (Iaboni, Ibanez, Gladman, Urowitz, & Moldofsky, 2006; Valencia-Flores et al., 1999).

Factors Contributing to Sleep Disturbances

Sleep disturbance in arthritis may be associated with a variety of factors including disease activity which may elicit pain and the release of cytokines that can affect sleep regulation (Krueger, Obál, Fang, Kubota, & Taishi, 2001) and other variables not associated with disease activity, such as depressive symptoms, and other sleep disorders such as obstructive sleep apnea and restless leg syndrome (Abad, Sarinas, & Guilleminault, 2008). Several studies in RA populations have demonstrated a significant positive association between disease activity and sleep disturbances (Crosby, 1988; Drewes et al., 2000; Drewes, Svendsen, et al., 1998; Westhovens et al., 2014; Wolfe, Michaud, & Li, 2006), except for one study reporting no correlation between disease activity and objective sleep parameters (Hirsch et al., 1994). Increased disease activity (pain, joint tenderness, and morning stiffness) during a mean follow-up period of 175.8±70.9 days resulted in increased time in slow wave sleep and Stage Wake and decrease time in Stage 2 NREM sleep suggesting increased time spent awake and nonrestorative sleep (Drewes et al., 2000). In a cross-sectional study of 305 RA patients, increased disease activity determined by the 28-joint Disease Activity Score and C-reactive protein levels (DAS28-CRP) was independently associated with poor sleep quality based on the PSQI (Westhovens et al., 2014). The studies examining the association between disease activity and sleep disturbances in patients with SLE are conflicting (Chandrasekhara et al., 2009; Costa et al., 2005; Gudbjornsson & Hetta, 2001; Kasitanon et al., 2013; Palagini et al., 2014; Valencia-Flores et al., 1999; Vina et al., 2013). Several studies found disease activity to be a significant determinant of subjective and objective sleep disturbances (Chandrasekhara et al., 2009; Gudbjornsson & Hetta, 2001; Valencia-Flores et al., 1999), whereas others found no association between disease activity and poor sleep quality (Costa et al., 2005; Kasitanon et al., 2013; Palagini et al., 2014; Vina et al., 2013).

Pain is a cardinal symptom of arthritis and is associated with self-reported sleep disturbances and sleep architecture (Drewes et al., 2000; Power, Perruccio, & Badley, 2005; Sasaki et al., 2013). Pain has been shown to have a significant indirect effect, through disease activity, on sleep quality in RA (Westhovens et al., 2014). The relationship between arthritis and insomnia symptoms and unrefreshing sleep is partly mediated by pain as evidenced by a reduced effect of arthritis on these sleep problems after adjustment for pain (reductions of 64 % and 53 %, respectively) (Power et al., 2005). Nocturnal knee pain is a significant predictor of poor sleep quality in knee OA (Sasaki et al., 2013).

According to a recent meta-analysis, the prevalence of depression in patients with RA ranges from 17 to 29 %, depending on the method of defining depression (Matcham, Rayner, Steer, & Hotopf, 2013). Among adults with RA, those with depression or anxiety are three times more likely to report sleep disturbance than those without depression or anxiety (Louie et al., 2011). Depression and pain are strong predictors of sleep complaints (Wolfe et al., 2006). Data from studies in RA suggest interactions between pain, depression, and sleep disturbances (Cakirbay, Bilici, Kavakcio, Guler, & Tan, 2004; Nicassio et al., 2012; Nicassio & Wallston, 1992). RA patients with clinically diagnosed major depression reported higher pain levels and poorer sleep quality than RA patients without major depression (Cakirbay et al., 2004). In a longitudinal study of 242 RA patients followed for two years (Nicassio & Wallston, 1992), cross-sectional multiple regression analysis revealed a significant correlation between pain and self-reported sleep problems. Pain at baseline was shown to exacerbate sleep problems at follow-up, but prior sleep problems did not affect subsequent pain. In a more recent cross-sectional study of 106 RA patient, Nicassio, Ormseth, Kay, et al. (2012) explored whether pain may lead to sleep disturbance through its effect on depression. Both pain and depressive symptoms were independently associated with greater PSQI scores and depressive symptoms partially mediated the effects of pain on sleep quality. Depression is very common in patients with SLE, with up to 75 % having a diagnosis of depression or reporting depressive symptoms (Palagini et al., 2013). Depression appears to be a determinant of sleep disturbances in patients with SLE, such that depressive symptoms remained a significant predictor of poor sleep even after adjustment for demographics, medications, and disease activity (Costa et al., 2005; Kasitanon et al., 2013; Palagini et al., 2014). In a study of 50 patients with SLE, the association between depression and poor sleep quality was significant in bivariate analysis but not in the full model regression analysis (Chandrasekhara et al., 2009).

Impact of Sleep Disturbances on Health and Well-Being

Sleep disturbances can lead to changes in pain, mood, fatigue, and disability in patients with arthritis, although studies in both RA and OA populations suggest that these relationships are complex (Luyster et al., 2011; Nicassio et al., 2012; Nicassio, Ormseth, Kay, et al., 2012; Parmelee, Tighe, & Dautovich, 2015). The relationship between sleep and pain is likely bidirectional, and it has been proposed that sleep disturbance may increase pain perception via direct influences on central pain processing leading to exacerbations in daily pain and, in turn, contributing to sleep disturbances (Smith, Quartana, Okonkwo, & Nasir, 2009). Among 59 women with RA, greater sleep problems were associated with a lower pain threshold at all three sites assessed in the study (i.e., wrists, thumbnails, and trapezius), which suggested a defect in central pain processing (Lee et al., 2009). Irwin et al. (2012) conducted an experimental study to examine the effects of partial night sleep deprivation on pain perception in 27 patients with RA and 27 healthy controls and on arthritis-specific joint pain. Partial sleep deprivation followed a baseline night and occurred prior to a recovery night. In the morning following sleep loss, patients with RA reported exaggerated increases in symptoms of pain as compared to controls. Sleep loss exacerbated RA-related joint pain indicated by an increase in number of painful joints and joint pain severity (Irwin et al., 2012). Diminished conditioned pain modulation (CPM), a mechanism of central nervous system pain amplification, and its association with sleep problems was evaluated in a study of 58 female RA patients and 54 age-matched pain-free controls (Lee et al., 2013). RA patients had an attenuated CPM induced using a cold water bath compared to controls. The association between RA and diminished CPM was mediated by sleep problems.

Sleep difficulties (e.g., insomnia) have been identified as a precipitating factor of depression in the general population (Baglioni et al., 2011) and in patients with arthritis (Ferguson & Cotton, 1996; Irwin et al., 2012; Nicassio & Wallston, 1992; Parmelee et al., 2015). Sleep loss due to experimental partial sleep deprivation resulted in higher levels of depression and anxiety in patients with RA as compared to controls (Irwin et al., 2012). Additionally, studies have reported interrelationships between sleep disturbances, pain, and depression in RA and OA. Nicassio and Wallston (1992) found self-reported sleep problems to be significantly associated with higher concomitant depression independent of pain in RA. The interaction of high pain and high sleep problems was independently associated with increased depression from baseline to 2-year follow-up. Those with high pain and high sleep problems were more depressed at follow-up than those with low pain and high sleep problems, suggesting that pain level changed the way in which sleep problems exacerbate depression over time (Nicassio & Wallston, 1992). Cross-sectional and longitudinal associations of sleep disturbance with pain and depression were examined in a sample of 367 patients with OA followed for 1 year (Parmelee et al., 2015). Sleep disturbance was defined as having trouble sleeping (e.g., difficulty initiating and maintaining sleep and early morning awakenings) indicative of insomnia based on a research diagnostic interview. Sleep disturbance and pain were independently associated with depression at baseline. There was a significant interaction of sleep and pain on concurrent depression symptoms, such that depressive symptoms were higher among those with greater sleep disturbance and high pain (Parmelee et al., 2015). Longitudinal analyses revealed sleep disturbance, but not pain, to be a predictor of depression over time.

Fatigue is a frequent yet unpredictable symptom of arthritis, including RA and OA, and can comprise both physical and cognitive fatigue. As compared to controls, patients with RA reported greater fatigue following a night of partial sleep deprivation, suggesting that sleep loss leads to increases in fatigue in RA (Irwin et al., 2012). In a study comparing correlates of fatigue between patients with RA and OA, sleep disturbance was found to be significantly associated with fatigue in adjusted analyses among OA patients, but not among RA patients (Stebbings, Herbison, Doyle, Treharne, & Highton, 2010). It is important to note that sleep disturbance was assessed using a visual analog scale with the question "How would you rate the average amount of sleep you have had over the last seven days," which may not have captured aspects of disturbed sleep in RA that may be more strongly associated with fatigue. A prospective study of women with RA or Sjögren's syndrome (n=25 RA and 14 Sjögren's syndrome) explored the roles of discomfort and disturbed sleep in next day fatigue (Goodchild, Treharne, Booth, & Bowman, 2010). For participants with either condition, greater discomfort in the evening was associated with more somatic and mental fatigue the following day, and this relationship was moderated by poor sleep defined by sleep quality/quantity and sleep efficiency based on sleep diary and actigraphy. In other words, on nights when sleep was more disturbed, evening's discomfort had a greater impact on next day's fatigue (Goodchild et al., 2010). In men and women with recent-onset (≤1 year) RA, the components of "physical disability" and "mental aspects" based on principal component analysis explained a larger amount of the variance in fatigue through the 3 years after study inclusion (Thyberg, Dahlström, & Thyberg, 2009). More specifically, the "physical disability" component included disease activity, activity limitation, and pain, whereas the "mental aspects" component included mental health and sleep disturbance. Sleep quality has been shown to account for 8 % of the variance in fatigue among older RA patients (Belza, Henke, Yelin, Epstein, & Gilliss, 1993). The interrelationships among poor sleep quality, disease activity, and mood as determinants of fatigue were examined in a recent study of 106 patients with RA and found poor sleep quality to play a significant role in explaining fatigue (Nicassio, Ormseth, Custodio, et al., 2012). Structural equation modeling revealed direct, positive independent effects of poor sleep quality (i.e., sleep efficiency, perceived sleep quality, and daily disturbances from the PSQI) and disease activity (i.e., joint pain and tenderness and RA disease activity) on fatigue (i.e., assessed by the Multidimensional Assessment of Fatigue Global Fatigue Index and Vitality subscale of the SF-36). Mood disturbance (i.e., assessed by the Center for Epidemiological Studies of Depression and the Perceived Stress Scale) directly and indirectly affected fatigue through poor sleep quality. In addition, disease activity indirectly influenced fatigue through mood disturbance and poor sleep quality (Nicassio, Ormseth, Custodio, et al., 2012).

Sleep disturbance may lead to functional declines in patients with arthritis. Self-reported arthritis-related sleep disruptions are associated with increased physician visits, use of prescriptions and over-the-counter medications, use of physical treatments such as heat, cold, massage, or splint, and resting or limiting activities, all of which are suggestive of impairments in functional status (Jordan et al., 2000). Improvements in sleep quality during 6 months of tocilizumab treatment were correlated with improvements in functional disability suggesting improving sleep may have positive effects on disability in RA (Fragiadaki, Tektonidou, Konsta, Chrousos, & Sfikakis, 2012). Cross-sectional analyses in patients with knee OA revealed no significant association between sleep disturbance and functional disability regarding mobility, walking and bending, hand and finger function, arm function, self-care, and household tasks (Parmelee et al., 2015). However, sleep disturbance predicted disability at 1 year even after controlling for baseline depressive symptoms and increases in pain during the 1-year follow-up. A study of 162 patients with RA found poor sleep quality to be significantly associated with greater functional disability, accounting for 7 % of the variance after controlling for sociodemographic, medical, and medication variables (Luyster et al., 2011). Additionally, sleep quality was shown to have an indirect effect on disability through its relationship with pain severity and fatigue.

Sleep disturbance is associated with inflammation, such that insufficient sleep can produce a pro-inflammatory response by increasing cytokine secretion (Simpson & Dinges, 2007). Studies of total and partial sleep deprivation in healthy individuals have found increases in both blood levels and genomic markers of pro-inflammatory cytokines, including interleukin-6 (IL-6), tumor necrosis factor-α (TNF-α), and C-reactive protein (CRP). After a night of total sleep deprivation in healthy men, there was an increase in next day IL-6 secretion and associated fatigue and sleepiness and a decrease in next night IL-6 secretion and deeper sleep that night (Vgontzas et al., 1999). Similar findings have been shown after 1 week of partial sleep deprivation (Vgontzas et al., 2004). Total (4 days) but not partial sleep deprivation (4 days but with 2 two-hour naps per day) significantly increased IL-6 plasma concentrations and TNF-α R1, a soluble receptor for TNF-α (Shearer et al., 2001). Following a morning of partial sleep deprivation in healthy adults, monocyte production of IL-6 and TNF-α and transcription of IL-6 and TNF-α messenger RNA were significantly increased (Irwin, Wang, Campomayor, Collado-Hidalgo, & Cole, 2006). As compared to controls, healthy adults exposed to total or partial sleep deprivation for 10 consecutive nights exhibited increases in high-sensitivity CRP (Meier-Ewert et al., 2004). Sleep quality, as well as quantity, also is associated with inflammation (Friedman et al., 2005; Hong, Mills, Loredo, Adler, & Dimsdale, 2005). These findings suggest that sleep disturbances can lead to increases in inflammation, and thus could contribute to increased disease activity in patients with RA.

Effects of Pharmacological and Nonpharmacological Treatments on Sleep Disturbances

Pharmacological

Although many patients with RA (19–25 %) and OA (18–29 %) report taking prescription or over-the-counter sleep medications (Taylor-Gjevre et al., 2011; Vitiello et al., 2013; Vitiello, Rybarczyk, Von Korff, & Stepanski, 2009; Westhovens et al., 2014), there is a dearth of studies that have examined the effect of hypnotics on sleep and other arthritis-related symptoms in patients with arthritis. Early pilot studies of a combination of an nonsteroidal anti-inflammatory drug (NSAID) and benzodiazepine hypnotic suggest that the effect of the two drugs on pain and sleep disturbance in RA may be superior to NSAID alone (Hobkirk, Rhodes, & Haslock, 1977; Sharma & Haslock, 1978). The efficacy of short-acting benzodiazepine hypnotics, temazepam and triazolam, in treating sleep disturbances has been explored in OA and RA patients (Leigh, Hindmarch, Bird, & Wright, 1987; Walsh, Muehlbach, Lauter, Hilliker, & Schweitzer, 1996). Temazepam resulted in significant improvements in objective sleep, including reductions in duration of awakenings and percentage of Stage Wake sleep and increases in percentage of NREM stage 2 sleep, sleep efficiency, and REM latency, in a sample of 15 male patients with OA (Leigh et al., 1987). In a double-blind crossover study of 15 RA patients with subjective complaints of difficulty falling asleep or maintaining sleep, triazolam or placebo was administered during two 7 night periods and PSG was conducted on the last two nights of each condition (Walsh et al., 1996). Significantly higher total sleep time, time spent in NREM stage 2 and slow wave sleep, and longer REM latency were found in the triazolam condition compared to placebo. However, there were no differences in measures of sleep fragmentation, including amount of NREM stage 1 sleep, number of awakenings, and arousal frequency, nor pain between the triazolam and placebo conditions.

The effect of zopiclone, a nonbenzodiazepine hypnotic used for the treatment of insomnia, on subjective and objective sleep parameters in 40 patients with RA was tested in a double-blind placebo-controlled trial (Drewes, Bjerregård, Taagholt, Svendsen, & Nielsen, 1998). Patients were randomly assigned to 14 days of treatment with either 7.5 mg zopiclone or placebo and underwent in-home PSG before and after treatment. As compared to the placebo group, the zopiclone group reported significant improvements in sleep quality after 1 and 2 weeks of treatment, despite no changes in pain. After 1 week of treatment, the zopiclone group had a reduction in self-reported number of awakenings and sleep latency, but these improvements did not persist after 2 weeks of treatment. Treatment with zopiclone had little effect on objective sleep parameters, except for an increase in time spent in NREM stage 2 sleep, a decrease in number of awakenings over 2 min, and a shift towards higher frequencies in the EEG (Drewes, Bjerregård, et al., 1998). A more recent double-blind placebo-controlled pilot study was conducted to evaluate the efficacy of eszopiclone 3 mg, a nonbenzodiazepine hypnotic, on sleep, pain, and joint stiffness in 153 patients with RA and comorbid insomnia (Roth et al., 2009). Patients were randomly assigned to receive eszopiclone 3 mg or placebo for 4 weeks, followed by a 2-week placebo discontinuation phase to assess possible rebound effects. Using a daily, morning interactive voice response system, patients reported on sleep characteristics and completed assessments of insomnia severity, RA-related pain, and swollen and tender joints. After 1 week of treatment, the eszopiclone group reported significantly lower WASO, lower sleep latency, greater total sleep time, and better sleep quality and depth of sleep than the placebo group. Eszopiclone treatment resulted in significant improvements in these sleep characteristics and insomnia severity from baseline to posttreatment, relative to placebo. Additionally, the eszopiclone group had greater reductions in pain and joint stiffness from baseline to 4 weeks compared to placebo. There was some evidence of rebound insomnia on the first night after discontinuation of eszopiclone (Roth et al., 2009). In a study of an over-the-counter sleep aid, Valerian, on sleep disturbances in 15 patients RA (Taibi, Bourguignon, & Taylor, 2008), a 600-mg dose of Valerian taken 1 h before bedtime for 5 days did not significantly improve self-report and actigraphy-measured total sleep time, WASO, sleep efficiency, sleep quality, or sleep latency when compared to placebo.

Nonpharmacological

Both aerobic and resistance exercise can improve sleep quality and sleep architecture (Driver & Taylor, 2000; Yang, Ho, Chen, & Chien, 2012). The effect of exercise on body temperature, autonomic, endocrine, and metabolic functioning, and mood have been proposed as mechanisms that may contribute to improved subsequent sleep (Uchida et al., 2012). In the case of arthritis, exercise reduces pain and fatigue and increases mobility, which may, in turn, lead to improvements in sleep (Roddy, Zhang, & Doherty, 2005; Stenström & Minor, 2003). A recent randomized controlled trial of a 12-week cardiovascular exercise (i.e., walking) and resistance training program evaluated the effect of exercise on sleep quality and fatigue in 78 patients with RA (Durcan, Wilson, & Cunnane, 2014). Those in the exercise group had significant improvements in sleep quality and fatigue after treatment, whereas sleep quality and fatigue did not increase in the control group who received only information about the benefits of exercise in RA. Compared to the control group, the exercise group had significantly greater improvements in sleep quality, fatigue, and pain (Durcan et al., 2014). Given previous studies reporting pain to be an independent predictor of sleep disturbances in RA (Nicassio, Ormseth, Kay, et al., 2012; Nicassio & Wallston, 1992), it is plausible that the improvements in sleep quality associated with exercise may be partly due to reductions in pain. In a randomized controlled trial of 321 older adults with self-reported arthritis, the effect of the 8-week People With Arthritis Can Exercise (PACE) program developed by the Arthritis Foundation on sleep disturbances was examined (Freburger, Callahan, Shreffler, & Mielenz, 2010). Individuals in the PACE intervention group were less likely to wake up at night and wake up tired at posttreatment as compared to the control group who did not receive the intervention. The intervention significantly decreased the number of days that individuals woke up tired, with 42 % reporting greater than 7 days of waking up tired at baseline and 25 % reporting waking up tired following the 8-week program; however, this effect was not maintained at 3 and 6 months (Freburger et al., 2010). Low-intensity aerobic exercise 3 days a week for 12 weeks for session durations of 15, 25, and 35 min among women with RA resulted in improvements in sleep quality (Harkcom, Lampman, Banwell, & Castor, 1985). These findings suggest that the benefits of exercise on sleep can be achieved in a short period of time.

Yoga is a multimodal complementary and alternative medicine practice that has been shown to improve insomnia symptoms and sleep quality in adults with insomnia (Afonso et al., 2012;

Khalsa, 2004). Recent pilot studies in patients with arthritis have explored the effects of yoga on sleep disturbances (Hansen, 2010; Taibi & Vitiello, 2011; Ward, Stebbings, Athens, Cherkin, & Baxter, 2014). Feasibility data from a pilot randomized controlled trial in 26 patients with RA revealed significantly greater improvements in sleep quality among those who completed an 8-week relaxation-based yoga program including one group practice session and three home practice sessions per week compared to usual care (Ward et al., 2014). Taibi and Vitiello (2011) conducted a pilot study of gentle yoga in a sample of 13 women with OA and complaints of poor sleep. Both objective (i.e., actigraphy) and subjective measures of sleep were collected at baseline and following the 8-week program of weekly group yoga and daily 20 min home yoga before bedtime. Insomnia symptom severity and sleep diary-reported sleep latency, sleep efficiency, and number of nights experiencing insomnia symptoms significantly improved from pretreatment to posttreatment (Taibi & Vitiello, 2011). No changes in sleep quality or actigraphy-obtained sleep parameters were found. Six-week sessions of 1-h group yoga sessions did not significantly improve sleep disturbances among 14 individuals with OA, although half of the participants reported improvement in sleep disturbances at post-intervention (Hansen, 2010). Further research is needed to examine the effects of yoga on sleep disturbances in arthritis.

Biofeedback has been used in both RA and OA populations and has had positive effects on sleep (Achterberg, McGraw, & Lawlis, 1981; Yılmaz et al., 2010). Biofeedback provides visual and audible signals to patients of their body functions to help them learn to control and change these functions, such as relaxing muscles, in an effort to improve pain or other ailments. Yilmaz et al. randomly assigned patients with knee OA to receive a strengthening exercise program ($n = 20$) or strengthening exercise program plus EMG-biofeedback ($n = 20$), which provided feedback on muscle contraction during exercise enabling stronger contractions, for 3 weeks (Yılmaz et al., 2010). Sleep was assessed by the sleep subscale of the Nottingham Health Profile that asked about sleep medications, difficulty initiating and maintaining sleep, early morning awakenings, and sleeping badly at night. Sleep was found to improve only in the EMG-biofeedback plus exercise group, and this group had significantly greater improvements in sleep as compared to the strengthening exercise only group. In an early study in women with RA (Achterberg et al., 1981), 12 patients were given physiotherapy (i.e., heat packs or cryotherapy, home exercise program, and instructions for proper body mechanics and posture) for 12 sessions 30–40 min each and 17 patients received EMG-biofeedback for skin temperature training and relaxation. Although there were no changes in hours of sleep between the groups, the EMG-biofeedback and relaxation group had a significantly greater improvement in the number of awakenings, such that the biofeedback and relaxation group showed a decline of 2.08 times pretreatment to 1.54 times posttreatment, whereas the physiotherapy group reported an average of 3.5 awakenings at pretreatment and 3.17 awakenings at posttreatment. Although the data are limited, these preliminary findings suggest that biofeedback may be a beneficial adjunctive treatment to exercise that can improve sleep, likely due to decreases in pain.

Cognitive-behavioral therapy (CBT) for pain management helps patients develop pain coping skills through relaxation and distraction techniques, activity pacing, and cognitive restructuring aimed at identifying negative pain-related thoughts and replacing them with more adaptive coping thoughts (Keefe, 1996). Patients are then encouraged to apply these learned coping skills in everyday situations and to develop plans for dealing with difficult situations such as pain flares. CBT for pain management has been utilized in arthritis populations (Dixon, Keefe, Scipio, Perri, & Abernethy, 2007) and has been shown to have beneficial effects not only on pain and disability but also sleep (O'Leary, Shoor, Lorig, & Holman, 1988). More recent studies have begun to explore the utility of CBT for insomnia (CBT-I) in patients with OA (Rybarczyk et al., 2005; Vitiello et al., 2009, 2013, 2014). Multicomponent CBT-I uses behavioral and psychological techniques such as sleep education, restriction of time in bed, stimulus control (strengthening associations between bed and sleep), and cognitive restructuring and relaxation training to address anxiety-provoking beliefs about sleep (Edinger & Means, 2005; Morin, 2004). Older adults with insomnia and comorbid conditions, OA, coronary artery disease, or chronic obstructive pulmonary disease, were randomly assigned to either 8 weekly CBT-I group sessions or an attention control stress management and wellness intervention (SMW) (Rybarczyk et al., 2005). Sleep was assessed by sleep diary and PSQI. Regardless of type of condition, those in the CBT-I group showed significant improvements in sleep quality as compared to the attention control. A secondary analysis of data from this randomized controlled trial examined the impact of improved sleep on pain for OA participants only (Vitiello et al., 2009). Twenty-three patients with OA were randomly assigned to CBT-I and 28 patients with OA to SMW. Measures of sleep and pain assessed 1 year after treatment in the CBT-I group only were also included in these analyses. Patients with OA in the CBT-I intervention reported significantly decreased WASO and sleep latency and increased sleep efficiency and corresponding reductions in pain after treatment and these changes in sleep persisted at 1-year follow-up, whereas there was a nonsignificant trend for reduced pain (Vitiello et al., 2009). The SMW group did not report significant changes in sleep or pain from before to after treatment. These findings suggest that CBT-I has both short-term and long-term benefits for sleep quality in OA patients with comorbid insomnia, and that CBT-I, despite not addressing pain management, may also improve pain in these patients. It has been proposed that CBT-I may help to break the vicious cycle of arthritis pain and sleep disturbance by increasing the pain threshold and reducing the amplification of the pain-signal transmission through improvements in sleep, which in turn, can lead to less perceived pain, increased activity levels, and more positive emotions and cognitions (Vitiello et al., 2009) (Fig. 9.1). A recent randomized controlled trial of a 6-week CBT for insomnia and pain (CBT-PI) examined the effects of CBT-PI on sleep and pain outcomes in patients with OA and comorbid insomnia ($n=367$) (Vitiello et al., 2013). Patients were randomly assigned to cognitive-behavioral pain coping skills intervention (CBT-P), CBT-PI which added the standard components of CBT for insomnia, or an educational attention control. CBT-PI participants had significantly greater improvements in insomnia severity over a 9-month assessment period (baseline, posttreatment at 2 months, and 9-month follow-up) than both the CBT-P and attention control groups. CBT-PI and CBT-I had significantly greater sleep efficiency measured by actigraphy than the attention control group, but sleep efficiency was

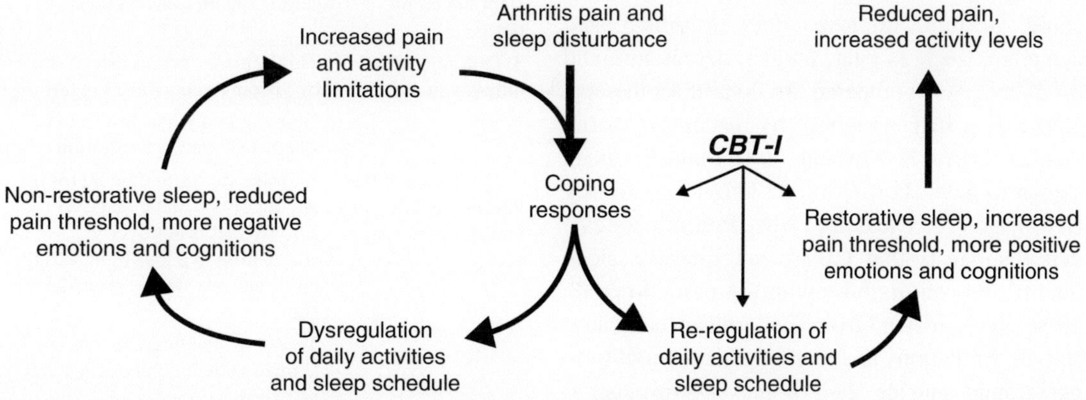

Fig. 9.1 Cognitive behavioral therapy for insomnia improves sleep and decreases pain in older adults with comorbid insomnia and osteoarthritis. J Clin Sleep Med. 2009;5(4):355–62 (from Vitiello MV, Rybarczyk B, Von Korff M, Stepanski EJ)

similar between the two CBT groups. There were no differences in pain severity from baseline to 9-month follow-up between the three groups. Additional analyses were conducted using 18-month follow-up data to examine the relationship between short-term improvements in sleep and long-term improvements in sleep and pain (Vitiello et al., 2014). Sleep quality and pain assessed at 9-month and 18-month follow-ups were compared between improvers who had decreased insomnia severity at posttreatment across the three treatment groups and nonimprovers whose insomnia severity did not improve at posttreatment regardless of treatment assignment. Improvers showed significant, sustained improvements across 9 and 18 months compared to nonimprovers in sleep quality. Although there was no difference in pain severity between improvers and nonimprovers at posttreatment, improvers reported sustained improvements in pain severity at 9 and 18 months. These findings suggest that the benefits of improved sleep on pain may result from sustained improvements in sleep over time (Vitiello et al., 2014).

Management of Sleep in Patients with Arthritis

Since many patients with arthritis report sleep disturbances (Louie et al., 2011), inquiring about sleep problems is important for identifying and subsequently treating sleep disturbances that could, in turn, improve other arthritis-related symptoms such as pain, fatigue, depression, and disability. As compared to pharmacotherapy, CBT-I is often preferred by patients (Morin, Gaulier, Barry, & Kowatch, 1992) and has been shown to have short-term and long-term efficacy (Irwin, Cole, & Nicassio, 2006). Preliminary evidence suggests that CBT-I can improve sleep quality and pain in those with OA (Vitiello et al., 2009, 2013, 2014). Given that arthritis can cause activity limitations and restrict patients' ability to get around outside their homes (Verbrugge & Juarez, 2006), patients may be reluctant to undergo CBT-I which requires 6–8 weekly face-to-face individual sessions. Thus, alternative nonpharmacological insomnia treatment options that are less intensive may be more appealing to patients and have more widespread dissemination.

Brief behavioral treatment for insomnia (BBTI) is a manualized, behavioral treatment program involving two in-person sessions and two telephone booster sessions. BBTI can be delivered by healthcare professionals without specialized training. BBTI emphasizes the behavioral components of CBT-I, in particular sleep restriction and stimulus control, by modifying waking behaviors to increase and regulate the duration of wakefulness to increase homeostatic sleep drive and provide an individualized sleep and wake prescription to optimize the circadian sleep drive (Troxel, Germain, & Buysse, 2012). The intervention provides patients with four main "rules" for better sleep (Table 9.1): (1) reduce time in bed, (2) get up at the

Table 9.1 Brief behavioral sleep for insomnia (BBTI): four rules for better sleep

Rules	Description
1. Reduce time in bed	Decrease the amount of time awake in bed to habitual sleep time (based on sleep diary) plus 30 min
	Cutting down time in bed will increase how long spent awake and will lead to quick, deeper, more solid sleep
2. Get up the same time every day of the week, no matter how poorly you slept the night before	Getting up at the same time helps set the biological clock and regulates exposure to morning light, also an important cue for setting the biological clock
3. Don't go to bed unless you are sleepy	This helps to increase sleep drive by keeping you awake longer
	Going to bed when you're not sleepy can lead to frustration
4. Don't stay in bed unless you are asleep	If awake for more than 30 min, get out of bed and engage an activity that is not overly stimulating in a low-light setting. Once you are sleepy, return to bed
	This helps the brain develop a learned association between bed and sleep
	Have activities planned ahead of time that you can do when you get out of bed

same time of day every day, regardless of sleep duration, (3) do not go to bed unless sleepy, and (4) do not stay in bed unless asleep. BBTI has been shown to have short-term efficacy in a sample of 79 older adults with insomnia and comorbid conditions (Buysse et al., 2011). In brief, participants were randomly assigned to either BBTI or an information control consisting of printed sleep education materials. As compared to the IC group, patients receiving BBTI reported significant improvements in sleep diary- and actigraphy-measured sleep outcomes and had greater rates of treatment response (defined as PSQI score of ≥3 points or change in sleep diary sleep efficiency of ≥10 %) at posttreatment. Of the 25 patients with a favorable treatment response, 64 % no longer met insomnia criteria at 6-month follow-up.

Only one study has directly tested the effects of a sleep intervention in patients with arthritis (Vitiello et al., 2013, 2014). The favorable effects of CBTI on sleep and pain in this study warrant future research to explore cognitive and behavioral treatments for insomnia in patients with arthritis. BBTI may be a viable treatment option due to its brief design requiring limited in-person sessions and the advantage of treatment delivery by nurses and other professionals with limited experience in sleep medicine or behavioral therapies.

References

Abad, V. C., Sarinas, P. S., & Guilleminault, C. (2008). Sleep and rheumatologic disorders. *Sleep Medicine Reviews, 12*(3), 211–228.

Achterberg, J., McGraw, P., & Lawlis, G. F. (1981). Rheumatoid arthritis: A study of relaxation and temperature biofeedback training as an adjunctive therapy. *Biofeedback and Self Regulation, 6*(2), 207–223.

Afonso, R. F., Hachul, H., Kozasa, E. H., de Souza Oliveira, D., Goto, V., Rodrigues, D., Tufik, S., & Leite, J.R. (2012). Yoga decreases insomnia in postmenopausal women: A randomized clinical trial. *Menopause, 19*(2), 186–193.

Baglioni, C., Battagliese, G., Feige, B., Spiegelhalder, K., Nissen, C., Voderholzer, U., Lombardo, C., & Riemann, D. (2011). Insomnia as a predictor of depression: A meta-analytic evaluation of longitudinal epidemiological studies. *Journal of Affective Disorders, 135*(1), 10–19.

Belza, B. L., Henke, C. J., Yelin, E. H., Epstein, W. V., & Gilliss, C. L. (1993). Correlates of fatigue in older adults with rheumatoid arthritis. *Nursing Research, 42*(2), 93–99.

Budhiraja, R., Roth, T., Hudgel, D. W., Budhiraja, P., & Drake, C. L. (2011). Prevalence and polysomnographic correlates of insomnia comorbid with medical disorders. *Sleep, 34*(7), 859.

Buysse, D. J., Ancoli-Israel, S., Edinger, J. D., Lichstein, K. L., & Morin, C. M. (2006). Recommendations for a standard research assessment of insomnia. *Sleep, 23*(9), 1155–1173.

Buysse, D. J., Germain, A., Moul, D. E., Franzen, P. L., Brar, L. K., Fletcher, M. E., Begley, A., Houck, P.R., Mazumdar, S., Reynolds, C.F., & Monk, T.H. (2011). Efficacy of brief behavioral treatment for chronic insomnia in older adults. *Archives of Internal Medicine, 171*(10), 887–895.

Buysse, D. J., Reynolds, C. F., III, Monk, T. H., Berman, S. R., & Kupfer, D. J. (1989). The Pittsburgh Sleep Quality Index: A new instrument for psychiatric practice and research. *Psychiatry Research, 28*(2), 193–213.

Cakirbay, H., Bilici, M., Kavakcio, C. A., Guler, M., & Tan, Ü. (2004). Sleep quality and immune functions in rheumatoid arthritis patients with and without major depression. *The International Journal of Neuroscience, 114*(2), 245–256.

Chandrasekhara, P. K. S., Jayachandran, N. V., Rajasekhar, L., Thomas, J., & Narsimulu, G. (2009). The prevalence and associations of sleep disturbances in patients with systemic lupus erythematosus. *Modern Rheumatology, 19*(4), 407–415.

Costa, D. D., Bernatsky, S., Dritsa, M., Clarke, A. E., Dasgupta, K., Keshani, A., & Pineau, C. (2005). Determinants of sleep quality in women with systemic lupus erythematosus. *Arthritis Care & Research, 53*(2), 272–278.

Crosby, L. J. (1988). EEG sleep variables of rheumatoid arthritis patients. *Arthritis and Rheumatism, 1*(4), 198 204.

Dixon, K. E., Keefe, F. J., Scipio, C. D., Perri, L. M., & Abernethy, A. P. (2007). Psychological interventions for arthritis pain management in adults: A meta-analysis. *Health Psychology, 26*(3), 241–250.

Drewes, A. M., Bjerregård, K., Taagholt, S. J., Svendsen, L., & Nielsen, K. D. (1998). Zopiclone as night medication in rheumatoid arthritis. *Scandinavian Journal of Rheumatology, 27*(3), 180–187.

Drewes, A. M., Nielsen, K. D., Hansen, B., Taagholt, S. J., Bjerregård, K., & Svendsen, L. (2000). A longitudinal study of clinical symptoms and sleep parameters in rheumatoid arthritis. *Rheumatology (Oxford), 39*(11), 1287–1289.

Drewes, A. M., Svendsen, L., Nielsen, K. D., Taagholt, S. J., & Bjerregård, K. (1994). Quantification of alpha-EEG activity during sleep in fibromyalgia: A study based on ambulatory sleep monitoring. *Journal of Musculoskelatal Pain, 2*(4), 33–53.

Drewes, A. M., Svendsen, L., Taagholt, S. J., Bjerregård, K., Nielsen, K. D., & Hansen, B. (1998). Sleep in rheumatoid arthritis: A comparison with healthy subjects and studies of sleep/wake interactions. *Rheumatology (Oxford), 37*(1), 71–81.

Driver, H. S., & Taylor, S. R. (2000). Exercise and sleep. *Sleep Medicine Reviews, 4*(4), 387–402.

Durcan, L., Wilson, F., & Cunnane, G. (2014). The effect of exercise on sleep and fatigue in rheumatoid arthritis: A randomized controlled study. *The Journal of Rheumatology, 41*(10), 1966–1973.

Edinger, J. D., Fins, A. I., Glenn, D. M., Sullivan, R. J., Jr., Bastian, L. A., Marsh, G. R., Dailey, D., Hope, V.T., Young, M., Shaw, E. & Vasilas, D. (2000). Insomnia and the eye of the beholder: Are there clinical markers of objective sleep disturbances among adults with and without insomnia complaints? *Journal of Consulting and Clinical Psychology, 68*(4), 586–593.

Edinger, J. D., & Means, M. K. (2005). Cognitive-behavioral therapy for primary insomnia. *Clinical Psychology Review, 25*(5), 539–558.

Ferguson, S. J., & Cotton, S. (1996). Broken sleep, pain, disability, social activity, and depressive symptoms in rheumatoid arthritis. *Australian Journal of Psychology, 48*(1), 9–14.

Fragiadaki, K., Tektonidou, M. G., Konsta, M., Chrousos, G. P., & Sfikakis, P. P. (2012). Sleep disturbances and interleukin 6 receptor inhibition in rheumatoid arthritis. *The Journal of Rheumatology, 39*(1), 60–62.

Freburger, J. K., Callahan, L. F., Shreffler, J. H., & Mielenz, T. J. (2010). The effects of a physical activity program on sleep-and health-related quality of life in older persons with arthritis. *Journal of Applied Gerontology, 29*(4), 395–414.

Friedman, E. M., Hayney, M. S., Love, G. D., Urry, H. L., Rosenkranz, M. A., Davidson, R. J., Singer, B.H., & Ryff, C.D. (2005). Social relationships, sleep quality, and interleukin-6 in aging women. *Proceedings of the National Academy of Sciences of the United States of America, 102*(51), 18757–18762.

Goodchild, C., Treharne, G., Booth, D., & Bowman, S. (2010). Daytime patterning of fatigue and its associations with the previous night's discomfort and poor sleep among women with primary Sjögren's syndrome or rheumatoid arthritis. *Musculoskeletal Care, 8*(2), 107–117.

Greenwood, K. M., Lederman, L., & Lindner, H. D. (2008). Self-reported sleep in systemic lupus erythematosus. *Clinical Rheumatology, 27*(9), 1147–1151.

Gudbjornsson, B., & Hetta, J. (2001). Sleep disturbances in patients with systemic lupus erythematosus: A questionnaire-based study. *Clinical and Experimental Rheumatology, 19*(5), 509–514.

Hansen, E. G. (2010). Yoga for seniors with arthritis: A pilot study. *The International Journal of Yoga Therapy, 1*(1), 55–60.

Harkcom, T. M., Lampman, R. M., Banwell, B. F., & Castor, C. W. (1985). Therapeutic value of graded aerobic exercise training in rheumatoid arthritis. *Arthritis and Rheumatism, 28*(1), 32–39.

Hirsch, M., Carlander, B., Vergé, M., Tafti, M., Anaya, J. M., Billiard, M., & Sany, J. (1994). Objective and subjective sleep disturbances in patients with rheumatoid arthritis. *Arthritis and Rheumatism, 37*(1), 41–49.

Hobkirk, D., Rhodes, M., & Haslock, I. (1977). Night medication in rheumatoid arthritis: II. Combined therapy with indomethacin and diazepam. *Rheumatology (Oxford), 16*(2), 125–127.

Hong, S., Mills, P. J., Loredo, J. S., Adler, K. A., & Dimsdale, J. E. (2005). The association between interleukin-6, sleep, and demographic characteristics. *Brain, Behavior, and Immunity, 19*(2), 165–172.

Iaboni, A., Ibanez, D., Gladman, D. D., Urowitz, M. B., & Moldofsky, H. (2006). Fatigue in systemic lupus erythematosus: Contributions of disordered sleep, sleepiness, and depression. *The Journal of Rheumatology, 33*(12), 2453–2457.

Irwin, M. R., Cole, J. C., & Nicassio, P. M. (2006). Comparative meta-analysis of behavioral interventions for insomnia and their efficacy in middle-aged adults and in older adults 55+ years of age. *Health Psychology, 25*(1), 3–14.

Irwin, M. R., Olmstead, R., Carrillo, C., Sadeghi, N., FitzGerald, J. D., Ranganath, V. K., & Nicassio, P.M. (2012). Sleep loss exacerbates fatigue, depression, and pain in rheumatoid arthritis. *Sleep, 35*(4), 537–543.

Irwin, M. R., Wang, M., Campomayor, C. O., Collado-Hidalgo, A., & Cole, S. (2006). Sleep deprivation and activation of morning levels of cellular and genomic markers of inflammation. *Archives of Internal Medicine, 166*(16), 1756–1762.

Jordan, J. M., Bernard, S. L., Callahan, L. F., Kincade, J. E., Konrad, T. R., & DeFriese, G. H. (2000). Self-reported arthritis-related disruptions in sleep and daily life and the use of medical, complementary, and self-care strategies for arthritis: The National Survey of Self-care and Aging. *Archives of Family Medicine, 9*(2), 143–149.

Kasitanon, N., Achsavalertsak, U., Maneeton, B., Wangkaew, S., Puntana, S., Sukitawut, W., & Louthrenoo, W. (2013). Associated factors and psychotherapy on sleep disturbances in systemic lupus erythematosus. *Lupus, 22*(13), 1353–1360.

Keefe, F. J. (1996). Cognitive behavioral therapy for managing pain. *Clinical Psychologist, 49*(3), 4–5.

Khalsa, S. B. S. (2004). Treatment of chronic insomnia with yoga: A preliminary study with sleep–wake diaries. *Applied Psychophysiology and Biofeedback, 29*(4), 269–278.

Kirwan, J., Heiberg, T., Hewlett, S., Hughes, R., Kvien, T., Ahlmèn, M., Boers, M., Minnock, P., Saag, K., Shea, B., Almazor, M.S., & Taal, E. (2003). Outcomes from the patient perspective workshop at OMERACT 6. *The Journal of Rheumatology, 30*(4), 868–872.

Krueger, J. M., Obál, F., Fang, J., Kubota, T., & Taishi, P. (2001). The role of cytokines in physiological sleep regulation. *The Annals of the New York Academy of Sciences, 933*(1), 211–221.

Lavie, P., Epstein, R., Tzischinsky, O., Gilad, D., Nahir, M., Lorber, M., & Scharf, Y. (1992). Actigraphic measurements of sleep in rheumatoid arthritis: Comparison of patients with low back pain and healthy controls. *The Journal of Rheumatology, 19*(3), 362–365.

Lee, Y. C., Chibnik, L. B., Lu, B., Wasan, A. D., Edwards, R. R., Fossel, A. H., Helfgott, S.M., Solomon, D.H., Clauw, D.J., & Karlson, W. (2009). The relationship between disease activity, sleep, psychiatric distress and pain sensitivity in rheumatoid arthritis: A cross-sectional study. *Arthritis Research & Therapy, 11*(5), R160.

Lee, Y. C., Lu, B., Edwards, R. R., Wasan, A. D., Nassikas, N. J., Clauw, D. J., Solomon, D.H., & Karlson, E. (2013). The role of sleep problems in central pain processing in rheumatoid arthritis. *Arthritis and Rheumatism, 65*(1), 59–68.

Leigh, T., Hindmarch, I., Bird, H., & Wright, V. (1987). Temazepam as a hypnotic in osteoarthritic patients. *Human Psychopharmacology: Clinical and Experimental, 2*(1), 35–41.

Leigh, T., Hindmarch, I., Bird, H., & Wright, V. (1988). Comparison of sleep in osteoarthritic patients and age and sex matched healthy controls. *Annals of the Rheumatic Diseases, 47*(1), 40–42.

Louie, G. H., Tektonidou, M. G., Caban-Martinez, A. J., & Ward, M. M. (2011). Sleep disturbances in adults with arthritis: Prevalence, mediators, and subgroups at greatest risk. Data from the 2007 National Health Interview Survey. *Arthritis Care & Research, 63*(2), 247–260.

Luyster, F. S., Chasens, E. R., Wasko, M. C. M., & Dunbar-Jacob, J. (2011). Sleep quality and functional disability in patients with rheumatoid arthritis. *Journal of Clinical Sleep Medicine, 7*(1), 49–55.

Mahowald, M. W., Mahowald, M. L., Bundlie, S. R., & Ytterberg, S. R. (1989). Sleep fragmentation in rheumatoid arthritis. *Arthritis and Rheumatism, 32*(8), 974–983.

Matcham, F., Rayner, L., Steer, S., & Hotopf, M. (2013). The prevalence of depression in rheumatoid arthritis: A systematic review and meta-analysis. *Rheumatology (Oxford), 52*(12), 2136–2148.

Mckinley, P. S., Ouellette, S. C., & Winkel, G. H. (1995). The contributions of disease activity, sleep patterns, and depression to fatigue in systemic lupus erythematosus. *Arthritis and Rheumatism, 38*(6), 826–834.

Meier-Ewert, H. K., Ridker, P. M., Rifai, N., Regan, M. M., Price, N. J., Dinges, D. F., & Mullington, J.M. (2004). Effect of sleep loss on C-reactive protein, an inflammatory marker of cardiovascular risk. *Journal of the American College of Cardiology, 43*(4), 678–683.

Moldofsky, H. (1989). Sleep influences on regional and diffuse pain syndromes associated with osteoarthritis. *Seminars in Arthritis and Rheumatism, 18*(4), 18–21.

Moldofsky, H., Lue, F., & Smythe, H. (1983). Alpha EEG sleep and morning symptoms in rheumatoid arthritis. *The Journal of Rheumatology, 10*(3), 373–379.

Morin, C. M. (2004). Cognitive-behavioral approaches to the treatment of insomnia. *The Journal of Clinical Psychiatry, 65*(Suppl 16), 33–40.

Morin, C. M., Gaulier, B., Barry, T., & Kowatch, R. A. (1992). Patients' acceptance of psychological and pharmacological therapies for insomnia. *Sleep, 15*(4), 302–305.

Nicassio, P. M., Ormseth, S. R., Custodio, M. K., Irwin, M. R., Olmstead, R., & Weisman, M. H. (2012). A multidimensional model of fatigue in patients with rheumatoid arthritis. *The Journal of Rheumatology, 39*(9), 1807–1813.

Nicassio, P. M., Ormseth, S. R., Kay, M., Custodio, M., Irwin, M. R., Olmstead, R., & Weisman, M.H. (2012). The contribution of pain and depression to self-reported sleep disturbance in patients with rheumatoid arthritis. *Pain, 153*(1), 107–112.

Nicassio, P. M., & Wallston, K. A. (1992). Longitudinal relationships among pain, sleep problems, and depression in rheumatoid arthritis. *Journal of Abnormal Psychology, 101*(3), 514–520.

O'Leary, A., Shoor, S., Lorig, K., & Holman, H. R. (1988). A cognitive-behavioral treatment for rheumatoid arthritis. *Health Psychology, 7*(6), 527–544.

Palagini, L., Mosca, M., Tani, C., Gemignani, A., Mauri, M., & Bombardieri, S. (2013). Depression and systemic lupus erythematosus: A systematic review. *Lupus, 22*(5), 409–416.

Palagini, L., Tani, C., Bruno, R., Gemignani, A., Mauri, M., Bombardieri, S., Riemann, D., & Mosca, M. (2014). Poor sleep quality in systemic lupus erythematosus: Does it depend on depressive symptoms? *Lupus, 23*(13). doi:10.1177/0961203314540762.

Parmelee, P. A., Tighe, C. A., & Dautovich, N. D. (2015). Sleep disturbance in osteoarthritis: Linkages with pain, disability and depressive symptoms. *Arthritis Care & Research, 67*(3), 358–365.

Power, J. D., Perruccio, A. V., & Badley, E. M. (2005). Pain as a mediator of sleep problems in arthritis and other chronic conditions. *Arthritis Care & Research, 53*(6), 911–919.

Roddy, E., Zhang, W., & Doherty, M. (2005). Aerobic walking or strengthening exercise for osteoarthritis of the knee? A systematic review. *Annals of the Rheumatic Diseases, 64*(4), 544–548.

Roth, T., Price, J. M., Amato, D. A., Rubens, R. P., Roach, J. M., & Schnitzer, T. J. (2009). The effect of eszopiclone in patients with insomnia and coexisting rheumatoid arthritis: A pilot study. *The Primary Care Companion—Journal of Clinical Psychiatry, 11*(6), 292–301.

Rybarczyk, B., Stepanski, E., Fogg, L., Lopez, M., Barry, P., & Davis, A. (2005). A placebo-controlled test of cognitive-behavioral therapy for comorbid insomnia in older adults. *Journal of Consulting and Clinical Psychology, 73*(6), 1164–1174.

Sariyildiz, M. A., Batmaz, I., Bozkurt, M., Bez, Y., Cetincakmak, M. G., Yazmalar, L., Ucar, D., & Celepkolu, T. (2014). Sleep quality in rheumatoid arthritis: Relationship between the disease severity, depression, functional status and the quality of life. *Journal of Clinical Medicine Research, 6*(1), 44–52.

Sasaki, E., Tsuda, E., Yamamoto, Y., Maeda, S., Inoue, R., Chiba, D., Okubo, N., Takahashi, I., Nakaji, S., & Ishibashi, Y. (2013). Nocturnal knee pain increases with the severity of knee osteoarthritis, disturbing patient sleep quality. *Arthritis Care & Research, 66*(7), 1027–1032.

Sharma, B., & Haslock, I. (1978). Night medication in rheumatoid arthritis. III. The use of sulindac. *Current Medical Research and Opinion, 5*(6), 472–475.

Shearer, W. T., Reuben, J. M., Mullington, J. M., Price, N. J., Lee, B.-N., Smith, E. B., Szuba, M.P., Van Dongen, H.P.A., & Dinges, D.F. (2001). Soluble

TNF-α receptor 1 and IL-6 plasma levels in humans subjected to the sleep deprivation model of spaceflight. *The Journal of Allergy and Clinical Immunology, 107*(1), 165–170.

Simpson, N., & Dinges, D. F. (2007). Sleep and inflammation. *Nutrition Reviews, 65*(s3), S244–S252.

Smith, M. T., Quartana, P. J., Okonkwo, R. M., & Nasir, A. (2009). Mechanisms by which sleep disturbance contributes to osteoarthritis pain: A conceptual model. *Current Pain and Headache Reports, 13*(6), 447–454.

Stebbings, S., Herbison, P., Doyle, T. C., Treharne, G. J., & Highton, J. (2010). A comparison of fatigue correlates in rheumatoid arthritis and osteoarthritis: Disparity in associations with disability, anxiety and sleep disturbance. *Rheumatology (Oxford), 49*(2), 361–367.

Stenström, C. H., & Minor, M. A. (2003). Evidence for the benefit of aerobic and strengthening exercise in rheumatoid arthritis. *Arthritis Care & Research, 49*(3), 428–434.

Taibi, D. M., Bourguignon, C., & Taylor, A. (2008). A feasibility study of valerian extract for sleep disturbance in person with arthritis. *Biological Research for Nursing, 10*(4), 409–417.

Taibi, D. M., & Vitiello, M. V. (2011). A pilot study of gentle yoga for sleep disturbance in women with osteoarthritis. *Sleep Medicine, 12*(5), 512–517.

Taylor-Gjevre, R., Gjevre, J., Nair, B., Skomro, R., & Lim, H. (2011). Components of sleep quality and sleep fragmentation in rheumatoid arthritis and osteoarthritis. *Musculoskeletal Care, 9*(3), 152–159.

Tench, C., McCurdie, I., White, P., & D'Cruz, D. (2000). The prevalence and associations of fatigue in systemic lupus erythematosus. *Rheumatology (Oxford), 39*(11), 1249–1254.

Thyberg, I., Dahlström, Ö., & Thyberg, M. (2009). Factors related to fatigue in women and men with early rheumatoid arthritis: The Swedish TIRA study. *Journal of Rehabilitation Medicine, 41*(11), 904–912.

Troxel, W. M., Germain, A., & Buysse, D. J. (2012). Clinical management of insomnia with brief behavioral treatment (BBTI). *Behavioral Sleep Medicine, 10*(4), 266–279.

Uchida, S., Shioda, K., Morita, Y., Kubota, C., Ganeko, M., & Takeda, N. (2012). Exercise effects on sleep physiology. *Frontiers in Neurology, 3*, 48.

Valencia-Flores, M., Resendiz, M., Castãno, V. A., Santiago, V., Campos, R. M., Sandino, S., Valencia, X., Alcocer, J., Ramos, G.G., & Bliwise, D.L. (1999). Objective and subjective sleep disturbances in patients with systemic lupus erythematosus. *Arthritis and Rheumatism, 42*(10), 2189–2193.

Verbrugge, L. M., & Juarez, L. (2006). Profile of arthritis disability: II. *Arthritis Care & Research, 55*(1), 102–113.

Vgontzas, A. N., Papanicolaou, D. A., Bixler, E. O., Lotsikas, A., Zachman, K., Kales, A., Prolo, P., Wong, M., Licinio, J., Gold, P.W., Hermida, R.C., Mastorakos, G., & Chrousos, G.P. (1999). Circadian interleukin-6 secretion and quantity and depth of sleep. *The Journal of Clinical Endocrinology and Metabolism, 84*(8), 2603–2607.

Vgontzas, A., Zoumakis, E., Bixler, E., Lin, H.-M., Follett, H., Kales, A., & Chrousos, G.P. (2004). Adverse effects of modest sleep restriction on sleepiness, performance, and inflammatory cytokines. *The Journal of Clinical Endocrinology and Metabolism, 89*(5), 2119–2126.

Vina, E. R., Green, S. L., Trivedi, T., Kwoh, C. K., & Utset, T. O. (2013). Correlates of sleep abnormalities in systemic lupus: A cross-sectional survey in an urban, academic center. *Journal of Clinical Rheumatology, 19*(1), 7–13.

Vitiello, M. V., McCurry, S. M., Shortreed, S. M., Baker, L. D., Rybarczyk, B. D., Keefe, F. J., & Von Korff, M. (2014). Short-term improvement in insomnia symptoms predicts long-term improvements in sleep, pain, and fatigue in older adults with comorbid osteoarthritis and insomnia. *Pain, 155*(8), 1547–1554.

Vitiello, M. V., McCurry, S. M., Shortreed, S. M., Balderson, B. H., Baker, L. D., Keefe, F. J., Rybarczyk, B.D., & Von Korff, M. (2013). Cognitive-behavioral treatment for comorbid insomnia and osteoarthritis pain in primary care: The lifestyles randomized controlled trial. *Journal of the American Geriatrics Society, 61*(6), 947–956.

Vitiello, M. V., Rybarczyk, B., Von Korff, M., & Stepanski, E. J. (2009). Cognitive behavioral therapy for insomnia improves sleep and decreases pain in older adults with co-morbid insomnia and osteoarthritis. *Journal of Clinical Sleep Medicine, 5*(4), 355–362.

Walsh, J., Muehlbach, M., Lauter, S., Hilliker, N., & Schweitzer, P. (1996). Effects of triazolam on sleep, daytime sleepiness, and morning stiffness in patients with rheumatoid arthritis. *The Journal of Rheumatology, 23*(2), 245–252.

Ward, L., Stebbings, S., Athens, J., Cherkin, D., & Baxter, G. D. (2014). Yoga for pain and sleep quality in rheumatoid arthritis: A pilot randomized controlled trial. *Journal of Alternative and Complementary Medicine, 20*(5), A87. doi:10.1089/acm.2014.531.abstract.

Westhovens, R., Van der Elst, K., Matthys, A., Tran, M., & Gilloteau, I. (2014). Sleep problems in patients with rheumatoid arthritis. *The Journal of Rheumatology, 41*(1), 31–40.

Wolfe, F., Michaud, K., & Li, T. (2006). Sleep disturbance in patients with rheumatoid arthritis: Evaluation by medical outcomes study and visual analog sleep scales. *The Journal of Rheumatology, 33*(10), 1942–1951.

Yang, P.-Y., Ho, K.-H., Chen, H.-C., & Chien, M.-Y. (2012). Exercise training improves sleep quality in middle-aged and older adults with sleep problems: A systematic review. *Journal of Physiotherapy, 58*(3), 157–163.

Yılmaz, O. O., Senocak, O., Sahin, E., Baydar, M., Gulbahar, S., Bircan, C., & Alper, S. (2010). Efficacy of EMG-biofeedback in knee osteoarthritis. *Rheumatology International, 30*(7), 887–892.

Disability, Limitations, and Function for People with Arthritis

10

Kristina A. Theis

Abbreviations

AAAL	Arthritis-attributable activity limitation
AAVL	Arthritis-attributable volunteer limitation
AAWL	Arthritis-attributable work limitation
ADL	Activities of daily living
CDC	Centers for Disease Control and Prevention
DALY	Disability-adjusted life years
DSM IV	Diagnostic and Statistical Manual of Mental Disorders 4th edition
IADL	Instrumental activities of daily living
ICF	International Classification of Functioning, Disability, and Health
K-6	Kessler 6
NHIS	National Health Interview Survey
SIPP	Survey of Income and Program Participation
SPD	Serious psychological distress
SPR	Social participation restriction
WHO	World Health Organization
YLD	Years lived with disability
YLL	Years of life lost

The findings and conclusions in this report are those of the author and do not necessarily represent the official position of the Centers for Disease Control and Prevention.

K.A. Theis, PhD (✉)
Division of Population Health, Arthritis Program, Centers for Disease Control and Prevention, 4770 Buford Highway, NE, Mailstop F-78, Atlanta, GA, 30341, USA
e-mail: KTheis@cdc.gov

The ICF framework is used as a lens through which to examine several summary measures of disability (e.g., DALYs, ADLs/IADLs), arthritis-attributable limitations (work, activity, volunteer), and population-level surveillance of function among people with arthritis. Other impacts, including mental health among people with arthritis, health-related quality-of-life, participation restriction, and disparities in arthritis effects are also addressed.

It is important to remember that all people can be healthy and live well with or without a disability. It is also important to estimate the number of people with disabilities or limitations and the types of difficulties that can occur in order to improve planning for programs, interventions, clinical management, and accommodations.

By virtually any method used to describe disabilities and limitations, arthritis has substantial negative consequences, particularly related to function and mobility.

In this chapter, I aim to provide a broad overview of conceptions of arthritis disability and its impacts, using the ICF framework as a lens to understand how arthritis fits in across continuums of function, person–environment interactions, and the adult life-span (World Health Organization, 2001).

Disabilities and limitations can be measured in many ways. There is no single definition for "disability," and many programs, surveillance systems, and studies use different definitions based on specific needs and/or available data.

P.M. Nicassio (ed.), *Psychosocial Factors in Arthritis*, DOI 10.1007/978-3-319-22858-7_10

As such, a condition or limitation considered to be a disability in one context may not be classified likewise in other situations. An additional difficulty for researchers is that the presence of a specific underlying cause of a disability, such as arthritis, can affect different people in different ways and may not always result in similar disability across individuals.

Beyond the difficulties of definitions and ascertainment, it is important to remember that all people can be healthy and live well with or without a disability. At the same time, there is value in estimating the number of people with disabilities and limitations and the types of restrictions that can occur in order to improve planning for programs, interventions, accommodations, clinical practice, and other important purposes. By virtually any method used to describe disabilities and limitations, arthritis has substantial negative consequences, particularly related to function and mobility.

Disability Measurement

Because there are so many ways to define and describe disability, and because concepts and understanding of disability have changed so drastically in the past several decades, a brief discussion of the evolution of thinking about disability is warranted here. The last half century has seen some dramatic shifts in thinking about and describing disability. For example, the disability-adjusted life year (DALY), intended to be a neutral equalizer, has faced criticism for its implicit premise that quality-of-life with a disability is automatically less than living without a disability (Groce, Chamie, & Me, 1999). The World Health Organization (WHO) revised its own International Classification of Impairment, Disability, and Health twice before moving away from a model that created a "healthy" vs. "disabled" dichotomy, finally developing the more widely accepted International Classification of Function, Disability, and Health (ICF) in 2001 (World Health Organization, 2001). Recent years have seen refinement of the concept of disability that has been more inclusive on the whole.

Models of disability over a 50-year period reflect the transformation from understanding disability as a personal, limiting characteristic (handicap) to one of an interaction between a person and his or her environment. Importantly, each of these newer models explicitly recognizes that, whatever the organic cause of impact, it influences three distinct levels: body, person, and society. Starting in the late 1990s, the interaction of an individual with society and his/her environment has also been a more frequent and broadly accepted contextual element when defining, describing, and understanding disability.

The International Classification of Function, Disability, and Health (ICF)

Figure 10.1 illustrates the current conceptualization of disability, as promoted by the WHO. Moving the emphasis away from an individual deficit to an interaction between person and environment has made this a widely accepted model of disability. Notably, the ICF allows for examination of the consequences of a disorder or a disease on one or more of physical impairments (body functions and structures), activity limitations, and participation restriction in the context of sweeping environmental and individual personal factors. Each of these levels of impact is discussed as applicable in the sections that follow.

The current ICF framework was unanimously endorsed by all WHO member states in May 2001 as "the international standard to describe and measure health and disability" (World Health Organization, 2015). The ICF emphasizes that disability is a universal experience as part of a continuum of health and function, which are influenced by environmental factors. Applications of the ICF include national and international surveillance, reporting, and evaluation, as well as clinical and epidemiological uses at a variety of population levels. A breakthrough of the ICF, and a departure from some previous frameworks, is the focus on the impact of biology and impairment on the function of the individual in personal and environmental contexts (World Health Organization, 2015).

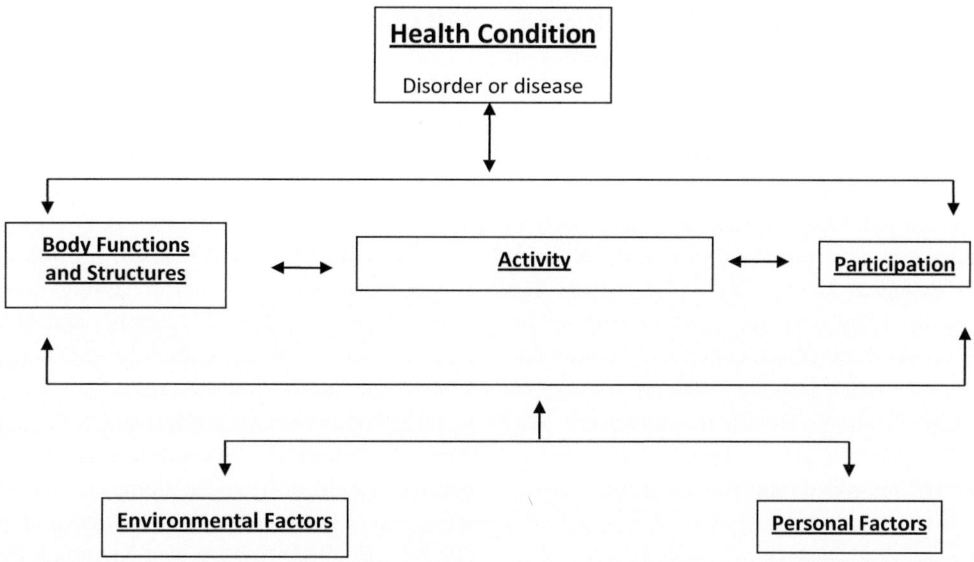

Fig. 10.1 The World Health Organization's International Classification of Function, Disability, and Health (ICF) (reproduced with permission)

Arthritis Background and Definitions

Arthritis is reported by 1-in-5 (52.5 million) US adults ages 18 or older (Barbour et al., 2013). The case-finding definition for self-reported, doctor-diagnosed arthritis used by the Centers for Disease Control and Prevention is a "yes" to "Have you ever been told by a doctor or other health professional that you have some form of arthritis, rheumatoid arthritis, gout, lupus, or fibromyalgia?" (Barbour et al., 2013). Due to the complexities of gathering and tracking arthritis data as well as time and resource constraints, most population-based studies of arthritis prevalence and impact (e.g., national surveys) must rely on the efficiency of self-report. While clinical and population-based studies suggest that individuals often have limited knowledge of their specific rheumatic condition and frequently cannot report their diagnosis accurately (Barlow, Turner, & Wright, 1998; Lawrence et al., 1989; Rasooly, Papageorgiou, & Badley, 1995), self-report of a medical diagnosis of an arthritis condition (without information on sub-type) has been demonstrated to have adequate sensitivity (66–76 %) and specificity (75–96 %) compared to a clinically assessed diagnosis (Busija, Hollingsworth, Buchbinder, & Osborne, 2007; Sacks et al., 2005).

Although self-reports often lack diagnostic specificity, they are meaningful from a population perspective in that they frequently capture symptomatic disease and, because of unequal access to and use of health care providers to treat arthritis symptoms, likely capture burden more completely than relying on a patchwork of clinical data for population estimates. Ascertaining arthritis prevalence by self-report is congruent with the reporting for many other diseases and conditions (e.g., asthma, heart disease), and case-finding questions that ask respondents to self-report a doctor-diagnosis of arthritis likely increase accuracy of the reports, i.e., improved specificity and fewer false-positives for an actual arthritis diagnosis (Bolen, Helmick, Sacks, Gizlice, & Potter, 2011). The term "arthritis" describes more than 100 conditions; most of which are characterized by pain, aching, stiffness, and/or swelling in or around the joints or elsewhere in the musculoskeletal system (Theis, Helmick, & Hootman, 2007). Due to the population-based emphasis of this chapter, "arthritis" refers to the case-finding definition described above; deviations from this definition are noted and/or cited.

Arthritis is a large and growing problem throughout the world (Helmick et al., 2008; Lawrence et al., 2008; WHO Scientific Group, 2003), and musculoskeletal and rheumatic diseases are recognized as the most common cause of morbidity globally (WHO Scientific Group, 2003). To define and describe disability, function, and limitations for people with arthritis, this chapter is organized first by describing major summary measures of disability, specific functional limitations, and related mental health measures among people with arthritis, followed by arthritis-attributable measures.

Major Summary Measures of Disability

DALYs, YLLs, and YLDs

Several measures have been proposed to capture summaries of disability, particularly to make comparisons across conditions and populations. One of the most frequently cited measure, the DALY, has been especially promoted in the multiple iterations of the Global Burden of Disease (GBD) Study (Murray et al., 2012). DALYs themselves are somewhat of a summary measure as they are derived by summing a measure of years of life lost (YLLs) and years lived with disability (YLDs) (Murray et al., 2012). Given the gargantuan undertaking of the GBD, it is understandable that only three (osteoarthritis, rheumatoid arthritis, and gout) of the more than 100 conditions that comprise "arthritis" are examined and reported. In the most recent analysis, the examined musculoskeletal conditions comprised 6.8 % of total DALYs, of which osteoarthritis alone accounted for 10 % (Murray et al., 2012). Estimates for 2010 indicated that gout, rheumatoid arthritis, and osteoarthritis globally produced 2 (95 % CI = 1–2), 70 (54–88), and 249 (172–352) DALYs per 100,000, respectively (Murray et al., 2012). (For some context, these values were 174 (167–184) for breast cancer and 222 (186–268) for hypertensive heart disease (Murray et al., 2012)).

ADLs/IADLs

Activities of daily living (ADLs) and instrumental activities of daily living (IADLs) actually represent summary measures of function and activity limitations and, for some IADLs, participation restriction, as defined by the ICF. ADLs are broadly defined as "basic tasks of everyday life" and represent activities such as bathing, dressing, transferring, using the toilet, continence, and eating; IADLs were subsequently developed to incorporate more activities necessary for independent community living and include managing personal finances, preparing meals, shopping, getting around outside the home, doing housework, using a telephone, and taking medication (Wiener, Hanley, Clark, & Van Nostrand, 1990).

Most population-based US studies measuring ADLs or IADLs among people with arthritis have focused on older adults (Martin & Schoeni, 2014; Song, Chang, & Dunlop, 2006). Song et al. found that, even after adjusting for other risk factors, older adults (age ≥65 years) with arthritis at baseline had higher incidence of ADL disability compared with those without arthritis (9.3 % vs. 4.5 %) over two years of follow-up, and that approximately 1-in-4 new cases of ADL disability in the population were due to arthritis, with an adjusted population-attributable fraction of 23.7 % (Song et al., 2006). Another study examining causes of ADL and IADL disability in US adults between 1997 and 2010 found that arthritis/rheumatism ranked second (behind back/neck problem) among adults ages 40–64 and first among adults ≥65 years; importantly, in the younger group limitations increased over the study period (Martin & Schoeni, 2014). A recent Dutch study had very similar findings in terms of ADL disability, including the greater emphasis on arthritis vs. back pain as a cause among older adults, and reported that high prevalence, moderately disabling conditions, specifically arthritis, make the greatest contributions to population disability among older adults (Klijs, Nusselder, Looman, & Mackenbach, 2011).

There has been some criticism of ADLs/IADLs as being too focused on narrow functional limitations at the expense of other important areas of life that may have more meaning to some individuals (such as personal relationships), and broader evaluation of disability in advanced or valued activities beyond activities that are necessary for survival or self-sufficiency have been suggested (Katz, 2004).

Main Cause of Disability

Another source of general disability surveillance in the USA has been the Survey of Income and Program Participation (SIPP). Over a period of 15 years, three independent cross-sectional ascertainments of the prevalence and causes of disability among US adults were conducted through the SIPP by the U.S. Census Bureau. Each of these analyses demonstrated that arthritis or rheumatism is the most common cause of disability, and, in the most recent of these analyses, the top three most common causes of disability were found to be (1) arthritis or rheumatism (8.6 million), (2) back or spine problems (7.6 million), and (3) heart trouble (3.0 million) (Brault, Hootman, Helmick, Theis, & Armour, 2009).

SIPP used a broad and comprehensive set of questions to identify disability. Because of the breadth of the scope of disability as defined by SIPP, it is not possible to classify this measure in one of the ICF categories; the SIPP definition includes impairments, activity limitations, and participation restrictions, making it a thorough definition for surveillance and planning purposes. Respondents were classified as having a disability if they answered "yes" to at least one of the queried limitation categories: (1) use of an assistive aid (cane, crutches, walker, or wheelchair), (2) difficulty performing activities of daily living (getting around inside the home, getting in/out of a bed/chair, bathing, dressing, eating, and toileting) or instrumental activities of daily living (getting around outside the home, taking care of money/bills, preparing meals, doing light housework, managing prescriptions, and using the telephone), or specified functional activities (seeing letters/words in newsprint, hearing normal conversation, having speech understood, walking three city blocks, climbing a flight of stairs, grasping objects, lifting/carrying 10 lb), (3) one or more selected impairments (learning disability, mental retardation, other developmental disability, Alzheimer's disease/senility/dementia, or other emotional/mental disability), or (4) limitation in the ability to work around the house or at a job or business. Effects of temporary conditions (less than 5 months duration) were excluded. Individuals who reported any of these limitations (except those with only "use of an assistive aid" or "selective impairments") were also asked "Which condition or conditions cause these difficulties?" and shown a list of 30 conditions from which they were asked to identify the cause of their disability. Respondents indicating more than one condition were asked to identify a main condition.

Arthritis or rheumatism was cited as the main cause of disability most often overall (19.0 %, 95 % CI = 18.0–20.0), for men (11.5 %, 95 % CI = 10.3–12.7), and for women (24.3, 95 % CI = 22.9–25.7) (Brault et al., 2009). Back or spine problems was the next most common cause of disability, cited by 16.8 %, which was statistically significantly lower than for arthritis or rheumatism. The same is true for all remaining mutually exclusive reported causes, which ranged in prevalence from 0.2 % (AIDS or AIDS-related condition and, separately, speech disorder) to 12.9 % (other) to sum to 100 % (Brault et al., 2009).

Specific Functional Limitations

Surveillance of nine specific functional limitations is also conducted in the USA through the National Health Interview Survey (NHIS), which is an ongoing multistage, probability sample survey conducted by in-person interview representative of the civilian, non-institutionalized population (National Center for Health Statistics, 2009). These functional limitations would be considered activity limitations in the ICF framework and are useful clinical targets for intervention as many of them represent critical capacities for independent living. The prevalence of functional limitations is high among people with arthritis. When the root question "By yourself, and without using any special equipment, how difficult is it for you to …" was queried with a 5-point scale ((1) Not at all difficult, (2) Only a little difficult, (3) Somewhat difficult, (4) Very difficult, (5) Can't do at all) among respondents with self-reported, doctor-diagnosed arthritis, limitations restricted to responses of "very difficult" and "can't do at all" ranged from 5.5 % (grasp/handle small objects) to 27.3 % (stand or be on feet for about 2 h) (Theis, Murphy, Hootman, & Wilkie, 2013). The remaining functional limitations were stoop, bend, or kneel (27.2 %), walk a quarter of a mile or three city blocks (21.0 %), push/pull large objects (e.g., living room chair) (18.2 %), climb up ten steps without resting (15.3 %), carry/lift something as heavy as 10 lb (e.g., bag of groceries) (12.4 %), reach up over head (7.0 %), and sit for 2 h (9.8 %) (Theis et al., 2013). Findings from this study also indicated that slightly greater than 2-in-5 (43 %) adults with arthritis report at least one functional limitation (Theis et al., 2013). The range of prevalence of functional limitations among people with arthritis, from 1-in-20 to 2-in-5, suggests substantial disability in many basic and necessary activities for everyday life.

Mental Health Measures

Mental health impacts are important components of disease consequences and the study of disability because of the complex relationship between mental and physical conditions, coping ability, pain perception, and interference with compliance and responsiveness to treatment and self-management behaviors, such as physical activity (Burnett, Coverdale, Pickens, & Dyer, 2006; Dimatteo, Lepper, & Croghan, 2000; Graves, Scott, Lempp, & Weinmann, 2009; Lowe et al., 2004; McFarlane & Brooks, 1988; Parker & Wright, 1995; Rosemann, Laux, & Kuehlein, 2007; Scopaz, Piva, Wisniewski, & Fitzgerald, 2009; Soderlin, Hakala, & Nieminen, 2000). Specifically, functional disabilities among people with arthritis can be worsened by depression (Rosemann et al., 2007), and impaired mental health itself can increase disability and decrease quality-of-life and physical function (Crotty et al., 1994; Lowe et al., 2004; McFarlane & Brooks, 1988; Parker & Wright, 1995; Rupp, Boshuizen, Dinant, Jacobi, & van den Bos, 2006).

For people with arthritis, symptoms often affect mood, and negative mental health impacts are common. For example, a nationally representative US study found that both serious psychological distress (as measured by the K-6 (Kessler et al., 2002) and frequent anxiety or depression were significantly and substantially higher in adults with arthritis compared with those without (5.6 % vs. 1.8 % and 26.2 % vs. 10.7 %, respectively) (Shih, Hootman, Strine, Chapman, & Brady, 2006). The K-6, which measures non-specific serious psychological distress in populations and has been shown to discriminate DSM-IV cases from non-cases (Kessler et al., 2010), uses a six-question scale to assess how often in the past 30 days respondents felt each of: sad, worthless, nervous, restless, hopeless, and that everything was an effort (Kessler et al., 2002). Frequent anxiety or depression in this study was defined as a "yes" response to: "During the past 12 months have you been frequently depressed or anxious?" (Shih et al., 2006). Shih et al. also found that, among adults with arthritis, younger age, recurrent pain, physical inactivity, functional or social limitations, comorbid medical conditions, lower socioeconomic status, and divorce/separation were significantly associated with serious psychological distress. In fact, serious psychological distress was 6.5 times more prevalent in adults ages 18–44 years compared with those 65 years or older (Shih et al., 2006). Because this study was cross-sectional in nature, the temporal sequence between functional or social limitations and serious psychological distress could not be assessed, but the strong, significant relationship between them was established (Shih et al., 2006).

Another nationally representative US study of adults with arthritis ages 45 or older found that one-third of respondents reported at least one episode of anxiety or depression, anxiety was significantly more common than depression (31 % vs. 18 %), and that most respondents with depression (84 %) also reported anxiety (Murphy, Sacks,

Brady, Hootman, & Chapman, 2012). This study used the Arthritis Impact Measurement Scales to assess anxiety and depression separately (Meenan, Mason, Anderson, Guccione, & Kazis, 1992). Importantly, conclusions from this study indicated that, despite greater focus on depression among people with arthritis, anxiety is almost twice as common; due to the lack of a distinct profile of people with arthritis reporting anxiety and/or depression that all people with arthritis should be screened and treated for both conditions; and low prevalence of help-seeking for mental health among people with arthritis suggests unmet treatment need in this area (Murphy et al., 2012).

Health-Related Quality-of-Life

Health-Related Quality-of-Life (HRQOL), while not strictly a measure of disability, is a useful reflection of how overall health states, and the absence of acceptable levels of health, influence perceived physical and mental health. Among adults ages 18 years or older, those with arthritis report fair/poor health, mean numbers of physically unhealthy, mentally unhealthy, and activity-limited days in the past month substantially and significantly more often than those without arthritis (Furner, Hootman, Helmick, Bolen, & Zack, 2011). For fair/poor health, 27 % of US adults with arthritis report this outcome compared with only 12 % of those without arthritis (Furner et al., 2011). For mean numbers of mentally unhealthy days (5.4 vs. 2.8), physically unhealthy days (6.6 vs. 2.5), and activity-limited days (4.3 vs. 1.4) adults with arthritis report 1.9, 2.6, and 3.0 times more affected days, respectively, than their non-arthritis counterparts (Furner et al., 2011).

Social and Community Participation Restriction

Arthritis affects many important components of life, including social participation (Wilkstrom, Book, & Jacobson, 2006), which itself can be associated with well-being (Zimmer, Hickey, & Searle, 1997). Barriers imposed by the physical impairments of arthritis may cause some people with arthritis to reduce or cease social participation and may lead to negative mental health consequences and reduced quality-of-life (AIHW, 2008). While many individuals are able to alter their lives successfully to live with arthritis, it can cause tremendous interruptions for others. For example, many people with arthritis report giving up hobbies, social groups, and volunteer activities to accommodate their symptoms (Gignac, Coot, & Badley, 2008; Katz & Morris, 2007; Katz, Morris, Trupin, Yazdany, & Yelin, 2008; Prady, Vale, & Hill, 1998; Theis, Murphy, Hootman, Helmick, & Sacks, 2010). Frequent pain, which is common in under-managed arthritis, is an "extremely demotivating and depressing condition" for both the individual and the friends and family with whom they try to engage (Prady et al., 1998). Yelin et al. suggest that up to two-thirds of people with rheumatoid arthritis experience losses in social relationships, disrupted leisure activities, work limitations, and transportation problems as a result of the condition (Yelin, Henke, & Esptein, 1987). Effects on social contact, limitations on family role, functioning, isolation, and role alteration have also been demonstrated to be negative psychosocial consequences of arthritis (Ryan, 1998).

Many of the consequences of arthritis on social and community engagement can be captured through the "participation" domain of the ICF. According to the WHO, participation is reflected at the societal level and represents "involvement in a life situation," while participation restriction represents "problems an individual may experience in involvement in life situations," which can indicate difficulties in such areas as visiting friends, leisure activities, and running errands (World Health Organization, 2001). Participation can be examined in a variety of domains that include engagement in interpersonal situations. Social participation restriction (SPR) has been estimated at 1-in-9 or 11 % of US adults with arthritis (Theis et al., 2013). SPR included limitations in shopping, going to movies or sporting events, and participating in social activities like visiting friends, attending clubs and meetings, or going to parties (Theis et al., 2013). In this study, which took a comprehensive ICF approach to examining disability, severe joint pain and functional limitations were among the most strongly associated characteristics with SPR in multivariable-adjusted analyses (Theis et al., 2013).

A separate study examining community participation restriction among older adults (≥50 years) with chronic conditions found that adults with fairly low prevalence conditions (e.g., stroke, serious psychological distress, neurological conditions) reported generally high community participation restriction (9–20 %), while individuals with high prevalence conditions (e.g., arthritis) had comparatively lower proportions of community participation restriction (5–10 %) but made up the greatest burden in terms of absolute numbers (~1 million per condition) (Theis & Furner, 2011). When arthritis was considered as a comorbidity, community participation restriction was reported by at least 10 % of respondents with all studied conditions, except hypertension (Theis & Furner, 2011). When queried about the perceived environmental barrier causes of their restriction, people with arthritis often cited accessibility (e.g., building design) and mobility barriers (e.g., sidewalks/curbs) (Theis & Furner, 2011), illustrating the person–environment interaction perspective promoted by the ICF.

Arthritis-Attributable Impact Measures

National and state-specific health surveillance systems in the USA have, in recent years, afforded the opportunity to examine specific arthritis-attributable impacts, sometimes as part of the monitoring of Healthy People 2010 and 2020 national health objective initiatives (U.S. Department of Health and Human Services, 2010, 2013). Among these are several measures that can be considered to represent various aspects of disability among adults with arthritis and that reflect impairments, activity limitations, and participation restriction in terms of ICF domains.

Arthritis-Attributable Work Limitation

An important Healthy People 2020 arthritis objective is to "reduce the proportion of people with doctor-diagnosed arthritis who are limited in their ability to work for pay due to arthritis" (U.S. Department of Health and Human Services, 2013). Arthritis-attributable work limitation (AAWL) is defined for Healthy People 2020 and U.S. public health surveillance purposes as a "yes" to "In this next question, we are referring to work for pay. Do arthritis or joint symptoms now affect whether you work, the type of work you do, or the amount of work you do?" Nationally, the prevalence of AAWL is 30 % among working-age (18–64 year old) adults with arthritis, which equates to 1-in-20 or 5 % of the entire US working-age population (Theis, Murphy, Hootman, Helmick, & Yelin, 2007).

Holding a job has valuable benefits in terms of identity, status, and feelings of self-worth and self-esteem, while both a person's economic situation and mental health can be adversely affected by joblessness (Prady et al., 1998). Workforce participation provides opportunities to contribute productively to society and to remain financially independent (ABS, 2005). As described by Armstrong and Wilkie, workforce participation is necessary for individual prosperity and full participation in society as well as being "central to identity, social roles, and social status" (Armstrong & Wilkie, 2009). On the other hand, being outside the labor force may have a negative impact on a person's health (ABS, 2005). Burgard et al. established via analysis of two longitudinal datasets that involuntary job loss is associated with significantly poorer overall self-rated health and more depressive symptoms; moreover, among involuntary job losers whose job loss was for health-related reasons, the declines in health are even more severe (Burgard, Brand, & House, 2007). Job loss also represents more than the loss of wage and non-wage economic benefits. It is the loss of a major social role and of on-the-job social networks (Burgard et al., 2007; Hayes & Nutman, 1981). In addition, being unemployed is a stigmatized condition in many countries, which brings the potential of anxiety, insecurity, shame, and the worsening of psychological symptoms such as depression (Burgard et al., 2007; Gallo, Bradley, Siegel, & Kasl, 2000). The high prevalence of AAWL among adults with arthritis puts them at greater risk for these negative outcomes and provides an important target population for intervention.

Arthritis-Attributable Volunteer Limitations

Volunteering can be a meaningful personal pursuit; particularly for older adults, volunteering can also be a meaningful social role. Increased life satisfaction, as well as positive changes in psychological and physical well-being, has been demonstrated to be associated with volunteering in longitudinal studies (Meier & Stutzer, 2004; Musick & Wilson, 2003; Pilliavin & Siegel, 2007; van Willigen, 2000). Some evidence suggests that "volunteering may be more beneficial to older adults with functional limitations" (Morrow-Howell, Hinterlong, Rozario, & Tang, 2003). Taken together, this evidence suggests that limitations in the ability to volunteer, particularly due to arthritis, may be a consequential marker of participation restriction, as defined by the ICF, in a population that already experiences excess disability and functional and activity limitations. It is also true that volunteers contribute substantially to the economy, with some estimates of volunteer output equal to 0.8–1.3 % of the gross domestic product (Pho, 2004), making volunteering a valuable social and economic good beyond personal benefits.

A study of middle and older age (≥45 years) US adults with arthritis found that 32.5 % of this population reported volunteering, of whom 2-in-5 (40.5 %) indicated that arthritis limits the type and/or amount of volunteering that they do (Theis, Murphy, Hootman, Helmick, & Sacks, 2010). An additional 26.7 % of US adults ≥45 years with arthritis reported that, while they do not volunteer, arthritis is their main barrier for not doing so (Theis et al., 2010). Associations with arthritis-attributable volunteer limitations and arthritis as the main barrier to volunteering were largely intuitive. For example, the highest prevalence of arthritis-attributable volunteer limitations and arthritis as a main barrier to volunteering was among those who were unable to work/disabled (70.1 % and 59.5 %, respectively). And, in multivariable-adjusted logistic regression models, poor physical function was the most strongly associated correlate with each outcome (AOR = 8.0 and 4.3, respectively) (Theis et al., 2010). A strength of this study was the ascertainment of respondent attribution of arthritis impact on their volunteering activities, which provides consequential insight into how these individuals perceive effects of arthritis on their lives and participation opportunities.

Arthritis-Attributable Activity Limitation

Verbrugge et al. classified human activities into three categories: (1) discretionary (e.g., socializing, leisure activities, volunteering, and activities for relaxation or pleasure); (2) committed (associated with social identity and "principle productive roles," e.g., paid work, family care); (3) obligatory (required for self-sufficient survival, e.g., activities of daily living, self-care, and hygiene) (Verbrugge, Gruber-Baldini, & Fozard, 1996). There is evidence that people with arthritis often employ the adaptive strategy of reducing discretionary activities to conserve time and energy for committed and obligatory activities (Gignac, Coot & Badley, 2008; Katz et al., 2008; Katz & Morris, 2007; Theis et al., 2010). Whether by conscious choice or not, arthritis is known to reduce or restrict activities, including a range of what individuals consider "valued life activities" (Katz et al., 2009; Katz & Morris, 2007). The most recent (2010–2012) national estimates indicate that 42.3 % of US adults with arthritis report arthritis-attributable activity limitations, defined as "yes" to "Are you now limited in any way in any of your usual activities because of arthritis or joint symptoms? (Barbour et al., 2013)."

Arthritis-Attributable activity limitations already affect 1-in-10 (9.8 %) of the ≥18-year-old population in the USA, an estimated 22.7 million people. Previous projections estimated that arthritis-attributable activity limitations would not affect that number of people until at least 2020 (Hootman & Helmick, 2006). Therefore, the current prevalence of arthritis-attributable activity limitations is outpacing projections and may reach the 2030 projected prevalence (25 million) much sooner than anticipated (Barbour et al., 2013; Hootman & Helmick, 2006). Because of the inclusive nature of the arthritis-attributable activity limitations question, it is not possible to determine whether respondents are reporting activity limitations, participation restrictions, or both, when viewed through the framework of the ICF; however, it is clear that substantial, population-wide limitations due to arthritis are being reported. The rapidly increasing prevalence of these limitations suggests an unmet need in managing arthritis and its symptoms to limit the extent of disability caused by the condition.

Arthritis-Attributable Interference in Routine Life Activities

Roles and activities that are important to people with chronic conditions are getting more attention from researchers, as are their effects on health and health outcomes (Ahlstrand, Bjork, Thyberg, Borsbo, & Falkmer, 2012; Gignac et al., 2008; Katz et al., 2009; Katz & Yelin, 2001). Expanding traditional clinical endpoints to more outcomes with patient-centered meaning and value is congruent with the 2012 Institute of Medicine (IOM) report *Living well with chronic disease: public health action to reduce disability and improve functioning and quality-of-life*, which recommends greater emphasis on quality-of-life measures among people with chronic conditions and improving peoples' capacity to live well over the life course (Institute of Medicine, 2012). The broad measure of arthritis-attributable activity limitations is described above. The measures that comprise arthritis-attributable interference in routine life activities provide an understanding of arthritis-specific impacts on selected domains of activity, which can help both further characterize effects of arthritis and identify those in need of intervention.

In a population-based survey of adults ages ≥45 with arthritis, a series of questions assessing arthritis-attributable interference in routine life activities was asked for the domains of: (1) household chores, (2) recreational and leisure activities, (3) social activities, and (4) shopping (Theis & Murphy, 2011). Response categories were "a lot," "a little," and "not at all." At least some interference (a lot or a little) was reported by greater than half of respondents for each domain; interference was greatest for household chores (68 %) and recreation and leisure activities (65 %) (Theis, Brady, Helmick, Murphy, & Barbour, 2012). Overall, only 21 % reported no arthritis-attributable interference in routine life activities. These interferences were significantly higher in women compared with men (42 % vs. 31 %) but similar by age and race/ethnicity. Substantial arthritis-attributable interference in routine life activities ("a lot" of interference in one or more domain) was >50 % for several subgroups, including those reporting severe arthritis-related fatigue (74 %), severe joint pain (68 %), anxiety (61 %), depression (68 %), and low confidence in managing arthritis symptoms (65 %) (Theis et al., 2012). These domains of routine life activities reflect activity limitation and participation restriction under the ICF framework and demonstrate substantial arthritis impacts in fairly nuanced life domains. As more patient-driven health outcomes gain in importance, disability in these areas should be recognized and addressed more often.

Racial and Ethnic Disparities in Arthritis-Attributable Limitations

While arthritis causes substantial disability in terms of population impact, some racial/ethnic groups are affected disproportionately (Bolen et al., 2010; Murphy et al., 2011).

For example, based on national data, arthritis-attributablework limitation, arthritis-attributable activity limitation, and severe joint pain were higher among Non-Hispanic blacks, Hispanics, and multiracial or other respondents with arthritis compared with Non-Hispanic whites with arthritis, despite sometimes lower population prevalence of arthritis (i.e.,. among Non-Hispanic blacks and Hispanics) (Bolen et al., 2005). The magnitude of these differences was 7.0–13.3 percentage points higher for arthritis-attributable work limitations; 10.9–17.6 percentage points higher for arthritis-attributable activity limitations, and 13.3–15.2 percentage points higher for severe joint pain among Non-Hispanic blacks, Hispanics, and multiracial or other respondents with arthritis compared with Non-Hispanic whites with arthritis (Bolen et al., 2005).

Another study demonstrated that, while Hispanics have lower population prevalence of arthritis than Non-Hispanic whites or blacks, there is substantial variation in arthritis impacts among Hispanic subgroups (Murphy et al., 2011). In this study, the prevalence of arthritis-attributable work limitations ranged from 33.9 % (Other/Multi-Hispanic subgroups) to 52.8 % (Dominican/Dominican American); prevalence of arthritis-attributable activity limitations ranged from 34.2 % (Cuban/Cuban American) to 50.8 % (Puerto Rican); and prevalence of severe joint pain ranged from 29.9 % (Other/Multi-Hispanic subgroups) to 46.1 % (Dominican/Dominican American) (Murphy et al., 2011).

Quantifying differential impacts by racial/ethnic groups may be useful for planning interventions and making concerted efforts to reduce disability and limitations in specific, disproportionately affected populations.

Interventions

Interventions are discussed in detail elsewhere in this book. However, it is worth mentioning here that clinical, public health, and policy interventions are all relevant and useful tools for reducing disability and improving quality-of-life, function, and participation among people with arthritis. As demonstrated in the findings and summaries reported above, pain and poor physical function, while limitations in their own right, are strongly associated with and contribute to additional measures of disability, limitation, and participation restriction. Better management and pain control among patients with arthritis and more aggressive intervention intensity and timing for function preservation may result in substantial health gains and reductions in disability (Theis et al., 2013). Addressing modifiable environmental barriers, improving clinical management, aligning financial and tax incentives to support efforts to remain in the workforce, and much broader and comprehensive use of evidence-based public health physical activity and self-management intervention programs are all promising strategies (Brady et al., 2013; Brady, Jernick, Hootman, & Sniezek, 2009; Holland, Burström, et al., 2011; Holland, Nylén, et al., 2011; Theis et al., 2013; Theis & Furner, 2011; Theis, Murphy, et al., 2007).

Conclusion

As mentioned in the introduction, arthritis, by any definition, can be profoundly disabling, whether the metric is a specific functional or activity limitation, a general impact measure like ADLs, or the comprehensive concept of participation restriction. Beyond the individual, personal consequences of arthritis disability, there are considerable societal and economic impacts of arthritis as well. The unique contributions of arthritis and its symptoms to mental health, well-being, and quality-of-life are also important to remember in the context of disability estimates and questions about measurement and outcomes.

There will never be a single definition of disability. There will never be a conceptualization or framework of disability, no matter how well intentioned, that pleases everyone or meets everyone's needs. That said, there will still be a very real need to describe and address health condition consequences and to plan for and manage conditions like arthritis that threaten the lives people want and need to lead. This chapter has attempted to provide a broad overview of conceptions of arthritis disability and its impacts, using the ICF framework as a lens to understand how arthritis fits in across continuums of function, person–environment interactions, and the lifespan. It is worth reiterating that good health and quality-of-life are available to all, regardless of chronic conditions or functional status. It is worth charging clinicians, public health professionals, researchers, policymakers, individuals, and society as a whole with taking a broad and comprehensive view of disability and taking steps to reduce, delay, and address it in order to promote physical and mental health for all.

References

Ahlstrand, I., Bjork, M., Thyberg, I., Borsbo, B., & Falkmer, T. (2012). Pain and daily activities in rheumatoid arthritis. *Disability and Rehabilitation, 34*(15), 1245–1253.

Armstrong, R., & Wilkie, R. (2009). Musculoskeletal problems and work in the UK—Time for a new approach? *Rheumatology, 48*, 709–710.

Australian Bureau of Statistics [ABS]. (2005). *Health, disability, age and labour force participation* (Cat. no. 6105.0). Canberra, Australian Capital Territory: ABS.

Australian Institute of Health and Welfare [AIHW]. (2008). *Arthritis and osteoporosis in Australia 2008* (Cat. no. PHE 106). Canberra, Australian Capital Territory: AIHW.

Barbour, K. E., Helmick, C. G., Theis, K. A., Murphy, L. B., Hootman, J. M., Brady, T. J., Cheng, Y. J. (2013). Prevalence of doctor-diagnosed arthritis and arthritis-attributable activity limitation—United States, 2010–2012. *MMWR, 62*(44), 869–873.

Barlow, J. H., Turner, A. P., & Wright, C. C. (1998). Comparison of clinical and self-reported diagnoses for participants on a community-based arthritis self-management programme. *British Journal of Rheumatology, 37*(9), 985–987.

Bolen, J., Helmick, C. G., Sacks, J. J., Gizlice, Z., & Potter, C. (2011). Should people who have joint symptoms, but no diagnosis of arthritis from a doctor, be included in surveillance efforts? *Arthritis Care & Research, 63*(1), 150–154.

Bolen, J., Scheib, L., Hootman, J. M., Helmick, C. G., Theis, K., Murphy, L. B., et al. (2010). Differences in the prevalence and impact of arthritis among racial/ethnic groups in the United States, National Health Interview Survey, 2002, 2003, 2004. *Preventing Chronic Disease, 7*(3). Retrieved January 21, 2014, from http://www.cdc.gov/pcd/issues/2010/may/10_0035.htm

Bolen, J., Sniezek, J., Theis, K., Helmick, C., Hootman, J., Brady, T., et al. (2005). Racial/ethnic differences in the prevalence and impact of doctor-diagnosed arthritis—United States, 2002. *MMWR, 54*(5), 119–123.

Brady, T. J., Jernick, S. L., Hootman, J. M., & Sniezek, J. E. (2009). Public health interventions for arthritis: Expanding the toolbox of evidence-based interventions. *Journal of Women's Health, 18*(12), 1905–1917.

Brady, T. J., Murphy, L., O'Colmain, B. J., Beauchesne, D., Daniels, B., Greenberg, M., et al. (2013). A meta-analysis of health status, health behaviors, and health care utilization outcomes of the chronic disease self-management program. *Preventing Chronic Disease, 10*, 120112. Retrieved from http://dx.doi.org/10.5888/pcd10.120112

Brault, M. W., Hootman, J., Helmick, C. G., Theis, K. A., & Armour, B. S. (2009). Prevalence and most common causes of disability among adults, United States, 2005. *MMWR, 58*(16), 421–426.

Burgard, S. A., Brand, J. E., & House, J. S. (2007). Toward a better estimation of the effect of job loss on health. *Journal of Health and Social Behavior, 48*, 369–384.

Burnett, J., Coverdale, J. H., Pickens, S., & Dyer, C. B. (2006). What is the association between self-neglect, depressive symptoms and untreated medical conditions? *Journal of Elder Abuse & Neglect, 18*, 25–34.

Busija, L., Hollingsworth, B., Buchbinder, R., & Osborne, R. H. (2007). Role of age, sex, and obesity in the higher prevalence of arthritis among lower socioeconomic groups: A population-based survey. *Arthritis and Rheumatism, 57*(4), 553–561.

Crotty, M., McFarlane, A. C., Brooks, P. M., Hopper, J. L., Bieri, D., & Taylor, S. J. (1994). The psychosocial and clinical status of younger women with early rheumatoid arthritis: A longitudinal study with frequent measures. *British Journal of Rheumatology, 33*(8), 754–760.

Dimatteo, M. R., Lepper, H. S., & Croghan, T. W. (2000). Depression is a risk factor for noncompliance with medical treatment: Meta-analysis of the effects of anxiety and depression on patient adherence. *Archives of Internal Medicine, 160*, 2101–2107.

Furner, S., Hootman, J. M., Helmick, C. G., Bolen, J., & Zack, M. M. (2011). Health-related quality of life of US adults with arthritis: Analysis of data from the Behavioral Risk Factor Surveillance System, 2003, 2005, and 2007. *Arthritis Care & Research, 63*(6), 788–799.

Gallo, W. T., Bradley, E. H., Siegel, M., & Kasl, S. V. (2000). Health effects of involuntary job loss among older workers: Findings from the Health and Retirement Study. *Journal of Gerontology: Social Sciences, 55B*, S131–S140.

Gignac, M., Backman, C., Davis, A., Lacaille, D., Mattison, C., Montie, P., et al. (2008). Understanding social role participation: What matters to people with arthritis? *The Journal of Rheumatology, 35*(8), 1655–36.

Gignac, M. A. M., Coot, C., & Badley, E. M. (2008). Adaptation to chronic illness and disability and its relationship to perceptions of independence and dependence. *Psychology and Aging, 55B*, P362–P372.

Graves, H., Scott, D., Lempp, H., & Weinmann, J. (2009). Illness beliefs predict disability in rheumatoid arthritis. *Journal of Psychosomatic Research, 67*(5), 417–423.

Groce, N. E., Chamie, M., & Me, A. (1999). Measuring the quality of life: Rethinking the World Bank's disability-adjusted life years. *International Rehabilitation Review, 49*, 12–15.

Hayes, J., & Nutman, P. (1981). *Understanding the unemployed: The psychological effects of unemployment*. London, UK: Tavistock.

Helmick, C. G., Felson, D. T., Lawrence, R. C., Gabriel, S., Hirsch, R., Kwoh, C. K., et al. (2008). Estimates of the prevalence of arthritis and other rheumatic conditions in the United States. Part I. *Arthritis and Rheumatism, 58*(1), 15–25.

Holland, P., Burström, B., Whitehead, M., Diderichsen, F., Dahl, E., Barr, B., et al. (2011). How to macro-level contexts and policies affect the employment changes of chronically ill and disabled people? Part I: The impact of recession and deindustrialization. *International Journal of Health Services, 41*(3), 395–413.

Holland, P., Nylén, L., Thielen, K., van der Wel, K. A., Chen, W., Barr, B., et al. (2011). How do macro-level contexts and policies affect the employment chances of chronically ill and disabled people? Part II: The impact of active and passive labor market policies. *International Journal of Health Services, 41*(3), 415–430.

Hootman, J. M., & Helmick, C. G. (2006). Projections of U.S. prevalence of arthritis and associated activity limitations. *Arthritis and Rheumatism, 54*(1), 226–229.

Institute of Medicine. (2012). *Living well with chronic disease: Public health action to reduce disability and improve functioning and quality-of-life*. Washington, DC: Institute of Medicine.

Katz, P. (2004). Function, disability, and psychological well-being. *Advances in Psychosomatic Medicine, 25*, 41–62.

Katz, P. P., & Morris, A. (2007). Use of accommodations for valued life activities: Prevalence and effects on disability scores. *Arthritis and Rheumatism, 57*, 730–737.

Katz, P., Morris, A., Gregorich, S., Yazdany, J., Eisner, M., Yelin, E., et al. (2009). Valued life activity disability played a significant role in self-rated health among adults with chronic health conditions. *Journal of Clinical Epidemiology, 62*(2), 158–166.

Katz, P. P., Morris, A., Trupin, L., Yazdany, J., & Yelin, E. (2008). Disability in valued life activities among individuals with systemic lupus erythematosus. *Arthritis and Rheumatism, 59*, 465–473.

Katz, P., & Yelin, E. H. (2001). Activity loss and the onset of depressive symptoms. *Arthritis and Rheumatism, 44*(5), 1194–1202.

Kessler, R. C., Andrews, G., Colpe, L. J., Hiripi, E., Mroczek, D. K., Normand, S. L., et al. (2002). Short screening scales to monitor population prevalences and trends in non-specific psychological distress. *Psychological Medicine, 32*(6), 959–976.

Kessler, R. C., Green, J. G., Gruber, M. J., Sampson, N. A., Bromet, E., Cuitan, M., et al. (2010). Screening for serious mental illness in the general population with the K6 screening scale: Results from the WHO World Mental Health (WMH) survey initiative. *International Journal of Methods in Psychiatric Research, 19*(Suppl 1), 4–22.

Klijs, B., Nusselder, W. J., Looman, C. W., & Mackenbach, J. P. (2011). Contribution of chronic disease to the burden of disability. *PLoS One, 6*(9), e25325.

Lawrence, R. C., Felson, D. T., Helmick, C. G., Arnold, L. M., Choi, H., Devo, R. A., et al. (2008). Estimates of the prevalence of arthritis and other rheumatic conditions in the United States. Part II. *Arthritis and Rheumatism, 58*(1), 26–35.

Lawrence, R. C., Hochberg, M. C., Kelsey, J. L., et al. (1989). Estimates of the prevalence of selected arthritic and musculoskeletal diseases in the United States. *The Journal of Rheumatology, 16*, 427–441.

Lowe, B., Willand, L., Eich, W., Zipfel, S., Ho, A. D., Herzog, W., et al. (2004). Psychiatric comorbidity and work disability in patients with inflammatory rheumatic diseases. *Psychosomatic Medicine, 66*, 395–402.

Martin, L. G., & Schoeni, R. F. (2014). Trends in disability and related chronic conditions among the forty-and-over population: 1997–2010. *Disability and Health Journal, 7*(2014), S4–S14.

McFarlane, A. C., & Brooks, P. M. (1988). Determinates of disability in rheumatoid arthritis. *British Journal of Rheumatology, 27*, 7–14.

Meenan, R. F., Mason, J. H., Anderson, J. J., Guccione, A. A., & Kazis, L. E. (1992). AIMS2: The content and properties of a revised and expanded Arthritis Impact Measurement Scales health status questionnaire. *Arthritis and Rheumatism, 35*, 1–10.

Meier, S., & Stutzer, A. (2004). *Is volunteering rewarding in itself?* Retrieved from http://ssrn.com/abstract505042

Morrow-Howell, N., Hinterlong, J., Rozario, P. A., & Tang, F. (2003). Effects of volunteering on the well-being of older adults. *The Journals of Gerontology Series B: Psychological Sciences and Social Sciences, 58B*, S137–S145.

Murphy, L. B., Bolen, J., Schieb, L., Hootman, J. M., Langmaid, G. A., & Cheng, Y. J. (2011). Prevalence of doctor-diagnosed arthritis and arthritis-attributable effects among Hispanic adults by Hispanic subgroup—United States, 2002, 2003, 2006, and 2009. *MMWR, 60*(6), 167–171.

Murphy, L. B., Sacks, J., Brady, T. J., Hootman, J. M., & Chapman, D. P. (2012). Anxiety and depression among US adults with arthritis: Prevalence and correlates. *Arthritis Care & Research, 64*(7), 968–976.

Murray, C. J. L., Vos, T., Lozano, R., Naghavi, M., Flaxman, A. D., Michaud, C., et al. (2012). Disability-adjusted life years (DALYs) for 291 diseases and injuries in 21 regions, 1990–2010: A systematic analysis for the Global Burden of Disease Study 2010. *Lancet, 380*, 2197–2223.

Musick, M. A., & Wilson, J. (2003). Volunteering and depression: The role of psychological and social resources in different age groups. *Social Science & Medicine, 56*, 259–269.

National Center for Health Statistics. (2009). *Data file documentation, National Health Interview Survey, 2009 (machine readable data file and documentation)*. Hyattsville, MD: National Center for Health Statistics, Centers for Disease Control and Prevention.

Parker, J. C., & Wright, G. E. (1995). The implications of depression for pain and disability in rheumatoid arthritis. *Arthritis Care & Research, 8*, 279–283.

Pho, Y. H. (2004). *Volunteer output and the national accounts: An empirical analysis*. Retrieved from http://www.beagov/papers/pdf/Volunteer_output_paperpdf
Pilliavin, J. A., & Siegel, E. (2007). Health benefits of volunteering in the Wisconsin Longitudinal Study. *Journal of Health and Social Behavior, 48*, 450–464.
Prady, J., Vale, A., & Hill, J. (1998). Body image and sexuality. In J. Hill (Ed.), *Rheumatology nursing: A creative approach* (pp. 109–123). Sydney, New South Wales, Australia: Churchill Livingston.
Rasooly, I., Papageorgiou, A. C., & Badley, E. M. (1995). Comparison of clinical and self reported diagnosis for rheumatology outpatients. *Annals of the Rheumatic Diseases, 52*, 850–852.
Rosemann, T., Laux, G., & Kuehlein, T. (2007). Osteoarthritis and functional disability: Results of a cross-sectional study among primary care patients in Germany. *BMC Musculoskeletal Disorders, 8*, 79.
Rupp, I., Boshuizen, H., Dinant, H. J., Jacobi, C., & van den Bos, G. (2006). Disability and health-related quality of life among patients with rheumatoid arthritis: Association with radiographic joint damage, disease activity, pain, and depressive symptoms. *Scandinavian Journal of Rheumatology, 35*(3), 175–181.
Ryan, S. (1998). The social implications of rheumatic disease. In J. Hill (Ed.), *Rheumatology nursing: A creative approach* (pp. 125–136). Sydney, New South Wales, Australia: Churchill Livingston.
Sacks, J. J., Harrold, L. R., Helmick, C. G., Gurwitz, J. H., Emani, S., & Yood, R. A. (2005). Validation of a surveillance case definition for arthritis. *The Journal of Rheumatology, 32*(2), 340–347.
Scopaz, K. A., Piva, S. R., Wisniewski, S., & Fitzgerald, G. K. (2009). Relationships of fear, anxiety, and depression with physical function in patients with knee osteoarthritis. *Archives of Physical Medicine and Rehabilitation, 90*, 1866–1873.
Shih, M., Hootman, J. M., Strine, T. W., Chapman, D. P., & Brady, T. J. (2006). Serious psychological distress in U.S. adults with arthritis. *Journal of General Internal Medicine, 21*(11), 1160–1166.
Soderlin, M. K., Hakala, M., & Nieminen, P. (2000). Anxiety and depression in a community-based rheumatoid arthritis population. *Scandinavian Journal of Rheumatology, 29*, 177–183.
Song, J., Chang, R. W., & Dunlop, D. D. (2006). Population impact of arthritis on disability in older adults. *Arthritis and Rheumatism, 55*(2), 248–255.
Theis, K. A., Brady, T. J., Helmick, C. G., Murphy, L., & Barbour, K. E. (2012). Arthritis-attributable interference in routine life activities. *Arthritis and Rheumatism, 64*(10), S1018.
Theis, K. A., & Furner, S. (2011). Shut-in? Impact of chronic conditions on community participation restriction among older adults. *J Aging Res. 2011*. Article ID 759158 [Epub 2011 Aug 3].
Theis, K. A., Helmick, C. G., & Hootman, J. M. (2007). Arthritis burden and impact are greater among U.S. women than men: Intervention opportunities. *Journal of Women's Health, 16*(4), 441–453.
Theis, K. A., & Murphy, L. (2011). Arthritis Conditions Health Effects Survey (ACHES) Data Documentation.
Theis, K. A., Murphy, L., Hootman, J. M., Helmick, C. G., & Sacks, J. J. (2010). Arthritis restricts volunteer participation: Prevalence and correlates of volunteer status among adults with arthritis. *Arthritis and Rheumatism, 62*(7), 907–916.
Theis, K. A., Murphy, L., Hootman, J. M., Helmick, C. G., & Yelin, E. (2007). Prevalence and correlates of arthritis-attributable work limitation in the U.S. population among persons ages 18–64: 2002 National Health Interview Survey Data. *Arthritis and Rheumatism, 57*(3), 355–363.
Theis, K. A., Murphy, L., Hootman, J. M., & Wilkie, R. (2013). Social participation restriction among U.S. adults with arthritis: A population-based study using the International Classification of Functioning, Disability, and Health (ICF). *Arthritis Care & Research, 65*(7), 1059–1069.
U.S. Department of Health and Human Services. (2010). *Healthy people 2010. With understanding and improving health and objectives for improving health* (2nd ed., 2 Vols.). Washington, DC: Government Printing Office.
U.S. Department of Health and Human Services. (2013). *Healthy people 2020*. Washington, DC: Office of Disease Prevention and Health Promotion. Retrieved December 5, 2013, from http://www.healthypeople.gov/2020/topicsobjectives2020/objectiveslist.aspx?topicId=3
van Willigen, M. (2000). Differential benefits of volunteering across the life course. *The Journals of Gerontology. Series B, Psychological Sciences and Social Sciences, 55B*, S308–S318.
Verbrugge, L. M., Gruber-Baldini, A. L., & Fozard, J. L. (1996). Age differences and age changes in activities: Baltimore Longitudinal Study of Aging. *The Journal of Gerontology: Social Sciences, 51B*, S30–S41.
WHO Scientific Group. (2003). *The burden of musculoskeletal conditions at the start of the new millennium*. Geneva, Switzerland: World Health Organization.
Wiener, J. M., Hanley, R. J., Clark, R., & Van Nostrand, J. F. (1990). Measuring the activities of daily living: Comparisons across national surveys. *Journal of Gerontology, 45*(6), S229–S237.
Wilkstrom, I., Book, C., & Jacobson, L. T. (2006). Difficulties in performing leisure activities among persons with newly diagnosed rheumatoid arthritis: A prospective, controlled study. *Rheumatology, 45*, 1162–1166.
World Health Organization. (2001). *International classification of functioning, disability, and health*. Geneva, Switzerland: World Health Organization.
World Health Organization. (2015). International Classification of Functioning, Disability and Health (ICF) [updated 2015; cited April 1, 2015]. Retrieved from http://www.who.int/classifications/icf/icf_more/en/
Yelin, E., Henke, C., & Esptein, W. (1987). Work dynamics of the person with rheumatoid arthritis. *Arthritis and Rheumatism, 30*, 507–512.
Zimmer, Z., Hickey, T., & Searle, M. S. (1997). The pattern of change in leisure activity behavior among older adults with arthritis. *Gerontologist, 37*, 384–392.

Revisiting Unequal Treatment: Disparities in Access to and Quality of Care for Arthritis

11

Adria N. Armbrister and Ana F. Abraído-Lanza

Introduction

Racism and social discrimination harm health (Krieger, 1999; Williams & Jackson, 2005). That is the conclusion to which health disparities research has come over the last two decades based on the finding that in the United States, blacks, American Indians, and Latinos of all races suffer disproportionately from both chronic and acute illness (Williams & Jackson, 2005). According to the Centers for Disease Control and Prevention (CDC, 2015), American Indians who comprise 2 % of the US population, have the highest prevalence of arthritis (25.2 %) of any racial or ethnic group in the United States (Dall'Era, Snipes, Cisternas, Gordon, & Helmick, 2014). The arthritis prevalence rate is 11.1 % among Latinos, compared with 19.4 % for non-Hispanic blacks and 23.8 % for non-Latino whites. Despite lower prevalence of arthritis, arthritis-attributable limitations are greater among non-Hispanic blacks (44.6 %) and Hispanics (43.2 %) compared to non-Hispanic whites (36.2 %). Blacks, American Indians, and Latinos also report a higher prevalence of activity limitations in work (almost 42 % for non-Latino blacks) and more severe pain than do non-Latino whites with arthritis (CDC, 2015).

Black, American Indian, and Latina women also experience higher morbidity and mortality from autoimmune diseases such as Systemic Lupus Erythematosus (SLE) (Alarcón et al., 1999; CDC, 2013; Society for Women's Health Research) that, in 90 % of cases, includes some acute or severe arthritic inflammation and resultant activity limitation.[1] Among black women in the United States, SLE incidence is almost eight times that of the general population (8.1–11.4/100,000 population per year)[2] and Latina, American Indian, Native Hawaiian, and Asian[3]

The opinions expressed in this publication are those of the authors and do not necessarily reflect the views of the Inter-American Development Bank, its Board of Directors, or the countries they represent.

A.N. Armbrister, PhD
Gender and Diversity Division, Social Sector, Inter-American Development Bank, 1300 New York Avenue, NW, Mail Stop W0608, Washington, DC 20577, USA
e-mail: adriaa@iadb.org

A.F. Abraído-Lanza, PhD (✉)
Department of Sociomedical Sciences, Mailman School of Public Health, Columbia University, 722 West 168th Street, New York, NY, 11530, USA
e-mail: aabraido@columbia.edu

[1] SLE affects women disproportionately (8 women:1 man) and is usually diagnosed during women's child bearing years (ages 15–45) (Domino, 2011).

[2] Caucasian men have the least common incidence of SLE (0.3–0.9/100,000 per year) (Domino, 2011).

[3] The fourfold increase in risk for Native Hawaiian and Asian women was found for Hawaii only.

P.M. Nicassio (ed.), *Psychosocial Factors in Arthritis*, DOI 10.1007/978-3-319-22858-7_11

women have almost four times the risk of diagnosis when compared with Caucasian women (Domino, 2011; Nass, 2001; Richards, 2003).

The reasons for this increased risk and severity among Black, American Indian, and Latino arthritis patients have been examined in a range of studies, from genetic (Bomback & Gharavi, 2013; Molokhia et al., 2003; Raman & Mohan, 2003; Tsao, 2003) and biomedical (Eudy, Vines, Dooley, Cooper, & Parks, 2014; Kim-Howard et al., 2014; Schulman et al., 1999) to environmental (Williams, Watkins, Anderson, & Tumiel-Berhalter, 2011) and sociocultural (Allen et al., 2010; González, Toloza, McGwin, & Alarcón, 2013). The search for the genetic underpinnings of health disparities for blacks and other minority groups has a long history in the United States. In the late nineteenth century, diseases from which blacks seemed to suffer disproportionately were deemed "black" diseases and were considered evidence of "inherent black frailty," inferiority, and immutable elements of blacks' evolutionary lot (Washington, 2006). However, the advent of *health disparities* research in the 1990s led to an exploration of social and cultural explanations for the disparate health outcomes seen between blacks and whites. Public health research on *health disparities* reached a fever pitch in the late 1990s and early 2000s following closely the economic, political science, and sociological work on income inequality within and among countries and across social domains including employment, education, housing, health, and social stratification (Beckfield, 2004; Kawachi, 2000; Ryscavage, 1999; Sen, 1992).

In one of the earliest statements defining the health disparities movement, "Social Conditions as Fundamental Causes of Disease," Link and Phelan (1995) assert that socioeconomic status (SES), treated largely until that time as a confounding variable in risk factor-based epidemiologic research, must be evaluated contextually rather than tangentially if we are to understand the distribution of disease. In addition to contextualizing, they suggest that researchers take into account the "fundamental causes" of disease, that is, factors that affect access to resources that promote health. These fundamental causes do not change despite the elimination of the mechanisms that link these causes to disease (Link & Phelan, 1995). For Link and Phelan (1995), class (in conjunction with gender and race/ethnicity) is the most important "fundamental cause" of inequality in the United States, deserving of independent attention by public health problem-solvers. They conclude:

> Specifically, if the social factor is a fundamental cause, one cannot claim to have accounted for its effects by having "explained" its association with the inclusion of intervening variables in a path or regression model. Second, to understand associations between fundamental causes and disease, medical sociologists need to examine the broader determinants of the resources that fundamental causes entail. This distinctly sociological enterprise will link medical sociologists to the broader discipline in a productive way as we seek to understand how general resources like knowledge, money, power, prestige, and social connections are transformed into the health-related resources that generate patterns of morbidity and mortality. (Link & Phelan, 1995, p. 88)

As a result of these theories and related research, national public health priorities turned toward testing and identifying the central aspects of class, gender, and race/ethnicity that are most relevant to addressing the health of disadvantaged groups in the United States (Link & Phelan, 2000; Marmot, 2004). At the federal level, in 2003 at the request of the U.S. Congress, the Institute of Medicine (IOM) of the National Academies of Medicine issued a landmark report on health inequalities called *Unequal Treatment: Confronting Racial and Ethnic Disparities in Health Care* (Smedley et al., 2003). The report was striking in that it shed light on disparities between racial and non-English speaking ethnic groups across a wide spectrum of health care including (but not limited to) treatment of cancer, cardiovascular disease, management of chronic diseases such as diabetes, referrals for a variety of tests, and mental health services. The report concluded that there are important differences between racial/ethnic groups in their rates of receipt of medical procedures, even when insurance status, income, age, and severity of conditions were comparable among patients. In addition to identifying multiple disparities in health care, the IOM report highlighted the importance of considering access to health care as a multicomponent concept. Specifically, it described factors that contribute to disparities, such as features of health care systems and settings, of physicians and the clinical encounter, and of patients.

In sum, the IOM report showed clearly that in the United States, racial and ethnic minorities received less optimal treatment and lower quality health services than did whites (Smedley et al., 2003). Later, in 2010, the U.S. Department of Health and Human Services' (DHHS) *Healthy People 2010*, "a long-term national agenda aimed at improving health in the United States" (National Research Council, 2004), named elimination of health disparities across gender, race, ethnicity, education, income, geography, and sexual orientation as one of its two main goals.[4] Interestingly, at the international level, the Pan American Health Organization (PAHO) also issued goals for the study and eradication of health inequalities based on poverty, education, ethnicity, and gender (Alleyne et al., 2002). Finally, it is also widely understood that the fulfillment of the Millennium Development Goals (MDGs) will require a concerted effort to address disparities in health (Busso, Cicowiez, & Gasparini, 2005).

Chapter Overview

Drawing from some of the levels of influence outlined in the IOM report, this chapter provides a discussion of disparities in health care among people with arthritis by focusing on the clinical encounter and patient factors. We first describe groundbreaking research on physician bias (much of which focuses on cardiovascular disease). We highlight experimental studies and other novel methodologies that include conversation and interactional analyses. We then turn to classic sociological concepts, including power, privilege, and stigma, as analytic tools for understanding these disparities. We propose that the interplay of power, prestige, and stigma create a thorny relationship between physicians and patients. Next, we highlight research and issues relevant to arthritis, with a particular focus on rheumatoid arthritis, osteoarthritis, and systemic lupus erythematosus, common forms of arthritis for which a growing body of research exists on health disparities. Finally, we conclude with research and policy recommendations. Although we acknowledge the population differences inherent in the terms Black and African American, we use these terms interchangeably and in accordance with the terminology employed in the studies we cite. The same convention is adopted for the use of the terms Hispanic and Latino.

Research on Physician Bias

Experimental Studies

In this section, we highlight briefly three notable biomedical and medical sociological health disparities experiments that explored whether physicians' biases may account for differences by race in use of life-saving interventions. A fourth study (Armbrister, 2014), the only of its kind to focus on arthritis-related disease, is described later in the chapter. Given the strengths of experimental methods in drawing causal inferences, these studies merit mention.

To date, the most groundbreaking clinical work on the effect of racism, sexism, and classism on health has been conducted through studies of cardiovascular disease (CVD) and coronary heart disease (CHD) (Arber et al., 2006; Ayanian & Epstein, 1991; Giles et al., 1995; Schulman et al., 1999). These studies find that women and blacks often are overlooked as candidates for potentially life-saving interventions and receive lower quality care than whites.

In a novel study, Schulman et al. (1999) measured physicians' propensity to refer patients for cardiac catheterization by patient race and gender. Patient confederates were presented to

[4]The first goal of Health People 2010 is "to help individuals of all ages increase life expectancy and improve their quality of life" (U.S. Department of Health and Human Services, 2010).

physicians in video vignettes in which scripts and performances were strictly controlled and all patients had the same income, insurance coverage, and personality affects. Physicians were randomly assigned to watch one of eight videos of "patients," who varied only in age (middle-aged versus older), gender (male versus female), and race (Black versus White). The study found that physicians were least likely to refer black women for the procedure:

> our finding that the race and sex of the patient influence the recommendations of physicians independently of other factors may suggest bias on the part of the physicians. However, our study could not assess the form of bias…. [it] may represent overt prejudice on the part of physicians or…could be the result of subconscious perceptions rather than deliberate actions or thoughts. Subconscious bias occurs when a patient's membership in a target group automatically activates a cultural stereotype in the physician's memory regardless of the level of prejudice the physician has. (Schulman et al., 1999, p. 625.

This study and others that followed underline the potential importance of the physician's own personal characteristics (e.g., length of experience, medical specialty, race, gender, and personality) in his or her decision-making process (McKinlay, 1996; McKinlay, Potter, & Feldman, 1996; Sabin et al., 2009).

Using case vignettes, Sabin, Rivara, and Greenwald (2008) explored whether (1) quality of care would vary by patient race; and (2) strength of implicit race bias would be related to quality care for pediatric patients. The web-based study, conducted with 95 pediatric faculty, fellows, and residents from one department at a research university, presented the Race Attitude Implicit Association Test (IAT); the Race and Compliant Patient IAT; and the Race and Quality of Medical Care IAT as measures of implicit discriminatory beliefs. The IAT is a measure of unconscious bias. Participants were also asked to respond to two explicit bias items: "'*My feelings towards African Americans are…*' and '*My feelings towards European Americans are…*' (*Answer options ranged from* 0 = cold *to* 10 = warm)" (Sabin et al., 2008, p. 680). Finally, participants were presented with two of four possible pediatric case vignettes in which patient confederates were either African American or white. They then assessed whether treatment recommendations for pain control, management of urinary tract infection (UTI), Attention Deficit Hyperactivity Disorder, and asthma control varied by patient race. Specifically, following the vignettes, participants were asked to indicate the appropriateness of a series of treatment options using a 5-item Likert scale that ranged from: *I strongly disagree, this is clearly the wrong treatment option* to *I strongly agree. This is clearly a good treatment option*. One of the treatment options included the ideal care for the case depicted, but none of the options represented negligent or inadequate care.

Their analyses revealed little evidence of overall implicit bias as measured by responses to the IAT tests administered. However, results indicated mild implicit stereotypes about race and compliance skewed toward African Americans, who were conceived as more compliant than European American patients (76 % versus 19 %) and more likely to receive "preferred" medical care (88 % versus 0 %). In addition, the authors also found that for all cases except asthma care, participants identified the ideal treatment recommendation more frequently. In contrast to the earlier work of Schulman et al. (1999), treatment recommendations did not vary by patient race except for management of UTI, for which ideal care occurred more often for African Americans than whites (Sabin et al., 2008, p. 681). The study concluded that the small sample size, use of a convenience sample, a physician sample skewed toward women, and the newness of the *Compliant Patient IAT* and the *Quality of Medical Care IAT* may have influenced their findings. In a similar 2005 study, Sabin and Greenwald found that increasing pro-white bias scores of physicians on a measure of implicit attitudes about race were associated with less optimal recommendations for narcotic pain medication for black pediatric patients, but found no other significant treatment associations (Sabin & Greenwald, 2012).

A third study by Green and Carney (2007) asked 202 internal and emergency medical residents in four academic medical hospitals in

Massachusetts and Georgia to consider a written patient vignette and photograph of a 50-year-old man suffering chest pain. Participants were asked to read the vignette and indicate whether they would recommend thrombolysis (clot busting techniques) and to specify the strength of their recommendation. Physician participants were then asked to comment on their patient's personal characteristics (e.g., patient cooperativeness) and were given an explicit discrimination measure and three Implicit Association Tests (IATs). The study found that physicians exhibited slight pro-white bias and that they indicated the need for thrombolysis equally between black and white patients. The authors emphasized that, given the large body of evidence of black men's increased likelihood of coronary artery disease, equal treatment constitutes a disparity. They also found that, compared to those with lower IAT scores, respondents with higher IATs (more pro-white bias) were less likely to recommend thrombolysis to black patients. In sum, two of the three studies described above found racial bias in physicians' decision-making and stereotyping of patients.

Other Methodological Approaches

In complement to the results of the biomedical studies of physician decision-making, studies of patient perceptions of racial bias have also led to the conclusion that physicians' implicit and explicit biases may play an important role in health disparities. For example, Berrios-Rivera et al. (2006) found that for the RA and SLE study participants both their ethnicity and physician's communication style (the amount of information provided, sensitivity and patient-centeredness) were associated with satisfaction with the medical encounter. In explanation, Berrios et al. suggest that "perhaps physicians (and/or patients) have subconscious biases, stereotypes, perceptions, or misconceptions…that interfere with open communication, empathy, and the development of trust" (p. 391). They base this hypothesis on the same studies of cardiovascular disease (CVD) and coronary heart disease (CHD) summarized above.

Cruz-Flores et al. (2011) reviewed the stroke care literature from 1972 to 2010 and found differences in the burden of stroke risk and stroke care between racial and ethnic minorities in the United States and whites. The disparities include among the myriad explanations for these disparities patient mistrust and physician bias. They explain that "differences in socioeconomic status and insurance coverage, mistrust of the healthcare system, the relatively limited number of providers who are members of minority groups, and system limitations, may contribute to disparities in access to or quality of care" (Cruz-Flores et al., 2011, p. 2103).

Another type of study, led by epidemiologists using some microsociological tools (e.g., conversation and interaction analysis), has sought to examine physician–patient communication in depth. These studies analyzed differences in physicians' interaction styles and behaviors with black and white patients, finding that many times, physicians' conversations with black patients differed in content and quality from their conversations with white patients. Specifically, physicians were more likely to lecture black patients and "adopt a narrowly biomedical communication pattern with African Americans, a pattern associated with low satisfaction ratings for patients as well as doctors" (Ashton et al., 2003).

Power, Prestige, and Stigma

The literature on social interactions in the medical encounter offers some explanation for physicians' behavior, implicating *power* imbalance and stigma as the main driver of continued health inequalities in medical treatment. Talcott Parsons (1951), for example, presents illness not only as a biological phenomenon, but also as a social role ("sick role") whose boundaries are dictated by social expectations. Specifically, the "sick role" is an expression of social deviance with the express purpose of exempting the sick person from her prescribed social duties for the duration of the illness, absolving her of responsibility for the illness. To perform the role successfully, the patient must additionally desire to get well, seek professional help in recovering from the illness and cooperate with the prescribed treatment. In Parson's conception, the power differential between physician and patient is needed to absolve the patient of her responsibility for accomplishing her duties.

Another branch of the power literature focuses on relations between patient and physician as a reflection of traditional power structures (Conrad, 1992, 2001; Pappas, 1990; Todd, 1989), the "embodiment" of culture and the established moral order (Alexander, 1982; Farmer, 1992; Kleinman, Eisenberg, & Good, 1978; Krieger, 1999). Farmer (2005) views this "embodiment" as a reflection of structural violence. Social constructionists legitimize explanations for disease based on the lived experiences of the sufferer that are often at odds with biomedical findings and methods that purport objectivity (Taussig, 1980).

Swidler (1986) takes the analysis of social interaction and its manifestation in culture in a different direction—away from the power of individuals or groups and toward the power of culture itself. She analyzes the relationship between cultural influence and action offering a view of culture as "a 'tool kit' of symbols, stories, rituals, and world-views which people may use to solve problems (Swidler, 1986). The tool kit imagery serves to emphasize that the organizing functions of culture are not uniform…but actors select relevant tools to construct their behaviors.

Prestige and status are often used interchangeably to indicate "*the esteem, respect, or approval that is granted by an individual or a collectivity for performances or qualities they consider above average*…[p]restige (negative or positive) may also be granted for *qualities* with which the individual is endowed at birth, such as nobility, membership in an ethnic group, or perhaps musical genius" (Goode, 1978). Prestige can also be earned by granting the "*right kind of approval*" to others (i.e., learning from the response of those around us that we have reacted "correctly").

At the same time as societies grant praise and esteem, they also remove it through dispraise and disapproval. Dispraise can be communicated through gesture, facial expression or verbally, and has perceptible effects. In fact, social psychological studies show that the more an individual's identity falls below the norm set by those in interaction with him or her, the greater the *frequency* of any performance below the norm (Goode, 1978). This cycle spirals downward as it repeats, increasing the likelihood of receiving more direct dispraise and the probability that others will join in the heaping on of disapproval. The repetition of low performance also increases the chance that "other sanctions or controls will be applied against the offender…[and] that the criticism will contain moral overtones or be expressed in moralistic rhetoric; and that the critic will display anger" (Goode, 1978). Steele and Aronson (1995) have termed this phenomenon stereotype threat, the feeling that one is at risk of confirming stereotypes of one's group and the consequent ingroup underperformance when reminded of these stereotypes.

In sum, prestige (esteem) and its converse, disapproval, function to control and correct behavior, both of the criticized and of the group to whom the criticized belongs. In this social order, this type of negative control is applied inequitably: the more powerful (socially superior group) being less likely to receive strong overt sanctions than the less powerful (socially inferior group) (Goode, 1978). Furthermore, many times sanctions are based solely on stereotypes about a socially inferior group. For example, as Rubio and Williams (2004) assert, negative stereotypes about Blacks and other minorities "are likely to have profound implications in situations ranging from personal day-to-day interactions to public policy. Research on stereotypes indicates that the endorsement of negative racial stereotypes leads to discrimination against minority groups" (Rubio & Williams, 2004).

Closely related to the concepts of prestige or status is stigma, a phenomenon that occurs when the labeling of human differences results in negative stereotyping and the categorization of people into "us" and "them" (Link & Phelan, 2001). Not only do societies recognize and shy away from the stigmatized, they actively reduce the life chances of the stigmatized person (Goffman, 1963).

Kwate et al. (2006)) and others argue that racism is a form of stigma for two reasons: (1)

"blackness" and black people are linked to a set of undesirable characteristics; and (2) the experience of residential and social segregation constitutes a de facto demarcation of "us" and "them." Stigma is revealed in several pervasive, though neither necessarily logical nor consistent, stereotypes. These include among others: the ascription of inferior intellects to black people that "in school settings…underlies peer perceptions of undeservedness, inequalities in educational placement, and attacks on affirmative action"; the ongoing message that black people, especially black men, are dangerous and prone to criminality; the perception of blacks as lazy and uninterested in work; that black people, especially black women, are servants; and are able to "withstand extremes of heat, physician labor, and pain." Recent studies suggest the continued reliance on this latter stereotype in medicine, as African Americans are still less likely than whites to be prescribed analgesic medication (Heins et al., 2006). Moreover, the application of these stereotypes in and of themselves can harm the health of African Americans as "stereotypes of African Americans fuel a moral economy that not only takes an intrapsychic toll on Black minds, but also subtly interweaves policies and practices that subordinate Black people" (Kwate & Meyer, 2011).

We propose that power, prestige, and stigma converge to create a thorny relationship between physicians and patients. Physicians, in a place of authority and thus greater prestige, have and are exhorted to gain the compliance of patients, perhaps members of a stigmatized racial or ethnic group to which all manner of negative stereotypes have been ascribed (Zola, 1972).

Research on Arthritis Populations

In the following sections, we provide an overview of two overarching classifications of direct and indirect causes of disparities in the sociocultural arm of arthritis, research in which issues of power, prestige, and stigma contribute to the creation and perpetration of health disparities—studies focused on patient-level factors (such as medical mistrust, adherence to medications, and health literacy) and research that highlights elements of the clinical encounter (focusing on physician biases in medication prescriptions and other forms of treatment). Given recent reviews of research on disparities in arthritis (see McBurney & Vina, 2012; McIlvane, 2009), we selected issues which we see as key for further research.

Patient Factors

Patient-level factors that have been measured to provide an explanation of disparities in SLE and forms of arthritis include: lack of compliance with drug regimens; inadequate or abnormal coping with illness; less frequent health care visits due to lack of private health insurance coverage; low educational attainment; family wealth and social capital (Alarcón et al., 1999, 2004; Kim-Howard et al., 2014; McIlvane, 2009; Ward et al., 2003). Among these factors, only poverty and insurance status have been found consistently to influence duration and severity of disease for black and Latino patients (González et al., 2013).

Medical Mistrust

Among other patient-level variables, medical mistrust emerges as key in the context of patient–physician interactions and general satisfaction with health care. Medical mistrust stems from a variety of sources that include historic, salient cases of mistreatment of ethnic minorities, and racism and discrimination experienced in the health care system (Smedley et al., 2003). Although the vast majority of research on these issues focuses on African Americans, there is growing evidence that Latinos report that racism is a significant problem in health care, express concerns about being mistreated due to their ethnic background, and they are more likely than whites to believe that Hispanics receive poorer quality healthcare than do whites (Lillie-Blanton et al., 2000). As the Institute of Medicine report notes, medical mistrust may create significant problems in health settings: "if patients convey mistrust, refuse treatment, don't adhere to or comply poorly with treatment, providers may become less engaged in the treatment process, and patients are less likely to be provided alternative treatments and services" (Smedley et al., 2003, p.174). Thus, medical mistrust could lead to a vicious cycle in which physicians (consciously or unconsciously) provide less quality care, which serves to reinforce patient's negative perceptions of the medical system.

Goodin et al. (2013) examined whether pain was associated with medical mistrust and racial discrimination in sample of 130 community-dwelling adults (67 African Americans, 63 non-Hispanic whites) with symptomatic knee osteoarthritis. Racial differences were found such that, relative to non-Hispanic whites, African Americans had more sensitivity to heat pain. In addition, they reported more racial discrimination and greater mistrust of medical research compared with non-Hispanic whites. Importantly, among African Americans but not whites, greater racial discrimination predicted lower heat pain tolerance. Mistrust of medical researchers did not significantly predict heat pain tolerance for either racial group. The researchers concluded that racial discrimination may influence the clinical pain severity of African Americans via the nociceptive processing of painful stimuli.

Although medical mistrust refers more broadly to general feelings of distrust of the institution of medicine, physician trust is another important but more narrow concept. Physician trust more narrowly encompasses patients' perceptions of their physicians. Few studies of arthritis populations focus on patient characteristics and aspects of the patient–physician relationship that predict trust in physicians. In their study of 102 patients (74 % of whom were Black or Latino) being treated in publicly funded hospitals in Houston, Texas for systemic lupus erythematosus (SLE) or rheumatoid arthritis (RA) patients, Berrios-Rivera et al. (2006) found that ethnicity was associated with trust. Specifically, Black and Latino ethnicity predicted decreased trust of physicians. Moreover, a sex-by-race interaction indicated that African American and Latino males reported lower trust in physicians than nonwhite females. Decreased trust was also associated with greater disease activity, as did decreased trust in the US health system. However, several physician interaction variables were associated with greater trust: doctors' informativeness, sensitivity to concerns, and patient-centeredness. No other sociodemographic variables (age, education, marital status) predicted trust.

Sleath et al.'s (2008) study of 1063 people with arthritis illustrates the importance of physician's interactions with patients. A large proportion of their sample (92 %) reported using CAM for their arthritis. Of these, only about half (54 %) discussed CAM with their rheumatologist. Patient sociodemographic characteristics of age, education, and race did not predict CAM discussions, and neither did medical skepticism (defined as doubts about the ability of conventional medicine to significantly alter health). However, women, patients who used more types of CAM, and those who rated their rheumatologist as engaging in more participatory decision-making style, were significantly more likely to tell their physicians about their CAM use. Because a participatory style may lead patients to feel at ease, and facilitate communications with their rheumatologists, they are more likely to share important information about CAM and perhaps other treatment issues openly with their physicians. These findings are similar to those of Berrios-Rivera et al. (2006), who reported that patients' willingness to disclose concerns was greater among those with physicians who used a patient-centered communication style.

Overall, it remains unclear the extent to which medical mistrust and physician trust impact patient–physician interactions and medical outcomes among people with arthritis. The IOM concluded that despite levels of mistrust, minority patients express satisfaction with their healthcare providers, and that mistrust alone is not likely to lead minority patients to reject or refuse treatment or preventative care (Smedley et al., 2003). Research is lacking on these issues among people with RA. As McIlvane (2009) notes, more research is needed to better understand the experiences and perceptions of Blacks and Latinos as they interact with health care providers and navigate the health care system.

Health Literacy

Given the importance of self-management in the rheumatic diseases, health literacy has emerged as an important concept. Health literacy, defined according to The Patient Protection and Affordable Care Act of 2010, Title V, refers to the capacity of individuals to obtain, communicate, process, and understand basic health information and services to make appropriate health decisions. Health literacy, however, encompasses more than simple comprehension of health-related material. It includes the capacity to act on health information (National Library of Medicine, 2015).

Quinlan et al. (2013) note that studies of patients with RA report rates of low health literacy ranging from 5 % to as high as 35 %. There is evidence that health literacy varies across SES and ethnic minority groups. For example, greater health literacy is associated with higher education, white race, and younger age. After adjusting for potential confounders, there is also some evidence that health literacy is associated with medication knowledge but not medication adherence in RA patients (Quinlan et al., 2013).

Despite the importance of health literacy and its association with indicators of social disadvantage, there is limited research on the relationship between health literacy and physical outcomes among people with rheumatic diseases. Only a handful of research has been conducted on this issue, most with small sample sizes. However, a large, recent study of over 6000 patients with RA recruited from the practices of over 800 rheumatologists across the nation, found a significant relationship between health literacy and better functional outcomes (Caplan, Wolfe, Michaud, Quinzanos, & Hirsh, 2014). In fact, the size of the association exceeded that of prednisone use, smoking history, and biologic agent use, and it was independent of education.

Drug Therapy and Adherence

Disparities in prescriptions for medications (discussed below) may account for some of the observed differences in disease outcomes between various groups. On the other hand, adherence to medications may vary by group.

There is some evidence of ethnic differences in adherence to medications, such that African American patients have lower adherence than whites. Overall, there is limited research examining differences in rates of adherence among racial/ethnic groups (see McBurney & Vina, 2012).

African American and Latino patients report a variety of barriers to adherence. These include language difficulties communicating with health professionals, cost, disease severity leading to missed appointments, difficulties taking medications at specified times, and perceptions that medications are toxic or harmful (see McBurney & Vina, 2012). In addition, low level of education and income, and side effects from medications, are associated with less adherence.

It would be important to further study the extent to which patient–physician relationship factors affect adherence to medical regimens among various ethnic/racial groups with arthritis. Relatively little is known about the association between adherence to drug regimens as a function of or reaction to health provider attitudes or actions (Walsh, Algert, & Rothfield, 1996).

Other Patient Factors: Treatment Preferences, Health Behaviors, and Psychosocial Variables

In this section, we have focused specifically on patient factors relevant to access to and quality of health care—medical mistrust and interactions with physicians, health literacy, and adherence to medications—which require further study. However, a wide literature exists on other patient or individual-level factors that could contribute to health disparities. For example, previous reviews and commentaries on health disparities point to a host of research on cognitive and psychosocial factors, including patient preferences (see Escalante, 2007; McBurney & Vina, 2012; McIlvane, 2009). In general, these studies show that even among samples with medical insurance, African Americans, and Latinos have lower preferences for surgery than do whites.

As McIlvane (2009), notes, however, African Americans and Latinos may present with more severe symptoms and advanced disease prior to undergoing surgical procedures for arthritis.

Finally, we point readers to other chapters in this book that focus on socioeconomic status, differences in health behaviors, and other psychosocial factors, including stress that could play a role in producing disparities (Baldassari and Callahan).

The Clinical Encounter

Most studies of physician-level factors in health disparities focus on issues of racial, ethnic, and gender discrimination because studies indicate that white physicians, compared to their counterparts of other races and ethnicities, report higher levels of pro-white bias (Sabin et al., 2009). Bias against minority groups affects not only interpersonal interactions but may also support the subtle interweaving of policies and practices that influence provider assessment and decision-making (Kwate & Meyer, 2011; Rubio & Williams, 2004).

These studies include indicators of discrimination, such as: communication style (verbal hostility; over-talking the patient and physical distance from the patient, language barriers) (Ashton et al., 2003; Bradshaw, Tomany-Korman, & Flores, 2007); and racial or ethnic affinity (race-concordance between patient and physician and empathy) (Drwecki, Moore, Ward, & Prkachin, 2011; Kaseweter, Drwecki, & Prkachin, 2012; Saha, Komaromy, Koepsell, & Bindman, 1999; Xu, Zuo, Wang, & Han, 2009). Other research explicitly explores the correlation between implicit or explicit bias assessed by available psychosocial measurement tools with medical decision-making (Suarez-Almazor et al., 2005).

Though nascent and thus less extensive than the cardiovascular literature on physician bias (Arber et al., 2006; Green et al., 2007; Schulman et al., 1999) and pain management (Staton et al., 2007; Tate & Chibnall, 2014), the arthritis literature has developed around measuring physician-mediated differences in prescriptions for medications, and life-saving or quality of life enhancing interventions, such as Total Joint Replacement (Cisternas, Murphy, & Helmick, 2009; Emejuaiwe, Jones, Ibrahim, & Kwoh, 2007; Suarez-Almazor et al., 2005) and treatment of solid organ involvement in SLE (Armbrister, 2014).

Prescriptions for Medications

McBurney and Vina's (2012) review of ethnic and racial disparities in RA indicates that ethnic minorities and socioeconomically disadvantaged groups are less likely than whites and those of higher social status to receive medications, such as disease-modifying antirheumatic drugs (DMARDs). For example, national data of all Medicare managed care plans indicate that relative to whites and nonwhites, those with low personal incomes, and residents of certain geographic regions (e.g., low-SES zip codes), were less likely to receive DMARDs (Schmajuk et al., 2011).

Additional evidence from a study of patients in public and private clinics in Texas showed significant delays in initiation of DMARD therapy (Suarez-Almazor et al., 2005). For African American and Latino patients, there was a median of 7 years prior to receiving DMARDs compared to only 1 year for whites.

McBurney and Vina (2012) pointed to these patterns as evidence of a potentially disturbing cycle. Specifically, inadequate treatment of RA may lead to further deterioration of health among populations who are already disadvantaged by their active RA.

Surgery and Other Treatments

Emejuaiwe et al.'s (2007) review of 9 studies on TJR indicates that African Americans and Latinos are less likely than whites to undergo Total Knee Replacement (TKR), hip Joint Replacement (JR), and Total Hip Arthroplasty (THR). Furthermore, relative to whites, these groups are less willing to consider these procedures, perhaps due to higher incidence of familiarity with people who have reported poor experiences with TJR. The same racial disparities have been reported for the Medicare population (Cisternas et al., 2009).

Suarez-Almazor et al. (2005) surveyed 198 white, African American, and Latino patients with advanced knee osteoarthritis to assess their knowledge of Total Knee Replacement (TKR), and to investigate whether their physicians had recommended TKR. African American and Latino patients had less knowledge of TKR and perceived the procedure as more risky than did white patients. They found no evidence of physician bias in recommendations of TKR.

Armbrister (2014) used face-to-face and internet-based instruments to survey 94 rheumatologists and used patient symptom vignettes and closed- and open-ended treatment questions to measure physicians' bias and its relation to treatment decisions for fictional women SLE patients presenting with symptoms of lupus nephritis (LN), a fairly common organ involvement for people with SLE. The study question centered on how and whether decisions about medical treatment and follow-up differ among patients as a function of several variables: the patient's race; the severity of symptoms; the physician's perception of the patient's personal characteristics (e.g., personality, mood); the physician's demographic characteristics; and the physician's score on the discriminatory belief measures named above. Overall, this study did not find evidence that physicians recommended less optimal treatment to black patients. However, given black women's increased likelihood of developing End Stage Renal Disease (ESRD) and to experience early mortality from lupus nephritis (LN) (Lea, 2002; Rivera et al., 2009), the study concluded that a finding of no difference in treatment between black and white patients may constitute an important treatment disparity.

To further explore disparities in treatment, patient–physicians interactions merit more research attention. As others have concluded, the relationship between medical provider and patient may serve to explain "disparities in the use of surgical or other invasive interventions, in which trust and effective communication play a larger role in decision-making" (Saha, 1999, p. 1718).

Though none of the studies reviewed in this section included physician-level factors in health disparities for arthritis and related illnesses, they have provided blueprints for policy, institutional, and personal reform.

Further Research and Policy Recommendations

Several of the physician-level studies have recommended the implementation of cultural-sensitivity training and culturally responsive institutional practices to improve physician–patient communication and patient education around availability and effectiveness of treatments such as TJR (Suarez-Almazor et al., 2005). The studies reviewed also recommend improvements in measurement of bias among physicians, as current measures may be dated and thus could either activate stereotype threat or promote vigilance that could lead to over-compensatory behaviors among white physicians. For example, Schulman et al.'s (1999) study is now widely known in academic medicine. As a result, physicians' bias may be either under- or overestimated.

Kwate also suggests that "future research should continue to specify the domain of observables for the construct of racism, and develop or refine [perceived racism] scale items to attend more closely to experiences of gendered stigma" (Kwate et al., 2006). There is additionally a need to focus on women's health outcomes as separate and different from men's. The results of studies into diseases that affect men and women fairly equally show gender and racial bias in treatment recommendations (Arber et al., 2006; Schulman et al., 1999). However, this body of work focuses on the expressions of these disparities as though race and gender are mutually exclusive. Moreover, this research does not delve deeply into the intersectional nature of race and gender in their findings. Thus, the specific experience of black women and other women of color with physician-mediated health disparities has been overlooked. Future research should focus not only on understanding how health disparities function for women patients, particularly those with chronic illnesses that affect women disproportionately, but also on the creation of methods to reduce disparities specific to these diseases that go beyond cultural-sensitivity training.

At an institutional policy level, Armbrister (2014) recommends that in the case of SLE, rheumatologists and family practitioners/general practitioners be required to justify reasons for not following guidelines in prescription and testing recommendations, like those spelled out for SLE (Yazdany et al., 2009). Similarly, Bornstein and Emler suggest that the use of these types of accountability tools could improve health outcomes for minority patients by "providing the most relevant and objective empirical information available, and incorporating it with clinical expertise, test results and patient preferences, [so that] many of the biases associated with doctors relying too heavily on intuition and selectively attending to some information while ignoring other relevant information could be avoided" (Bornstein & Emler, 2002). Bornstein and Emler also recommend the use of decision analytic aids, often computerized, to improve physicians' decision-making performance and reduce any possible differentiation between patients due to race, gender, or other personal characteristics.

Finally, 20 more years of research into health inequalities without the financing and implementation of empirically based interventions will do little to reduce health disparities. The research community must translate the current body of studies into a working agenda for piloting models of physician-led disparity reduction programs. These programs should test the feasibility of the recommendations above: the use of accountability systems; sharing of up-to-date empirical evidence with clinicians; and the use of diagnostic aids. They should also employ a gender focus in their design: both physicians treating diseases common to the general population and those treating "women's" illnesses need to understand the implications of both the physician's interaction style and the impact of the disease and its treatment on both women and men in order to make recommendations that will enhance compliance (Granger et al., 2009). Government programs in countries with national health systems and even the U.S.' Patient Protection and Affordable Care Act (known also as "Obamacare") afford optimal contexts in which to test the effectiveness of these strategies.

References

Alarcón, G., Gerald, M., Jr., Ámerica U., Friedman, A. W., Roseman, J. M., Fessler, B.J., … Reveille, J. D. (2004). Systemic lupus erythematosus in a multiethnic lupus cohort (LUMINA) XVII. Predictors of self-reported health-related quality of life early in the disease course. *Arthritis Care and Research, 51*(3), 465–74.

Alarcón, G. S., Rodríguez, J.L., Benavides, G., Brooks, K., Kurusz, H., Reveille, J.D. (1999). Systemic lupus erythematosus in three ethnic groups. V. Acculturation, health-related attitudes and behaviors, and disease activity in hispanic patients from the LUMINA cohort. *Arthritis Care & Research, 12*(4), 267–276.

Alexander, L. (1982). Illness maintenance and the new American sick role. In Chrisman, D., & Maretzki, T. (Eds.), Clinically applied anthropology (pp. 351–367). New York: Reidel.

Allen, K. D., Oddone, E. Z., Coffman, C. J., Keefe, F. J., Lindquist, J. H., & Bosworth, H. B. (2010). Racial differences in osteoarthritis pain and function: Potential explanatory factors. *Osteoarthritis and Cartilage, 18*, 160–167.

Alleyne, G., Castillo-Salgado, C., Schneider, M. C., Enrique, L. & Vidaurre, M. (2002). Overview of social inequalities in health in the region of the Americas, using various methodological approaches. *Pan American Journal of Public Health, 12*(6), 388–397.

Arber, S., McKinlay, J., Adams, A., Marceau, L., Link, C., O'Donnell, A. (2006). Patient characteristics and inequalities in doctors' diagnostic and management strategies relating to CHD: A video-simulation experiment. *Social Science and Medicine, 62*, 103–115.

Armbrister, A. N. (2014). *The influence of discriminatory beliefs on practice: Racial disparities in the treatment of women with systemic lupus erythematosus (SLE).* Dissertation, Columbia University.

Ashton, C. M., Haidet, P., Paterniti, D. A., Collins, T. C., Gordon, H. S., O'Malley, K., Petersen, L.A., Sharf, B.F., Suarez-Almazor, M.E., Wray, N.P., & Street, R. L. (2003). Racial and Ethnic Disparities in the Use of Health Services: Bias, Preferences, or Poor Communication? *Journal of General Internal Medicine, 18*(2), 146-152.

Ayanian, J., & Epstein, A. (1991). Differences in the use of procedures between women and men hospitalized for coronary heart disease. *New England Journal of Medicine, 325*(4), 221–225.

Beckfield, J. (2004). Does income inequality harm health? New cross-national evidence. *Journal of Health and Social Behavior, 45*(3), 231–248.

Berrios-Rivera, J. P., Street, R. L., Jr., Garcia Popa-Lisseanu, M. G., Kallen, M. A., Richardson, M. N.,

Janssen, N. M., … Suarez-Almazor, M. E. (2006). Trust in physicians and elements of the medical interaction in patients with rheumatoid arthritis and systemic lupus erythematosus. *Arthritis & Rheumatism, 55*(3), 385–393. doi:10.1002/art.21988.

Bomback, A. S., & Gharavi, A. G. (2013). Lupus nephritis: Ancestry, genetic risk and health disparities. *Nature Reviews. Nephrology, 9*(12), 699–700.

Bornstein, B., & Emler, A. (2002). Rationality in medical decision-making: A review of the literature on doctors' decision-making biases. *Journal of Education in Clinical Practice, 7*(2), 97–107.

Bradshaw, M., Tomany-Korman, S., & Flores, G. (2007). Language barriers to prescriptions for patients with limited English proficiency: A survey of pharmacies. *Pediatrics, 120*, e225–e235.

Busso, M., Cicowiez, M., & Gasparini, L. (2005). *Ethnicity and the millennium development goals. Facultad de Ciencias Económicas Universidad Nacional de la Plata (CEDLAS)*. Retrieved January 25, 2015, from http://cedlas.econo.unlp.edu.ar/eng/pantalla.php?seccion=special_studies&idP=128

Caplan, L., Wolfe, F., Michaud, K., Quinzanos, I., & Hirsh, J. M. (2014). Strong association of health literacy with functional status among rheumatoid arthritis patients: A cross sectional study. *Arthritis Care & Research, 66*, 508–514. doi:10.1002/acr.22165.

Centers for Disease Control and Prevention [CDC]. (2013). *FastStats: Health of Black or African-American Non-Hispanic population*. 2013 January 11, 2013. Retrieved March 13, 2013, from http://www.cdc.gov/nchs/fastats/black_health.htm

Centers for Disease Control and Prevention [CDC]. (2015). *Arthritis data*. Retrieved January 23, 2015, from http://www.cdc.gov/arthritis/data_statistics/race.htm

Cisternas, M. G., Murphy, L., & Helmick, C. G. (2009). Racial disparities in total knee replacement among medicare enrollees United States, 2000 2006. *Morbidity and Mortality Weekly, 58*, 133–138.

Conrad, P. (1992). Medicalization and social control. *Annual Reviews, 18*, 209–232.

Conrad, P. (2001). The meaning of mediations: Another look at compliance. In P. Conrad (Ed.), *The sociology of health and illness: Critical perspectives* (pp. 137–148). New York, NY: Worth.

Cruz-Flores, S., Rabinstein, A., Biller, J., Elkind, M. S., Griffith, P., Gorelick, P. B., Howard, G., Leira, E. C., Morgenstern, L.B., Ovbiagele, B., Peterson, E., Rosamond, W., Trimble, B., Valderrama, A. L.; American Heart Association Stroke Council; Council on Cardiovascular Nursing; Council on Epidemiology and Prevention; Council on Quality of Care and Outcomes Research. (2011). Racial-ethnic disparities in stroke care: The American experience a statement for healthcare professionals from the American heart association/American stroke association. *Stroke, 42*(7), 2091–2116.

Dall'Era, M. C., Snipes, K., Cisternas, M., Gordon, C., & Helmick, C. G. (2014). Preliminary population-based incidence and prevalence estimates of systemic lupus erythematosus: The California Lupus Surveillance Project. *Arthritis Research & Therapy, 16*(Suppl 1), A38.

Domino, F. J. (2011). *5-Minute clinical consult 2012*. Baltimore, MD: The Lippincott Williams & Wilkins.

Drwecki, B. B., Moore, C. F., Ward, S. E., & Prkachin, K. M. (2011). Reducing racial disparities in pain treatment: The role of empathy and perspective-taking. *Pain, 152*, 1001–1006.

Emejuaiwe, N., Jones, A. C., Ibrahim, S. A., & Kwoh, C. K. (2007). Disparities in joint replacement utilization: A quality of care issue. *Clinical and Experimental Rheumatology, 25*(Suppl 47), S44–S49.

Escalante, A. (2007). Health disparities in the rheumatic diseases. *Arthritis & Rheumatism, 57*(4), 547–552. doi:10.1002/art.22677.

Eudy, A. M., Vines, A. I., Dooley, M. A., Cooper, G. S., & Parks, C. G. (2014). Elevated C-reactive protein and self-reported disease activity in systemic lupus erythematosus. *Lupus, 23*(14), 1460–1467.

Farmer, P. (1992). *AIDS and accusation: Haiti and the geography of blame*. Los Angeles, CA: University of California Press.

Farmer, P. (2005). *Pathologies of power: Health human rights, and the new war on the poor*. Los Angeles, CA: University of California Press.

Giles, W., Kittner, S. J., Hebel, J. R., Losonczy, K. G., & Sherwin, R. W. (1995). Determinants of black-white differences in the risk of cerebral infarction. The National Health and Nutrition Examination Survey Epidemiologic Follow-Up Study. *Archives of Internal Medicine, 155*(12), 1319–1324.

Goffman, E. (1963). *Stigma: Notes on the management of spoiled identity*. Prentice Hall: Englewood Cliffs, NJ.

González, L. A., Toloza, S. M. A., McGwin, G., & Alarcón, G. S. (2013). Ethnicity in systemic lupus erythematosus (SLE): Its influence on susceptibility and outcomes. *Lupus, 22*(12), 1214 1224.

Goode, W. J. (1978). *The celebration of heroes: Prestige as a social control system*. Los Angeles: University of California Press.

Goodin, B. R., Pham, Q. T., Glover, T. L., Sotolongo, A., King, C. D., Sibille, K. T., & Fillingim, R. B. (2013). Perceived racial discrimination, but not mistrust of medical researchers, predicts the heat pain tolerance of African Americans with symptomatic knee osteoarthritis. *Health Psychology, 32*(11), 1117–1126. doi:10.1037/a0031592.

Granger, B. B., Ekman, I., Granger, C. B., Ostergren, J., Olofsson, B., Michelson, E., McMurray, J. J., Yusuf, S., Pfeffer, M. A., & Swedberg, K. (2009). Adherence to medication according to sex and age in the CHARM programme. *European Journal of Heart Failure, 11*(11), 1092–1098.

Green, A. R., Carney, D. R., Pallin, D. J., Ngo, L. H., Raymond, K. L., Iezzoni, L. I., Banaji, M. R. (2007). Implicit bias among physicians and its prediction of thrombolysis decisions for black and white patients. *Journal of General Internal Medicine, 22*, 1231–1238.

Heins, J., Heins, A., Grammas, M., Costello, M., Huang, K., & Mishra, S. (2006). Disparities in analgesia and opioid prescribing practices for patients with musculoskeletal pain in the emergency department. *Journal of Emergency Nursing, 32*(2), 219–224.

Kawachi, I. (2000). Income inequality and health. In I. Kawachi & L. Berkman (Eds.), *Social epidemiology* (pp. 76–94). New York, NY: Oxford University Press.

Kaseweter, K.A., Drwecki, B.B., Prkachin, K.M. (2012). Racial differences in pain treatment and empathy in a Canadian sample. Pain Research & Management, 17(6), 381-384.

Kim-Howard, X., Sun, C., Molineros, J. E., Maiti, A. K., Chandru, H., Adler, A., … & Musuruana, J. (2014). Allelic heterogeneity in NCF2 associated with systemic lupus erythematosus (SLE) susceptibility across four ethnic populations. *Human Molecular Genetics, 23*(6), 1656–1668.

Kleinman, A., Eisenberg, L., & Good, B. (1978). Culture illness and care: Clinical lessons from anthropologic and cross-cultural research. *Annals of Internal Medicine, 88*, 257–258.

Krieger, N. (1999). Embodying inequality: A review of concepts, measures, and methods for studying health consequences of discrimination. *International Journal of Health Services, 29*(2), 295–352.

Kwate, N. O. A., & Meyer, I. H. (2011). On sticks and stones and broken bones. *Du Bois Review, 8*(1), 191–198.

Kwate, N. O. A., Davis, N., Hatch, S., & Meyer, I. H. (2006). What do we mean by racism? Conceptual and measurement issues in discrimination and stigma among African Americans. In *The Robert Wood Johnson Health & Society Scholars-Stigma, Prejudice and Discrimination Conference 2006*, New York, NY.

Lea, J. P. (2002). Lupus nephritis in African Americans. *The American Journal of the Medical Sciences, 323*(2), 85–89.

Lillie-Blanton M., Brodie M., Rowland D., Altman D., & McIntosh M. (2000). Race, ethnicity, and the health care system: Public perceptions and experiences. *Medical Care Research and Review, 57* (Suppl 1), 218-234.

Link, B. G., & Phelan, J. (1995). Social conditions as fundamental causes of disease. *Journal of Health and Social Behavior*. Spec No.: 80–94.

Link, B. G., & Phelan, J. (2000). Evaluating the fundamental cause explanation for social disparities in health. In C. E. Bird, P. Conrad, & A. Fremont (Eds.), *Handbook of medical sociology*. Princeton, NJ: Prentice-Hall.

Link, B. G., & Phelan, J. C. (2001). Conceptualizing stigma. *Annual Review of Sociology, 27*, 363–385.

Marmot, M. (2004). *The Status Syndrome: How Social Standing Affects Our Health and Longevity.* New York: Henry Holt and Company.

McBurney, C. A., & Vina, E. R. (2012). Racial and ethnic disparities in rheumatoid arthritis. *Current Rheumatology Reports, 14*, 463–471. doi:10.1007/s11926-012-0276-0.

McIlvane, J. (2009). Arthritis and health inequalities in Blacks and Latinos. *Annual Review of Gerontology & Geriatrics, 29*, 181–202. doi:10.1891/0198-8794.29.181. R13.

McKinlay, J. B. (1996). Some contributions from the social system to gender inequalities in heart disease. *Journal of Health and Social Behavior, 37*(1), 1–26.

McKinlay, J., Potter, D., & Feldman, H. (1996). Non-medical influences on medical decision-making. *Social Science & Medicine, 42*(5), 769–776.

Molokhia, M., Hoggart, C., Patrick, A. L., Shriver, M., Parra, E., Ye, J., Silman, A. J., & McKeigue, P. M. (2003). Relation of risk of systemic lupus erythematosus to west african admixture in a caribbean population. *Human Genetics, 112*, 310–318.

Nass, T. (2001). Lupus: A patient care guide for nurses and other health professionals. In D.o.H.a.H.S. (DHHS) (Ed.). Bethesda, MD: National Institutes of Health.

National Library of Medicine. (2015). *Health literacy*. Bethesda, MD: National Institutes of Health, US Department of Health and Human Services. Retrieved January 22, 2015, from http://nnlm.gov/outreach/consumer/hlthlit.html

National Research Council. (2004). Eliminating health disparities: Measurement and data needs. In M. V. Ploeg & E. Perrin (Eds.), *Panel on DHHS collection of race and ethnicity data*. Washington, DC: The National Academies Press.

Pappas, G. (1990). Some implications for the study of the doctor-patient interaction: power, structure, and agency in the works of Howard Waitzkin and Arthur Kleinman. *Social Science and Medicine, 30*(2), 199–204.

Parsons, T. (1951). *The social system*. Glencoe, IL: Free Press.

Quinlan, P., Price, K. O., Magid, S. K., Lyman, S., Mandl, L. A., & Stone, P. W. (2013). The relationship among health literacy, health knowledge, and adherence to treatment in patients with rheumatoid arthritis. *Hospital for Special Surgery, 9*, 42–49. doi:10.1007/s11420-012-9308-6.

Raman, K., & Mohan, C. (2003). Genetic underpinnings of autoimmunity—Lessons from studies in arthritis, diabetes, lupus and multiple sclerosis. *Current Opinion in Immunology, 15*, 651–659.

Richards, J. S. (2003). The global impact of systemic lupus erythematosus. *Ethnicity & Disease, 13*, 175–176.

Rivera, T. L., Belmont, H. M., Malani, S., Latorre, M., Benton, L., Weisstuch, J., Barisoni, L., Tseng, C. E., Izmirly, P. M., Buyon, J. P., & Askanase, A. D. (2009). Current therapies for lupus nephritis in an ethnically heterogeneous cohort. *The Journal of Rheumatology, 36*(2), 298–305.

Rubio, M., & Williams, D. R. (2004). The social dimension of race. In B. M. B. A. Maurine and Goodman (Eds.), Race and research (pp. 1–26). Washington, DC: American Public Health Association.

Ryscavage, P. (1999). *Income inequality in America.* Armonk: Sharpe.

Sabin, J. A., & Greenwald, A. G. (2012). The influence of implicit bias on treatment recommendations for 4 common pediatric conditions: Pain, urinary tract infection, attention deficit hyperactivity disorder, and asthma. *American Journal of Public Health, 102*, 988–995. doi:10.2105/AJPH.2011.300621.

Sabin, J., Rivara, F. P., & Greenwald, A. G. (2008). Physician implicit attitudes and stereotypes about race and quality of medical care. *Medical Care, 46*(7), 678–685.

Sabin, J. A., Nosek, B. A., Greenwald, A., & Rivara, F. P. (2009). Physicians' implicit and explicit attitudes about race by MD race, ethnicity and gender. *Journal of Healthcare for the Poor and Underserved, 20*, 896–913.

Saha, S., Komaromy, M., Koepsell, T. D., & Bindman, A. B. (1999). Patient–physician racial concordance and the perceived quality and use of health care. *Archives of Internal Medicine, 159*, 997–1004.

Schmajuk, G., Trivedi, A. N., Solomon, D. H., Yelin, E., Trupin, L., Chakravarty, E. F., & Yazdany, J. (2011). Receipt of disease-modifying antirheumatic drugs among patients with rheumatoid arthritis in medicare managed care plans. *JAMA, 305*, 480–486.

Schulman, K. A., Berlin, J. A., Harless, W., Kerner, J. F., Sistrunk, S., Gersh, B. J., Dube, R., Taleghani, C. K., Burke, J. E., Williams, S., Eisenberg, J. E., Ayers, W., & Escarce, J. J. (1999). The effect of race and sex on physicians' recommendations for cardiac catheterization. *New England Journal of Medicine, 340*(8), 618–626.

Sen, A. (1992). *Inequality reexamined.* New York, NY: Russel Sage Foundation.

Sleath, B., Callahan, L. F., Devellis, R. F., & Beard, A. (2008). Arthritis patients' perceptions of rheumatologists' participatory decision making style and communication about complementary and alternative medicine. *Arthritis & Rheumatism, 59*, 416–421. doi:10.1002/art.23307.

Smedley, B. D., Stith, A., & Nelson, A., (Eds.), & The Committee on Understanding and Eliminating Racial and Ethnic Disparities in Health Care. (2002). *Unequal treatment: Confronting racial and ethnic disparities in health care*. Washington, DC: National Academy Press.

Society for Women's Health Research and the National Women's Health Resource Center, Inc. (2002). *Autoimmune diseases in women.*

Staton, L. J., Panda, M., Chen, I., Genao, I., Kurz, J., Pasanen, M., & Cykert, S. (2007). When race matters: Disagreement in pain perception between patients and their physicians in primary care. *Journal of the National Medical Association, 99*, 532–538.

Steele, C. M., & Aronson, J. (1995). Stereotype threat and the intellectual test performance of African Americans. *Journal of Personality and Social Psychology, 69*, 797–811.

Suarez-Almazor, M. E., Julianne, S., Adam Kelly, P., O'Malley, K., Byrne, M., Richardson, M., & Pak, C. (2005). Ethnic variation in knee replacement: Patient preferences or uninformed disparity? *Archives of Internal Medicine, 165*(10), 1117–1124.

Swidler, A. (1986). Culture in action: Symbols and strategies. *American Sociological Review, 51*(2), 273–286.

Tate, R. C., & Chibnall, J. T. (2014). Racial/ethnic disparities in the assessment and treatment of pain. *American Psychologist, 69*(2), 131–141.

Taussig, M. T. (1980). Reification and the consciousness of the patient. *Social Science and Medicine, 14B*, 3–13.

Todd, A. D. (1989). *Delusions in discourse, in intimate adversaries: Cultural conflict between doctors and women patients.* Philadelphia: University of Pennsylvania Press.

Tsao, B. (2003). The genetics of human systemic lupus erythematosus. *Trends in Immunology, 24*(11), 595–599.

U.S. Department of Health and Human Services (2010). *Healthy people 2010: Understanding and improving health.* Washington, DC: U.S. Government Printing Office.

Walsh, S. J., Algert, C., & Rothfield, N. F. (1996). Racial aspects of comorbidity in systemic lupus erythematosus. *Arthritis Care and Research, 96*, 509–516.

Ward, M. M., Sundaramurthy, S., Lotstein, D., Bush, T. M., Neuwelt, C. M., & Street, R. L. (2003). Participatory patient-physician communication and morbidity in patients with systemic lupus erythematosus. *Arthritis & Rheumatism, 49*(6), 810–818.

Washington, H. A. (2006). *Medical apartheid: The dark side of medical experimentation on Black Americans from colonial times to the present.* New York, NY: Doubleday.

Williams, D. R., & Jackson, P. B. (2005). Social sources of racial disparities in health. *Health Affairs, 24*(2), 325–331.

Williams, E. M., Watkins, R., Anderson, J., & Tumiel-Berhalter, L. (2011). A geographic information assessment of exposure to a toxic waste site and development of systemic lupus erythematosus (SLE): Findings from the buffalo lupus project. *Journal of Toxicology and Environmental Health Sciences, 3*(3), 52.

Xu, X., Zuo, X., Wang, X., & Han, S. (2009). Do you feel my pain? Racial group membership modulates empathic neural responses. *Journal of Neuroscience, 29*, 8525–8529.

Yazdany, J., Panopalis, P., Gillis, J.Z., Schmajuk, G., MacLean, C. H., Wofsy, D., Yelin, E., & Systemic Lupus Erythematosus Quality Indicators Project Expert Panels. (2009). A quality indicator set for systemic lupus erythematosus. *Arthritis & Rheumatism, 61*(3), 370–377.

Zola, I. (1972). Medicine as an institution of social control. *Sociological Review, 20*, 487–504.

Part II

Management

Evaluation of Psychological Distress in the Rheumatology Clinic

12

Desiree R. Azizoddin, Cinnamon Westbrook, Angelyna M. Lowe, and Perry M. Nicassio

Introduction

For patients with chronic illness, seeking and receiving satisfactory healthcare can be extremely frustrating. This is particularly true for patients with rheumatic conditions due to the waxing and waning of symptoms and their debilitating effects on functional adaptation. Additionally, some of the primary symptoms that occur in these conditions such as chronic fatigue, numbness, and pain can be hard to quantify and manage. In many instances, patients may experience difficulty in adequately describing their symptoms, contributing to barriers in communication that may lead to misunderstandings regarding the meaning of their symptoms and underlying psychological issues. A further complication in treating patients with arthritis is that they present with high rates of psychiatric comorbidity (see Chaps. 3, 4), particularly depression and anxiety. The primary focus of this chapter is to address the evaluation of depression and anxiety in the rheumatology setting.

In 2010, adults visited their physician's office an average of 3.9 times (United States Census Bureau, 2013). Moreover, 7 out of 10 visits to a primary care physician are for treatment of chronic illnesses (Chapman, Perry, & Strine, 2005). The average number of visits to a general practitioner increases for patients who present with psychological symptoms. Primary care patients with even mild depression have been noted to use healthcare services up to two to three times more than their non-depressed counterparts (Strosahl, 2001). The treatment of psychological distress in patients receiving medical care is critical for maintaining patients' psychological and physical well-being. Importantly, depression, psychological stress, and deficient coping skills have been shown to increase the risk for early morbidity, mortality, and relapse among patients with chronic illness (Fawzy et al., 1993; Frasure-Smith, 1991).

D.R. Azizoddin, MA (✉) • C. Westbrook, MA
A.M. Lowe, MA
Department of Psychology, Loma Linda University, Loma Linda, CA, USA
e-mail: Dazizoddin@LLU.edu; Dazizodd@gmail.com

P.M. Nicassio, PhD
Department of Psychiatry, School of Medicine, University of California, Los Angeles, CA, USA

Prevalence of Depression and Anxiety in Arthritis

Depression and anxiety are highly prevalent in arthritis populations. Estimates of depression range from 20 to 54 % in patients with systemic lupus erythematosus (SLE), 10 to 46 % in patients with rheumatoid arthritis (RA), and 10 to 46 % in

P.M. Nicassio (ed.), *Psychosocial Factors in Arthritis*, DOI 10.1007/978-3-319-22858-7_12

patients with osteoarthritis (OA) (Blixen & Kippes, 1999; Isik, Koca, Ozturk, & Mermi, 2007; Keefe et al., 2002; Söderlin, Hakala, & Nieminen, 2000; Somers, Kurakula, Criscione-Schreiber, Keefe, & Clowse, 2012; Tayer, Nicassio, Radojevic, & Krall, 1996). Additionally, RA patients are twice as likely to experience depression compared to the general population (Kojima et al., 2009).

Anxiety has been reported in approximately 20–30 % of individuals with arthritis (Ødegård, Finset, Mowinckel, Kvien, & Uhlig, 2007; Söderlin et al., 2000; VanDyke et al., 2004). A longitudinal study assessing the 10-year progression of disease activity, depression, anxiety, and pain in a sample of patients with RA indicated that depression and elevated pain were associated with increased anxiety over time (Ødegård et al., 2007). Over 30 % of participants had clinically significant levels of pain, depression, and even greater levels of anxiety (Ødegård et al., 2007). In a sample of 80 patients with RA, 70.8 % reported symptoms of anxiety and depression; 41.5 % met criteria for a diagnosis of depression, and 13.4 % met criteria for a diagnosis of anxiety (Isik et al., 2007). The prevalence of depression is elevated for individuals with arthritis and deserves appropriate assessment and intervention for successful patient-centered care.

In arthritis and several other chronic disease patient populations, depression and anxiety have been found to contribute to a variety of negative health outcomes. Both disorders demonstrate a positive, linear relationship with C-reactive protein levels, indicative of increased inflammation and with higher perceived pain (Kojima et al., 2009). Individuals with RA experiencing current depressive symptoms are more likely to experience increased pain, and those with a previous history of major depression are at even higher risk for having pain (Fifield, Tennen, Reisine, & McQuillan, 1998; (Keefe, Abernethy, & Campbell, 2005). Daily diary-based assessments of pain, coping, and mood in a sample of women and men with arthritis indicated that patients with RA reported 42 % more pain than patients with OA, related to mood and coping changes (Affleck et al., 1999). Furthermore, mood disturbance in arthritis has been linked to increased fatigue, increased disability, and lower quality of life (Nery et al., 2007; Nyklíček, Hoogwegt, & Westgeest, 2015; Somers et al., 2009; Stebbings, Herbison, Doyle, Treharne, & Highton, 2010).

Depression in rheumatic disease is associated with poor medical adherence, more emergency room visits, and higher medical costs (DiMatteo, Lepper, & Croghan, 2000; Egede, Zheng, & Simpson, 2002; Julian et al., 2009; Mcnamara, 2007; Partridge et al., 2008; Vermeire, Hearnshaw, Van Royen, & Denekens, 2001). RA specifically has been noted as the second most costly illness among all other chronic medical conditions (Ozminkowski, Burton, Goetzel, Maclean, & Wang, 2006). A review by Bruce (2008) indicated that depression is related to increased healthcare costs as a consequence of increased physician and hospital visits, medication expenses, missed work, and overall employer costs.

Depression and anxiety in patients with chronic illness can lead to increased engagement in negative health behaviors and ineffective coping mechanisms (Bruce, 2008; Choi, 2013; Park & Gaffey, 2007; Lin et al., 2004). A longitudinal study assessing a sample of patients with RA, conducted by Ang et al., concluded that comorbid depression resulted in twice the likelihood of early mortality (Ang, Choi, Kroenke, & Wolfe, 2005). This relationship could be potentially explained by lack of treatment adherence, engagement in negative coping mechanisms, increased disability, and increased disease activity. Together, these findings emphasize the importance of screening and treating depression and psychological distress in patients with arthritis. The absence of screening and treatment protocols represents a major limitation in rheumatology care (Nicassio, 2008).

Challenges Involved in Evaluating Psychological Distress in Medical Patients

The burden of evaluating and treating mental health symptoms in medical patients is often assumed by primary care physicians. Many patients with mental health concerns receive at least part of their treatment through their general practitioner (Wittchen, Muhlig, & Beesdo, 2003). The reduced stigma associated with visiting a primary care physician, lack of understanding regarding psychiatric disorders, or other barriers patients face regarding seeking mental health treatment may all be contributing factors. Accordingly, the prospect of patients getting specialized treatment from a mental health practitioner may be quite low.

The time constraints faced by physicians in rendering clinical care may inhibit opportunities for addressing psychological distress. Furthermore, the organized interview structure most healthcare systems have adopted during patient encounters increases the difficulty in developing and maintaining patient rapport. In order to establish a more organized and streamlined patient visit, medical professionals are being trained to follow preset algorithms and structured practice guidelines (Groopman, 2008). This linear framework includes initiating the session, gathering information, a physical examination, ordering tests, analyzing results, formulating a hypothesis following data collection, providing an explanation, and planning and closing the session (Epstein et al., 2009; Groopman, 2008). However, while this strategy is efficient for healthcare practitioners who must treat their patients under time pressures, this streamlined process may interfere with the capacity to evaluate patients' emotional functioning. With physician–patient interactions averaging approximately 18 min, there is little opportunity for meaningful communication surrounding patients' psychological status (Mauksch, Dugdale, Dodson, & Epstein, 2008). During the clinical interview, patients may leave clues about their current emotional state, but rarely have an opportunity to provide a thorough narrative about their emotional experiences. Furthermore, when medical personnel hear the feelings expressed by patients, there may be little recognition or validation of those feelings (Platt & Hardee, 2013). In oncology settings, for example, several studies have found that the psychological care of patients is insufficiently addressed or ignored (Mitchell, Hussain, Grainger, & Symonds, 2011; Okuyama et al., 2011; Rodriguez et al., 2010; Söllner et al. 2001).

Listening intently and acknowledging and summarizing a patient's experience are invaluable. Effective doctor–patient interactions contribute to greater satisfaction with medical care, the ability to share pertinent information for an accurate diagnosis, follow advice, and adhere to the prescribed treatment (Ha, Anat, & Longnecker, 2010; Osterberg & Blaschke, 2005). Moreover, research has shown that effective doctor–patient relationships may contribute to greater perceived control, the ability to tolerate pain, recover from illness, decreased tumor growth, improved daily functioning, and enhanced psychological adjustment (Eccleston, 2001; Gatchel, Peng, Peters, Fuchs, & Turk, 2007; Ha et al., 2010; Holzemer et al., 1999).

One of the most important steps in comprehensive medical treatment for individuals with rheumatic disease involves the ability to address the level of psychological distress frequently experienced by this population. How can successful doctor–patient communication be promoted with the goal of treating the whole patient effectively within the time-limited clinical interactions that occur in the rheumatology setting? The initial approach to whole-person care begins with efficient and time-sensitive screening tools that accurately identify depression and anxiety in this population (Murphy, Sacks, Brady, Hootman, & Chapman, 2012; Nicassio, 2010; Shih, Hootman, Strine, Chapman, & Brady, 2006; Stang et al., 2006).

Evaluating Psychological Distress in Arthritis

Assessing levels of depression, anxiety, and distress may provide important information relevant to determining patients' overall quality of life and disease trajectory (Quinten et al., 2011). Having an interdisciplinary team address the multifactorial nature of distress symptoms may improve health outcomes and cost-effectiveness (Walker et al., 2014; Whitmer, Pruemer, Nahleh, & Jazieh, 2006). Addressing psychological symptoms early and providing effective treatment may lead to better quality of life and medical management (Holland et al., 2013; Julian et al., 2009). Through the early detection of emotional distress, open communication regarding a patient's psychological needs arises that allows for the implementation of psychosocial interventions by mental health specialists or, in some instances, by the medical team (Bidstrup, Johansen, & Mitchell, 2011; Davidson et al., 2006; Holland et al., 2013; Lichtman et al., 2008; Meijer et al., 2013; US Preventive Services Task Force, 2009). Screening measures that can detect elevated levels of anxiety and depression are most beneficial when combined with compatible intervention resources for managing patients presenting with distress (Bidstrup et al., 2011; Carlson, Groff, Maciejewski, & Bultz, 2010; Lichtman et al., 2008). Clinic barriers for adopting screening practices include lack of resources, difficulties implementing change to the traditional medical model, provider challenges, communication problems, and patient factors (Holland, 2004; Dolbeault, Boistard, Meuric, Copel, & Brédart, 2011; Jacobsen et al., 2005; Whitmer, Pruemer, Wilhelm, McCaig, & Hester, 2006).

Procedural factors must be considered in order to be effective in screening psychological distress in patients with arthritis. Screening can theoretically lead to the inclusion of patients who experience distress that would otherwise be missed and only detected when severity of symptoms increases (Mitchell et al., 2011). Alternatively, application of screening tools that lack sensitivity can lead to the inclusion of patients who experience "short-lived" and expected levels of psychological distress that do not require treatment (Bidstrup et al., 2011). With the inclusion of patients experiencing subclinical levels of distress, referral resources can be misused. All patients screened for presenting distress do not need further psychosocial services (Meijer et al., 2013). Screening tools, however, should not be relied on exclusively. It is essential that during the doctor–patient interaction, doctors attend to the "whole" person, noticing the patients' presentation and being sensitive to the underlying clues patients provide when they do not explicitly share feelings.

Depression and anxiety have distinct symptoms that may be apparent through observation of patients' clinical presentation. Knowing what symptoms to detect can be helpful in guiding physicians' evaluations. More than half of outpatient medical visits are for somatic complaints, many of which are associated with underlying depression or anxiety (Culpepper, Clayton, Lieberman, & Susman, 2008; Kroenke, Spitzer, Williams, Monahan, & Lowe, 2007). Unfortunately, physicians and patients sometimes engage in an unspoken understanding that physical symptoms are the only legitimate reason for help-seeking and treatment (Eisenberg, 1992). While many patients with depression or anxiety may feel more comfortable focusing on the occurrence of somatic symptoms, patients will more than likely answer questions about the presence of symptoms related to depression or anxiety when they are queried.

The *Diagnostic and Statistical Manual of Mental Disorders,* Fifth edition (DSM-5) lists the symptoms related to depression as including low, sad, or depressed mood for most of the day, nearly every day, loss of interest or pleasure in activities that were once enjoyable (anhedonia), significant changes in appetite and/or weight that were unintentional, sleep disturbances, psychomotor agitation or retardation, fatigue or loss of energy, feelings of hopelessness, worthlessness or inappropriate guilt, and cognitive changes such as difficulty thinking or concentrating, and recurrent thoughts of death or suicide. In order to be diagnosed with depression, the patient must experience at least five or more of the symptoms for at least a 2-week period. These symptoms also must reflect a change from the patient's baseline mood (American Psychiatric Association, 2013). Generally, symptoms for anxiety include excessive anxiety or worry (apprehensive expectation), difficulty controlling the worry, restlessness or feeling keyed up or on edge, being easily fatigued, difficulty concentrating or the mind going blank, irritability, muscle tension (headache, intestinal discomfort, and aching of extremities), sleep disturbance, and the patient's level of anxiety causes significant distress in areas of daily functioning including relational, occupational, and social domains (DSM-5).

While many of the symptoms of depression or anxiety will likely be shared by patients during intake questions, observing the behavior of the patient during the interview is also important. The more noticeable symptoms of unstated depression that may arise during an interaction with patients include tearfulness, appearing fatigued, a softer tone of voice (hypophonia), diminished prosody, shortened responses to questions, reduced facial expressions, reduced smiling, response themes of hopelessness and loss of control, diminished eye contact, and psychomotor retardation which may be reflected in the patient moving slower, demonstrating a slower reaction time or taking longer to respond to a question due to difficulties thinking or reduced speech (Sobin & Sackeim, 1997). For some patients, psychomotor agitation may be evident, manifested as general restlessness, including rapid arm and leg movements and rapid and scattered speech. Patients with more serious depression may demonstrate inadequate self-care, which may be noticeable during the encounter in the form of a disheveled appearance (i.e. unclean nails, wrinkled clothes, unkempt hair, body odor, etc.).

Anxiety may include symptoms that overlap with symptoms of depression as the disorders often co-occur. Symptoms specific to anxiety that may be noticeable during the interaction include excessive worry, avoidance, sympathetic arousal such as sweating, trembling or shaking, chest palpitations or pain, shortness of breath, and gastrointestional distress (Culpepper et al., 2008).

Screening tools are increasingly helpful in assessing patients' current level of functioning during the clinical interview, but when many practitioners report finding screening questionnaires for mood disorders cumbersome and time-consuming (Arroll, Khin, & Kerse, 2003), taking the time to listen to patients as well as noticing any nonverbal clues that patients provide will provide important information about their current emotional state. There are actions that a clinician can take that will ease both the patient and the physician during the encounter, which take little to no additional time. For example, paying attention, listening well, and then providing patients with evidence and a brief verbal summary of what they reported demonstrate that they were heard (Platt & Hardee, 2013).

Doctors with better communication and interpersonal skills are able to detect problems sooner, prevent medical crises and expensive, unnecessary interventions, and provide better support to their patients (Ha et al., 2010). This may lead to higher quality outcomes and better satisfaction, lower costs of care, greater patient understanding of health issues, and better adherence to the treatment process as a whole. Appreciating the comorbidity of anxiety and depression found in arthritis patients and knowing what to look for through effective clinical and interpersonal skills used in tandem with efficient screening tools will allow the medical practitioner to be able to address the whole person and develop knowledgeable and successful treatment plans.

A meta-analysis by Luoma, Martin, and Pearson (2002) assessing contact with healthcare professionals and individuals before death by suicide concluded that 58 % (range 42–70 %) of patients who committed suicide had seen a primary care physician in the previous month and 77 % (58–90 %) had seen a primary care physician in the last year. Using screening measures sensitive to mood symptoms and correlates of suicide can provide valuable information and tailor interventions to prevent suicide and manage risk. Changes in mood are expected in populations with autoimmune disorders, at diagnosis and throughout the disease experience, and consistent screening and follow-up are essential to ensure that patients' needs are being met. Importantly, early screening and intervention can prevent worsening of mood symptoms. Even for patients who are not currently suicidal or experiencing severe mood symptoms, using a screening tool for psychological health can help identify patients for proactive intervention before symptoms develop further. Screening tools also may promote a discussion regarding mental health-related problems, which may be overlooked by both patients and providers due to stigma. Screening tools can facilitate a conversation of mental health-related concerns, normalizing the experience of patients with autoimmune diseases and leading to the provision of direct and effective referrals for psychological and/or behavioral interventions (see Chap 16).

The following section reviews the most commonly used and validated measures for assessing depression and anxiety in medical settings that are applicable to patients with arthritis.

Assessing Depression

Patient Health Questionnaire-9

Developed for use in primary care settings for patients of all ages and medical diagnoses with a third-grade reading level, the PHQ-9 is a self-report measure with widespread use in acute and chronic conditions. A significant advantage of the PHQ-9 is that its items align with diagnostic criteria for depression (Kroenke, Spitzer, & Williams, 2001). It comes in two versions, the PHQ-9 and the PHQ-2, which includes the first two items (depressed mood and anhedonia). It has been found to be reliable with $\alpha = 0.89$ and a sensitivity of 84 % and specificity of 72 % (Mulrow et al., 1995). It has been translated and widely used in languages including, but not limited to, Spanish, French, Arabic, German, Czech, Dutch, Russian, German, Hindi, Italian, Japanese, Portuguese, and Polish and takes about 5 min to complete.

Strengths. The PHQ-9 is short, easy to administer and interpret, and is psychometrically strong. It directly corresponds with the diagnostic criteria for depression from the DSM-V, and therefore can be used to establish an interim diagnosis. It has been found to be reliable and valid across various cultures (Martin, Rief, Klaiberg, & Braehler, 2006; Monahan et al., 2009; Wulsin, Somoza, & Heck, 2002). The scale is sensitive to change, with a change of five points as an indicator of significant change in depression. It is free and publically available at http://www.phqscreeners.com/. This measure is a great tool for clinical and research purposes.

Weaknesses. If the PHQ-2 is administered and a score of 3 or greater is obtained, it should not be interpreted alone. Rather the entire PHQ-9 should be administered.

Center for Epidemiologic Studies-Depression

The CES-D scale is a 20-item self-report measure designed to assess depression severity over the past week in the general population with at least a third-grade reading level and has also been used in clinical populations (Radloff 1997). Previous research has demonstrated high reliability and internal consistency of $\alpha = 0.87$, as well as high specificity 88 %, and sensitivity 100 % (Beekman et al., 1997). It assesses four factors of functioning, including depressed affect, positive affect, somatic problems, and psychomotor retardation and takes about 10 min to complete. The measure has been translated into Arabic, Chinese, Dutch, French, German, Greek, Korean, Italian, Japanese, Portuguese, Russian, Spanish, Turkish, and Vietnamese.

Strengths. The CES-D is brief and easy to administer and score, with a recommended cutoff score of 19 as indication of clinically relevant depression, specifically in patient populations with chronic pain (Martens et al., 2003; Turk & Okifuji, 1994). It comes in multiple versions, including a 9-item version designed for screening in arthritis patients (Martens et al., 2006). This measure is also publically available and free to use at www.chcr.brown.edu/pcoc/cesdscale.pdf.

Weaknesses. The CES-D has a high false positive rate when using the cutoff score of 16 as recommended, and with 20 items, missing data are common. Use of shortened versions can help mitigate these difficulties, but these versions may over-classify those with multiple health conditions as depressed (Smarr & Neefer, 2011). While responses on the CES-D have not been shown to differ significantly between cultural or ethnic groups (Roberts, 1980), it is important to note that the positive affect and interpersonal dimensions of the scale have been received differently, particularly in some Asian cultures (Mui, Burnette, & Chen, 2002). It was also found that what Westerners might cite as psychological complaints, non-Westerners may attribute to somatic complaints (Mui et al., 2002). This scale is not sensitive to change in scores over time and does not assess appetite, anhedonia, psychomotor agitation or retardation, guilt, or suicidality, which are all diagnostic criteria for depression. Because it does not address all diagnostic criteria, it is not optimal for making a diagnosis or for research purposes. Lastly, due to its high correlation with measures for anxiety, it may not be specific for depression and may measure general distress instead.

Beck Depression Inventory-II

The BDI, originally published in 1961, is a self-report scale created to assess depression over the past 2 weeks in patients aged 13 years and older with a fifth-grade reading level and has undergone various revisions. The revisions were made to improve wording and to assess symptoms that corresponded with the DSM for a depressive disorder, including cognitive, vegetative, somatic, and affective symptoms (Beck, Rush, Shaw, & Emery, 1979). It has been validated for adult clinical, psychiatric, and general populations. Research indicates a high reliability and internal consistency of $\alpha = 0.92$ for outpatient populations (Smarr & Neefer, 2011). It was also found to have a sensitivity of 82 % and specificity of 82 % in a study of primary care patients (Beck, Guth, Steer, & Ball, 1997). This measure is also available in a wide range of translations, Arabic, Chinese, Dutch, Finnish, French, German, Icelandic, Italian, Japanese, Persian, Spanish, Swedish, Turkish, and Xhosa. This measure can be used both clinically and for research purposes.

Strengths. The BDI-II is easy to administer and score with minimal training required and has high predictive validity (Smarr & Neefer, 2011). It can be self-administered or given orally, with a completion time of 5–15 min. Scores are determined by summing severity ratings and using the recommended cutoff scores (0–13: minimal; 14–19: mild; 20–28: moderate; 29–63: severe) to indicate severity of depression. It has been validated across many cultures (Ghassemzadeh, Mojtabai, Karamghadiri, & Ebrahimkhani, 2005; Kojima et al., 2002). The BDI-II has been found to be sensitive to changes in depression (5-point change: minimal difference; 10–19: moderate; ≥20: large) in cross-cultural studies (Viljoen, Iverson, Griffiths, & Woodward, 2003).

Weaknesses. The BDI-II is longer than other measures, consisting of 21 items. There have been concerns about overlapping symptoms with medical conditions and depression, thus confounding diagnostic formulations. Assessments of depression in elderly populations should include somatic complaints, but this practice may not apply for all populations (Norris, Arnau, Bramson, & Meagher, 2003). Caution should be used in interpreting scores to determine the etiology of somatic complaints. While the BDI FastScreen for Medical Patients was developed to be a shorter measure for use in primary care, it requires the same amount of time to complete. The measure omits items related to somatic complaints (Beck, Steer, & Brown, 2000). This measure is not available to the public and needs to be purchased from Pearson Assessments.

Geriatric Depression Scale

The GDS is a 30-item self-report measure developed to assess depression symptoms in older adults and has been used to differentiate between depression and dementia. It is also available in a short form, consisting of only 15 items. Both formats have been used widely in most medical populations and diverse populations. The measure assesses both affective and cognitive symptoms of depression. The GDS is psychometrically sound with a reliability of $\alpha = 0.94$ (Yesavage et al., 1983). The original form has a sensitivity of 77.4 % and specificity of 65.4 %, while the short form has a sensitivity of 81.3 % and specificity of 78.4 % (Mitchell, Bird, Rizzo, & Meader, 2010). Versions are also available in Arabic, Chinese, Creole, Danish, Dutch, Farsi, French, French Canadian, German, Greek, Hebrew, Hindi, Hungarian, Icelandic, Italian, Japanese, Korean, Lithuanian, Malay, Maltese, Norwegian, Portuguese, Romanian, Russian, Serbian, Spanish, Swedish, Thai, Turkish, Vietnamese, and Yiddish.

Strengths. The GDS is well-studied in elderly populations, is easy to administer, and has strong psychometric properties. It is sensitive to change in depression with a notable change of 6–11 points in arthritis patients (Radloff & Teri, 1986). The scale's strong psychometric properties make it a great option for research purposes. This scale offers a separate short form that consists of only 15 items to reduce test-taking fatigue when necessary. It is free to use and is available at www.Stanford.edu/~yesavage/GDS.html.

Weaknesses. The validity of the GDS has been a cause for concern if used with patients under 65 or over 85. It may also measure general distress rather than depression, as some of the items reflect anxiety symptoms. The GDS has been shown to be reliable for assessing depression in those with mild neurocognitive disorders, but should be used cautiously with those with moderate to severe cognitive disorders (Stiles & McGarrahan, 1998). This measure also should be used with caution when assessing patients from non-Western cultures as it has been noted that depression is viewed differently in elderly populations from varying cultures. The GDS may not account for these differences and, therefore, may not be as sensitive of a measure as it is in Western cultures (Chang, 1996; Jang, Small, & Haley, 2001). It does not assess somatic complaints common in elderly populations, so it would be necessary to evaluate the effects of depressed mood on their physical functioning, which could be essential in measuring depression in patients with arthritis.

Hospital Anxiety and Depression Scale-Depression

The HADS is a 14-item self-report scale used to assess anxiety and depression in patients in the general medical population between the ages of 16 and 65 years old. The subscales are often used separately. Seven of the items measure cognitive and affective symptoms of depression (HADS-D); somatic items are not included. The depression subscale has been found to be internally reliable with α ranging from 0.82 to 0.90 (Bjelland, Dahl, Haut, & Neckelmann, 2002). It was also found that sensitivity ranged from 56 to 100 % and specificity ranged from 73 to 94 %. The scale has been translated into many languages, including, but not limited to: Arabic, Chinese, Danish, Dutch, Finnish, French, German, Hebrew, Hungarian, Italian, Japanese, Korean, Norwegian, Portuguese, Spanish, Swedish, Thai, and Urdu.

Strengths. The HADS-D has been widely used in various medical populations, is time-efficient, requires no training, and is easy to administer and score with recommended cutoff scores for severity. It is easily divided to assess depression and anxiety separately.

Weaknesses. Research has demonstrated that the HADS contains items that are not culturally sensitive, i.e. "Sit at ease and feel relaxed". Items such as these are anxiety-related, but in various cultures, may load onto the depression scale (Leung, Wing, Kwong, Lo, & Shum, 1999). Clinical judgment should be used when administering this measure to culturally diverse patients. The HADS-D is only to be used as a screening tool for emotional distress and does not demonstrate good predictive validity when making a diagnosis (Goldberg, 1985). This scale is available for purchase at http://www.glassessment.co.uk/health_and_psychology/resources/hospital_anxiety_scale/hospital_anxiety_scale.asp?css=1.

Assessing Anxiety

Beck Anxiety Inventory

The BAI is a 21-item self-report measure aimed at assessing anxiety, with a focus on somatic complaints (i.e., shaking, dizziness, feeling hot, etc.) rather than cognitive complaints of anxiety (i.e., excessive worry, rumination, etc.). It is reliable, with $\alpha = 0.94$ (Fydrich, Dowdall, & Chambless, 1993). The BAI has varying specificity and sensitivity depending on the cutoff score used. Using a recommended cutoff score of 10 for mild anxiety, the BAI has specificity of 45 % and sensitivity of 94 % (Kabacoff, Segal, Hersen, & Van Hasselt, 1997). It has been translated into many languages, including but not limited to: Spanish, French, German, African languages, and Norwegian.

Strengths. The BAI includes somatic symptoms of anxiety, is brief, easy to administer and score, sensitive to change, and can also be administered via a computer program. It has also been shown to have good reliability across other cultures (Ulusoy, Sahin, & Erkmen, 1998; Wetherell & Arean, 1997).

Weaknesses. The BAI has not been validated in arthritis. Because it does focus on somatic complaints, there may be overlap of symptoms reported by chronically ill patients. This measure does not assess for cognitive symptoms of anxiety, which can be essential for understanding patient needs and concerns, and therefore may need to be supplemented by other measures. It is not publically available and can be purchased at www.pearsonassessments.com.

General Anxiety Disorder-7

The GAD-7 is a self-report measure designed for, and validated with, medical patients in primary care settings. Although it focuses primarily on symptoms of Generalized Anxiety Disorder, it possesses sufficient sensitivity, 82 % and specificity 89 %, to assess general anxiety and has been validated in a diverse range of medical settings in patients ranging in age from 15 to 95 (Spitzer, Kroenke, Williams, & Lowe, 2006). It has been translated and validated in various other languages, including German, Turkish, Spanish, French, Filipino, Chinese, Greek, Hindi, and many others.

Strengths. The GAD-7 is time-efficient, easy to administer and score, and useful for assessing anxiety severity over time. It assesses for core criteria necessary for diagnoses, but should only be used as screener, indicating the need for further clinical evaluation (Spitzer et al., 2006). The GAD-7 has been validated for use in various cultures (Garcia-Campayo et al., 2010; Lowe et al., 2008; Ruiz et al., 2011). Its strong psychometric properties make it an excellent tool for clinical and research purposes. It is free and publically available at http://www.phqscreeners.com/pdfs/03_GAD-7/English.pdf.

Weaknesses. This measure focuses on one type of anxiety disorder, generalized anxiety disorder, and may not be sensitive to the specific types of anxiety that can present differently in chronic pain populations.

Hospital Anxiety and Depression Scale-Anxiety

As previously mentioned, the HADS is a 14-item scale used to measure depression and anxiety in the general medical population aged 16–65. Often, in arthritis populations the measure is split to measure depression and anxiety separately (Julian, 2011). The seven items used to measure anxiety, referred to as HADS-A target symptoms of tension, worry, fear, panic, difficulties in relaxing, and restlessness. The HADS-A has been found reliable as a separate scale with α ranging from 0.84 to 0.90 (Dagnan, Chadwick, & Trower, 2000). The scale is translated into many languages, including but not limited to: Arabic, Chinese, Danish, Dutch, Finnish, French, German, Hebrew, Hungarian, Italian, Japanese, Korean, Norwegian, Portuguese, Spanish, Swedish, Thai, and Urdu.

Strengths. The HADS-A is brief, easy to administer and score, and is sensitive to change over time. It is commonly used in arthritis patients and provides an adequate measure of general anxiety in clinical populations.

Weaknesses. The HADS-A may not be valid in elderly patients and does not identify specific anxiety disorders (Julian, 2011). The anxiety subscale captured more depressed elderly patients than patients with anxiety and therefore may not have discriminant validity when used with the elderly (Davies, Burn, McKenzie, Brothwell, & Wattis, 1993). As previously mentioned, this scale should be used with caution in culturally diverse patients as some anxiety-related items are not culturally sensitive (Leung et al., 1999). This scale is available for purchase at http://www.glassessment.co.uk/health_and_psychology/resources/hospital_anxiety_scale/hospital_anxiety_scale.asp?css=1.

State-Trait Anxiety Inventory

The State-Trait Anxiety Inventory (Spielberger, 1983) is a 40-item self-report measure designed to measure anxiety in both the state form (defined as a current state of anxiety) and the trait form (defined as a general propensity to experience anxiety) in both adults and children. There are 20 items in both the State and Trait anxiety subscales. The Trait Anxiety scale is widely used and has a high reliability ranging from $\alpha=0.86$ to 0.95 (Spielberger, 1983). The measure is available in 48 languages.

Strengths. This measure has been used extensively in chronic pain patients and is useful in identifying patients more prone to anxiety. It is well studied, psychometrically sound, and thus great for clinical and research applications.

Weaknesses. Due to its length, this measure takes about 10 min to complete, which may make it a poor choice in a busy clinic environment. Because the T-Anxiety subscale identifies pervasive traits, it is not as appropriate for use as the S-Anxiety when evaluating changes in anxiety over time (Julian, 2011). This measure has been validated in many cultures, but there has been evidence to show that translated versions in some cultures result in higher anxiety scores. This may be due to translation issues, as demonstrated by the tendency of monolingual patients to have higher scores than those who are bilingual in English and their national language (Bergeron, 1983). Other cultural groups, such as the Japanese, that are more likely to inhibit positive feelings appear to have higher levels of anxiety on the STAI (Iwata & Higuchi, 2010). Lastly, this measure is not available publically and can be purchased at http://www.mindgarden.com/index.htm.

Administration of the Screening and Referral Process

The major goals of the screening process are the following: (1) to ensure that all patients are screened, (2) to identify patients who are in need of psychological or behavioral treatment, and (3) to facilitate follow-up care to a mental health provider or a behavioral medicine specialist. Including all patients in the screening process promotes the view that screening is an integral component of the evaluation process and not the result of idiosyncratic transactions within the clinical encounter that may cause patients to feel stigmatized or self-conscious (Thombs et al., 2008). Importantly, the screening must include mechanisms and procedures for organizing and managing data and a referral process to enhance quality management for patients needing psychological treatment (Pignone et al., 2002). Screening should occur at intake and during standard appointments and can be administered by nurses, medical assistants, or other trained professionals on the rheumatology team. Screening measures can be administered to patients in the waiting room or elsewhere in the medical office prior to the medical appointment, provided that confidentiality is maintained (Holland, 2004). This model of screening has been adopted in some oncology settings which have included the following elements: verbal dialogue in which nurses openly ask patients screening questions in instances in which patients may need assistance, a paper format in which patients complete the questionnaires themselves, or an electronic handheld tablet format in which patients complete questionnaires electronically which are automatically transported to the medical record (Carlson et al., 2010; Dudgeon et al., 2012; Jacobsen, 2007).

Figure 12.1 outlines the essential components for a screening and a triage referral template.

It is important for the medical team to stay connected and supportive with patients and flexible through the implementation of the screening and referral process. While screening measures serve the purpose of objectively assessing depression and anxiety, addressing these symptoms with patients and the need for intervention will be most effective if patients are met with respect, are given the opportunity to take advantage of individualized treatment plans, and are monitored consistently through follow-up. Importantly, while many screening measures have cutoff points that increase the odds of a psychiatric diagnosis, these data should not be used alone in determining the need for follow-up care. Other verbal information obtained during interactions with professionals performing the screening or the medical visit may suggest the need for additional evaluation and management. For example, patients may report problems with sleep, diet or family and work-related issues that are distressing and merit clinical attention. Difficulties of

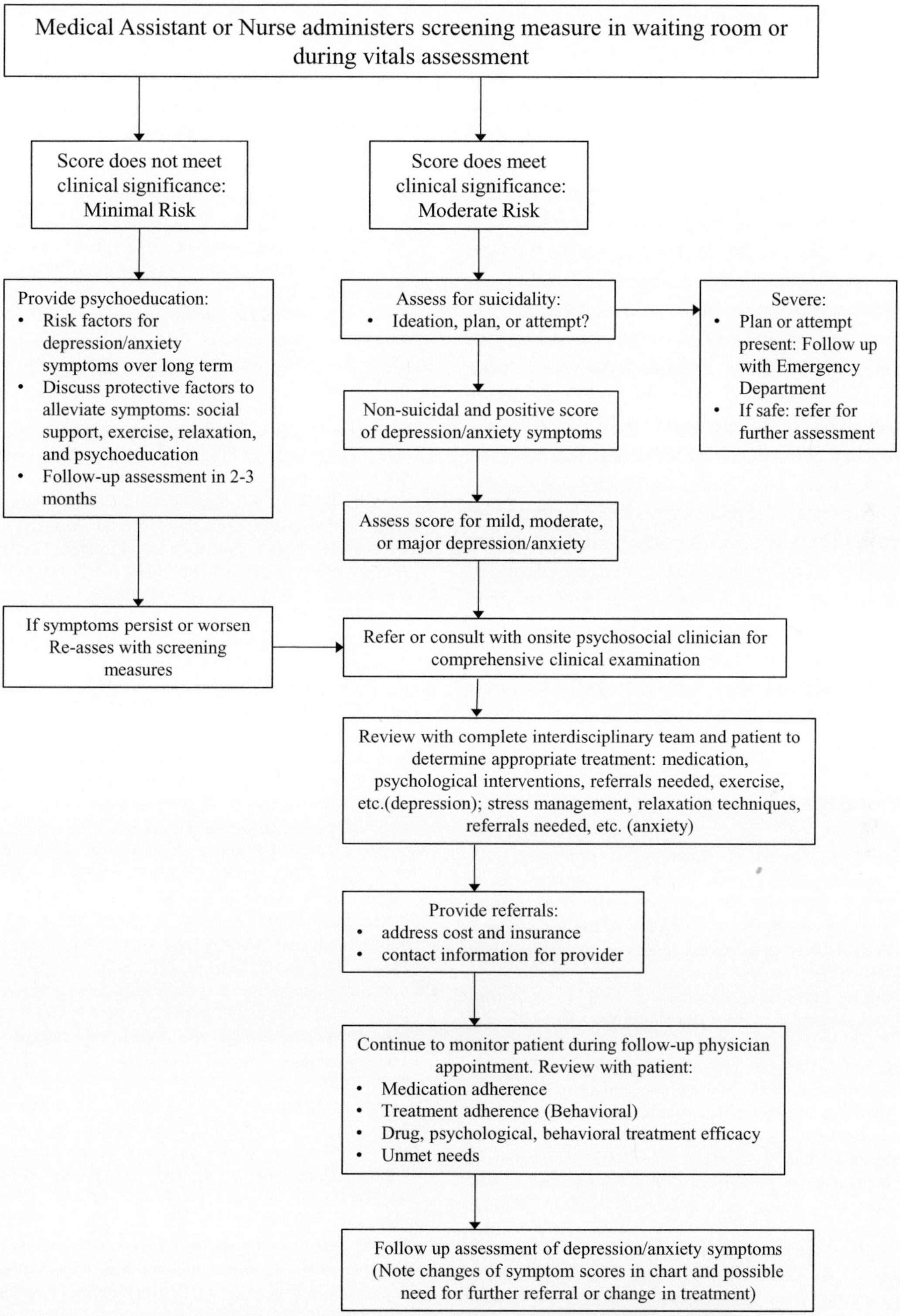

Fig. 12.1 Example procedure for assessing depression and anxiety within a rheumatology clinic

this nature are important to identify since they may compromise quality of life and interfere with medical treatment and adherence.

Several evidence-based interventions are available for managing depression, anxiety, and the difficult symptoms of arthritis. The screening and evaluation process plays a major role in identifying those patients who are in the greatest need for psychosocial care. Matching patients with the appropriate intervention is essential for the successful improvement of symptoms. Chapters 13, 14, 15, and 16 of this text provide an overview of potentially effective interventions for arthritis patients. Importantly, the support and active involvement of the medical team is crucial to the screening and referral process and the adoption of integrated care in the rheumatology setting. While depression and anxiety create a significant burden for many arthritis patients, these are very treatable disorders that must first be identified and evaluated as patients receive their medical care. Successful treatment requires coordinated treatment between mental health professionals and the rheumatology team and the willingness to broaden the focus of medical care.

References

Affleck, G., Tennen, H., Keefe, F. J., Lefebvre, J. C., Kashikar-Zuck, S., Wright, K., … Caldwell, D. S. (1999). Everyday life with osteoarthritis or rheumatoid arthritis: Independent effects of disease and gender on daily pain, mood, and coping. *Pain, 83*(3), 601–609.

American Psychiatric Association. (2013). *Diagnostic and statistical manual of mental disorders* (5th ed.). Washington, DC: Author.

Ang, D. C., Choi, H., Kroenke, K., & Wolfe, F. (2005). Comorbid depression is an independent risk factor for mortality in patients with rheumatoid arthritis. *Journal of Rheumatology, 32*, 1013–1019.

Arroll, B., Khin, N., & Kerse, N. (2003). Screening for depression in primary care with two verbally asked questions: Cross sectional study. *British Medical Journal, 327*(7424), 1144–1146. http://dx.doi.org/10.1136/bmj.327.7424.1144.

Beck, A. T., Guth, D., Steer, R., & Ball, R. (1997). Screening for major depression disorders in medical inpatients with the beck depression inventory for primary care. *Behaviour Research and Thearpy, 35*(8), 785–791.

Beck, A. T., Rush, A. J., Shaw, B. F., & Emery, G. (1979). *Cognitive therapy of depression*. New York, NY: Guilford Press.

Beck, A. T., Steer, R. A., & Brown, G. K. (2000). *BDI: Fast screen for medical patients manual*. San Antonio, TX: The Psychological Corporation.

Beekman, A. T. F., Deeg, D. J. H., Limbeek, J. V., Braam, A. W., De Vries, M. Z., & Tilburg, W. V. (1997). Brief communication: Criterion validity of the Center for Epidemiologic Studies Depression scale (CES-D): Results from a community-based sample of older subjects in the Netherlands. *Psychological Medicine, 27*(1), 231–235.

Bergeron, J. (1983). State-trait anxiety in French-English bilinguals: Cross-cultural considerations. *Series in Clinical & Community Psychology: Stress & Anxiety, 2*, 157–176.

Bidstrup, P. E., Johansen, C., & Mitchell, A. J. (2011). Screening for cancer-related distress: Summary of evidence from tools to programmes. *Acta Oncologica, 50*(2), 194–204.

Bjelland, I., Dahl, A. A., Haut, T. T., & Neckelmann, D. (2002). The validity of the Hospital Anxiety and Depression Scale: An updated literature review. *Journal of Psychosomatic Research, 52*(2), 69–77.

Blixen, C. E., & Kippes, C. (1999). Depression, social support, and quality of life in older adults with osteoarthritis. *Image: The Journal of Nursing Scholarship, 31*(3), 221–226.

Bruce, T. O. (2008). Comorbid depression in rheumatoid arthritis: Pathophysiology and clinical implications. *Current Psychiatry Reports, 10*(3), 258–264.

Carlson, L. E., Groff, S. L., Maciejewski, O., & Bultz, B. D. (2010). Screening for distress in lung and breast cancer outpatients: A randomized controlled trial. *Journal of Clinical Oncology, 28*(33), 4884–4891.

Chang, A. C. (1996). Clinical validation of the Geriatric Depression Scale (GDS) Chinese version. *Journal of Aging and Health, 8*(2), 238–253.

Chapman, D., Perry, G., & Strine, T. (2005). The vital link between chronic disease and depressive disorders. *Preventing Chronic Disease, 2*(1), 1–10.

Choi, J. H., Chung, K. M., & Park, K. (2013). Psychosocial predictors of four health-promoting behaviors for cancer prevention using the stage of change of Transtheoretical Model. *Psycho-Oncology, 22*(10), 2253–2261.

Culpepper, L., Clayton, A., Lieberman, J., III, & Susman, J. (2008). Treating depression and anxiety in primary care. *The Primary Care Companion to the Journal of Clinical Psychiatry, 10*(2), 145–152. Retrieved May 20, 2015

Dagnan, D., Chadwick, P., & Trower, P. (2000). Psychometric properties of the Hospital Anxiety and Depression Scale with a population of members of a depression self-help group. *British Journal of Medical Psychology, 73*(1), 129–137.

Davidson, K. W., Kupfer, D. J., Bigger, J. T., Califf, R. M., Carney, R. M., Coyne, J. C., … Suls, J. M. (2006).

Assessment and treatment of depression in patients with cardiovascular disease: National Heart, Lung, and Blood Institute Working Group Report. *Annals of Behavioral Medicine, 32*(2), 121–126.

Davies, K. N., Burn, W. K., McKenzie, F. R., Brothwell, J. A., & Wattis, J. P. (1993). Evaluation of the hospital anxiety and depression scale as a screening instrument in geriatric medical inpatients. *International Journal of Geriatric Psychiatry, 8*(2), 165–169.

DiMatteo, M. R., Lepper, H. S., & Croghan, T. W. (2000). Depression is a risk factor for noncompliance with medical treatment: Meta-analysis of the effects of anxiety and depression on patient adherence. *Archives of Internal Medicine, 160*(14), 2101–2107.

Dolbeault, S., Boistard, B., Meuric, J., Copel, L., & Brédart, A. (2011). Screening for distress and supportive care needs during the initial phase of the care process: A qualitative description of a clinical pilot experiment in a French cancer center. *Psycho-Oncology, 20*(6), 585–593.

Dudgeon, D., King, S., Howell, D., Green, E., Gilbert, J., Hughes, E., ... Sawka, C. (2012). Cancer Care Ontario's experience with implementation of routine physical and psychological symptom distress screening. *Psycho - Oncology, 21*(4), 357–364.

Eccleston, C. (2001). Role of psychology in pain management. *British Journal of Anaesthesia, 87*(1), 144–152.

Egede, L. E., Zheng, D., & Simpson, K. (2002). Comorbid depression is associated with increased health care use and expenditures in individuals with diabetes. *Diabetes Care, 25*(3), 464–470.

Eisenberg, L. (1992). Treating depression and anxiety in primary care: Closing the gap between knowledge and practice. *New England Journal of Medicine, 326*, 1080–1084.

Epstein, O., Perkin, D., Cookson, J., Watt, I., Rakhit, R., Robbins, A., & Hornett, G. (2009). *Pocket guide to clinical examination* (4th ed.). Edinburgh: Mosby Elsevier.

Fawzy, F. I., Fawzy, N. W., Hyun, C. S., Elashoff, R., Guthrie, D., Fahey, J. L., & Morton, D. L. (1993). Malignant melanoma: Effects of an early structured psychiatric intervention, coping, and affective state on recurrence and survival 6 years later. *Archives of General Psychiatry, 50*, 681–689.

Fifield, J., Tennen, H., Reisine, S., & McQuillan, J. (1998). Depression and the long-term risk of pain, fatigue, and disability in patients with rheumatoid arthritis. *Arthritis & Rheumatism, 41*, 1851–1857.

Frasure-Smith, N. (1991). In-hospital symptoms of psychological stress as predictors of long-term outcome after acute myocardial infarction in men. *The American Journal of Cardiology, 67*(2), 121–127.

Fydrich, T., Dowdall, D., & Chambless, D. L. (1993). Reliability and validity of the beck anxiety inventory. *Journal of Anxiety Disorders, 6*(1), 55–61.

Garcia-Campayo, J., Zamorano, E., Ruiz, M., Pardo, A., Perez-Paramo, M., Lopez-Gomez, V., ... Rejas, J. (2010). Cultural adaptation into Spanish of the generalized anxiety disorder-7 (GAD-7) scale as a screening tool. *Health and Quality of Life Outcomes, 8*(8), 1–11.

Gatchel, R. J., Peng, Y. B., Peters, M. L., Fuchs, P. N., & Turk, D. C. (2007). The biopsychosocial approach to chronic pain: Scientific advances and future directions. *Psychological Bulletin, 133*(4), 581.

Ghassemzadeh, H., Mojtabai, R., Karamghadiri, N., & Ebrahimkhani, N. (2005). Psychometric properties of a Persian-language version of the Beck Depression Inventory—Second edition: BDI-II-PERSIAN. *Depression and Anxiety, 21*(4), 185–192.

Goldberg, D. (1985). Identifying psychiatric illness among general medical patients. *British Medical Journal (Clinical Research Edition), 29*, 161–162.

Groopman, J. (2008). *How Doctors think.* New York, NY: Houghton Mifflin.

Ha, J. F., Anat, D., & Longnecker, N. (2010). Doctor-patient communication: A review. *The Ochsner Journal, 10*(1), 38–43.

Holland, J. C. (2004). IPOS Sutherland Memorial Lecture: An international perspective on the development of psychosocial oncology: Overcoming cultural and attitudinal barriers to improve psychosocial care. *Psycho-Oncology, 13*(7), 445–459.

Holland, J. C., Andersen, B., Breitbart, W. S., Buchmann, L. O., Compas, B., Deshields, T. L., ... Freedman-Cass, D. A. (2013). Distress management. *Journal of the National Comprehensive Cancer Network, 11*(2), 190–209.

Holzemer, W. L., Corless, I. B., Nokes, K. M., Turner, J. G., Brown, M. A., Powell-Cope, G. M., ... Portillo, C. J. (1999). Predictors of self-reported adherence in persons living with HIV disease. *AIDS Patient Care and STDs, 13*(3), 185–197.

Isik, A., Koca, S. S., Ozturk, A., & Mermi, O. (2007). Anxiety and depression in patients with rheumatoid arthritis. *Clinical Rheumatology, 26*(6), 872–878.

Iwata, N., & Higuchi, H. R. (2010). Responses of Japanese and American university students to the STAI items that assess the presence or absence of anxiety. *Journal of Personality Assessment, 74*(1), 48–62.

Jacobsen, P. B. (2007). Screening for psychological distress in cancer patients: Challenges and opportunities. *Journal of Clinical Oncology, 25*(29), 4526–4527.

Jacobsen, P. B., Donovan, K. A., Trask, P. C., Fleishman, S. B., Zabora, J., Baker, F., & Holland, J. C. (2005). Screening for psychologic distress in ambulatory cancer patients. *Cancer, 103*(7), 1494–1502.

Jang, Y., Small, B. J., & Haley, W. E. (2001). Cross-cultural comparability of the Geriatric Depression Scale: Comparison between older Koreans and older Americans. *Aging & Mental Health, 5*(1), 31–37.

Julian, L. J. (2011). Measures of anxiety: State-Trait Anxiety Inventory (STAI), Beck Anxiety Inventory (BAI), and Hospital Anxiety and Depression Scale-Anxiety (HADS-A). *Arthritis Care & Research, 63*(11), 467–472.

Julian, L. J., Yelin, E., Yazdany, J., Panopalis, P., Trupin, L., Criswell, L. A., & Katz, P. (2009).

Depression, medication adherence, and service utilization in systemic lupus erythematosus. *Arthritis Care & Research, 61*(2), 240–246.

Kabacoff, R., Segal, D., Hersen, M., & Van Hasselt, V. (1997). *Journal of Anxiety Disorders, 11*(1), 33–47.

Keefe, F. J., Abernethy, A. P., & Campbell, L. C. (2005). Psychological approaches to understanding and treating disease-related pain. *Annual Review of Psychology, 56*, 601–630.

Keefe, F. J., Smith, S. J., Buffington, A. L., Gibson, J., Studts, J. L., & Caldwell, D. S. (2002). Recent advances and future directions in the biopsychosocial assessment and treatment of arthritis. *Journal of Consulting and Clinical Psychology, 70*(3), 640.

Kojima, M., Furukawa, T., Takahashi, H., Kawai, M., Nagaya, T., & Tokudome, S. (2002). Cross-cultural validation of the Beck Depression Inventory-II in Japan. *Psychiatry Research, 110*(3), 291–299.

Kojima, M., Kojima, T., Suzuki, S., Oguchi, T., Oba, M., Tsuchiya, H., … Ishiguro, N. (2009). Depression, inflammation, and pain in patients with rheumatoid arthritis. *Arthritis Care & Research, 61*(8), 1018–1024.

Kroenke, K., Spitzer, R., Williams, J., Monahan, P., & Lowe, B. (2007). Anxiety disorders in primary care: Prevalence, impairment, comorbidity, and detection. *Annals of Internal Medicine, 146*(5), 317–325.

Kroenke, K., Spitzer, R. L., & Williams, J. B. (2001). The PHQ-9: Validity of a brief depression severity measure. *Journal of General Internal Medicine, 16*(9), 606–613.

Leung, C. M., Wing, Y. K., Kwong, P. K., Lo, A., & Shum, K. (1999). Validation the Chinese-Cantonese version of the Hospital Anxiety and Depression Scale and comparison with the Hamilton Rating Scale of Depression. *Acta Psychiatrica Scandinavica, 100*(6), 456–461.

Lichtman, J. H., Bigger, J. T., Blumenthal, J. A., Frasure-Smith, N., Kaufmann, P. G., Lespérance, F., … Froelicher, E. S. (2008). Depression and coronary heart disease recommendations for screening, referral, and treatment: A science advisory from the American Heart Association Prevention Committee of the Council on Cardiovascular Nursing, Council on Clinical Cardiology, Council on Epidemiology and Prevention, and Interdisciplinary Council on Quality of Care and Outcomes Research: Endorsed by the American Psychiatric Association. *Circulation, 118*(17), 1768–1775.

Lin, E. H., Katon, W., Von Korff, M., Rutter, C., Simon, G. E., Oliver, M., … Young, B. (2004). Relationship of depression and diabetes self-care, medication adherence, and preventive care. *Diabetes care, 27*(9), 2154–2160.

Lowe, B., Decker, O., Muller, S., Brahler, E., Schellberg, D., Herzog, W., Herzberg, P. Y. (2008). Validation and standardization of the Generalized Anxiety Disorder Screener (GAD-7) in the general population. *Medical Care, 46*(3), 266–274.

Luoma, J. B., Martin, C. E., & Pearson, J. L. (2002). Contact with mental health and primary care providers before suicide: A review of the evidence. *The American Journal of Psychiatry, 159*(6), 909–916.

Martens, M. P., Parker, J. C., Smarr, K. L., Hewett, J. E., Ge, B., Slaughter, J. R., & Walker, S. E. (2006). Development of a shortened Center for Epidemiological Studies Depression Scale for assessment of depression in rheumatoid arthritis. *Rehabilitation Psychology, 51*(2), 135–139.

Martens, M. P., Parker, J. C., Smarr, K. L., Hewett, J. E., Slaughter, J. R., & Walker, S. E. (2003). Assessment of depression in rheumatoid arthritis: A modified version of the Center for Epidemiologic Studies Depression Scale. *Arthritis & Rheumatology, 49*(4), 549–555.

Martin, A., Rief, W., Klaiberg, A., & Braehler, E. (2006). Validity of the Brief Patient Health Questionnaire Mood Scale (PHQ-9) in the general population. *General Hospital Psychiatry, 28*, 71–77.

Mauksch, L., Dugdale, D., Dodson, S., & Epstein, R. (2008). Relationship, communication, and efficiency in the medical encounter creating a clinical model from a literature review. *Archives of Internal Medicine, 168*(13), 1387–1395.

Mcnamara, D. (2007). Depressed interferes with anti-TNF-alpha therapy. *Rheumatology News, 6*(6), 54–59.

Meijer, A., Roseman, M., Delisle, V. C., Milette, K., Levis, B., Syamchandra, A., … Thombs, B. D. (2013). Effects of screening for psychological distress on patient outcomes in cancer: A systematic review. *Journal of Psychosomatic Research, 75*(1), 1–17.

Mitchell, A. J., Bird, V., Rizzo, M., & Meader, N. (2010). Diagnostic validity and added value of the Geriatric Depression Scale for depression in primary care: A meta-analysis of the GDS-30 and GDS-15. *Journal of Affective Disorders, 125*(1), 10–17.

Mitchell, A. J., Hussain, N., Grainger, L., & Symonds, P. (2011). Identification of patient-reported distress by clinical nurse specialists in routine oncology practice: A multicentre UK study. *Psycho-Oncology, 20*(10), 1076–1083.

Monahan, P., Shacham, E., Reece, M., Kroenke, K., Ong'or, W., Omollo, O., … Ojwang, C. (2009). Validity/reliability of PHQ-9 and PHQ-2 depression scales among adults living with HIV/AIDS in western Kenya. *Journal of General Internal Medicine, 24*(2), 189–197.

Mui, A., Burnette, D., & Chen, L. (2002). Cross-cultural assessment of geriatric depression: A review of the CES-D and GDS. In J. H. Skinner (Ed.), *Multicultural measurement in older populations*. New York, NY: Springer.

Mulrow, C. D., Williams, J. W., Gerety, M. B., Ramirez, G., Montiel, O. M., & Kerber, C. (1995). Case-finding instruments for depression in primary care settings. *Annals of Internal Medicine, 122I*(12), 913–921.

Murphy, L., Sacks, J., Brady, T., Hootman, J., & Chapman, D. (2012). Anxiety and depression among US adults with arthritis: Prevalence and correlates. *Arthritis Care and Research, 64*(7), 968–976.

Nery, F. G., Borba, E. F., Hatch, J. P., Soares, J. C., Bonfá, E., & Neto, F. L. (2007). Major depressive disorder and disease activity in systemic lupus erythematosus. *Comprehensive Psychiatry, 48*(1), 14–19.

Nicassio, P. M. (2008). The problem of detecting and managing depression in the rheumatology clinic. *Arthritis Care & Research, 59*(2), 155–158.

Nicassio, P. (2010). Arthritis and psychiatric disorders: Disentangling the relationship. *Journal of Psychosomatic Research, 68*(2), 183–185.

Norris, M. P., Arnau, R. C., Bramson, R., & Meagher, M. W. (2003). The efficacy of somatic symptoms in assessing depression in older primary care patients. *Clinical Gerontology, 27*(1), 43–57.

Nyklíček, I., Hoogwegt, F., & Westgeest, T. (2015). Psychological distress across twelve months in patients with rheumatoid arthritis: The role of disease activity, disability, and mindfulness. *Journal of Psychosomatic Research, 78*(2), 162–167.

Ødegård, S., Finset, A., Mowinckel, P., Kvien, T. K., & Uhlig, T. (2007). Pain and psychological health status over a 10-year period in patients with recent onset rheumatoid arthritis. *Annals of the Rheumatic Diseases, 66*(9), 1195–1201.

Okuyama, T., Akechi, T., Yamashita, H., Toyama, T., Nakaguchi, T., Uchida, M., & Furukawa T. A. (2011). Oncologists' recognition of supportive care needs and symptoms of their patients in a breast cancer outpatient consultation. *Japanese Journal of Clinical Oncology, 41*(11), 1251–1258.

Osterberg, L., & Blaschke, T. (2005). Adherence to medication. *New England Journal of Medicine, 353*(5), 487–497.

Ozminkowski, R. J., Burton, W. N., Goetzel, R. Z., Maclean, R., & Wang, S. (2006). The impact of rheumatoid arthritis and medical expenditures, absenteeism, and short-term disability benefits. *Journal of Occupational and Environmental Medicine, 48*, 135–148.

Park, C. L., & Gaffey, A. E. (2007). Relationships between psychosocial factors and health behavior change in cancer survivors: An integrative review. *Annals of Behavioral Medicine, 34*(2), 115–134.

Partridge, A. H., LaFountain, A., Mayer, E., Taylor, B. S., Winer, E., & Asnis-Alibozek, A. (2008). Adherence to initial adjuvant anastrozole therapy among women with early-stage breast cancer. *Journal of Clinical Oncology, 26*(4), 556–562.

Pignone, M. P., Gaynes, B. N., Rushton, J. L., Burchell, C. M., Orleans, C. T., Mulrow, C. D., & Lohr, K. N. (2002). Screening for depression in adults: A summary of the evidence for the US Preventive Services Task Force. *Annals of Internal Medicine, 136*(10), 765–776.

Platt, F., & Hardee, J. (2013). How are you feeling? I mean emotionally, how are you feeling? *Journal of Clinical Outcomes Management, 20*(12), 555–558.

Quinten, C., Maringwa, J., Gotay, C. C., Martinelli, F., Coens, C., Reeve, B. B., ... Bottomley, A. (2011). Patient self-reports of symptoms and clinician ratings as predictors of overall cancer survival. *Journal of the National Cancer Institute, 103*(24), 1851–1858.

Radloff, L. S. (1997). The CES-D scale: A self-report depression scale for research in the general population. *Applied Psychological Measurement, 1*, 385–401.

Radloff, L. S., & Teri, L. (1986). Use of the Center for Epidemiological Studies-Depression Scale with older adults. *Clinical Gerontology, 5*, 119–136.

Roberts, R. E. (1980). Reliability of the CES-D Scale in different ethnic contexts. *Psychiatry Research, 2*(2), 125–143.

Rodriguez, K. L., Bayliss, N., Alexander, S. C., Jeffreys, A. S., Olsen, M. K., Pollak, K. I., ... Arnold, R. M. (2010). How oncologists and their patients with advanced cancer communicate about health-related quality of life. *Psycho-Oncology, 19*(5), 490–499.

Ruiz, M., Zamorano, E., Garcia-Campayo, J., Pardo, A., Freire, O., & Rejas, J. (2011). Validity of the GAD-7 scale as an outcome measure of disability in patients with generalized anxiety disorders in primary care. *Journal of Affective Disorders, 128*(3), 277–286.

Shih, M., Hootman, J., Strine, T., Chapman, D., & Brady, T. (2006). Serious psychological distress in US adults with arthritis. *Journal of General Internal Medicine, 21*, 1160–1166.

Smarr, K. L., & Neefer, A. L. (2011). Meaures of depression and depressive symptoms. *Arthritis Care & Research, 63*(11), 454–466.

Sobin, C., & Sackeim, H. (1997). Psychomotor symptoms of depression. *American Journal of Psychiatry, 154*, 4–17.

Söderlin, M. K., Hakala, M., & Nieminen, P. (2000). Anxiety and depression in a community-based rheumatoid arthritis population. *Scandinavian Journal of Rheumatology, 29*(3), 177–183.

Söllner, W., DeVries, A., Steixner, E., Lukas, P., Sprinzl, G., Rumpold, G., & Maislinger, S. (2001). How successful are oncologists in identifying patient distress, perceived social support, and need for psychosocial counseling? *British Journal of Cancer, 84*(2), 179.

Somers, T. J., Keefe, F. J., Pells, J. J., Dixon, K. E., Waters, S. J., Riordan, P. A. ... Rice, J. R. (2009). Pain catastrophizing and pain-related fear in osteoarthritis patients: Relationships to pain and disability. *Journal of Pain & Symptom Management, 37*, 863–872.

Somers, T. J., Kurakula, P. C., Criscione-Schreiber, L., Keefe, F. J., & Clowse, M. E. (2012). Self-efficacy and pain catastrophizing in systemic lupus erythematosus: Relationship to pain, stiffness, fatigue, and psychological distress. *Arthritis Care & Research, 64*(9), 1334–1340.

Spielberger, C. (1983). *Manual for the State-Trait Anxiety Inventory* (rev. ed.). Palo Alto, CA: Consulting Psychologists Press.

Spitzer, R. L., Kroenke, K., Williams, J. B. W., & Lowe, B. (2006). A brief measure for assessing generalized anxiety disorder. *Archives of Internal Medicine, 166*, 1092–1097.

Stang, P., Brandenburg, N., Lane, M., Merikangas, K., Von Korff, M., & Kessler, R. (2006). Mental and physical comorbid conditions and days in role among persons with arthritis. *Psychosomatic Medicine, 68*, 152–158.

Stebbings, S., Herbison, P., Doyle, T. C., Treharne, G. J., & Highton, J. (2010). A comparison of fatigue correlates in rheumatoid arthritis and osteoarthritis: Disparity in associations with disability, anxiety and sleep disturbance. *Rheumatology, 49*(2), 361–367.

Stiles, P. G., & McGarrahan, J. F. (1998). The Geriatric Depression Scale: A comprehensive review. *Journal of Clinical Geropsychology, 4*(2), 89–110.

Strosahl, K. (2001). The integration of primary care and behavioral health: Type II change in the era of managed care. In N. Cummings, W. O'Donohoe, S. Hayes, & V. Follette (Eds.), *Integrated behavioral healthcare: Positioning mental health practice with medical/surgical practice* (pp. 45–70). New York: Academic Press.

Tayer, W. G., Nicassio, P. M., Radojevic, V., & Krall, T. (1996). Pain and helplessness as correlates of depression in systemic lupus erythematosus. *British Journal of Health Psychology, 1*(3), 253–262.

Thombs, B. D., de Jonge, P., Coyne, J. C., Whooley, M. A., Frasure-Smith, N., Mitchell, A. J., … Ziegelstein, R. C. (2008). Depression screening and patient outcomes in cardiovascular care: A systematic review. *Journal of the American Medical Association, 300*(18), 2161–2171.

Turk, D. C., & Okifuji, A. (1994). Detecting depression in chronic pain patients: Adequacy of self-reports. *Behaviour Research and Therapy, 32*(1), 9–16.

Ulusoy, M., Sahin, N. H., & Erkmen, H. (1998). Turkish version of the Beck Anxiety Inventory: Psychometric properties. *Journal of Cognitive Psychotherapy, 12*(2), 163–171.

United States Census Bureau. (2013, July). *Health status, health insurance, and medical services utilization: 2010* (B. O'Hara & K. Caswell, Authors).

US Preventive Services Task Force. (2009). Screening for depression in adults: US preventive services task force recommendation statement. *Annals of Internal Medicine, 151*(11), 784–792.

VanDyke, M. M., Parker, J. C., Smarr, K. L., Hewett, J. E., Johnson, G. E., Slaughter, J. R., & Walker, S. E. (2004). Anxiety in rheumatoid arthritis. *Arthritis Care & Research, 51*(3), 408–412.

Vermeire, E., Hearnshaw, H., Van Royen, P., & Denekens, J. (2001). Patient adherence to treatment: Three decades of research. A comprehensive review. *Journal of Clinical Pharmacy and Therapeutics, 26*(5), 331–342.

Viljoen, J., Iverson, G., Griffiths, S., & Woodward, T. (2003). Factor structure of the Beck Depression Inventory-II in a medical outpatient sample. *Journal of Clinical Psychology in Medical Settings, 10*(4), 289–291.

Walker, S., Walker, J., Richardson, G., Palmer, S., Wu, Q., Gilbody, S., … Sharpe, M. (2014). Cost-effectiveness of combining systematic identification and treatment of co-morbid major depression for people with chronic diseases: The example of cancer. *Psychological medicine, 44*(07), 1451–1460.

Wetherell, J., & Arean, P. (1997). Psychometric evaluation of the Beck Anxiety Inventory with older medical patients. *Psychological Assessment, 9*(2), 136–144.

Whitmer, K. M., Pruemer, J. M., Nahleh, Z. A., & Jazieh, A. R. (2006). Symptom management needs of oncology outpatients. *Journal of Palliative Medicine, 9*(3), 628–630.

Wittchen, H., Muhlig, S., & Beesdo, K. (2003). Mental disorders in primary care. *Dialogues in Clinical Neuroscience, 5*(2), 115–128.

Wulsin, L., Somoza, E., & Heck, J. (2002). The feasibility of using the Spanish PHQ-9 to screen for depression in primary care in Honduras. *The Primary Care Companion to the Journal of Clinical Psychology, 4*(5), 191–195.

Yesavage, J.A., Brink, T.L., Rose, T.L., Lum, D., Huang, V., Adey, M., & Leirer, V.O. (1983). Development and validation of a geriatric depression screening scale: a preliminary report. *Journal of Psychiatric Research, 17*(1), 37–49.

Physical Activity and Psychosocial Aspects of Arthritis

13

Patricia Katz

The evidence is clear that physical activity and exercise offer health benefits such as improvements in cardiovascular risk factors, reduction of obesity and metabolic syndrome, and reduction in cancer risk. For individuals with arthritis, it also offers reductions in pain and improvements in function. In addition, a great deal of evidence indicates that physical activity improves mood and reduces the risk of depression and cognitive impairment. While the majority of the evidence comes from studies in the general population, a substantial body of literature also comes from studies of individuals with rheumatic diseases. This chapter will review the evidence linking physical activity and exercise to psychological and cognitive well-being and then present information to help practitioners guide patients in initiating physical activity.

Exercise, Physical Activity, Physical Inactivity, Sedentary Time

Most physical activity interventions in the general population and in rheumatology have used structured *exercise*programs as the intervention. These programs have varied in content (e.g., aerobic conditioning, resistance exercise, stretching), level of supervision (e.g., group setting or unsupervised), location (e.g., community center, gym, home-based), intensity (low, moderate, or vigorous activity), frequency (number of sessions per week), and duration (length of sessions and length of program), but have in common that the programs were defined. More recently, less structured programs have been developed with the intent of increasing *physical activity*. These programs often focus on walking.

Observational and epidemiologic studies of physical activity have previously relied primarily on self-report. While there are a number of validated and widely used self-report measures, there is a general tendency for people to over-report their activity and exercise time. Over the last decade or so, the use of accelerometers or other activity monitoring devices has become more common in research, reducing the need for self-report measures. These devices can provide data on the amount of activity and METs[1] or kilocalories expended, and often have other features.

[1] MET refers to "metabolic equivalent of task," and is used to express the energy cost of physical activities. One MET is considered the energy required for quiet sitting. Sample values: sleeping (0.9 MET), walking at 2.5 mph (2.9 MET), pushing a stroller (4.0 MET), running at 6 mph (9.8 MET), jumping rope (12.3 MET). These are average values; actual METs vary by age, sex, height, and body mass (Matthews et al., 2012). Activity is often expressed as MET minutes, representing the time expended at a certain level of activity.

P. Katz, PhD (✉)
Department of Medicine, School of Medicine, University of California, San Francisco, CA, USA
e-mail: Patti.Katz@ucsf.edu

P.M. Nicassio (ed.), *Psychosocial Factors in Arthritis,* DOI 10.1007/978-3-319-22858-7_13

Some studies have shifted focus from physical activity toward examining the impact of *physical inactivity*, or lack of moderate-to-vigorous activity (MVA) (Matthews et al., 2012; Pate, O'Neill, & Lobelo, 2008), and *sedentary*, or "sitting," time (Bankoski et al., 2011; Owen, Healy, Matthews, & Dunstan, 2010; Owen, Sparling, Healy, Dunstan, & Matthews, 2010; Pate et al., 2008). Epidemiologic studies of self-reported sitting time estimate that US adults spend an average of 4.7 h per day sitting (Harrington, Barreira, Staiano, & Katzmarzyk, 2014). Researchers acknowledge, however, that this is probably an underestimate. Unlike many unhealthy behaviors, sitting time is greater among individuals with more education, probably reflecting the prevalence of increasingly sedentary occupations as education increases. Sitting time includes TV viewing, time in cars, and, in some studies, computer time. There is compelling evidence that sedentary time is an independent risk for mortality, cardiovascular disease, obesity, metabolic syndrome, and cancer, even after accounting for MVA (Bankoski et al., 2011; Matthews et al., 2012).

The Centers for Disease Control and Prevention (CDC) has defined minimum standards for physical activity to improve health and reduce risk of disease: 150 min/week of moderate-to-vigorous activity, or 75 min/week of vigorous activity (http://www.cdc.gov/physicalactivity/everyone/guidelines/adults.html). Moderate-intensity activities are those that require 3–6 METs, or an individual would rate as a 5 or 6 on 0–10 scale of intensity. Vigorous-intensity activities require >6 METs. Converting the CDC recommendations to MET minutes yields about 600 MET minutes per week.

Physical Activity Levels in People with Rheumatic Diseases

While exercise was once thought to exacerbate inflammation and disease activity, it has now been recognized as safe and has been recommended for individuals with rheumatic diseases for several decades (Bennell, Dobson, & Hinman, 2014; Bennell & Hinman, 2011; Hochberg et al., 2012; Iversen, Brawerman, & Iversen, 2012; Stenstrom & Minor, 2003). Until recently, the majority of research on exercise in rheumatic diseases has been conducted among people with osteoarthritis (OA) and rheumatoid arthritis (RA). Exercise is a cornerstone of the management of OA symptoms and is recommended in all clinical guidelines, regardless of disease severity, pain, and functional status (Bennell et al., 2014). A recent Cochrane review (Hurkmans, van der Giesen, Vliet Vlieland, Schoones, & Van den Ende, 2009) reported no deleterious effects of aerobic training for persons with RA and concluded that exercise should be recommended for them.

In spite of recommendations, studies among individuals with rheumatic diseases have typically found low levels of physical activity (Mancuso, Perna, Sargent, & Salmon, 2011; Mancuso, Rincon, Sayles, & Paget, 2007; Semanik, Wilbur, Sinacore, & Chang, 2004; Sokka et al., 2008; Volkmann et al., 2010). For example, the QUEST-RA study including 5235 rheumatoid arthritis patients from 21 countries found that only 13.8 % reported exercise ≥3 times/week (Sokka et al., 2008). Inactivity was higher among women, persons who were older, had lower education, were obese, had comorbidities, or had low functional capacity, high disease activity, pain, and fatigue. The Osteoarthritis Initiative (OAI), a large population-based study of people with or at risk of developing osteoarthritis, measured physical activity by accelerometer over 7 days and found that 45 % of 1908 adults were inactive, 42 % insufficiently active, and only 13 % met physical activity guidelines (≥150 min of MVA/week), a proportion similar to that found in QUEST-RA (Sun et al., 2014). These results were confirmed in a systematic review that concluded that only a small-to-moderate proportion of individuals with hip and knee OA met current physical activity guidelines (Wallis, Webster, Levinger, & Taylor, 2013). Physical activity has been less studied in other rheumatic conditions, but existing data suggest similar trends (Kaleth, Slaven, & Ang, 2014; Katz et al., 2012; Swinnen, Scheers, Lefevre, Dankaerts, & deVlam, 2014).

In contrast, CDC surveillance studies report that 48 % of US adults meet current physical activity recommendations (http://www.cdc.gov/physicalactivity/data/facts.html)—a rate that is disappointing, but is still higher than among individuals with arthritis. It is important to consider that the inflammatory backgrounds of some of the rheumatic diseases, such as rheumatoid arthritis (RA), as well as their treatments, may magnify the negative effects of inactivity.

Psychological Impact of Physical Activity

Studies of physical activity and psychological well-being have focused predominantly on depression. These studies have used measures of depressive symptoms, such as the Centers for Epidemiological Studies Depression scale (CESD), Beck Depression Inventory (BDI), Geriatric Depression Scale (GDS), or Hospital Anxiety and Depression Scale (HADS), as the primary measure of mood. Scores are often used to define "depression." Actual diagnostic interviews to identify depression are used less often. Measures of positive mood states are rarely examined. There is evidence that physical activity and exercise interventions are beneficial in alleviating symptoms of anxiety, as well as depression (Anderson & Shivakumar, 2013), but anxiety has received less attention in rheumatic conditions, so will not be addressed here. This section focuses on studies of depression or high levels of depressive symptoms, and will use the term "depression" to refer to depressive symptom scores meeting cut points.

Physical Activity and Depression

General Population

Observational studies have consistently found an inverse relationship between physical activity and depression. Two recent examples are from large epidemiological studies. Researchers examined 10 years of data on 2891 women in the Study of Women's Health Across the Nation (SWAN) and found an incremental effect of physical activity (Dugan, Bromberger, Segawa, Avery, & Sternfeld, 2015). Compared to women who were inactive, women with activity below the CDC guidelines had 20 % decreased risk of depression over 10 years; women who met the CDC physical activity guidelines had a 52 % decreased risk of depression. A study of men found similar trends (Sieverdes et al., 2012). Compared to an inactive group, men in the low (1–499 MET min/week of leisure physical activity), medium (500–999 MET min/week), and high (≥1000 MET min/week) groups were 24, 51, and 51 % less likely to be depressed. Most of the benefit was seen by attaining at least medium-intensity activity levels (i.e., ≥500 MET min/week), which is roughly consistent with CDC guidelines.

From a slightly different perspective, physical *inactivity*and sedentary behavior, particularly time spent watching TV, also contribute significant risk for depression (Bruundsgaard, 2005; Poole et al., 2011; Teychenne, Ball, & Salmon, 2010a, 2010b; Vallance et al., 2011). Sui and colleagues examined the longitudinal relationship between sedentary behaviors, specifically TV time and time spent riding in a car, and depression in a group of almost 5000 adults (Sui et al., 2015). Over a mean follow-up period of 9.3 years, 15 % developed depression. After adjusting for a variety of baseline factors including MVA, more than 9 h/week in a car (compared to <5 h), more than 10 h per week of TV time (compared to ≤5 h), and more than 19 h of combined TV and car time yielded 28 %, 52 %, and 74 % increased risk of depression, respectively (Fig. 13.1). There was an important caveat to these findings—the increased risk was much greater among people who did not meet the recommended physical activity guidelines. In other words, adequate levels of MVA offered some protection from the potentially deleterious effects of sedentary behavior.

The evidence for sedentary time for computer and internet use is somewhat mixed, suggesting that such time may not be a strong risk factor for depression. There may also be a circular pattern between sedentary time and depression. Not only does sedentary time appear to increase the risk of depression, but depression may lead to further increases in sedentary time (Teychenne, Abbott, Ball, & Salmon, 2014).

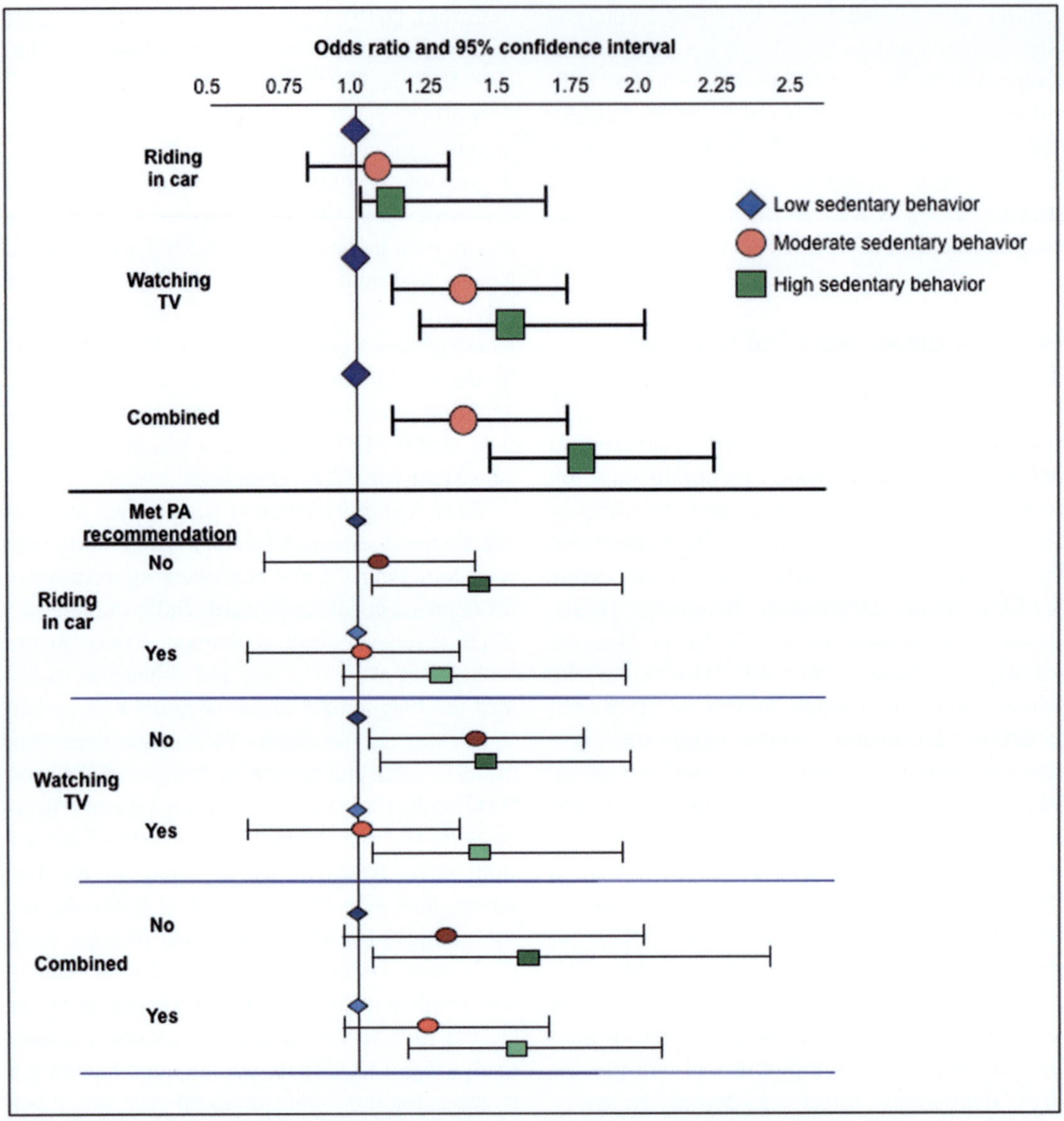

Fig. 13.1 Association between sedentary time (watching television and riding in a car) and development of depression. Adapted from Sui et al. (2015). The *top panel* shows the overall odds ratios and 95 % confidence intervals for risk of developing depression at 9.3 years of follow-up conferred by hours riding in a car, watching TV, and combined time riding in a car and watching TV at the baseline assessment. The *lower section* shows the risk (odds ratios and 95 % confidence intervals) for respondents who did and did not meet CDC physical activity guidelines at the baseline assessment. Low, moderate, and high levels of sedentary behavior were identified based on tertiles within the distribution. For riding in a car, low <5 h/week, moderate 5–8.9 h/week, high ≥9 h/week. For watching TV, low <5 h/week, moderate 5–10 h/week, high >10 h/week. For combined, low <12 h/week, moderate 12–18.9 h/week, high ≥19 h/week

Physical activity and exercise interventions show positive effects on depression, and a number of reviews have been published summarizing study results. The American Psychiatric Association guidelines for treatment of patients with major depressive disorder cite physical activity as beneficial, particularly for individuals with co-occurring medical problems (American Psychiatric Association Work Group on Major Depressive Disorder, 2010). A review by Conn reported that physical activity interventions reduced depressive symptoms, even among adults who were not clinically depressed (Conn, 2010). Interventions ranged in duration, frequency, and session length, but typically were designed as 30–60 min sessions, 3 times a week, for a mean of 62 sessions. Standardized mean effect sizes were 0.372 and 0.522 for supervised and unsupervised physical activity interventions, respectively. Meta-analyses of interventions for adults who were clinically depressed have shown larger effect sizes, ranging from 0.72 to 1.42 (Conn, 2010). In a Cochrane review, exercise was associated with a greater reduction in depression than controls (standardized mean difference [SMD] −0.62, 95 % CI −0.81, −0.42) (Cooney et al., 2013; Cooney, Dwan, & Mead, 2014). A review by Teychenne concluded that both moderate- and vigorous-intensity interventions were effective, and that both center-based and home-based interventions were effective (Teychenne, Ball, & Salmon, 2008).

In the most recent review of randomized controlled trials of exercise interventions for depression, Stanton and Reaburn identified seven trials that met criteria for evaluation (included adults with depression diagnosed by DSM IV criteria or a validated depression scale; had an aerobic or resistance training program intervention of any duration; included a comparison group including pharmacotherapy, education, psychotherapy, other type of exercise [e.g., stretching], or no intervention; and used a validated depression scale as the outcome measure) (Stanton & Reaburn, 2014). The authors concluded that aerobic exercise programs at low-to-moderate intensity, performed 3–4 times per week, with sessions from 30 to 40 min, and a program duration of at least 9 weeks were beneficial in treating depression. They also noted that program adherence rates varied from 50 to 100 %, which may be due to the exercise format (group vs. individual), type of exercise, exercise intensity, or some combination of these factors. One of the reviewed studies did find that their higher intensity exercise had lower adherence (Trivedi et al., 2011); however, that same study found that the higher intensity program had higher depression remission rates. An earlier study found effects on depression only for a higher intensity exercise intervention that was equivalent to the CDC public health exercise guidelines (Dunn, Trivedi, Kampert, Clark, & Chambliss, 2005).

Reviewing exercise interventions among individuals with a variety of chronic conditions, including chronic pain and fibromyalgia, Herring also found that exercise reduced depressive symptoms (Herring, Puetz, O'Connor, & Dishman, 2012). Larger effects were noted when baseline depressive symptoms were higher and physical activity levels were moderate or vigorous (compared to low).

The effects of physical activity interventions on depression may be equivalent to the effects of psychological therapy and pharmacological treatment. In the Cochrane review previously cited, seven trials compared exercise with psychological therapy, and no difference was seen between the two interventions (SMD −0.03, 95 % CI −0.32, 0.26). Four trials compared exercise with pharmacological treatment, and again, no significant difference was seen between the two types of interventions (SMD −0.11, 95 % CI −0.34, 0.12) (Cooney et al., 2013, 2014).

Rheumatic Conditions

The findings in general population studies are replicated in studies of persons with arthritis. Kelley and colleagues conducted a systematic review of exercise intervention studies in rheumatic conditions that targeted depression (Kelley, Kelley, & Hootman, 2015). To be included in the review, studies had to report randomized controlled trials, include an exercise-only intervention of at least 4 weeks and a comparable control group, and include adults with osteoarthritis (OA), rheumatoid arthritis (RA), fibromyalgia, or lupus. Interventions needed to be "community-deliverable," defined as an intervention that could be performed in a community setting including home, recreation centers, and the like. Studies published from 1981 through 2012 were included. A total of 29 studies were identified that met inclusion criteria, representing 2499 participants (1470 in exercise interventions and 979 in control interventions). The majority of studies (20 of 29, or 69 %) targeted individuals with fibromyalgia, 5 targeted OA, 2 RA, and 1 each included participants with either RA or lupus or OA and RA (Fig. 13.2). The median length of the intervention periods was 16 weeks, with a median of 3 sessions per week, and a median of 30 min per session. For the majority of studies in which the information was included, the intensity of training was classified as moderate. Drop-out from exercise groups ranged from 0 to 50 %, with a mean dropout rate of 16.2 ± 12.5 %; dropout from control groups was similar, ranging from 0 to 46 %, mean 14.1 ± 13.3 %. Interventions were both supervised and unsupervised, and took place in a variety of settings. Overall, the interventions demonstrated statistically and clinically significant reductions in depressive symptoms (SMD –0.42, 95 % CI –0.58 to –0.26), an effect similar to those found in general population studies. Because no clear evidence was found for a dose–response relationship, the authors suggest that the CDC physical activity guidelines are an appropriate starting point for activity recommendations.

Why Might Physical Activity Influence Depression?

Interventions have provided evidence that physical activity may reduce depressive symptoms in rheumatic diseases indirectly through reduced pain and better function. More recent evidence suggests that activity may also affect depression through mechanisms that are especially relevant to rheumatic conditions, based on the increasing rec-

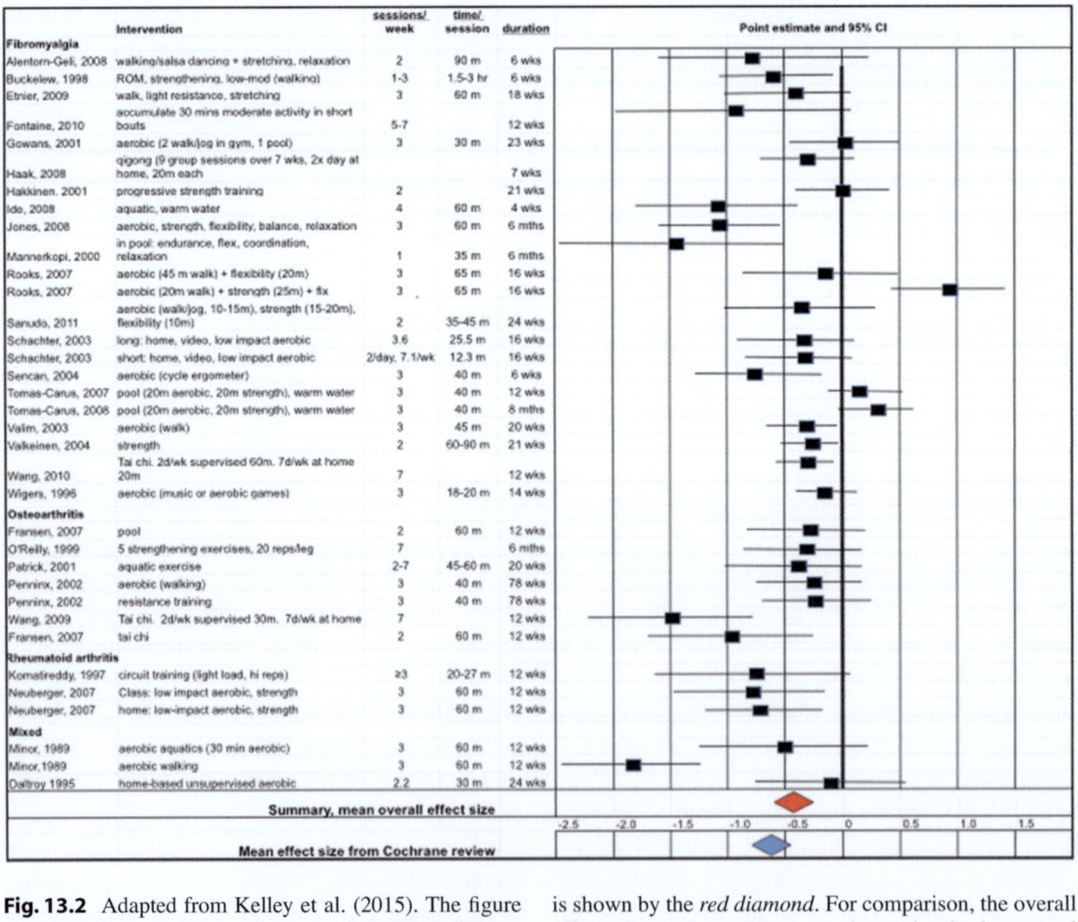

Fig. 13.2 Adapted from Kelley et al. (2015). The figure shows the point estimates (*boxes*) and 95 % confidence intervals (*lines*) for the reduction in depression conferred by the exercise intervention. The overall estimate of effect is shown by the *red diamond*. For comparison, the overall effect of exercise programs on depression in the general population, as estimated by Cooney et al. (2013), is shown as the *blue diamond*

ognition that depression is a pro-inflammatory state. Physical activity can directly lower systemic inflammation. Individuals who are more active also tend to have lower levels of adipose tissue and to report better sleep, both of which are also linked to lower levels of systemic inflammation and have well-established links with depression. Figure 13.3 illustrates potential pathways through which physical activity might influence depression. These pathways are interrelated—for example, pain can disturb sleep or increase fatigue, obesity increases systemic inflammation—so that physical activity may work through more than one pathway or may create synergistic effects.

There are additional effects of physical activity that are relevant to depression, such as effects on neurotransmitters in the brain and endorphins. These will not be discussed in this chapter because the effects are less specific to rheumatic conditions, but the reader is directed to recent reviews by Eyre and Prakash (Eyre, Papps, & Baune, 2013; Prakash, Voss, Erickson, & Kramer, 2015).

Pain. Higher levels of pain are consistently associated with a greater risk of depression (Goesling, Clauw, & Hassett, 2013; Kroenke et al., 2011). Previous exercise interventions among adults with arthritis have generally shown reductions in pain (Baillet et al., 2010; Conn, Hafdahl, Minor, & Nielsen, 2008). In fact, exercise had effects comparable to cognitive behavioral therapy in improving global health assessments among patients with chronic widespread pain (McBeth et al., 2012). The effects of exercise on pain seem to occur regardless of the type of exercise or activity. For example, muscle strengthening with or without aerobic exercise was found to be effective for pain relief in knee OA (Tanaka, Ozawa, Kito, & Moriyama, 2013), and consistent participation in the Arthritis Foundation's People with Arthritis Can Exercise (PACE) and Walk with Ease programs resulted in reductions in pain (Callahan et al., 2008, 2011). In fibromyalgia, accumulating at least 30 min of lifestyle physical activity through the day are associated with improvements in pain (Fontaine, Conn, & Clauw, 2010), and people with fibromyalgia who are physically active appear more able to modulate pain (Ellingson, Shields, Stegner, & Cook, 2012; McLoughlin, Stegner, & Cook, 2011).

The reasons that exercise affects pain are less clear. There have been suggestions that exercise increases the production of endorphins, which inhibit the transmission of pain. There is also evidence that exercise may modify central pain processing (Walsh & McWilliams, 2014), and that the intensity of activity may influence pain sensitivity (Andrzejewski, Kassolik, Bzozowski, & Cymer, 2010). In one study, meeting the CDC physical activity recommendations was associated with a reduction in experimentally tested pain sensitivity (Ellingson, Colbert, & Cook, 2012). Only actual levels of physical activity (i.e., activity measured with an actigraph), as opposed to self-reported activity, showed an association, and the strongest association, with lower pain thresholds was noted with accumulation of vigorous activity.

Function. Function may be one especially potent pathway through which activity affects mood. Williamson demonstrated the impact of activity restriction on development of depression (Williamson, 2000; Williamson & Schulz, 1992, 1995). Among individuals with a range of chronic illnesses, exercise was shown to be most effective in reducing depressive symptoms when it also improved functional status (Herring et al., 2012).

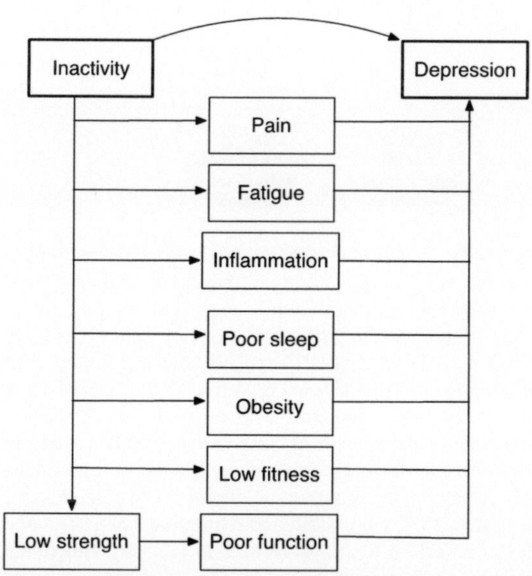

Fig. 13.3 Potential pathways through which physical inactivity might influence depression

In rheumatology, research has demonstrated that declines in functioning are strong predictors of subsequent onset of depression (Katz & Yelin, 1995, 2001). The declines in function that appear most important to the development of depression are losses of discretionary activities that are valued by individuals, particularly the loss of recreational and leisure activities and social interactions (Katz & Yelin, 2001). In contrast, the type of functioning usually measured in rheumatology, a lower level of functioning, is less predictive of the onset of depression (Fig. 13.4).

Physical activity can reduce functional limitations and reduce the risk of onset and progression of disability. Using data from the OAI, Dunlop demonstrated that greater time in light-intensity physical activity, measured by accelerometer, reduced the risk of disability onset and progression (Dunlop et al., 2014). Additional data from OAI showed that being less sedentary was associated with better function (Lee et al., 2015). Individuals who participated in the Arthritis Foundation's PACE and Walk with Ease programs experienced improvements in function

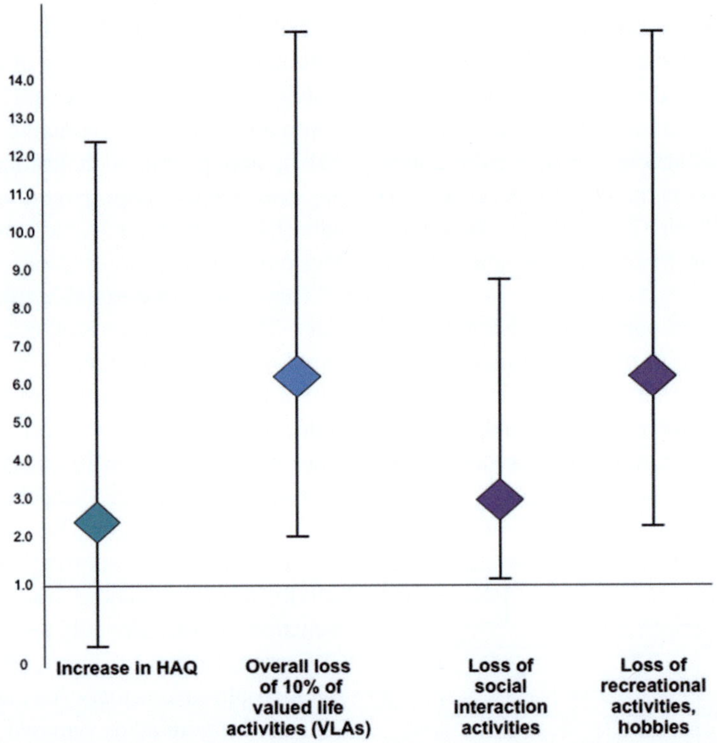

Fig. 13.4 Relationship of functional decline, measured by the Health Assessment Questionnaire (HAQ), and valued life activity (VLA) loss with subsequent onset of depression. Valued life activities (VLAs) are the wide array of activities that are important to people. They range from self care to household tasks, family care, and work, to social and recreational activities (Katz, Morris, & Yelin, 2006). The VLA Disability scale asks respondents to rate the amount of difficulty they have in 26 specific activities. A short version of the VLA has also been developed (Katz et al., 2011). The Health Assessment Questionnaire (HAQ) was developed to measure function in rheumatoid arthritis (Fries, Spitz, Kraines, & Holman, 1980). It collects information on difficulty in actions such as standing up from a chair, cutting one's meat, walking on flat ground, arising from a toilet, reaching above one's head, and opening doors. This study examined losses of function and VLAs from Time 1 to Time 2, and the subsequent development of depression at Time 3 (Katz & Yelin, 2001). Loss of 10 % of VLAs was associated with an odds (95 % CI) of developing depression of 5.87 (2.10, 16.08). Losses in two specific domains also had significant elevated odds of subsequent development of depression: social interaction (OR 3.07, 1.04–8.89) and recreational activities and hobbies (OR 6.13, 2.04–18.82). In contrast, functional decline as measured by the HAQ was not a significant predictor of new depression

(Callahan et al., 2008, 2011). Higher levels of physical activity have been linked to greater improvements in functioning in rheumatoid arthritis, fibromyalgia, and ankylosing spondylitis (Baillet et al., 2010; Bennell & Hinman, 2011; Brophy, Cooksey, et al., 2013; Conn et al., 2008; Fontaine et al., 2010; Iversen et al., 2012; Kaleth, Saha, Jensen, Slaven, & Ang, 2013). Conversely, lack of exercise or low physical activity has been associated with increased disability and loss of muscle mass (Minor, 2004).

Fatigue and sleep disturbance. Fatigue and sleep disturbances may be both symptoms and predictors of depression. Fatigue is almost universally experienced by individuals with RA (Nikolaus, Bode, Taal, & van de Laar, 2013), and high levels of fatigue have been found in other rheumatic conditions, including osteoarthritis, systemic lupus erythematosus, psoriatic arthritis, ankylosing spondylitis, and fibromyalgia (Bergman et al., 2009; Brophy, Davies, et al., 2013; Clauw, 2014; Kim, Luedtke, Vincent, Thompson, & Oh, 2012; Murphy, Alexander, Levoska, & Smith, 2013; Sterling et al., 2014; Walsh et al., 2014; Wolfe, Hawley, & Wilson, 1996). Only a handful of studies have examined the impact of exercise on fatigue in RA, and in those, exercise training appeared to improve fatigue levels (Bilberg, Ahlmén, & Mannerkorpi, 2005; Hakkinen, Sokka, Leitsalmi, Kautianinen, & Hannonen, 2003; Neill, Belan, & Ried, 2006; Neuberger et al., 2007; Rongen-van Dartel et al., 2014). A meta-analysis of non-pharmacological interventions for RA fatigue concluded that exercise interventions appear to be effective in reducing fatigue in RA, with effect sizes slightly smaller than those of a well-designed cognitive behavioral program (~0.5 compared to 0.6–0.7) (Cramp et al., 2013). Physical activity or exercise interventions have been identified as effective interventions for fibromyalgia symptoms, including fatigue (Kaleth et al., 2014).

Self-reported sleep disturbances are also common in rheumatic conditions (Abad, Sarinas, & Guilleminault, 2008; Clauw, 2014; Luyster, Chasens, Wasko, & Dunbar-Jacob, 2011; Nicassio et al., 2012; Palagini et al., 2014; Reading et al., 2009; Roehrs et al., 2013; Taylor-Gjevre, Gjevre, Nair, Skomro, & Lim, 2010; Taylor-Gjevre, Nair, & Gjevre, 2013; Treharne et al., 2007). In the general population, higher levels of physical activity are linked to better sleep quality. Among a group of older women, higher levels of moderate–vigorous physical activity were associated with less sleep fragmentation and better sleep efficiency, even after adjusting for age, education, body mass index (BMI), depressive symptoms, and arthritis (Lambiasse, Gabriel, Kuller, & Matthews, 2013), and exercise interventions show improvements in sleep quality among depressed individuals (Rethorst et al., 2013).

In RA, Nicassio and Wallston found a cross-sectional association between sleep and depression (Nicassio & Wallston, 1992). Longitudinally, pain appeared to exacerbate sleep problems, which, in turn, increased depressive symptoms. Irwin and colleagues examined the impact of a partial night sleep deprivation, a proxy for a common form of sleep disturbance, on mood and RA symptoms (Irwin et al., 2012). Results indicated that such sleep disturbance induced significant changes in depressive symptoms (as well as pain) after a single night. An interventional study found a significant improvement in self-reported sleep quality after a 12-week exercise program among individuals with RA (Durcan, Wilson, & Cunnane, 2014).

Inflammation. Many rheumatic conditions are characterized by inflammatory states. For example, elevated levels of a number of inflammatory biomarkers, including tumor necrosis factor α (TNF-α) and interleukin-6 (IL-6), are often noted in SLE and RA and are considered indicators of increased disease activity (Arend, 2001; Froneck & Horowitz, 2002). Likewise, depression is increasingly recognized as a pro-inflammatory state. Evidence includes observations that individuals with inflammatory diseases have elevated rates of depression, and significant portions of individuals with depression exhibit elevations in inflammatory factors, including C-reactive protein (CRP), IL-6, and TNF-α (Alexopoulos & Morimoto, 2011; Hamer, Batty, Marmot, Singh-Manoux, & Kivimäki, 2011; Maes, 2011; Matheny et al., 2011; Pasco et al., 2010; Prather,

Rabinovitz, Pollock, & Lotrich, 2009). Increases in inflammatory factors often precede increases in depressive symptoms, and "cytokine-induced depression" is well documented in the literature (Dantzer, O'Connor, Freund, Johnson, & Kelley, 2008; Prather et al., 2009). Some recent studies have suggested that depression may be the causal factor for inflammation (Copeland, Shanahan, Worthman, Angold, & Costello, 2012; Shaffer et al., 2011; Stewart, Rand, Mudoon, & Kamarck, 2009), but the bulk of the research literature suggests the reverse—that inflammation increases the risk of depression (Krisknadas & Cavanagh, 2012; Leonard, 2010; Lotrich, El-Gabalawy, Guenther, & Ware, 2011; Miller, Maletic, & Raison, 2009; Raedler, 2011; Raison, Capuron, & Miller, 2006; Raison & Miller, 2011).

While acute, unaccustomed exercise may put a strain on the body, chronic physical activity improves immune function (Huang, Zourdos, Jo, & Ormsbee, 2013). Regular physical activity decreases inflammatory biomarkers, including CRP, IL-6, and TNF-α (Abramson & Vaccarino, 2002; Autenrieth et al., 2009; Colbert et al., 2004; Eyre et al., 2013; Ford, 2002; Lavie, Church, Milani, & Earnest, 2011; Reuben, Judd-Hamilton, Harris, & Seeman, 2003; Shanely et al., 2013). Sedentary behavior has been linked in recent studies with elevations in systemic inflammation biomarkers such as CRP, IL-6, and TNF-α (Allison, Jensky, Marshal, Bertoni, & Cushman, 2012; Yates et al., 2012). Benatti and Pedersen provide a comprehensive review of the evidence linking physical activity and systemic inflammation in rheumatic diseases (Benatti & Pedersen, 2015), highlighting the effects of physical activity on improvements in function and physical capacity and body composition (i.e., obesity), in addition to direct improvement in inflammatory biomarker profiles.

Obesity. Both obesity and physical inactivity have been linked to numerous negative health effects, including depression, in the general population (Herring et al., 2012; Luppino et al., 2010; Shelton & Miller, 2010, 2011; Simon et al., 2006; Teychenne et al., 2010a, 2010b). Adipose tissue is a known source of proinflammatory cytokines, including TNF-α and IL-6 (Coppack, 2001; Giles et al., 2008; Visser, Bouter, McQuillan, Wener, & Harris, 1999). Obesity, particularly abdominal obesity, is strongly associated with concurrent and incident depression (de Wit et al., 2010; Luppino et al., 2010; Rivenes, Harvey, & Mykletun, 2009; Vogelzangs et al., 2010, 2011; Zhao et al., 2009). There has even recently been suggestion that adipose tissue may be a causal pathway for the inflammation-depression link (Shelton & Miller, 2011). Regular physical activity generally decreases adipose tissue.

Obesity is common among individuals with rheumatic diseases. Rates approaching 50 % have been found in cohorts with RA and lupus (Katz et al., 2011, 2013), reported rates in fibromyalgia range from 33 to 45 % (Kim, Luedtke, Vincent, Thompson, & Oh, 2012; Segura-Jimenez et al., 2015), and elevated rates are seen in OA (Sturner, Gunther, & Brenner, 2000). Obesity has received little attention as a predictor or risk factor of depression in rheumatic diseases. Observational studies have found associations between obesity and depression in fibromyalgia (Aparicio et al., 2011; Kim et al., 2012). A recent study examined obesity as a risk factor for the development of depression among a group of approximately 500 women with lupus (Katz et al., 2014). Possible and probable depression were estimated using validated SLE-specific cut points on the CESD (20 and 24, respectively). Obesity was defined using a validated lupus-specific BMI[2] cut point (BMI ≥ 26.8). Mean follow-up time was 9 years (range 2–11 years). In the analysis for possible depression, 31.6 % of those who were not obese became depressed, compared to 48.1 % of those who were obese (Table 13.1). In the analysis of probable depression, 25.9 % of those not obese became depressed compared to 42.6 % of those who were obese. After adjustment for covariates, obesity conferred an increased risk of depression of more than 50 %. Using the standard BMI cut point for obesity (BMI ≥ 30) yielded similar results.

[2] Body mass index (BMI), calculated as $\text{weight}_{kg} / \text{height}_{m^2}$, is the most common estimation of body composition and obesity. The standard definition of obesity is BMI ≥ 30.

Table 13.1 Risk of depression onset associated with obesity among women with SLE

	Possible depression (CESD ≥20)	Probable depression (CESD ≥24)
Total *n* for analysis	471	515
Obese at baseline	38.9 %	39.2 %
Became depressed		
Not obese	31.6 % (91)	25.9 % (81)
Obese*	48.1 % (88)	42.6 % (86)
Multivariate HR (95 % CI) for obesity†	1.56 (1.15, 2.11)	1.69 (1.23, 2.30)

From Katz et al. (2014)

Among a group of women with lupus, obesity at baseline was associated with elevated risk of new depression longitudinally

Possible and probable depression were defined using validated lupus-specific cut points on the CESD (Julian et al., 2011). Obesity was also defined using a validated lupus-specific criterion (Katz, Gregorich et al., 2011). Women who were depressed at baseline were omitted from the analyses

Women who met criteria for depression at baseline were excluded

*Obesity defined as BMI ≥ 26.8

†*HR* hazard ratio. Multivariate Cox regression model adjusted for age, race, baseline disease activity, smoking, and baseline physical functioning

Physical Activity and Well-Being

Psychological well-being is not just the absence of depression, however; it also includes the presence of positive affect. Broadly, there is a wealth of literature supporting the links between physical activity and positive mood, vigor, general well-being (Asztalos, De Bourdeaudhuij, & Cardon, 2010; Elavsky & McAuley, 2007). Additional psychosocial effects of exercise include distraction from negative thoughts, enhancement of self-esteem, and provision of a sense of mastery or self-efficacy (Eyre et al., 2013). Except for self-efficacy, exercise interventions in rheumatic diseases have not measured positive affect.

A variety of exercise interventions in rheumatic diseases have shown improvements in self-efficacy, which is linked to a number of positive effects including adherence to medications and other health recommendations, health behaviors, ratings of symptoms such as pain and joint stiffness, and function. Interventions showing effects on self-efficacy have included walking interventions and a variety of community-based programs combining strength, flexibility, balance, and aerobic conditions (Callahan et al., 2008, 2011; Levy et al., 2012; Schlenk, Lias, Sereika, Dunbar-Jacob, & Kwoh, 2011).

Qualitative studies offer insight into the impact of physical activity on well-being. Individuals with RA who had participated in an exercise program found that the program changed their self-image and led to improvements in overall well-being and feeling more energetic (Demmelmaier, Lindkvist, Nordgren, & Opava, 2015). They reported being now able to participate in social and recreational activities with friends and families in a way that was not possible prior to engaging in the exercise program. In addition, changes in perceptions of exercise were also reported—it was viewed as fun and rewarding. In another qualitative study, exercise was viewed as a means to resist disability and stay healthy, experience sensations of well-being, and engage in social participation on par with non-arthritis populations (Loeppenthin et al., 2014).

Physical Activity and Cognitive Function

Almost all of the literature on physical activity and cognitive function comes from outside rheumatology, often from studies of older adults. Because of the strong and consistent relationships found in those studies, and because cognitive dysfunction is increasingly recognized in rheumatic diseases, this topic is included here.

Cognitive Impairment in Rheumatic Conditions

Individuals with SLE are at significant risk of cognitive impairment (Ainiala, Loukkola, Peltola, Korpela, & Hietaharju, 2001; Brey et al., 2002; Denburg, Carbotte, & Denburg, 1997; Hanly, Fisk, McCurdy, Fougere, & Douglas, 2005; Kozora, Hanly, Lapteva, & Filley, 2008; Kozora,

Thompson, West, & Kotzin, 1996; Petri et al., 2008; Unterman et al., 2011), and evidence is mounting that individuals with RA may also have elevated risk of cognitive dysfunction (Antonchak, Saoudian, Khan, Brunner, & Luggen, 2011; Appenzeller, Bertolo, & Costallat, 2004; Bartolini et al., 2002; Hanly et al., 2005; Shin, Julian, Katz, & Wallhagen, 2011). Examples of the prevalence of cognitive impairment in these two conditions may be drawn from studies by Julian (Julian et al., 2012) and Shin (Demmelmaier et al., 2015). Both studies used a neuropsychological battery spanning a range of cognitive domains and defined impairment on each domain as performance below −1 standard deviation of population normative data. For lupus, impairment ranged from 6 % (semantic fluency) to 30 % (visuospatial learning), and for RA, from 8 % (working memory) to 30 % (visuospatial learning). Using a summary definition of cognitive dysfunction (≥/3 indices impaired), 25 % of SLE patients, and 10 % of RA patients, met criteria for prevalent cognitive dysfunction. Cognitive dysfunction is also highly prevalent in fibromyalgia. Between 50 and 80 % of individuals with fibromyalgia have impairments in memory, attention, and/or executive function (Bertolucci & de Oliveira, 2013), and "fibro fog," a constellation of cognitive issues including mental slowness, memory loss, and lack of clarity, is often cited as a symptom (Glass, 2009; Kravitz & Katz, 2015).

Physical Activity and Cognitive Impairment in Population Studies

Inactivity is linked to cognitive impairment in the general population (Angevaren, Aufdemkampe, Verhaar, Aleman, & Vanhees, 2008; Weuve et al., 2004; Yaffe, Barnes, Nevitt, Lui, & Covinsky, 2001; Zhu et al., 2014), and, conversely, higher levels of physical activity and fitness are associated with better cognitive function, particularly executive function[3] (Baker et al., 2010; Colcombe & Kramer, 2003; Etgen et al., 2010; Middleton et al., 2011; Weuve et al., 2004; Yaffe et al., 2009). Data from the Coronary Artery Risk Development in Young Adults study (CARDIA) examined the impact of cardiorespiratory fitness, which can be viewed as the result of physical activity, on cognitive function 25 years after assessment of fitness, when participants were 43–55 years of age. Results indicated that compared to the lowest quartile of fitness, performance on each cognitive test was 21–34 % better in the highest fitness quartile. Effects were noted specifically for verbal memory and psychomotor speed (Zhu et al., 2014).

In reviewing physical activity and cognitive decline among older non-demented adults, Sofi concluded that individuals who performed high levels of physical activity gained significant protection against cognitive decline (HR 0.62, 95 % CI 0.54–0.70) (Sofi et al., 2011). The effect of low-to-moderate activity was only slightly less (HR 0.65, 95 % CI 0.57–0.75). Effects were slightly greater when longer follow-up periods were examined. Angevaren's Cochrane review concluded that exercise interventions resulted in improved cardiorespiratory fitness, which coincided with improvements in cognitive functioning among older adults without known cognitive impairment (Angevaren, Aufdemkampe, Verhaar, Aleman, & Vanhees, 2008). Another meta-analysis of aerobic exercise interventions and cognitive performance found modest improvements in attention and processing speed, executive functioning, and memory (Smith et al., 2010). While the effects of physical activity on cognitive function of older adults seems clear, there is less evidence for younger adults due to paucity of studies (Prakash et al., 2015). Like sedentary behavior and depression, there also seems to be a circular relationship between inactivity and cognitive function. In a study of over 4000 older adults, inactivity led to declines in executive function, but the impact of poor executive functioning on later physical activity was even stronger (Daly, McMinn, & Allan, 2015).

[3] Executive function refers to higher-level cognitive processes that are involved in planning, organization, and management of cognitive processes. It includes domains such as working memory, reasoning, task flexibility, processing speed, and problem solving.

Investigations into the mechanisms for physical activity's effect on cognitive function are relatively recent and appear to show structural effects on the brain from physical activity. Physical activity has been shown to be protective of structural volume in the prefrontal cortex at 21-year follow-up (Rovio et al., 2010). Participation in physical activity also appears to be linked to a lower volume of brain white matter changes of the type considered a primary mechanism of age-related cognitive decline (Burzynska et al., 2014). The authors of that study speculated that the effect on white matter was due to the beneficial effects of physical activity on blood vessel integrity and elasticity. A more comprehensive review on this topic can be found in Prakash et al. (2015).

Physical Activity and Cognitive Impairment in Rheumatic Conditions

Little work has explored the potential link between physical activity and cognitive impairment in rheumatology. Inactivity was significantly and independently associated with executive function in women with lupus (OR 9.4 [1.7, 52.8]), even after controlling for age, race, education, disease activity, oral glucocorticoid use, obesity, and depression (Katz et al., 2012) (Fig. 13.5). Kozora reported a significant inverse relationship between cognitive impairment and 6-minute walk distance in lupus, a measure of functional cardiorespiratory fitness (Kozora et al., 2015).

Examining interventional studies, participants in a 6-week walking program based on Walk with Ease reported significant improvement in their ability to concentrate (Nyrop et al., 2011). There is some evidence that physical activity interventions improve cognitive function in fibromyalgia (Bertolucci & de Oliveira, 2013). Warm water exercise 3 times a week for 16 weeks demonstrated improvements in cognitive function among women with fibromyalgia (Munguia-Izquierdo & Legaz-Arrese, 2007), and an 18-week physical activity program produced improvements in self-reported cognitive function (Etnier et al., 2009).

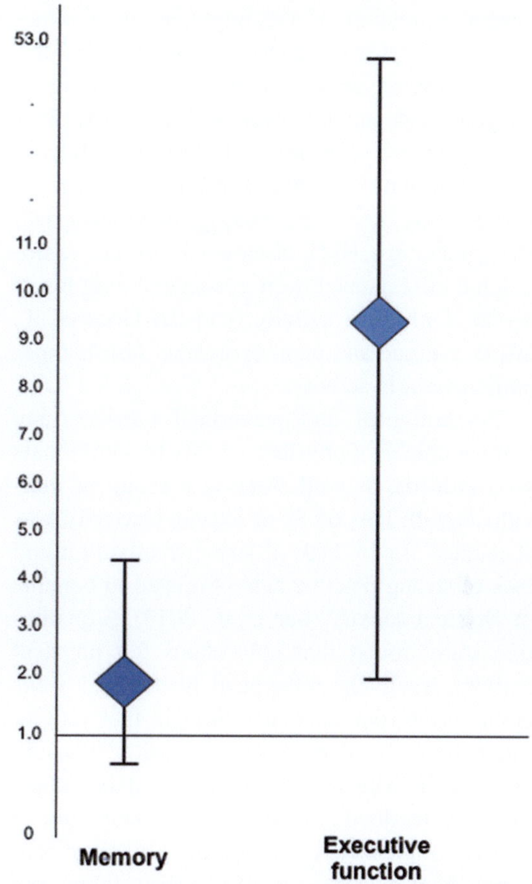

Fig. 13.5 Physical inactivity and risk of cognitive impairment. From Katz et al. (2012) Defining inactivity as <600 metabolic equivalent minutes per week, inactivity was associated with an significant elevated risk of impairment in executive function among women with systemic lupus erythematosus (Odds ratio = 9.4 [95 % confidence interval 1.7–52.8]). Inactivity was also associated with an elevated, but not statistically significant risk of impairment in memory function (OR = 1.8 [0.7, 4.4]). Activity was ascertained using the self-reported International Physical Activity Questionnaire (IPAQ) (Brown, Trost, Bauman, Mummery, & Owen, 2004; Craig et al., 2003). The definition of inactivity used was that specified in IPAQ scoring as "low activity"

Interventions and implementation

Barriers

In spite of the evidence supporting the benefits of physical activity, most studies show that individuals with arthritis are inactive. Some reasons for inactivity are similar to those expressed by the general population. For example, among the factors associated with inactivity in the QUEST-RA study, many are also associated with inactivity in the general population, such as female sex, older age, and less education (http://www.cdc.gov/physicalactivity/data/facts.html). Disease-specific barriers may also exist. Among individuals with RA, greater age, BMI, disease activity, and radiographic joint damage were associated with lower levels of physical activity (van der Goes et al., 2014). Fatigue and pain levels may also hamper participation in activity.

Psychological and perceptual barriers may hamper uptake of physical activity by individuals with arthritis, as well. Among a group of individuals with RA, 65 % of excess inactivity was accounted for by lack of strong motivation and lack of strong positive beliefs related to benefits of physical activity (Lee et al., 2012). A qualitative study found that individuals felt physical activity positively influenced health and well-being, but respondents also thought that activity might be a possible cause of arthritis (Kaptein et al., 2013). This group also discussed the impact of "role overload" in affecting decisions not to participate in activity. Patients have reported concerns about exercise causing harm to joints, not knowing what exercises to do, and not wanting to exercise because joints hurt (Law, Markland, Jones, Maddison, & Thom, 2013). Inactive individuals have been found to have negative disease-related outcome expectancies that were more distressing and that they believed were more likely to occur (Gyurcsik, Cary, Sessford, Flora, & Brawley, 2015). These issues are overlaid on barriers to activity caused by depression in general, such as loss of interest in activities and difficulty initiating activities.

Perhaps most importantly, individuals with rheumatic disease may not be getting the message from their physicians or other health care providers that physical activity is beneficial (Do, Hootman, Helmick, & Brady, 2011). Having a recommendation from a health professional may be the factor most strongly associated with engaging in physical activity or exercise (O'Donnell et al., 2013). This lack of advocacy for physical activity is not unique to rheumatology. An analysis of the 2011–2012 NHANES data found that over 50 % of adults who were completely sedentary had not been told by a health care profession to increase their exercise (Loprinzi & Beets, 2014).

Physicians and other providers may not have adequate information to guide their patients. In a survey from the Netherlands, rheumatologists, clinical nurse specialists, and physical therapists believed public health recommendations for moderate-intensity physical activity were attainable for persons with RA and that physical activity was an important health goal for RA, but most did not feel competent in offering advice about physical activity (Hurkmans et al., 2011). An additional barrier may be the advice individuals receive for how to manage disease symptoms. Pacing (e.g., taking breaks from activity) has traditionally been advocated as a way for people with arthritis to manage fatigue or pain (Murphy & Kratz, 2014). Yet one author writes, "Since patients with rheumatoid arthritis are already at risk for inactivity, further inactivation by activity pacing might potentially be harmful."(Cuperus, Hoogeboom, Neijland, van den Ende, & Keijsers, 2012).

Practical Solutions

Many types of programs have been developed to help people with arthritis increase physical activity. There is no strong evidence to favor one type of program over another. The primary criterion for success may be whether an individual will initiate and maintain it.

Some people may prefer the structure of an organized exercise program. The Arthritis Foundation's PACE and Walk with Ease programs are examples of such programs designed for people with arthritis. The Walk With Ease program (http://www.arthritis.org/we-can-help/community-programs/walk-with-ease) is offered in both a self-guided format or a group setting. Designed as a 6-week program to encourage people with arthritis to become and stay active, the group classes are structured around group walks. The home-based version includes online support such as video instruction, a message board and email alerts for meeting goals or milestones. Both versions encourage walking three times a week and include stretching and strengthening exercise, identifying barriers to exercise, and developing an individualized walking plan. The schedule of the WWE program would likely not meet the CDC activity recommendations without the addition of additional days or length of sessions, yet for inactive people, this type of program is a good place to start. Individuals who are depressed may benefit from the social contacts and support of group programs.

Participating in organized programs may be prohibitive for others due to logistic issues, cost, or other reasons. Walking may be the simplest way for many adults to increase their activity levels. Leisure walking, walking for transportation, or combination, are all effective means of increasing activity in older adults (Hekler, Castro, Buman, & King, 2012). Prescribing walking 5–7 days (vs. 3–5 days/week) a week at a moderate (vs. vigorous) pace, either in single or multiple sessions, may be the most effective way of increasing walking time (Williams, Matthews, Rutt, Napolitano, & Marcus, 2008). Importantly, walking interventions have shown statistically significant effects on depression (Robertson, Robertson, Jepson, & Maxwell, 2012), with effect sizes appearing to be within the same range as other exercise programs (SMD −0.86, 95 % CI −1.12, −0.61]). In contrast to other exercise programs, though, study completion rates of the 8 walking interventions reviewed were substantial higher, ranging from 75 to 100 %.

Use of pedometers is a simple means to measure and increase physical activity. A systematic review estimated that in a pedometer intervention of average duration (18 weeks), participants increased daily physical activity by almost 2500 steps more than controls by the end of the program (Bravata et al., 2007). Studies attempting to increase activity among older adults using pedometers and step diaries have found that individuals are able to use the devices easily and that compliance with pedometer and diary use is good (Bravata et al., 2007; Sugden et al., 2008). In an article reflecting on why pedometers work, Tudor-Locke points out that they are simple and accessible, low-literacy friendly, and the output is immediately understandable (Tudor-Locke & Lutes, 2009). Both self-monitoring by recording daily steps and having step goals appear to enhance the effectiveness of pedometer programs (Tudor-Locke & Lutes, 2009). In addition to the mechanical aspect of counting steps, many devices have online components to offer guidance in setting goals, activity tracking, and development of walking "buddies" or groups.

Physical activity guidelines for US adults call for 30 min per day of moderate-to-vigorous physical activity (MVPA) on at least 5 days per week (U.S. Department of Health and Human Services, 2008). Translating this to daily step counts yields a goal of approximately 8000 steps per day (Tudor-Locke, Leonardi, Johnson, Katzmarzyuk, & Church, 2011), about 3000 of which can be attributed to the 30-min exercise bout (assuming an average of 100 steps per minute) and the remaining 5000 to "background" daily activity (Tudor-Locke, Hatano, Pangrazi, & Kang, 2008). Research suggests that health benefits begin to accrue at 7500–9999 steps per day (Bravata et al., 2007; Jordan, Jurca, Tudor-Locke, Church, & Blair, 2005; Krum, Dessieux, Andrews, & Thompson, 2006; McKercher et al., 2009; Tudor-Locke et al., 2004, 2008). Increases of approximately 2800 steps on just 3 days a week have produced significant improvements in health outcomes (Church et al., 2009; Church, Earnest, Skinner, & Blair, 2007; Jordan et al., 2005; Martin, Church, Thompson, Earnest, & Blair, 2009). There is also evidence that <5000 steps per day is associated with health risk (Schmidt, Cleland, Shaw, Dwyer, & Venn, 2009).

Recognizing that the "background" levels of activity are likely to be lower for older adults and those with chronic illness, initial goals of 5500 steps per day have been suggested (Tudor-Locke et al., 2011). Even 5500 steps per day may be daunting for individuals who have been inactive. Setting lower initial targets, with the intention of gradual increases in steps over time, may seem more attainable, and lead to greater adherence to activity.

Walking-based interventions have been tested in rheumatic conditions to address symptoms, but not depression. In fibromyalgia, increasing physical activity through a "lifestyle physical activity" intervention (measured by steps/day) led to significant reductions in pain and perceived functional deficits after 12 weeks.(Fontaine et al., 2010) Another study of individuals with fibromyalgia demonstrated that increases of just 1000 steps per day predicted lower pain intensity, pain interference, and depressive symptoms (Kaleth et al., 2013). The author of that study recommended an accumulation of at least 5000 steps per day to reach clinically significant improvements, similar to the goal delineated by Tudor-Locke for adults with chronic illness.

A pedometer-based walking program for older adults with knee OA directed 10 % increases in steps every 4 weeks over 12 weeks and led to improved function, although depression was not measured (Talbot, Gaines, Huynh, & Metter, 2003). Walking ≥6000 steps day was found to protect against developing functional limitations in people with or at risk of knee OA (White et al., 2014). In fact, an analysis from the OAI suggests that if an intervention could move an individual from inactive to even insufficiently active and cost < $2900 over 2 years, it would be considered cost-effective based on quality-adjusted life years (QALYs) (Sun et al., 2014).

Table 13.2 provides some practical guidelines for introducing physical activity.

Summary

Evidence is accruing that exercise-based interventions are effective in preventing and treating depression in the general population (Babyak et al., 2000; Blumenthal et al., 1999, 2007; Conn, 2010; Dunn et al., 2005; Herring et al., 2012;

Table 13.2 Recommending physical activity and exercise for depression in people with arthritis

Type of activity	• There is no clear evidence on what type of exercise is the most beneficial for depression, although the best evidence supports aerobic activity. Aerobic activity can include activities such as walking, biking, or swimming
	• Walking may be the most approachable form of physical activity for currently inactive individuals. However, some individuals may prefer engagement with exercise groups, which can provide both structure and social interactions
	• There is also evidence that resistance exercise may be beneficial for mood. CDC guidelines recommend 2 or more days per week of muscle-strengthening exercise
Frequency	• Frequency should be at least three times per week, although there is some evidence that for depression, the recommendation should be at least five times per week
Duration	• Exercise bouts can be in segments of as little as 10 min. The goal is to accumulate a minimum of 150 min per week
	• New physical activity should be undertaken incrementally. Start with 10 min or so, and gradually increase
Intensity	• Activity should be of at least moderate intensity. Moderate intensity can be gauged using the "talk test." If an individual can talk, but not sing, during the activity, the intensity can be considered of moderate intensity. In vigorous activity, an individual will not be able to say more than a few words without pausing for breath (http://www.cdc.gov/physicalactivity/everyone/measuring/index.html)
Sit less	• "Sit less" is also an important message. Feehan and Westby point out that by standing up twice an hour during the 10 h most people are sitting during a day adds 40 min of light activity (Feehan & Westby, 2014). Other suggestions they provide are standing up and stretching during TV commercials or after a chapter in a book
Other	• Physical activity is safe for people with rheumatic conditions
	• Individuals who are depressed may need extra support in beginning a physical activity program and in maintaining it, at least in the initial stages
	• Pedometers or other activity monitors can serve as useful guides to help quantify activity and monitor progress. They can also serve as motivation. Many new activity monitoring devices include online communities and self-monitoring and motivational tools. Some activity monitors can track exercise other than walking or running
	• Careful selection of walking or other exercise shoes may be necessary for individuals with arthritis. Some individuals may benefit from shoe inserts or orthotics

Hoffman et al., 2011; Rosenberg et al., 2010). The American Psychiatric Association recognizes the importance of exercise as both a complement to traditional depression treatment, and as a first-line intervention for patients who have lower levels of depression and want to try alternatives to pharmaceutical intervention (American Psychiatric Association Work Group on Major Depressive Disorder, 2010). Immediate treatment effects are comparable to existing pharmacotherapy (Blumenthal et al., 2007), and there is some evidence that exercise therapy gains are maintained longer than those from traditional treatment modalities (Babyak et al., 2000; Hoffman et al., 2011). Activity-based interventions may be preferable depression intervention avenues for rheumatic disease for several reasons. Physical activity or exercise addresses the increased burden of obesity and physical inactivity in these conditions, avoids adding to patients' already substantial "pill burden," and provides an alternative to antidepressant medications that may increase cardiovascular risk (Hamer, Batty, Marmot et al., 2011; Hamer, Batty, Seldenrijk, & Kivimäki, 2011). Physical activity also promotes added health benefits with respect to overall functioning and general health beyond mood (e.g., decreased systemic inflammation, decreased fatigue, increased mobility and flexibility, decreased disability, and improved cardiovascular risk). Physical activity has few side effects and can be adapted to individuals' preferences and health status (Eyre et al., 2013). The key issue, particularly for individuals with depression, seems to be motivating patients to initiate and maintain physical activity.

The evidence supporting physical activity as an effective means of reducing cognitive decline, at least among older adults, is also robust. While there is little evidence of the effects of physical activity on cognitive function in rheumatic conditions, observational studies suggest a possible relationship. No treatments currently exist for cognitive impairment in rheumatic conditions, so further exploration of physical activity or exercise interventions may lead to improvements in patient outcomes. Clearly, this is an area where more research is needed.

Overall, physical activity and exercise interventions are safe for individuals with arthritis, and have the potential for improving mood and perhaps avoiding cognitive decline, in addition to well-documented cardiovascular and other health benefits. Even moderate increases in activity can have beneficial effects. While structural and psychological barriers to physical activity uptake exist, the most prominent barrier may be lack of recommendations to engage in physical activity by health professionals.

References

Abad, V. C., Sarinas, P. S., & Guilleminault, C. (2008). Sleep and rheumatologic disorders. *Sleep Medicine Reviews, 12*(3), 211–228.

Abramson, J., & Vaccarino, V. (2002). Relationship between physical activity and inflammation among apparently healthy middle-aged and older US adults. *Archives of Internal Medicine, 162*, 1286–1292.

Ainiala, H., Loukkola, J., Peltola, J., Korpela, M., & Hietaharju, A. (2001). The prevalence of neuropsychiatric syndromes in systemic lupus erythematosus. *Neurology, 57*, 496–500.

Alexopoulos, G., & Morimoto, S. (2011). The inflammation hypothesis in geriatric depression. *International Journal of Geriatric Psychiatry, 26*(11), 1109–1118.

Allison, M., Jensky, N., Marshal, S., Bertoni, A., & Cushman, M. (2012). Sedentary behavior and adiposity-associated inflammation: The multi-ethnic study of atherosclerosis. *American Journal of Preventive Medicine, 42*, 8 13.

American Psychiatric Association Work Group on Major Depressive Disorder. (2010). *Practice guideline for treatment of patients with major depressive disorder*. Retrieved February 10, 2015, from http://psychiatryonline.org/pb/assets/raw/sitewide/practice_guidelines/guidelines/mdd.pdf

Anderson, E., & Shivakumar, G. (2013). Effects of exercise and physical activity on anxiety. *Frontiers in Psychiatry, 4*, 46–49.

Andrzejewski, W., Kassolik, K., Bzozowski, M., & Cymer, K. (2010). The influence of age and physical activity on the pressure sensitivity of soft tissues of the musculoskeletal system. *Journal of Bodywork and Movement Therapies, 14*, 382–390.

Angevaren, M., Aufdemkampe, G., Verhaar, H. J., Aleman, A., & Vanhees, L. (2008). Physical activity and enhanced fitness to improve cognitive function in older people without known cognitive impairment. *Cochrane Database of Systematic Reviews, 3*, CD005381.

Antonchak, M., Saoudian, M., Khan, A., Brunner, H., & Luggen, M. (2011). Cognitive dysfunction in patients with systemic lupus erythematosus: A controlled study. *The Journal of Rheumatology, 38*(6), 1020–1025.

Aparicio, V., Ortega, F., Carbonell-Baeza, A., Camiletti, D., Ruiz, J., & Delgado-Fernandez, M. (2011). Relationship of weight status with mental and physical health in female fibromyalgia patients. *Obesity Facts, 4*, 443–448.

Appenzeller, S., Bertolo, M., & Costallat, L. (2004). Cognitive impairment in rheumatoid arthritis. *Methods and Findings in Experimental and Clinical Pharmacology, 26*, 339–343.

Arend, W. (2001). Mediators of inflammation, tissue destruction, and repair. B. Growth factors and cytokines. In J. Klippel (Ed.), *Primer on the rheumatic diseases* (12th ed.). Atlanta, GA: Arthritis Foundation.

Asztalos, M., De Bourdeaudhuij, I., & Cardon, G. (2010). The relationship between physical activity and mental health varies across activity intensity levels and dimensions of mental health among women and men. *Public Health Nutrition, 13*, 1207–1214.

Autenrieth, C., Schneider, A., Döring, A., Meisinger, C., Herder, C., Koenig, W., ... Thorand, B. (2009). Association between different domains of physical activity and markers of inflammation. *Medicine and Science in Sports and Exercise, 41*, 1706–1713.

Babyak, M., Blumenthal, J., Herman, S., Khatri, P., Doraiswamy, P., Moore, K., ... Krishnan, K. (2000). Exercise treatment for major depression: Maintenance of therapeutic benefit at 10 months. *Psychosomatic Medicine, 62*, 633–638.

Baillet, A., Zeboulon, N., Gossec, L., Combescure, C., Bodin, L., Juvin, R., ... Gaudin, P. (2010). Efficacy of cardiorespiratory aerobic exercise in rheumatoid arthritis: Meta-analysis of randomized controlled trials. *Arthritis Care & Research, 62*, 984–992.

Baker, L., Frank, L., Foster-Schubert, K., Green, P., Wilkinson, C., McTiernan, A., ... Craft, S. (2010). Effects of aerobic exercise on mild cognitive impairment. *Archives of Neurology, 67*, 71–79.

Bankoski, A., Harris, T., McClain, J., Brychta, R., Caserotti, P., Chen, K., ... Koster, A. (2011). Sedentary activity associated with metabolic syndrome independent of physical activity. *Diabetes Care, 34*, 497–503.

Bartolini, M., Candela, M., Brugni, M., Catena, L., Mari, F., Pomponio, G., ... Danieli, G. (2002). Are behaviour and motor performances of rheumatoid arthritis patients influenced by subclinical cognitive impairments? A clinical and neuroimaging study. *Clinical and Experimental Rheumatology, 20*, 491–497.

Benatti, F., & Pedersen, B. (2015). Exercise as an anti-inflammatory therapy for rheumatic diseases—Myokine regulation. *Nature Reviews. Rheumatology, 11*(2), 86–97.

Bennell, K., Dobson, F., & Hinman, R. (2014). Exercise in osteoarthritis: Moving from prescription to adherence. *Best Practice & Research. Clinical Rheumatology, 28*, 93–117.

Bennell, K., & Hinman, R. (2011). A review of the clinical evidence for exercise in osteoarthritis of the hip and knee. *Journal of Science and Medicine in Sport, 14*, 4–9.

Bergman, M., Shahouri, S., Shaver, T., Anderson, J., Weidensaul, D., Busch, R., ... Wolfe, F. (2009). Is fatigue an inflammatory variable in rheumatoid arthritis (RA)? Analyses of fatigue in RA, osteoarthritis, and fibromyalgia. *The Journal of Rheumatology, 36*, 2788–2794.

Bertolucci, P., & de Oliveira, F. (2013). Cognitive impairment in fibromyalgia. *Current Pain and Headache Reports, 17*, 344.

Bilberg, A., Ahlmén, M., & Mannerkorpi, K. (2005). Moderately intensive exercise in a temperate pool for patients with rheumatoid arthritis: A randomized controlled study. *Rheumatology, 44*, 502–508.

Blumenthal, J., Babyak, M., Doraiswamy, P., Watkins, L., Hoffman, B., Barbour, K., ... Sherwood, A. (2007). Exercise and pharmacotherapy in the treatment of major depressive disorder. *Psychosomatic Medicine, 69*, 587–596.

Blumenthal, J., Babyak, M., Moore, K., Craighead, W., Herman, S., Khatri, P., ... Krishnan, K. (1999). Effects of exercise training on older patients with major depression. *Archives of Internal Medicine, 159*, 2349–2356.

Bravata, D., Smith-Spangler, C., Sundaram, V., Gienger, A., Lin, N., Lewis, R., ... Sirard, J. (2007). Using pedometers to increase physical activity and improve health: A systematic review. *Journal of the American Medical Association, 298*, 2296–2304.

Brey, R., Holliday, S., Saklad, A., Navarrete, M., Hermosillo-Romo, D., Stallworth, C., ... McGlasson, D. (2002). Neuropsychiatric syndrome in lupus: Prevalence using standardized definitions. *Neurology, 58*, 1214–1220.

Brophy, S., Cooksey, R., Davies, H., Dennis, M., Zhou, S., & Siebert, S. (2013). The effect of physical activity and motivation on function in ankylosing spondylitis: A cohort study. *Seminars in Arthritis and Rheumatism, 42*, 619–626.

Brophy, S., Davies, H., Dennis, M., Cooksey, R., Husain, M., Irvine, E., & Siebert, S. (2013). Fatigue in ankylosing spondylitis: Treatment should focus on pain management. *Seminars in Arthritis and Rheumatism, 42*, 361–367.

Brown, W., Trost, S., Bauman, A., Mummery, K., & Owen, N. (2004). Test-retest reliability of four physical activity measures used in population surveys. *Journal of Science and Medicine in Sport, 7*, 205–215.

Bruundsgaard, H. (2005). Physical activity and modulation of systemic low-level inflammation. *Journal of Leukocyte Biology, 78*, 819–835.

Burzynska, A., Chaddock-Heyman, L., Voss, M., Wong, C., Gothe, N., Olson, E., ... Kramer, A. (2014). Physical activity and cardiorespiratory fitness are beneficial for white matter in low-fit older adults. *PLoS One, 9*, e107413.

Callahan, L., Mielenz, T., Freburger, J., Shreffler, J., Hootman, J., Brady, T., ... Schwartz, T. (2008). A randomized controlled trial of the people with arthritis can exercise programs: Symptoms, function, physical activity, and psychosocial outcomes. *Arthritis Care & Research, 59*, 92–101.

Callahan, L., Shreffler, J., Altpeter, M., Schoster, B., Hootman, J., Houenou, L., … Schwartz, T. (2011). Evaluation of group and self-directed formats of the Arthritis Foundations walk with ease program. *Arthritis Care & Research, 63*, 1098–1107.

Church, T., Earnest, C., Skinner, J., & Blair, S. (2007). Effects of different doses of physical activity on cardiorespiratory fitness among sedentary, overweight, or obese postmenopausal women with elevated blood pressure: A randomized controlled trial. *Journal of the American Medical Association, 297*, 2081–2091.

Church, T., Martin, C., Thompson, A., Earnest, C., Mikus, C., & Blair, S. (2009). Changes in weight, waist circumference and compensatory responses with different doses of exercise among sedentary, overweight postmenopausal women. *PLoS One, 4*, e4515.

Clauw, D. (2014). Fibromyalgia: A clinical review. *Journal of the American Medical Association, 311*, 1547–1555.

Colbert, L., Visser, M., Simonsick, E., Tracy, R., Newman, A., Kritchevsky, S., … Harris, T. (2004). Physical activity, exercise, and inflammatory markers in older adults: Findings from the health, aging, and body composition study. *Journal of American Geriatrics Society, 52*(7), 1098–1104.

Colcombe, S., & Kramer, A. (2003). Fitness effects on the cognitive function of older adults: A meta-analytic study. *Psychological Science, 14*, 125–130.

Conn, V. (2010). Depressive symptom outcomes of physical activity interventions: Meta-analysis findings. *Annals of Behavioral Medicine, 39*, 128–138.

Conn, V., Hafdahl, A., Minor, M., & Nielsen, P. (2008). Physical activity interventions among adults with arthritis: Meta-analysis of outcomes. *Seminars in Arthritis and Rheumatism, 37*, 307–316.

Cooney, G., Dwan, K., Greig, C., Lawlor, D., Rimer, J., Waugh, F., … Mead, G. (2013). Exercise for depression. *Cochrane Database Systematic Review*, Issue 9. Art. No. CD004366.

Cooney, G., Dwan, K., & Mead, G. (2014). Exercise for depression. *Journal of the American Medical Association, 311*, 2432–2433.

Copeland, W., Shanahan, L., Worthman, C., Angold, A., & Costello, E. (2012). Cumulative depression episodes predict later C-reactive protein levels: A prospective analysis. *Biological Psychiatry, 71*, 15–21.

Coppack, S. (2001). Pro-inflammatory cytokines and adipose tissue. *Proceedings of the Nutrition Society, 60*, 349–356.

Craig, C., Marshall, A., Sjöström, M., Bauman, A., Booth, M., Ainsworth, B., … Oja, P. (2003). International physical activity questionnaire: 12-country reliability and validity. *Medicine and Science in Sports and Exercise, 35*, 1381–1395.

Cramp, F., Hewlett, S., Almeida, C., Kirwan, K., Choy, E., Chalder, T., … Christensen, R. (2013). Non-pharmacological interventions for RA fatigue. *Cochrane Database of Systematic Reviews*, (8).

Cuperus, N., Hoogeboom, T., Neijland, Y., van den Ende, C., & Keijsers, N. (2012). Are people with rheumatoid arthritis who undertake activity pacing at risk of being too physically inactive? *Clinical Rehabilitation, 26*, 1048–1052.

Daly, M., McMinn, D., & Allan, J. (2015). A bidirectional relationship between physical activity and executive function in older adults. *Frontiers in Human Neuroscience, 13*, 1044.

Dantzer, R., O'Connor, J., Freund, G., Johnson, R., & Kelley, K. (2008). From inflammation to sickness and depression: When the immune system subjugates the brain. *Nature Reviews Neuroscience, 9*, 46–57.

de Wit, L., Fokkema, M., van Straten, A., Lamers, F., Cuijpers, P., & Penninx, B. (2010). Depressive and anxiety disorders and the association with obesity, physical, and social activities. *Depression and Anxiety, 27*, 1057–1065.

Demmelmaier, I., Lindkvist, A., Nordgren, B., & Opava, C. (2015). "A gift from heaven" or "this was not for me." A mixed methods approach to describe experiences of participation in an outsourced physical activity program for persons with rheumatoid arthritis. *Clinical Rheumatology, 34*(3), 429–439.

Denburg, S., Carbotte, R., & Denburg, J. (1997). Psychological aspects of systemic lupus erythematosus: Cognitive function, mood, and self-report. *The Journal of Rheumatology, 24*, 998–1003.

Do, B., Hootman, J., Helmick, C., & Brady, T. (2011). Monitoring health people 2010 arthritis management objectives: Education and clinician counseling for weight loss and exercise. *Annals of Family Medicine, 9*, 136–141.

Dugan, S., Bromberger, J., Segawa, E., Avery, E., & Sternfeld, B. (2015). Association between physical activity and depressive symptoms: Midlife women in SWAN. *Medicine and Science in Sports and Exercise, 47*, 335–342.

Dunlop, D., Song, J., Semanik, P., Sharma, L., Bathon, J., Eaton, C., … Chang, R. (2014). Relation of physical activity time to incident disability in community dwelling adults with or at risk of knee arthritis: Prospective cohort study. *British Medical Journal, 348*, g2472.

Dunn, A., Trivedi, M., Kampert, J., Clark, C., & Chambliss, H. (2005). Exercise treatment for depression: Efficacy and dose response. *American Journal of Preventive Medicine, 28*, 1–8.

Durcan, L., Wilson, F., & Cunnane, G. (2014). The effect of exercise on sleep and fatigue in rheumatoid arthritis: A randomized controlled study. *The Journal of Rheumatology, 41*, 1966–1973.

Elavsky, S., & McAuley, E. (2007). Physical activity and mental health outcomes during menopause: A randomized controlled trial. *Annals of Behavioral Medicine, 33*, 132–142.

Ellingson, L., Colbert, L., & Cook, D. (2012). Physical activity is related to pain sensitivity in healthy women. *Medicine and Science in Sports and Exercise, 44*, 1401–1406.

Ellingson, L., Shields, M., Stegner, A., & Cook, D. (2012). Physical activity, sustained sedentary behavior, and pain modulation in women with fibromyalgia. *The Journal of Pain, 13*, 195–206.

Etgen, T., Sander, D., Huntgeburth, U., Poppert, H., Först, H., & Bickel, H. (2010). Physical activity and incident cognitive impairment in elderly persons. *Archives of Internal Medicine, 170*, 186–193.

Etnier, J., Karper, W., Gapin, J., Barella, L., Chang, Y., & Murphy, K. (2009). Exercise, fibromyalgia, and fibrofog: A pilot study. *Journal of Physical Activity and Health, 6*, 239–246.

Eyre, H., Papps, E., & Baune, B. (2013). Treating depression and depression-like behavior with physical activity: An immune perspective. *Frontiers in Psychiatry, 4*, 1–27.

Feehan, L., & Westby, M. (2014). Exercise more and sit less: Two important health and lifestyle messages for people living with RA. *The Rheumatologist, 8*(1), 51–57.

Fontaine, K., Conn, L., & Clauw, D. (2010). Effects of lifestyle physical activity on perceived symptoms and physical function in adults with fibromyalgia: Results of a randomized trial. *Arthritis Research & Therapy, 12*, R55.

Ford, E. (2002). Does exercise reduce inflammation? Physical activity and C-reactive protein among US adults. *Epidemiology, 13*, 561–568.

Fries, J., Spitz, P., Kraines, R., & Holman, H. (1980). Measurement of patient outcome in arthritis. *Arthritis and Rheumatism, 23*, 137–145.

Froneck, M., & Horowitz, D. (2002). Cytokines in the pathogenesis of systemic lupus erythematosus. In D. Wallace & B. Hahn (Eds.), *Dubois' lupus erythematosus* (6th ed.). Philadelphia, PA: Lippincott Williams & Wilkins.

Giles, J., Bartlett, S., Andersen, R., Thompson, R., Fontaine, K., & Bathon, J. (2008). Association of body fat with C-reactive protein in rheumatoid arthritis. *Arthritis and Rheumatism, 58*, 2632–2641.

Glass, J. (2009). Review of cognitive dysfunction in fibromyalgia: A convergence on working memory and attentional control impairments. *Rheumatic Diseases Clinics of North America, 35*, 299–311.

Goesling, J., Clauw, D., & Hassett, A. (2013). Pain and depression: An integrative review of neurobiological and psychological factors. *Current Psychiatry Reports, 15*, 421.

Gyurcsik, N., Cary, M., Sessford, J., Flora, P., & Brawley, L. (2015). Pain anxiety and negative outcome expectations for activity: Do negative psychological profiles differ between the inactive and active? *Arthritis Care & Research, 67*, 58–64.

Hakkinen, A., Sokka, T., Leitsalmi, A., Kautianinen, H., & Hannonen, P. (2003). Effects of dynamic strength training on physical function, Valpar 9 work sample test, and working capacity in patients with recent-onset rheumatoid arthritis. *Arthritis Care & Research, 49*, 71–77.

Hamer, M., Batty, G., Marmot, M., Singh-Manoux, A., & Kivimäki, M. (2011). Anti-depressant medication use and C-reactive protein: Results from two population-based studies. *Brain, Behavior, and Immunity, 25*, 168–173.

Hamer, M., Batty, G., Seldenrijk, A., & Kivimäki, M. (2011). Antidepressant medication use and future risk of cardiovascular disease: The Scottish Health Survey. *European Heart Journal, 32*, 437–442.

Hanly, J., Fisk, J., McCurdy, G., Fougere, L., & Douglas, J. (2005). Neuropsychiatric syndromes in patients with systemic lupus erythematosus and rheumatoid arthritis. *The Journal of Rheumatology, 32*, 1459–1466.

Harrington, D., Barreira, T., Staiano, A., & Katzmarzyk, P. (2014). The descriptive epidemiology of sitting among US adults, NHANES 2009/2010. *Journal of Science and Medicine in Sport, 17*, 371–375.

Hekler, E., Castro, C., Buman, M., & King, A. (2012). The CHOICE study: A "taste-test" of utilitarian vs. leisure walking among older adults. *Health Psychology, 31*, 126–129.

Herring, M., Puetz, T., O'Connor, P., & Dishman, R. (2012). Effect of exercise training on depressive symptoms among patients with chronic illness: A systematic review and meta-analysis of randomized controlled trials. *Archives of Internal Medicine, 172*, 101–111.

Hochberg, M., Altman, R., April, K., Benkhalti, M., Guyatt, G., McGowan, J., … Tugwell, P. (2012). American College of Rheumatology 2012 recommendations for the use of nonpharmacologic and pharmacologic therapies in osteoarthritis of the hand, hip, and knee. *Arthritis Care & Research, 64*, 465–474.

Hoffman, B., Babyak, M., Chambliss, H., Sherwood, A., Doraiswamy, P., Coons, M., & Blumenthal, J. (2011). Exercise and pharmacotherapy in patients with major depression: One-year follow-up of the SMILE study. *Psychosomatic Medicine, 73*, 127–133.

Huang, C., Zourdos, M., Jo, E., & Ormsbee, M. (2013). Influence of physical activity and nutrition on obesity-related immune function. *Scientific World Journal, 2013*, 752071.

Hurkmans, E., de Gucht, V., Maes, S., Peeters, A., Ronday, H., & Vliet Vlieland, T. (2011). Promoting physical activity in patients with rheumatoid arthritis: Rheumatologists' and health professionals' practice and educational needs. *Clinical Rheumatology, 30*, 1603–1609.

Hurkmans, E., van der Giesen, F., Vliet Vlieland, T., Schoones, J., & Van den Ende, E. (2009). Dynamic exercise programs (aerobic capacity and/or muscle strength training) in patients with rheumatoid arthritis. *Cochrane Database of Systematic Reviews, 7*, CD006853.

Irwin, M., Olmstead, R., Carrillo, C., Sadeghi, N., Fitzgerald, J., Ranganath, V., & Nicassio, P. (2012). Sleep loss exacerbates fatigue, depression, and pain in rheumatoid arthritis. *Sleep, 35*, 537–543.

Iversen, M., Brawerman, M., & Iversen, C. (2012). Recommendations and the state of the evidence for physical activity interventions for adults with rheumatoid arthritis: 2007 to present. *International Journal of Clinical Rheumatology, 7*, 489–503.

Jordan, A., Jurca, G., Tudor-Locke, C., Church, T., & Blair, S. (2005). Pedometer indices for weekly physical activity recommendations in postmenopausal women. *Medicine and Science in Sports and Exercise, 37*, 1627–1632.

Julian, L., Gregorich, S., Tonner, C., Yazdany, J., Trupin, L., Criswell, L., … Katz, P. (2011). Using the Center for Epidemiologic Studies Depression scale to screen for depression in systemic lupus erythematosus. *Arthritis Care & Research, 63*, 884–890.

Julian, L., Yazdany, J., Trupin, L., Criswell, L., Yelin, E., & Katz, P. (2012). Validity of brief screening tools for cognitive impairment in RA and SLE. *Arthritis Care & Research, 64*, 448–454.

Kaleth, A., Saha, C., Jensen, M., Slaven, J., & Ang, D. (2013). Effect of moderate to vigorous physical activity on long-term clinical outcomes and pain severity in fibromyalgia. *Arthritis Care & Research, 65*, 1211–1218.

Kaleth, A., Slaven, J., & Ang, D. (2014). Does increasing steps per day predict improvement in physical function and pain interference in adults with fibromyalgia? *Arthritis Care & Research, 66*, 1887–1894.

Kaptein, S., Backman, C., Badley, E., Lacaille, D., Beaton, D., Hofstetter, C., & Gignac, M. (2013). Choosing where to put your energy: A qualitative analysis of the role of physical activity in the lives of working adults with arthritis. *Arthritis Care & Research, 65*, 1070–1076.

Katz, P., Gregorich, S., Yazdany, J., Trupin, L., Julian, L., Yelin, E., & Criswell, L. A. (2011). Obesity and its measurement in a community-based sample of women with systemic lupus erythematosus. *Arthritis Care & Research (Hoboken), 63*(2), 261–268.

Katz, P., Julian, L., Tonner, M., Yazdany, J., Trupin, L., Yelin, E., & Criswell, L. (2012). Physical activity, obesity, and cognitive impairment among women with systemic lupus erythematosus. *Arthritis Care & Research, 64*, 502–510.

Katz, P., Morris, A., & Yelin, E. (2006). Prevalence and predictors of disability in valued life activities among individuals with rheumatoid arthritis. *Annals of the Rheumatic Diseases, 65*, 763–769.

Katz, P., Radvanski, D., Allen, D., Buyske, S., Schiff, S., Nadkarni, A., … Hassett, A. (2011). Development and validation of a short form of the valued life activities disability questionnaire for rheumatoid arthritis. *Arthritis Care & Research, 63*, 1664–1671.

Katz, P., Rush, S., Trupin, L., Barton, J., Schmaju, G., Yazdany, J., … Margaretten, M. (2014). *Obesity is a risk factor for depression in systemic lupus erythematosus (SLE)*. Boston, MA: American College of Rheumatology.

Katz, P., Yazdany, J., Trupin, L., Schmajuk, G., Margaretten, M., Criswell, L., & Yelin, E. (2013). Sex differences in assessment of obesity in rheumatoid arthritis. *Arthritis Care & Research, 65*, 62–70.

Katz, P., & Yelin, E. (1995). The development of depressive symptoms among women with rheumatoid arthritis. *Arthritis and Rheumatism, 38*, 49–56.

Katz, P., & Yelin, E. (2001). Activity loss and the onset of depressive symptoms: Do some activities matter more than others? *Arthritis and Rheumatism, 44*, 1194–1202.

Kelley, G., Kelley, K., & Hootman, J. (2015). Effects of exercise on depression in adults with arthritis: A systematic review with meta-analysis of randomized controlled trials. *Arthritis Research & Therapy, 17*, 21.

Kim, C., Luedtke, C., Vincent, A., Thompson, J., & Oh, T. (2012). Association of body mass index with symptoms severity and quality of life in patients with fibromylagia. *Arthritis Care & Research, 64*, 222–228.

Kozora, E., Hanly, J. G., Lapteva, L., & Filley, C. M. (2008). Cognitive dysfunction in systemic lupus erythematosus: Past, present, and future. *Arthritis & Rheumatism, 58*(11), 3286–3298.

Kozora, E., Thompson, L., West, S., & Kotzin, B. (1996). Analysis of cognitive and psychological deficits in systemic lupus erythematosus patients without overt central nervous system disease. *Arthritis and Rheumatism, 39*, 2035–2045.

Kozora, E., Zell, J., Swigris, J., Strand, M., Duggan, E., Burleson, A., & Make, B. (2015). Cardiopulmonary correlates for cognition in systemic lupus erythematosus. *Lupus, 24*, 164–173.

Kravitz, H., & Katz, R. (2015). Fibrofog and fibromyalgia: A narrative review and implications for clinical practice. *Rheumatology International, 35*(7), 1115–1125.

Krisknadas, R., & Cavanagh, J. (2012). Depression: An inflammatory illness? *Journal of Neurology, Neurosurgery & Psychiatry, 83*, 495–502.

Kroenke, C., Wu, J., Bair, M., Krebs, E., Damush, T., & Tu, W. (2011). Reciprocal relationship between pain and depression: A 12-month longitudinal analysis in primary care. *The Journal of Pain, 12*, 964–973.

Krum, E., Dessieux, O., Andrews, P., & Thompson, D. (2006). The relationship between daily steps and body composition in postmenopausal women. *Journal of Women's Health, 15*, 202–210.

Lambiasse, M., Gabriel, K., Kuller, H., & Matthews, K. (2013). Temporal relationships between physical activity and sleep in older women. *Medicine and Science in Sports and Exercise, 45*, 2362–2368.

Lavie, C., Church, T., Milani, R., & Earnest, C. (2011). Impact of physical activity, cardiorespiratory fitness, and exercise training on markers of inflammation. *Journal of Cardiopulmonary Rehabilitation and Prevention, 31*, 137–145.

Law, R., Markland, D., Jones, J., Maddison, P., & Thom, J. (2013). Perceptions of issues relating to exercise and joint health in rheumatoid arthritis: A UK-based questionnaires study. *Musculoskeletal Care, 11*(3), 147–158.

Lee, J., Chang, R., Erhlich-Jones, L., Kwoh, C., Nevitt, M., Semanik, P., … Dunlop, D. (2015). Sedentary behavior and physical function: Objective evidence from the osteoarthritis initiative. *Arthritis Care Res (Hoboken), 67*(3), 366–373.

Lee, J., Dunlop, D., Ehrlich-Jones, L., Semanik, P., Manheim, L., & Chang, R. (2012). Public health impact of risk factors for physical inactivity in adults with rheumatoid arthritis. *Arthritis Care & Research, 64*, 488–493.

Leonard, B. (2010). The concept of depression as a dysfunction of the immune system. *Current Immunology Reviews, 6*(3), 205–212.

Levy, S., Macera, C., Hootman, J., Coleman, K., Lopez, R., Nichols, J., … Ji, M. (2012). Evaluation of a multicomponent group exercise program for adults with arthritis: Fitness and exercise with arthritis (FEPA). *Disability and Health Journal, 5*, 305–311.

Loeppenthin, K., Esbensen, B., Ostergaard, M., Jennum, P., Thomsen, T., & Midtgaard, J. (2014). Physical activity maintenance in patients with rheumatoid arthritis: A qualitative study. *Clinical Rehabilitation, 28*, 289–299.

Loprinzi, P., & Beets, M. (2014). Need for increased promotion of physical activity by health care professionals. *Preventive Medicine, 69*, 75–79.

Lotrich, F., El-Gabalawy, H., Guenther, L., & Ware, C. (2011). The role of inflammation in the pathophysiology of depression: Different treatments and their effects. *The Journal of Rheumatology, 38*(Suppl 88), 48–54.

Luppino, F., de Wit, L., Bouvy, P., Stijnen, T., Cuijpers, P., Penninx, B., & Zitman, F. (2010). Overweight, obesity, and depression: A systematic review and meta-analysis of longitudinal studies. *Archives of General Psychiatry, 67*, 220–229.

Luyster, F., Chasens, E., Wasko, M., & Dunbar-Jacob, J. (2011). Sleep quality and functional disability in patients with rheumatoid arthritis. *Journal of Clinical Sleep Medicine, 7*, 49–55.

Maes, M. (2011). Depression is an inflammatory disease, but cell-mediated immune activation is the key component of depression. *Progress in Neuro-Psychopharmacology & Biological Psychiatry, 35*(3), 664–675.

Mancuso, C., Perna, M., Sargent, A., & Salmon, J. (2011). Perceptions and measurements of physical activity in patients with systemic lupus erythematosus. *Lupus, 20*, 231–242.

Mancuso, C., Rincon, M., Sayles, W., & Paget, S. (2007). Comparison of energy expenditure from lifestyle physical activities between patients with rheumatoid arthritis and healthy controls. *Arthritis & Rheumatology, 57*, 672–678.

Martin, C., Church, T., Thompson, A., Earnest, C., & Blair, S. (2009). Exercise dose and quality of life: A randomized controlled trial. *Archives of Internal Medicine, 169*, 269–278.

Matheny, M., Miller, R., Shardell, M., Hawkes, W., Lenze, E., Magaziner, J., & Orwig, D. (2011). Inflammatory cytokine levels and depressive symptoms in older women in the year after hip fracture: Findings from the Baltimore Hip Studies. *Journal of the American Geriatrics Society, 59*, 2249–2255.

Matthews, C., George, S., Moore, S., Bowles, H., Blair, A., Park, Y., … Schatzkin, A. (2012). Amount of time spend in sedentary behaviors and cause-specfic mortality in US adults. *American Journal of Clinical Nutrition, 95*, 437–445.

McBeth, J., Prescott, G., Scotland, G., Lovell, K., Keeley, P., Hannaford, P., … Macfarlane, G. (2012). Cognitive behavior therapy, exercise, or both for treating chronic widespread pain. *Archives of Internal Medicine, 172*, 48–57.

McKercher, C., Schmidt, M., Sanderson, K., Patton, G., Dwyer, T., & Venn, A. (2009). Physical activity and depression in young adults. *American Journal of Preventive Medicine, 36*, 161–164.

McLoughlin, M., Stegner, A., & Cook, D. (2011). The relationship between physical activity and brain responses to pain in fibromyalgia. *The Journal of Pain, 12*, 640–651.

Middleton, L., Manini, T., Simonsick, E., Harris, T., Barnes, D., Tylavsky, F., … Yaffe, K. (2011). Activity energy expenditure and incident cognitive impairment in older adults. *Archives of Internal Medicine, 171*, 1251–1257.

Miller, A., Maletic, V., & Raison, C. (2009). Inflammation and its discontents: The role of cytokines in the pathophysiology of major depression. *Biological Psychiatry, 65*, 732–741.

Minor, M. (2004). Impact of exercise on osteoarthritis outcomes. *The Journal of Rheumatology, 70*, 81–86.

Munguia-Izquierdo, D., & Legaz-Arrese, A. (2007). Exercise in warm water decreases pain and improves cognitive function in middle-aged women with fibromyalgia. *Clinical and Experimental Rheumatology, 25*, 823–830.

Murphy, S., Alexander, N., Levoska, M., & Smith, D. (2013). The relationship between fatigue and subsequent physical activity among older adults with symptomatic osteoarthritis. *Arthritis Care & Research, 65*, 1617–1624.

Murphy, S., & Kratz, A. (2014). Activity pacing in daily life: A within-day analysis. *Pain, 155*, 2630–2637.

Neill, J., Belan, I., & Ried, K. (2006). Effectiveness of non-pharmacological interventions for fatigue in adults with multiple sclerosis, rheumatoid arthritis, or systemic lupus erythematosus: A systematic review. *Journal of Advanced Nursing, 56*, 617–635.

Neuberger, G., Aaronson, L., Gajewski, B., Embretson, S., Cagle, P., Loudon, J., & Miller, P. (2007). Predictors of exercise and effects of exercise on symptoms, function, aerobic fitness, and disease outcomes in rheumatoid arthritis. *Arthritis Care & Research, 57*, 943–952.

Nicassio, P., Ormseth, S., Kay, M., Custodio, M., Irwin, M., Olmstead, R., & Weisman, M. (2012). The contribution of pain and depression to self-reported sleep disturbance in patients with rheumatoid arthritis. *Pain, 153*, 107–112.

Nicassio, P., & Wallston, K. (1992). Longitudinal relationships among pain, sleep problems, and depression in rheumatoid arthritis. *Journal of Abnormal Psychology, 101*, 514–520.

Nikolaus, S., Bode, C., Taal, E., & van de Laar, M. (2013). Fatigue and factors related to fatigue in rheumatoid arthritis: A systematic review. *Arthritis Care & Research, 65*, 1128–1146.

Nyrop, K., Charnock, B., Martin, K., Lias, J., Altpeter, M., & Callahan, L. (2011). Effect of a six-week walking program on work place activity limitations among adults with arthritis. *Arthritis Care & Research, 63*, 1773–1776.

O'Donnell, S., Rusu, C., Bernatsky, S., Hawker, G., Canizares, M., Mackay, C., & Badley, E. (2013).

Exercise/physical activity and weight management efforts in Canadians with self-reported arthritis. *Arthritis Care & Research, 65*, 2015–2023.

Owen, N., Healy, G., Matthews, C., & Dunstan, D. (2010). Too much sitting: The population health science of sedentary behavior. *Exercise and Sport Sciences Reviews, 38*, 105–113.

Owen, N., Sparling, P., Healy, G., Dunstan, D., & Matthews, C. (2010). Sedentary behavior: Emerging evidence for a new health risk. *Mayo Clinic Proceedings, 85*, 1138–1141.

Palagini, L., Tani, C., Mauri, M., Carli, L., Vagnani, S., Bombardieri, S., … Mosca, M. (2014). Sleep disorders and systemic lupus erythematosus. *Lupus, 23*, 115–123.

Pasco, J., Nicholson, G., Williams, L., Jacka, F., Henry, M., Kotowicz, M., … Berk, M. (2010). Association of high-sensitivity C-reactive protein with de novo major depression. *The British Journal of Psychiatry, 197*, 372–377.

Pate, R., O'Neill, J., & Lobelo, F. (2008). The evolving definition of "sedentary". *Exercise and Sport Sciences Reviews, 36*, 173–178.

Petri, M., Nagibuddin, M., Carson, K., Sampedro, M., Wallace, D., Weisman, M., … Brey, R. (2008). Cognitive function in a systemic lupus erythematosus inception cohort. *The Journal of Rheumatology, 35*, 1776–1781.

Poole, L., Steptoe, A., Wawrzyniak, A., Bostock, S., Mitchell, E., & Hamer, M. (2011). Associations of objectively measured physical activity with daily mood ratings and psychophysiological stress responses in women. *Psychophysiology, 48*(8), 1165–1172.

Prakash, R., Voss, M., Erickson, K., & Kramer, A. (2015). Physical activity and cognitive vitality. *Annual Review of Psychology, 66*, 769–797.

Prather, A., Rabinovitz, M., Pollock, B., & Lotrich, F. (2009). Cytokine induced depression during IFN-α treatment: The role of IL-6 and sleep quality. *Brain, Behavior, and Immunity, 23*, 1109–1116.

Raedler, T. (2011). Inflammatory mechanisms in major depressive disorder. *Current Opinion in Psychiatry, 24*, 519–525.

Raison, C., Capuron, L., & Miller, A. (2006). Cytokines sing the blues: Inflammation and the pathogenesis of depression. *Trends in Immunology, 27*, 24–31.

Raison, C., & Miller, A. (2011). Is depression an inflammatory disorder? *Current Psychiatry Reports, 13*, 467–475.

Reading, S., Crowson, C., Rodeheffer, R., Fitz-Gibbon, P., Maradit-Kremers, H., & Gabriel, S. (2009). Do rheumatoid arthritis patients have a higher risk for sleep apnea? *The Journal of Rheumatology, 36*, 1869–1872.

Rethorst, C., Sunderajan, P., Greer, T., Grannemann, B., Nakonezny, P., Carmody, T., & Trivedi, M. (2013). Does exercise improve self-reported sleep quality in non-remitted major depressive disorder? *Psychological Medicine, 43*, 699–709.

Reuben, D., Judd-Hamilton, L., Harris, T., & Seeman, T. (2003). The associations between physical activity and inflammation markers in high-functioning older persons: MacArthur studies of successful aging. *Journal of American Geriatrics Society, 51*, 1125–1130.

Rivenes, A., Harvey, S., & Mykletun, A. (2009). The relationship between abdominal fat, obesity, and common mental disorders: Results from the HUNT study. *Journal of Psychosomatic Research, 66*, 269–275.

Robertson, R., Robertson, A., Jepson, R., & Maxwell, M. (2012). Walking for depression or depressive symptoms: A systematic review. *Mental Health and Physical Activity, 5*, 66–75.

Roehrs, T., Diederichs, C., Gillis, M., Burger, A., Stout, R., Lumley, M., & Roth, T. (2013). Nocturnal sleep, daytime sleepiness and fatigue in fibromyalgia patients compared to rheumatoid arthritis patients and healthy controls: A preliminary study. *Sleep Medicine, 14*, 109–115.

Rongen-van Dartel, S., Repping-Wuts, J., van Hoogmoed, D., Knoop, H., Bleijenberg, G., van Riel, P., & Fransen, J. (2014). Relationship between objectively assessed physical activity and fatigue in patients with rheumatoid arthritis: Inverse correlation of activity and fatigue. *Arthritis Care & Research, 66*, 852–860.

Rosenberg, D., Depp, C. A., Vahia, I. V., Reichstadt, J., Palmer, B. W., Kerr, J., … Jeste, D. V. (2010). Exergames for subsyndromal depression in older adults: A pilot study of a novel intervention. *American Journal of Geriatric Psychiatry, 18*(3), 221–226.

Rovio, S., Spulber, G., Niemen, L., Niskanen, E., Winblad, B., Tuomilheto, J., … Kivipelto, M. (2010). The effect of midlife physical activity on structural brain changes in the elderly. *Neurobiology of Aging, 31*, 1927–1936.

Schlenk, E., Lias, J., Sereika, S., Dunbar-Jacob, J., & Kwoh, C. (2011). Improving physical activity and function in overweight and obese older adults with osteoarthritis of the knee: A feasibility study. *Rehabilitation Nursing, 36*, 32–42.

Schmidt, M., Cleland, V., Shaw, K., Dwyer, T., & Venn, A. (2009). Cardiometabolic risk in younger and older adults across an index of ambulatory activity. *American Journal of Preventive Medicine, 37*, 278–284.

Segura-Jimenez, V., Aparicio, V., Alvarez-Gallardo, I., Carbonell-Baeza, A., Tornero-Quinones, I., & Delgado-Fernandez, M. (2015). Does body composition differ between fibromyalgia patients and controls? The Al-Andalus project. *Clinical and Experimental Rheumatology, 33*(1 Suppl 88), S25–S32.

Semanik, P., Wilbur, J., Sinacore, J., & Chang, R. (2004). Physical activity behavior in older women with rheumatoid arthritis. *Arthritis & Rheumatology, 51*, 246–252.

Shaffer, J., Edmondson, D., Chaplin, W., Schwartz, J., Shimbo, D., Burg, M., … Davidson, K. (2011). Directionality of the relationship between depressive symptoms and C-reactive protein in patients with acute coronary syndromes. *Psychosomatic Medicine, 73*, 370–377.

Shanely, R., Nieman, D., Henson, D., Jin, F., Knab, A., & Sha, W. (2013). Inflammation and oxidative stress are lower in physically fit and active adults. *Scandinavian Journal of Medicine & Science in Sports, 23*, 21–23.

Shelton, R., & Miller, A. (2010). Eating ourselves to death (and despair): The contribution of adiposity and inflammation to depression. *Progress in Neurobiology, 91*, 275–299.

Shelton, R., & Miller, A. (2011). Inflammation in depression: Is adiposity a cause? *Dialogues in Clinical Neuroscience, 13*, 41–54.

Shin, S., Julian, L., Katz, P., & Wallhagen, M. (2011). Cognitive impairment in persons with rheumatoid arthritis. *Arthritis and Rheumatism, 63*(10 Suppl), S975.

Sieverdes, J., Ray, B., Sui, X., Lee, D., Hand, G., Baruth, M., & Blair, S. (2012). Association between leisure time physical activity and depressive symptoms in men. *Medicine and Science in Sports and Exercise, 44*, 260–265.

Simon, G., Von Korff, M., Saunders, K., Miglioretti, D., Crane, P., Van Belle, G., & Kessles, R. (2006). Association between obesity and psychiatric disorders in the US adult population. *Archives of General Psychiatry, 63*, 824–830.

Smith, P., Blumenthal, J., Hoffman, B., Cooper, H., Strauman, T., Welsh-Bohner, K., … Sherwood, A. (2010). Aerobic exercise and neurocognitive performance: A meta-analytic review of randomized controlled trials. *Psychosomatic Medicine, 72*, 239–252.

Sofi, F., Valecchi, D., Bacci, D., Abbate, R., Gensini, G., Casini, A., & Macchi, C. (2011). Physical activity and risk of cognitive decline: A meta-analysis of prospective studies. *Journal of Internal Medicine, 269*, 107–117.

Sokka, T., Häkkinen, A., Kautiainen, H., Maillefert, J., Toloza, S., Mørk Hansen, T., … QUEST-RA Group. (2008). Physical inactivity in patients with rheumatoid arthritis: Data from twenty-one countries in a cross-sectional, international study. *Arthritis & Rheumatology, 59*, 42–50.

Stanton, R., & Reaburn, P. (2014). Exercise and the treatment of depression: A review of the exercise program variables. *Journal of Science and Medicine in Sport, 17*, 177–182.

Stenstrom, C., & Minor, M. (2003). Evidence for the benefit of aerobic and strengthening exercise in rheumatoid arthritis. *Arthritis & Rheumatology, 49*, 428–434.

Sterling, K., Gallop, K., Swinburn, P., Flood, E., French, A., Al Sawah, S., … Nixon, A. (2014). Patient-reported fatigue and its impact on patients with systemic lupus erythematosus. *Lupus, 23*, 124–132.

Stewart, J., Rand, K., Mudoon, M., & Kamarck, T. (2009). A prospective evaluation of the directionality of the depression-inflammation relationship. *Brain, Behavior, and Immunity, 23*, 936–944.

Sturner, T., Gunther, K., & Brenner, H. (2000). Obesity, overweight and patterns of osteoarthritis: The Ulm Osteoarthritis Study. *Journal of Clinical Epidemiology, 53*, 307–313.

Sugden, J., Sniehotta, F., Donnan, P., Boyle, P., Johnston, D., & McMurdo, M. (2008). The feasibility of using pedometers and brief advice to increase activity in sedentary older women—A pilot study. *BMC Health Services Research, 8*, 169.

Sui, X., Brown, W., Lavie, C., West, D., Pate, R., Payne, J., & Blair, S. (2015). Associations between television watching and car riding behaviors and development of depressive symptoms: A prospective studies. *Mayo Clinic Proceedings, 90*, 184–193.

Sun, K., Song, J., Lee, J., Chang, R., Eaton, C., Ehrlich-Jones, L., … Dunlop, E. (2014). Relationship of meeting physical activity guidelines with health-related utility. *Arthritis Care & Research, 66*, 1041–1047.

Swinnen, T., Scheers, T., Lefevre, J., Dankaerts, W., & deVlam, K. (2014). Physical activity assessment in patients with axial spondyloarthritis compared to healthy controls: A technology-based approach. *PLoS One, 9*, e85309.

Talbot, L., Gaines, J., Huynh, T., & Metter, E. (2003). A home-based pedometer-driven walking program to increase physical activity in older adults with osteoarthritis of the knee: A preliminary study. *Journal of the American Geriatrics Society, 51*, 387–392.

Tanaka, R., Ozawa, J., Kito, N., & Moriyama, H. (2013). Efficacy of strengthening or aerobic exercise on pain relief in people with knee osteoarthritis: A systematic review and meta-analysis of randomized controlled trials. *Clinical Rehabilitation, 27*, 1059–1071.

Taylor-Gjevre, R., Gjevre, J., Nair, B., Skomro, R., & Lim, H. (2010). Hypersomnolence and sleep disorders in a rheumatic disease population. *Journal of Clinical Rheumatology, 16*, 2555–2261.

Taylor-Gjevre, R., Nair, B., & Gjevre, J. (2013). Obstructive sleep apnoea in relation to rheumatoid disease. *Rheumatology, 52*, 15–21.

Teychenne, M., Abbott, G., Ball, K., & Salmon, J. (2014). Prospective associations between sedentary behavior and risk of depression in socio-economically disadvantaged women. *Preventive Medicine, 65*, 82–86.

Teychenne, M., Ball, K., & Salmon, J. (2008). Physical activity and likelihood of depression in adults: A review. *Preventive Medicine, 46*, 397–411.

Teychenne, M., Ball, K., & Salmon, J. (2010a). Physical activity, sedentary behavior and depression among disadvantaged women. *Health Education Research, 25*, 632–644.

Teychenne, M., Ball, K., & Salmon, J. (2010b). Sedentary behavior and depression among adults: A review. *International Journal of Behavioral Medicine, 17*, 246–254.

Treharne, G. J., Lyons, A. C., Hale, E. D., Douglas, K. M., Goodchild, C. E., Booth, D. A., & Kitas, G. D. (2007). Sleep disruption frequency in rheumatoid arthritis: Perceived stress predicts poor outcome over one year. *Musculoskeletal Care, 5*(1), 51–64.

Trivedi, M., Greer, T., Church, T., Carmody, T., Grannemann, B., Galper, D., … Blair, S. (2011). Exercise as an augmentation treatment for nonremitted major depressive disorder: A randomized, parallel dose comparison. *Journal of Clinical Psychiatry, 72*, 677–684.

Tudor-Locke, C., Bell, R., Myers, A., Harris, S., Ecclestone, N., Lauzon, N., & Rodger, N. (2004). Controlled outcome evaluation of the First Step Program: A daily physical activity intervention for individuals with type II diabetes. *International Journal of Obesity and Related Metabolic Disorders, 28*, 113–119.

Tudor-Locke, C., Craig, C., Aoyagi, Y., Bell, R., Croteau, K., De Bourdeaudhuij, I., ... Blair, S. (2011). How many steps/day are enough? For older adults and special populations. *International Journal of Behavioral Nutrition and Physical Activity, 8*, 80.

Tudor-Locke, C., Hatano, Y., Pangrazi, R., & Kang, M. (2008). Revisiting "how many steps are enough?". *Medicine & Science in Sports & Exercise, 40*(Suppl 7), S537–S543.

Tudor-Locke, C., Leonardi, C., Johnson, W., Katzmarzyuk, P., & Church, T. (2011). Accelerometer steps/day translation of moderate-to-vigorous activity. *Preventive Medicine, 53*, 31–33.

Tudor-Locke, C., & Lutes, L. (2009). Why do pedometers work? *Sports Medicine, 39*, 981–993.

U.S. Department of Health and Human Services. (2008). *Physical activity guidelines for Americans*. Retrieved November 27, 2012, from www.health.gov/paguidelines

Unterman, A., Nolte, J., Boaz, M., Abady, M., Shoenfeld, Y., & Zandman-Goddard, G. (2011). Neuropsychiatric syndromes in systemic lupus erythematosus: A meta-analysis. *Seminars in Arthritis and Rheumatism, 41*(1), 1–11.

Vallance, J., Winkler, E., Gardiner, P., Healy, G., Lynch, B., & Owen, N. (2011). Associations of objectively-assessed physical activity and sedentary time with depression: NHANES (2005-2006). *Preventive Medicine, 53*, 284–288.

van der Goes, M., Hoes, J., Cramer, M., van der Veen, M., van der Werf, J., Bijlsma, J., & Jacobs, J. (2014). Identifying factors hampering physical activity in longstanding rheumatoid arthritis: What is the role of glucocorticoid therapy? *Clinical and Experimental Rheumatology, 32*, 155–161.

Visser, M., Bouter, L., McQuillan, G., Wener, M., & Harris, T. (1999). Elevated C-reactive protein levels in overweight and obese adults. *Journal of the American Medical Association, 282*, 2131–2135.

Vogelzangs, N., Beekman, A., Boelhouwer, I., Bandinelli, S., Milaneschi, Y., Ferrucci, L., & Penninx, B. (2011). Metabolic depression: A chronic depressive subtype? Findings from the InCHIANTI study of older persons. *Journal of Clinical Psychiatry, 72*(5), 598–604.

Vogelzangs, N., Kritchevsky, S., Beekman, A., Brenes, G., Newman, A., Satterfield, S., ... Health ABC Study. (2010). Obesity and onset of significant depressive symptoms: Result from a prospective community-based cohort study of older men and women. *Journal of Clinical Psychiatry, 71*, 391–399.

Volkmann, E., Grossman, J., Sahakian, L., Skaggs, B., FitzGerald, J., Ragavendra, N., ... McMahon, M. (2010). Low physical activity is associated with proinflammatory high-density lipoprotein and increased subclinical atherosclerosis in women with systemic lupus erythematosus. *Arthritis Care & Research (Hoboken), 62*, 258–265.

Wallis, J., Webster, K., Levinger, P., & Taylor, N. (2013). What proportion of people with hip and knee osteoarthritis meet physical activity guidelines? A systematic review and meta-analysis. *Osteoarthritis and Cartilage, 21*, 1648–1659.

Walsh, J., McFadden, M., Morgan, M., Sawitzke, A., Duffin, K., Krueger, G., & Clegg, D. (2014). Work productivity loss and fatigue in psoriatic arthritis. *The Journal of Rheumatology, 41*, 1670–1674.

Walsh, J., & McWilliams, D. (2014). Mechanisms, impact and management of pain in rheumatoid arthritis. *Nature Reviews. Rheumatology, 10*, 581–592.

Weuve, J., Kang, J., Manson, J., Breteler, M. M. B., Ware, J., & Grodstein, F. (2004). Physical activity, including walking, and cognitive function in older women. *Journal of the American Medical Association, 292*(12), 1454–1461.

White, D., Tudor-Locke, C., Zhang, Y., Fielding, R., LaValley, M., Felson, D., ... Neogi, T. (2014). Daily walking and the risk of incident functional limitation in knee OA: An observational study. *Arthritis Care & Research (Hoboken), 66*(9), 1328–1336.

Williams, D., Matthews, C., Rutt, C., Napolitano, M., & Marcus, B. (2008). Interventions to increase walking behavior. *Medicine & Science in Sports & Exercise, 40*(Suppl 7), S567–S573.

Williamson, G. (2000). Pain, functional disability, and depressed affect. In G. Williamson, D. Shaffer, & P. Parmelee (Eds.), *Physical illness and depression in older adults* (pp. 51–64). New York: Kluwer Academic/Plenum Publishers.

Williamson, G., & Schulz, R. (1992). Pain, activity restriction, and symptoms of depression among community-residing elderly adults. *Journal of Gerontology: Psychological Sciences, 47*, P367–P372.

Williamson, G., & Schulz, R. (1995). Activity restriction mediates the association between pain and depressed affect: A study of younger and older adult cancer patients. *Psychology and Aging, 10*, 369–378.

Wolfe, F., Hawley, D., & Wilson, K. (1996). The prevalence and meaning of fatigue in rheumatic disease. *The Journal of Rheumatology, 23*, 1407–1417.

Yaffe, K., Barnes, D., Nevitt, M., Lui, L., & Covinsky, K. (2001). A prospective study of physical activity and cognitive decline in elderly women: Women who walk. *Archives of Internal Medicine, 161*, 1703–1708.

Yaffe, K., Fiocco, A., Lindquist, K., Vittinghoff, E., Simonsick, E., Newman, A., ... Health ABC Study. (2009). Predictors of maintaining cognitive function in older adults: The Health ABC study. *Neurology, 72*, 2029–2035.

Yates, T., Khunti, K., Wilmot, E., Brady, E., Webb, D., Srinivasan, B., ... Davies, M. (2012). Self-reported sitting time and markers of inflammation, insulin resistance, and adiposity. *American Journal of Preventive Medicine, 42*, 1–7.

Zhao, G., Ford, E., Dhingra, S., Li, G., Strine, T., & Mokdad, A. (2009). Depression and anxiety among US adults: Associations with body mass index. *International Journal of Obesity, 33*, 257–266.

Zhu, N., Jacobs, D. J., Schreiner, P., Yaffe, K., Bryan, N., Launer, L., … Sternfeld, B. (2014). Cardiorespiratory fitness and cognitive function in middle age: The CARDIA study. *Neurology, 82*, 1339–1346.

References for Figure 13.2

Alentorn-Geli, E., Padilla, J., Moras, G., Lazaro, H. C., & Fernandez-Sola, J. (2008). Six weeks of whole-body vibration exercise improves pain and fatigue in women with fibromyalgia. *Journal of Alternative and Complementary Medicine, 14*, 975–981.

Buckelew, S. P., Conway, R., Parker, J., Deuser, W. E., Read, J., Witty, T. E., … Kay, D. R. (1998). Biofeedback/relaxation training and exercise interventions for fibromyalgia: A prospective trial. *Arthritis and Rheumatism, 11*, 196–209.

Daltroy, L. H., Robb-Nicholson, C., Iversen, M. D., Wright, E. A., & Liang, M. H. (1995). Effectiveness of minimally supervised home aerobic training in patients with systemic rheumatic disease. *British Journal of Rheumatology, 34*, 1064–1069.

Fransen, M., Mairn, L., Winstanley, J., Lam, P., & Edmonds, J. (2007). Physical activity for osteoarthritis management: A randomized controlled clinical trial evaluating hydrotherapy or Tai Chi classes. *Arthritis and Rheumatism, 57*, 407–414.

Gowans, S. E., deHueck, A., Voss, S., Silaj, A., Abbey, S. E., & Reynolds, W. J. (2001). Effect of a randomized, controlled trial of exercise on mood and physical function in individuals with fibromyalgia. *Arthritis and Rheumatism, 57*, 407–414.

Haak, T., & Scott, B. (2008). The effect of Qigong on fibromyalgia (FMS): A controlled randomized study. *Disability and Rehabilitation, 30*, 625–633.

Hakkinen, A., Hakkinen, K., Hannonen, P., & Alen, M. (2001). Strength training induced adaptations in neuromuscular function of premenopausal women with fibromyalgia: Comparison with healthy women. *Annals of the Rheumatic Diseases, 60*, 21–26.

Ide, M. R., Laurindo, I. M. M., Rodrigues, A. L., & Tanaka, C. (2008). Effect of aquatic respiratory exercise-based program in patients with fibromyalgia. *International Journal of Rheumatic Diseases, 11*, 131–140.

Jones, K. D., Burckhardt, C. S., Deodhar, A. A., Perrin, N. A., Hanson, G. C., & Bennett, R. M. (2008). A six-month randomized controlled trial of exercise and pyridostigmine in the treatment of fibromyalgia. *Arthritis and Rheumatism, 58*, 612–622.

Komatireddy, G. R., Leitch, R. W., Cella, K., Browning, G., & Minor, M. (1997). Efficacy of low load resistive muscle training in patients with rheumatoid arthritis functional class II and III. *The Journal of Rheumatology, 24*, 1531–1539.

Mannerkorpi, K., Nyberg, B., Ahlmen, M., & Ekdahl, C. (2000). Pool exercise combined with an education program for patients with fibromyalgia syndrome. A prospective, randomized study. *The Journal of Rheumatology, 27*, 2473–2481.

Minor, M. A., Hewett, J. E., Webel, R. R., Anderson, S. K., & Kay, D. R. (1989). Efficacy of physical conditioning exercise in patients with rheumatoid arthritis and osteoarthritis. *Arthritis and Rheumatism, 32*, 1396–1405.

Neuberger, G. B., Aaronson, L. S., Gajewski, B., Embretson, S. E., Cagle, P. E., Loudon, J. K., & Miller, P. A. (2007). Predictors of exercise and exercise effects on symptoms, aerobic fitness, and disease outcomes of rheumatoid arthritis. *Arthritis and Rheumatism, 57*, 943–952.

O'Reilly, S. C., Muir, K. R., & Doherty, M. (1999). Effectiveness of home exercise on pain and disability from osteoarthritis of the knee: A randomized controlled trial. *Annals of the Rheumatic Diseases, 58*, 15–19.

Patrick, D. L., Ramsey, S. D., Spencer, A. C., Kinne, S., Belza, B., & Topolski, T. D. (2001). Economic evaluation of aquatic exercise for persons with osteoarthritis. *Medical Care, 39*, 413–424.

Rooks, D. S., Gautum, S., Romeling, M., Cross, M. L., Stratigakis, D., Evans, B., Goldenberg, D. L., Iversen, M. D., Katz, J. N. (2007). Group exercise, education, and combination self-management in women with fibromyalgia: A randomized trial. *Archives of Internal Medicine, 167*, 2192–2200.

Sanudo, B., Galiano, D., Carrasco, L., de Hoyo, M., & McVeigh, J. G. (2011). Effects of a prolonged exercise program on key health outcomes in women with fibromyalgia: A randomized controlled trial. *Journal of Rehabilitation Medicine, 43*, 521–526.

Schachter, C. L., Busch, A. J., Peloso, P. M., & Sheppard, M. S. (2003). Effects of short versus long bouts of aerobic exercise in sedentary women with fibromyalgia: A randomized controlled trial. *Physical Therapy, 83*, 340–358.

Sencan, S., Ak, S., Karan, A., Muslumanoglu, L., Ozcan, E., & Berker, E. (2004). A study to compare the therapeutic efficacy of aerobic exercise and paroxetine in fibromyalgia syndrome. *Journal of Back and Musculoskeletal Rehabilitation, 17*, 57–61.

Tomas-Carus, P., Gusi, N., Hakkinen, A., Hakkinen, K., Leal, A., & Ortega-Alonso, A. (2008). Eight months of physical training in warm water improves physical and mental health in women with fibromyalgia: A randomized controlled trial. *Journal of Rehabilitation Medicine, 40*, 248–252.

Tomas-Carus, P., Gusi, N., Leal, A., Garcia, Y., & Ortega-Alonso, A. (2007). The fibromyalgia treatment with physical exercise in warm water reduces the impact of the disease on female patients' physical and mental health. *Reumatologia Clinica, 3*, 33–37.

Valim, V., Oliveira, L., Suda, A., Silva, L., de Assis, M., Barros, N. T., … Natour, J. (2003). Aerobic fitness in fibromyalgia. *The Journal of Rheumatology, 30*, 1060–1069.

Valkeinen, H., Alen, M., Hannonen, P., Hakkinen, A., Airaksinen, O., & Hakkinen, K. (2004). Changes in knee extension and flexion force, EMG and functional capacity during strength training in older females with fibromyalgia and healthy controls. *Rheumatology (Oxford), 43*, 225–228.

Wang, C., Schmid, C. H., Hibberd, P. L., Kalish, R., Roubenoff, R., Rones, R., McAlindon, T. (2009). Tai Chi is effective in treating knee osteoarthritis: A randomized controlled trial. *Arthritis and Rheumatism, 61*, 1545–1553.

Wang, C., Schmid, C. H., Rones, R., Kalish, R., Yinh, J., Goldenberg, D. L., Lee, Y., McAlindon, T. (2010). A randomized trial of tai chi for fibromyalgia. *New England Journal of Medicine, 363*, 743–754.

Wigers, S. H., Stiles, T. C., & Vogel, P. A. (1996). Effects of aerobic exercise versus stress management treatment in fibromyalgia. A 4.5 year prospective study. *Scandinavian Journal of Rheumatology, 25*, 77–86.

Evidence-Based Complementary and Alternative Medical Approaches for Arthritis

14

Diana Taibi Buchanan

Complementary and Alternative Medicine: An Overview

Health practices that are not part of conventional, mainstream medicine are commonly referred to as complementary and alternative medical (CAM) modalities. Usually, persons use CAM modalities in conjunction with, rather than as alternative to, conventional medicine. However, persons may or may not disclose CAM use to their healthcare providers. In some settings, healthcare providers incorporate both conventional and CAM approaches, which is called integrative medicine. In the U.S., CAM research is mostly funded by the National Center for Complementary and Integrative Health (NCCIH), a center within the National Institutes of Health (NIH). Although "CAM" is the most familiar term (and is used throughout this chapter), NCCIH notes that their preferred term is "complementary health approaches". This term is appropriate because CAM modalities are not strictly medical. Furthermore, the term "approaches" is more appropriate than "medicine" or "therapies" given that many CAM modalities lack research evidence of therapeutic efficacy. For many modalities, physiological effects have been shown through research, but it cannot be assumed that these translate into clinical therapeutic effects.

Because CAM modalities are highly varied, it is helpful to categorize these by types. For many years, NCCIH assigned CAM approaches to five categories: (1) mind-body medicine, (2) biologically based therapies, (3) manipulative and body-based therapies, (4) energy therapies, and (5) alternative medical systems. More recently, however, NCCIH simplified this classification to only three categories: (1) natural products (e.g., herbs, vitamins, and probiotics); (2) mind-body practices (e.g., acupuncture, massage therapy, meditation, movement therapies, relaxation techniques, spinal manipulation, tai chi, and yoga); and (3) other complementary health approaches (e.g., traditional Chinese medicine [TCM], Ayurvedic medicine, and homeopathy) (National Center for Complementary and Integrative Health, 2008). Although this new classification is less descriptive, it removes somewhat forced categorization of therapies that logically belonged to more than one of the former categories. For instance, acupuncture could be considered a body-based therapy, an energy therapy, and part of an alternative medical system (TCM).

The widespread use of CAM approaches in the U.S. use gained attention in 1998, when an important survey by Eisenberg and colleagues

D.T. Buchanan, PhD, RN (✉)
Department of Biobehavioral Nursing and Health Systems, School of Nursing, University of Washington, 1959 NE Pacific Street, Box 327266, Seattle, WA 98195-7266, USA
e-mail: dmtaibi@uw.edu

P.M. Nicassio (ed.), *Psychosocial Factors in Arthritis*, DOI 10.1007/978-3-319-22858-7_14

was published in JAMA (Eisenberg et al., 1998). This survey showed that use of CAM in the U.S. increased from 34 % of adults in 1990 to 42 % in 1997. CAM approaches were most commonly used for chronic conditions. More recently, analysis of the 2007 National Health Interview Survey (NHIS) data showed about the same rate of CAM use as Eisenberg et al., with 38 % of surveyed individuals reporting CAM use in the past 12 months (Barnes, Bloom, & Nahin, 2007). Several surveys have shown a trend of greater CAM use among women than men in the general population (Barnes et al., 2007; Eisenberg et al., 1998) and among persons with arthritis (Callahan et al., 2009; Jawahar, Yang, Eaton, McAlindon, & Lapane, 2012).

Research on CAM use among persons with arthritis shows higher rates of use than the general population. In the 2007 NHIS data, musculoskeletal problems were the top reasons for CAM use, with arthritis being the fourth most common reason overall (Barnes et al., 2007). A survey of 2140 persons with various kinds of arthritis found that 91 % of those recruited from specialty care and 83 % of those recruited from primary care had ever used CAM for their arthritis; current use of at least one CAM modality was 76 % and 70 % in these groups, respectively (Callahan et al., 2009). The authors noted that particularly high rates of CAM use in this study compared to other research may be attributable to classifying prayer as a CAM modality. Another group that examined results from a longitudinal study of persons with knee osteoarthritis (OA) also found that a substantial proportion of the sample was regularly using CAM: 52 % at baseline and 47 % at year 4 (Yang, Dube, Eaton, McAlindon, & Lapane, 2013). The most commonly used CAM modalities among persons with arthritis included topical products, dietary supplements (especially glucosamine and chondroitin), chiropractic care, relaxation techniques, and movement practices (e.g., yoga, tai chi) (Callahan et al., 2009; Quandt et al., 2005; Yang et al., 2013).

Persons with arthritis use CAM approaches for many of the same reasons as conventional therapies: to manage pain, preserve function, and reduce the progression of joint damage. CAM may be appealing because of perceptions that these approaches are "natural" or safe and because they represent to the patient a holistic approach. Given the prevalence of CAM use among persons with arthritis, it is important for healthcare providers to address CAM in patient care. This chapter provides an overview of several of the most commonly used CAM approaches for osteoarthritis (OA) and rheumatoid arthritis (RA) and presents the current state of research evidence on these modalities.

Natural Products

Glucosamine and Chondroitin

Glucosamine and chondroitin are dietary supplements used by persons with arthritis both for symptom management and for modification of disease progression. These may be taken alone or in combination. Glucosamine and chondroitin are substances that naturally occur in joint and connective tissues. Research has shown that these substances can stimulate collagen synthesis in articular chondrocytes and reduce the production of pro-inflammatory mediators and proteases that contribute to joint degeneration (Henrotin, Marty, & Mobasheri, 2014). Currently, the American College of Rheumatology (ACR) guidelines for OA management do not recommend use of glucosamine and chondroitin (Hochberg et al., 2012). However, several recent reviews, including one by the lead author of the ACR guidelines, recommend that these substances may have small but significant benefits when taken over time (Gallagher et al., 2014; Henrotin et al., 2014; Hochberg, Chevalier, Henrotin, Hunter, & Uebelhart, 2013; Lee, Woo, Choi, Ji, & Song, 2010).

The majority of research on glucosamine and chondroitin has been conducted in persons with osteoarthritis, usually in the hip or knee. The largest trial to date, the Glucosamine/chondroitin Arthritis Intervention Trial (GAIT), was a randomized controlled trial (RCT) comparing five treatments (glucosamine, chondroitin, combination glucosamine and chondroitin, celecoxib, or placebo) given for 24 months in persons with knee OA (N=1583) (Clegg et al., 2006). A 20 % reduction in the pain subscale of the Western Ontario McMaster Osteoarthritis Index (WOMAC) was considered a significant treatment response. Glucosamine or chondroitin alone did not improve pain based on this response criterion, but the combination of glucosamine and chondroitin did improve pain (Clegg et al., 2006). Joint swelling was reduced in the chondroitin group only. Analyses of the 2-year follow-up showed that none of the treatments produced a significant improvements in WOMAC pain or joint space width, though celecoxib and glucosamine showed trends in WOMAC pain improvement that verged on significance (Sawitzke et al., 2008, 2010).

Two meta-analyses published in 2010 arrived at conflicting conclusions. Wandel et al. (2010) included 10 trials (6 glucosamine, 3 chondroitin, 1 combination), concluding that the evidence did not support the effectiveness of any of these supplements. Findings on pain showed little difference with glucosamine (standardized mean difference [SMD]=−.17), chondroitin (SMD=−.13), or combination (SMD=−.19). Effects on joint space narrowing (JSN) were also small (SMD not reported). Another meta-analysis by Lee et al. reported no effect of 1 year of glucosamine on JSN based on two trials (SMD=.078), but did find a small and significant effect at 3 years (SMD=.43), indicating the importance of treatment duration (Lee et al., 2010). Two years of chondroitin treatment (based on four trials) had a small but significant effect on JSN (SMD=.26). This review did not examine pain. Two recent reviews examined the highest quality research on glucosamine and chondroitin, but neither used meta-analysis (Gallagher et al., 2014; Henrotin et al., 2014). Henrotin et al. (2014) concluded that the evidence supports both supplements as promising treatments for OA, though the evidence presented in the review on glucosamine was particularly mixed. The evidence more consistently supported chondroitin for improving pain and preventing JSN. The authors also noted that glucosamine sulfate has been associated with more favorable outcomes than glucosamine hydrochloride. This is consistent with speculation that the benefits of glucosamine sulfate may be related to the sulfate component (Hoffer, Kaplan, Hamadeh, Grigoriu, & Baron, 2001). The other recent review noted that three of four studies of chondroitin meeting the criteria for inclusion in the review showed significant reduction of JSN versus placebo; however, only one of these studies showed reduction of pain (Gallagher et al., 2014). Of the three studies of glucosamine reviewed, two reported significant reduction of JSN, one reported improvement of the total WOMAC score, and one reported improved WOMAC pain. The one trial showing no effects for glucosamine or chondroitin was the GAIT study (Clegg et al., 2006).

Insufficient evidence on glucosamine for RA is available, and no studies have tested chondroitin. Only one recent trial has tested glucosamine (using glucosamine hydrochloride) in persons with RA (N=51) (Nakamura et al., 2007). Compared to placebo, 12 weeks of glucosamine resulted in no improvements in joint counts, pain, C-reactive protein, or erythrocyte sedimentation rate. The only improvement observed was reduced matrix metalloproteinase-3 levels. The only other study in this population was conducted in 1975, comparing glucosamine with indomethacin (Giordano, Capelli, & Chianese, 1975). Glucosamine improved joint tenderness; however, the findings are not particularly relevant due to major changes in RA treatment in the time since this study.

The overall safety profiles of glucosamine and chondroitin are favorable, though there is the potential for drug interactions and certain cautions are advisable. In the large GAIT study, the rate of adverse events did not differ between the supplements and placebo (Clegg et al., 2006). One serious adverse event that occurred after 2 years of treatment was possibly related to the glucosamine/chondroitin combination (myocardial infarction) (Sawitzke et al., 2010), but details are not provided. Persons with seafood allergies may react to glucosamine, which is derived from shellfish. Glucosamine has also been associated with photosensitivity and drowsiness; it should be used cautiously in persons with a history of topical allergy or depression (Natural Standard, 2014a, 2014b). Both glucosamine and chondroitin may increase risk of bleeding and should be used cautiously in persons taking anticoagulant medications (Natural Standard, 2014a). It has been suggested that glucosamine may alter carbohydrate metabolism, particularly in diabetics, but studies have only shown such effects at doses that grossly exceed regular use (Salazar et al., 2014). Evidence suggests that negative effects on carbohydrate metabolism are unlikely, but caution is still advisable.

In summary, despite a large trial that mostly failed to support the effectiveness of glucosamine and chondroitin for OA pain and joint structure, conclusions on the overall body of literature are difficult to reach. Some evidence shows reduced pain and joint protection (reduced JSN) in hip or knee OA, particularly with chondroitin. Evidence is currently insufficient to recommend glucosamine or chondroitin for RA. Any benefits of these supplements may take 2 or more years of treatment to become apparent (Lee et al., 2010). Benefits may also depend on product quality and dosing. Both supplements have favorable safety profiles. Therefore, glucosamine and chondroitin may be reasonable options for persons with OA, but this should be decided in consultation with a provider and understanding that benefits may be small.

Topical Products

There are a variety of CAM ointments and creams that are used for analgesic and anti-inflammatory effects, but few of these are supported by research. A recent Cochrane review examined topical agents, finding limited evidence supporting the benefits of arnica and comfrey, but not capsicum or stinging nettle (Cameron & Chrubasik, 2013). Arnica is a flower that is processed to produce topical analgesic products (and also as a homeopathic remedy, which is not discussed here). One study compared 21 days of arnica gel to ibuprofen gel in persons with hand OA ($N=175$) (Widrig, Suter, Saller, & Melzer, 2007). Both groups had similar improvements in hand pain and function. The rate of adverse events likely due to treatment was similar between groups ($n=6$ and 5 for ibuprofen and arnica, respectively), and most often involved skin irritation at the administration site. Arnica has not been compared to placebo. Arnica has been shown to inhibit platelet aggregation in vitro, but it is uncertain if this is a potential clinical side effect in humans (Natural Standard, 2014c). Additionally, persons allergic to flowers in the daisy family may also be allergic to arnica (Natural Standard, 2014c).

Comfrey is a plant that has been shown to have anti-inflammatory effects (Natural Standard, 2014d). A study of persons with knee OA ($N=220$) comparing 3 weeks of comfrey ointment to placebo found significant improvements in WOMAC pain, stiffness, and physical function with comfrey (Grube, Grunwald, Krug, & Staiger, 2007). Caution is warranted in the use of comfrey, which has been shown to be hepatotoxic (Natural Standard, 2014d). Absorption from prolonged topical use may cause risk of toxicity, but little is known about the risk. Persons might also experience allergic reactions to comfrey.

Capsicum (also called capsaicin) is derived from cayenne peppers. It reduces pain by depleting local nerve cells of substance P, thereby reducing pain transmission. Given this effect, topical capsicum is expected to cause a burning sensation as substance P is depleted (Cameron & Chrubasik, 2013). Although the Cochrane review concluded that capsaicin is not effective for OA (based on one study), a more recent review of five studies reported moderate effects on OA pain (Laslett & Jones, 2014). The authors reported a moderate effect on pain visual analog scale ratings (SMD=.44). The ACR recommendations for OA management conditionally recommend capsaicin for hand OA but not for knee OA (Hochberg et al., 2012).

In summary, arnica, comfrey, and capsaicin may be useful for OA pain, but research is scant. Topical agents may cause local irritation, and in some cases may cause systemic effects if absorbed, so monitoring of patient use is advisable. Finally, camphor and menthol, which are constituents of commonly available analgesic balms such as Tiger Balm and Elder Balm, have not been studied in person with arthritis, so there is no evidence available for recommendations.

Mind and Body Practices

Acupuncture

Acupuncture is a provider-based CAM approach. Although acupuncture is based in TCM, it is frequently administered without using the entire TCM system, or with incorporation of only parts of this system. The most characteristic aspect of acupuncture treatment involves insertion of small needles into specific points on the body to promote the flow of *qi* (life energy) along energy pathways called meridians. The flow of qi is considered vital to health, and blockages, excess, or deficits of qi are believed to cause symptoms and disease patterns. Treatments are based on traditional assessments of energy flow and symptom patterns. The patterns treated may or may not align with Western medicine diagnoses, depending on the condition being addressed. Other practices related to acupuncture include acupressure, which is manually applied pressure at acupuncture points, and electro-acupuncture, which is electrical stimulation of either surface acupuncture points or inserted needles. According to the 2007 NHIS data, 5.5 % of persons with arthritis had used acupuncture within the past 12 months (Hawk, Ndetan, & Evans, 2012). The effects of acupuncture on arthritis are suspected to occur through regulation of endogenous opioid mechanisms and modulation of central nervous system sensory processing in the limbic, subcortical, and brainstem structures (Amazaga Urruela & Suarez-almazor, 2012).

There is a fairly large, but highly varied, body of research on acupuncture for OA. There are fewer studies examining acupuncture for RA. In 2010, Manheimer et al. (2010) updated their previous Cochrane review of acupuncture for peripheral joint OA. The 16 RCTs examined, including 3498 participants, mostly addressed knee OA, with few addressing hip OA or both knee and hip OA. The meta-analysis showed significant effects of real acupuncture versus sham acupuncture at post-treatment on WOMAC pain (SMD = −.28) and WOMAC function (SMD = −.28), but the differences did not exceed the pre-determined threshold of clinical significance (SMD = −.39 and −.37 for pain and function, respectively). At a 6-month follow-up, these outcomes verged on significance, but were of smaller and clinically unimportant magnitude (WOMAC pain SMD = −.10, WOMAC function SMD = −.11). A more recent meta-analysis by Manyanga et al. (2014) examined 12 RCTs (1763 participants) of acupuncture for OA. This analysis reported similar findings; compared to sham acupuncture, real acupuncture was associated with significant post-treatment improvements in pain (SMD = −.29), functional mobility (SMD = −.34), and health-related quality of life (SMD = −.38). This analysis also examined the effect of intervention duration on the primary outcome of pain, finding stronger reduction of pain in treatments longer than 4 weeks versus those lasting 4 weeks or less. A novel network meta-analysis recently published by researchers for the Osteoarthritis Research Society International (OARSI) concurrently examined the effects of acupuncture and 21 other physical CAM and conventional approaches for OA (Corbett et al., 2013). This analysis demonstrated that reduction of pain with acupuncture was superior to usual care (SMD = −.89). The investigators also compared the other treatments directly to acupuncture, finding that acupuncture was superior for pain reduction compared to all treatments except inferential therapy, which was represented by only one study. The authors of all three of these meta-analyses noted a high risk of bias in most of the studies, especially due to uncertain or inadequate blinding of verum/sham treatment.

Research in persons with RA is much more limited and heterogeneous in terms of treatment (electro-acupuncture, acupuncture with moxibustion, etc.). A 2008 systematic review of acupuncture for RA found no effects of acupuncture treatments on pain or other outcomes (Lee, Shin, & Ernst, 2008). Another review published in the same year noted some favorable study outcomes, but also reported conflicting evidence (Wang, de Pablo, Chen, Schmid, & McAlindon, 2008). No major studies have been published since these reviews, though several studies have examined bee venom acupuncture, noting some promising results (Lee et al., 2014). Overall, high-quality research is needed before any confident recommendations can be made on the usefulness of acupuncture for RA.

Due to the nature of using a sham acupuncture comparison, it is possible that actual effects of acupuncture may be underestimated. It appears that sham acupuncture has effects on pain and function. In the OARSI network meta-analysis, sham acupuncture was shown superior to standard care for the outcome of pain (SMD = −.47) (Corbett et al., 2013). Sham acupuncture may involve full insertion of needles at a location that is not an actual acupuncture point, or it may involve retractable needles that are not actually inserted (Streitberger needles). It is suspected that needling non-meridian locations may produce analgesia through a diffuse noxious inhibitory (DNIC) mechanism, by which a local noxious stimulus may produce generalized analgesic effects (Manheimer et al., 2010). It is possible that even surface stimulation through non-inserted needles may produce a physiologic effect. On the other hand, it is also possible that sham acupuncture is an appropriate control for non-specific (placebo) effects that occur due to subjects' expectations of acupuncture. In sum, it remains unknown whether or not sham acupuncture is truly physiologically inert, but the effects do suggest that some of the efficacy of acupuncture is due to non-specific effects.

In regard to safety, acupuncture appears to be generally safe. Serious adverse events have been noted to occur with acupuncture, but these are rare. The most common serious adverse effects were pneumothorax and infections. The meta-analyses by Manheimer et al. (2010) and Manyanga et al. (2014) both reported no serious adverse events in any study, but they did note the occurrence of transient adverse events, including bleeding/bruising/swelling at the needle insertion sites, pain, sleepiness, faintness, and nausea.

In summary, the evidence suggests that acupuncture may be of some benefit for pain and function in persons with OA, but the effects appear small. The benefits of this treatment should be weighed against the cost of provider visits. For persons with RA, there is very limited evidence of benefit, but there is currently insufficient evidence to support recommendation of this treatment. Although it is generally safe, acupuncture does involve some risk of minor side effects and rare, but serious, side effects of which patients should be aware.

Massage Therapy

Massage therapy is a treatment that involves manual manipulation of soft tissues. There are a number of different styles of massage that vary in bodywork techniques and depth of tissue manipulation. In the U.S., Swedish massage is the most widely available style. The effects of massage that may benefit persons with arthritis include increased tissue circulation and reduced muscle tension (Field, 2014; Perlman et al., 2012). Some evidence also suggests that massage may produce the relaxation response through stimulation of the parasympathetic nervous system (Field, 2014; Perlman et al., 2012).

Only a few studies have examined massage for arthritis. In particular, Perlman and colleagues conducted two modestly sized, but well-designed trials of Swedish massage for knee OA (Perlman et al., 2012; Perlman, Sabina, Williams, Njike, & Katz, 2006). In the first RCT ($N = 68$), 8 weeks of massage versus a wait-list control produced significant improvement in WOMAC global, pain, stiffness, and physical function; pain ratings; and 50-ft timed walk (Perlman et al., 2006). The subsequent RCT ($N = 125$) not only compared massage to usual care, but also compared four doses of 8-week massage (30 min once or twice per week, 60 min once or twice per week) (Perlman et al., 2012). All massage groups showed improvement on WOMAC, pain, and functional outcomes, but results in the 60-min groups were more consistently significant than the 30-min groups. The researchers found that benefits plateaued at 60 min once per week. Effects in these studies persisted at follow-up assessments on week 16 (Perlman et al., 2006, 2012) and week 24 (Perlman et al., 2012). Field and colleagues conducted two studies of massage (style not noted) for hand OA (Field, Diego, Hernandez-Reif, & Shea, 2007; Field, Diego, & Solien-Wolfe, 2014). The initial study ($N=22$), which compared 4 weeks of massage to standard care, reported significantly improved pain, anxiety, and depression at post-treatment (Field et al., 2007). The follow-up study ($N=20$) compared 4 weeks of massage alone versus massage plus a menthol-based topical analgesic (Field et al., 2014). Both groups improved significantly on grip strength, pain, depression, and sleep disturbance, and the improvements were greater in the group receiving the topical analgesic. Finally, the same research group conducted a study of light versus medium pressure massage for 4 weeks in persons with RA (Field, Diego, Delgado, Garcia, & Funk, 2013). Compared to the light massage group, the medium massage group had significant improvements in pain, anxiety, depression, grip strength, and range of motion, but not sleep.

Overall, two well-designed trials with relevant clinical outcomes suggest that massage may be of benefit for persons with knee OA (Perlman et al., 2006, 2012). Research on the appropriate dose currently supports 60-min sessions once per week (Perlman et al., 2012). Although findings for hand OA and RA have shown some benefit, these studies were small and lacked standardized clinical outcome measures for these conditions (Field et al., 2007, 2013, 2014). Only one adverse event was reported in these studies (increased discomfort) (Perlman et al., 2006). A review of case reports of adverse events from massage found that, although adverse events may occur due to excessive pressure on nerves, circulatory tissues, and internal organs (e.g., hematoma, neuropathy), adverse events were rare, given the popularity of massage (Ernst, 2003). Furthermore, adverse events were rare when treatment was delivered by a trained professional therapist, especially using Swedish massage rather than a style using deeper pressure (e.g., rolfing).

Tai Chi

Tai chi was originally developed as a martial art in China, but today it is usually practiced as a gentle exercise and meditative practice. Tai chi involves sequences of fluid movements performed with mental awareness and deep breathing (National Center for Complementary and Integrative Medicine, 2006). The movement practice of tai chi is intended foremost to promote a state of tranquility or serenity. The foundation of tai chi lies in the traditional Chinese philosophy of energies within the body—yin and yang (opposing energies that should be in balance) and qi (one's overall life force). Tai chi is believed to aid the flow of qi by promoting the balance of yin and yang (National Center for Complementary and Integrative Health, 2006). There are five styles of tai chi that have variations in pose performance and sequencing, but the overall intent of tai chi practice is consistent across styles. Tai chi may benefit persons with arthritis through physical and psychological effects. The exercise involves standing and shifting balance between the feet. Thus, tai chi may improve quadriceps strength and bone mineral density, though evidence is mixed (Lee, Pittler, Shin, & Ernst, 2008). The performance of fluid motions in the upper and lower body may also improve joint mobility. However, tai chi may not be strenuous enough to improve aerobic capacity (Lee, Lee, & Ernst, 2009). The meditative component of tai chi may be helpful for reducing mood disturbances such as depression and anxiety. Finally, attending a class-based exercise may provide benefits through social contact.

Several small-to-moderate-sized studies have examined tai chi for OA, but the majority of these studies included persons with hip or knee OA only. Two recent meta-analyses concluded that evidence supports the benefits of tai chi for persons with OA. The meta-analysis by Lauche, Langhorst, Dobos, and Cramer (2013) included five studies of persons with knee OA only (with a total of 252 participants). Compared to attention control or usual care, 8–20 weeks of tai chi resulted in significant improvements in pain

(SMD=−.72), physical function (SMD=−.72), stiffness (SMD=−.59), and the physical component of quality of life (SMD=−.88). No serious adverse events were related to tai chi, and the only minor adverse event was transient muscle pain (Yan et al., 2013). Another recent meta-analysis found similar results, including seven studies of both hip and knee OA (348 participants) (Yan et al., 2013). Compared to controls, tai chi significantly improved pain (SMD=−.45), physical function (SMD=−.61), and stiffness (SMD=−.31).

Although numerous research studies have examined tai chi for RA, most of these studies have included only small samples, and findings were varied. A 2004 Cochrane review of tai chi for RA examined 4 studies (206 participants) (Han et al., 2004). The authors reported no effects on clinically important outcomes, but tai chi did not exacerbate RA, and in one study, it was viewed as more enjoyable than conventional exercise. A more recent systematic review including five trials found no effects of tai chi on pain or fatigue, but found some evidence suggesting improved quality of life, disability ratings, and mood (Lee, Pittler, & Ernst, 2007). Studies published since these reviews suggest benefit, but have continued to include very small study samples. In a 2008 pilot study ($N=20$), Wang and colleagues reported that a significantly greater proportion persons with RA completing 12 weeks of tai chi versus usual care met ACR responder criteria post-treatment (Wang, 2008). Most recently, Lee and colleagues tested 12 weeks of tai chi (with and without auricular acupressure) in 21 persons with RA. They found pre-post improvement across physical and symptom outcomes including balance, grip strength, pinch strength, 50 ft timed walk, joint pain, and swollen and tender joint counts (Lee, Hale, Hemingway, & Woolridge, 2012). A one-group study of 15 persons with RA showed significant improvements on some physical outcomes (swollen joint count, timed stand, pain during shoulder movement), but not on several other outcomes (disability ratings, fatigue, pain, quality of life, self-efficacy) (Uhlig, Fongen, Steen, Christie, & Odegard, 2010). In sum, evidence suggests that tai chi may be of benefit in RA, but larger, controlled studies are needed to determine whether or not this should be a recommended treatment.

In summary, evidence currently supports the usefulness and safety of tai chi for knee, and possibly hip, OA. Evidence is suggestive of benefit in RA, but the research literature is of inadequate quality to recommend tai chi for this group. Evidence supports the overall safety of tai chi. Transient muscle soreness is common (Wayne, Berkowitz, Litrownik, Buring, & Yeh, 2014), but this is not unexpected in persons with arthritis who may have muscle deconditioning.

Yoga

Yoga, like tai chi, is a movement-based mind-body practice. Traditional yoga, which originated in India around 200 BCE or earlier, involves eight "limbs" that provide physical, spiritual, and general lifestyle guidance (Sharma, 2014). Yoga in the U.S. generally involves only a few of these components, namely physical postures, breathing practices, and meditative mental focus. The purpose of the physical practice of yoga is ultimately to promote mental calm and awareness. Yoga may provide benefits by promoting muscle strength, flexibility, and balance (Roland, Jakobi, & Jones, 2011). The meditative component may help with mood, coping, and self-efficacy (Bartlett, Moonaz, Mill, Bernatsky, & Bingham, 2013).

Research on yoga for arthritis has been increasing in the past few years, but the field remains dominated by small, often uncontrolled or poorly controlled studies. Given the lack of RCTs, no meta-analyses on yoga for arthritis are available. Studies of persons with OA show mixed results on pain, stiffness, and function. Most of these studies were in persons with knee lower extremity OA (Ebnezar, Nagarathna, Yogitha, & Nagendra, 2012; Kolasinski et al., 2005; Taibi & Vitiello, 2011), though one study did not specify site (Park, McCaffrey, Dunn, & Goodman, 2011) and another examined yoga for hand OA (Garfinkel, Schumacher, Husain, Levy, & Reshetar, 1994). Three small uncontrolled studies ($N=11$–25) examined 8 weeks of yoga; two of these reported improvements in pain and function (Garfinkel et al., 1994; Kolasinski et al., 2005), whereas the other reported improvement in sleep but not pain or disability (Taibi & Vitiello, 2011). A small quasi-experimental study compared 8 weeks of chair yoga with Reiki or education ($N=21$) (Park et al., 2011). Pain and function improved in the yoga group, but did not significantly differ from the other groups. The largest trial of yoga for OA compared 3 months of yoga versus conventional physical therapy exercises in 250 persons with knee OA (Ebnezar et al., 2012). The yoga group had significantly greater improvements than the control group in walking pain, WOMAC disability, knee range of motion, and walking time. Despite the positive findings, this study (conducted in India) delivered an unusually intense treatment with daily yoga sessions. Finally, a recent RCT compared 8 weeks of yoga with wait-list control in women with knee OA ($N=35$). Results showed significantly greater improvements in WOMAC pain, WOMAC stiffness, and function (repeated chair stands) in the yoga group (Cheung, Wyman, Resnick, & Savik, 2014). In summary, the most recent and rigorous studies of yoga have provided results suggesting improved pain and function in persons with knee OA. However, no large trials have tested yoga in the manner in which it is typically used in the U.S., which is class attendance once or twice a week, perhaps including some home practice.

Several studies have tested yoga for persons with RA. A very small ($N=5$) uncontrolled trial of 6 weeks of yoga produced improved pain, depression, and self-efficacy in participants with RA (Evans et al., 2010). A later RCT by this research group ($N=26$) compared 6 weeks of yoga with usual care (Evans et al., 2013). Group comparisons showed improvement in pain disability, the Health Assessment Questionnaire (HAQ) general health subscale, and two SF-36 subscales (general health and vitality), but no differences in disease activity (DAS28), SF-36 mental or pain scales, or HAQ Disability. Another RCT of 7 weeks of yoga versus an unspecified control group ($N=80$) reported significant improvements in pain, morning stiffness, joint counts, and several physical measures, including C-reactive protein in the yoga group (Singh, Bhandari, & Rana, 2011). Finally, an uncontrolled study of 64 persons with RA tested 1 week of twice-daily yoga, finding improvement in HAQ Disability and rheumatoid factor, but not overall HAQ or C-reactive protein (Telles, Naveen, Gaur, & Balkrishna, 2011). Overall, research findings on yoga for RA are varied and result from studies lacking rigorous designs. As with OA, larger studies are needed testing yoga interventions that reflect the manner in which yoga is commonly used in the community.

Overall, yoga appears to be safe if practiced appropriately. No serious adverse events or overall disease exacerbations were reported in these studies (Bartlett et al., 2013), but some studies have reported exacerbation of pain with yoga (Park et al., 2011; Taibi & Vitiello, 2011). This may be related to deconditioning, but could also be related to inappropriateness of particular poses and practices for an individual's condition. Yoga instructors should be attentive to individual needs, and class sizes should be sufficiently small that persons with arthritis can receive individual instruction when needed. Another safety concern is the style of yoga. Some styles are inappropriate for persons with arthritis. Styles that are not recommended include Ashtanga (sometimes called "power yoga"), which is strenuous, and Bikram or "hot yoga", which is performed in a room heated to 100° or more (Bartlett et al., 2013). Vinyasa yoga moves quickly from one pose to the next, with little time to attend to joint alignment. This style should be used cautiously in persons with arthritis. Recommended styles that tend to be gentle include Anusara, Integral, Iyengar, Sivanda, and Viniyoga (Bartlett et al., 2013). Helpful information is available from researchers in the Johns Hopkins Arthritis Center (http://www.hopkinsarthritis.org/patient-corner/disease-management/yoga-for-arthritis/).

In summary, yoga may be beneficial for persons with arthritis, but there is currently insufficient evidence of good quality to recommend yoga as an effective treatment. Rigorous RCTs reflecting realistic interventions are needed. Yoga appears safe when practiced appropriately, but a gentle style and experienced instructor should be selected.

Discussing CAM with Patients

Research shows that up to about 70 % of patients may not disclose CAM use to their healthcare providers (Chao, Wade, & Kronenberg, 2008). Patients are more likely to disclose the use of CAM providers (e.g., chiropractic, acupuncture) than self-care practices (e.g., megavitamins, yoga or tai chi, relaxation) (Chao et al., 2008). In many cases, patients fear a negative response from their providers (Chang, Chang, & Siren, 2013; Robinson & McGrail, 2004). In other cases, patients feel that it is not important to disclose CAM use because they believe the approaches are natural and safe, or that their self-management is not pertinent to treatment by their providers. Finally, with the availability of information, patients may not feel the need to engage their providers for information about CAM modalities (Chang et al., 2013).

It is important for providers to broach the conversation about CAM use with their patients. NCCIH has provided helpful resources at the "Time to Talk" webpage (https://nccih.nih.gov/health/tips). This webpage includes tips for speaking with patients on this topic, as well as educational materials encouraging discussion of CAM use.

With the varieties of CAM modalities, it is a significant challenge for providers to maintain current knowledge of these modalities. It is helpful to know the effects and side effects of the most common approaches used by certain patient populations, such as those discussed in this chapter, and have resources ready for learning about other modalities. Table 14.1 lists some useful resources. In particular, NCCIH and the Longwood Herbal Task Force provide patient education materials available as well as summaries for providers. When assessing use of CAM modalities among persons with arthritis, it is important to note that persons with arthritis commonly use CAM for other conditions as well (Quandt et al., 2005).

Some recommendations for addressing CAM with patients are as follows:

- *Be approachable*. Many patients fear negatively impacting their relationship with their providers by disclosing CAM use. Even if a modality is not advisable for a patient, approach the matter in a sensitive, educational manner.
- *Find out where patients are getting their information.* Patients may or may not be using reputable sources of information. It may be helpful to have some sources ready to recommend, such as those listed in Table 14.1.
- *Emphasize that patients should not stop taking conventional treatments without discussion with their provider.* Most patients use CAM in conjunction with their conventional treatments. However, in some cases, patients may be hoping for an alternative with fewer side effects; in these cases, they also risk reduced efficacy. For patients with conditions such as RA, foregoing prescribed treatments may lead to irreversible disease progression. It is advisable to discuss the patient's reasons for using CAM and discuss adherence to conventional treatments.
- *Provide education and/or resources on potential side effects and interactions.* Patients may assume that CAM approaches are safe because they are perceived as "natural". It is important to discuss potential adverse effects, especially potential interactions between supplements and conventional medications.
- *Collaborate with the patient to meet care goals.* Patients have varied reasons for using CAM approaches. It is helpful to explore the patient's own goals to collaborate for effective care and symptom management.

In conclusion, certain CAM approaches hold promise as adjunct treatments for reducing arthritis progression and controlling symptoms. However, none of these modalities is currently supported by strong research evidence.

Table 14.1 Websites with evidence-based resources on CAM

Title	URL	Description
National Center for Complementary and Integrative Health (NCCIH)	https://nccih.nih.gov/	NCCIH is the center within the National Institutes of Health that funds CAM research. The website includes resources to disseminate research findings and to educate patients and providers on the current state of evidence on CAM modalities
Time to Talk	https://nccih.nih.gov/health/tips	The Time to Talk topics within the NCCIH website include resources to promote dialog on CAM between providers and patients
	https://nccih.nih.gov/health/tips/osteoarthritis-supplements	Within the Time to Talk webpages, there is a page specifically devoted to dietary supplements for OA
Longwood Herbal Task Force (LHTF)	http://www.longwoodherbal.org/	The LHTF is a collaborative project of Boston Children's Hospital, the Massachusetts College of Pharmacy and Health Sciences and the Dana Farber Cancer Institute. This project produces and disseminates evidence-based information on herbs and supplements, including brief provider summaries, patient information sheets, and in-depth monographs
Natural Standard	https://naturalmedicines.therapeuticresearch.com/	Natural standard is an independent collaboration that produces evidence-based monographs on a wide variety of CAM topics

Glucosamine, chondroitin, acupuncture, and tai chi have moderate evidence of benefit, but effects are also small. Limited research suggests that certain topical agents, massage therapy, and yoga may be helpful, but more research is needed. It is important for patients to discuss CAM use with providers for collaborative examination of cost and benefit, as well as safety, side effects, and potential interactions with conventional treatments. Given the widespread use of CAM approaches, this is clearly an important area in which collaboration with patients and consideration of their own care goals are important.

References

Amazaga Urruela, M., & Suarez-almazor, M. E. (2012). Acupuncture in the treatment of rheumatic diseases. *Current Rheumatology Reports, 14*, 589–597.

Barnes, P. M., Bloom, B., & Nahin, R. L. (2007). Complementary and alternative medicine use among adults and children: United States. *National Health Statistics Reports, 2008*, 1–23.

Bartlett, S. J., Moonaz, S. H., Mill, C., Bernatsky, S., & Bingham, C. O., 3rd. (2013). Yoga in rheumatic diseases. *Current Rheumatology Reports, 15*, 387. doi:10.1007/s11926-013-0387-2.

Callahan, L. F., Wiley-Exley, E. K., Mielenz, T. J., Brady, T. J., Xiao, C., Currey, S. S., Sleath, B. L., Sloane, P. D., DeVellis, R. F., & Sniezek, J. (2009). Use of complementary and alternative medicine among patients with arthritis. *Preventing Chronic Disease, 6*, A44.

Cameron, M., & Chrubasik, S. (2013). Topical herbal therapies for treating osteoarthritis. *Cochrane Database of Systematic Reviews, 5*, CD010538. doi:10.1002/14651858.CD010538.

Chang, H. Y., Chang, H. L., & Siren, B. (2013). Exploring the decision to disclose the use of natural products among outpatients: A mixed-method study. *BMC Complementary and Alternative Medicine, 13*, 319. doi:10.1186/1472-6882-13-319.

Chao, M. T., Wade, C., & Kronenberg, F. (2008). Disclosure of complementary and alternative medicine to conventional medical providers: Variation by race/ethnicity and type of CAM. *Journal of the National Medical Association, 100*, 1341–1349.

Cheung, C., Wyman, J. F., Resnick, B., & Savik, K. (2014). Yoga for managing knee osteoarthritis in older women: A pilot randomized controlled trial. *BMC Complementary and Alternative Medicine, 14*, 160. doi:10.1186/1472-6882-14-160.

Clegg, D. O., Reda, D. J., Harris, C. L., Klein, M. A., O'Dell, J. R., Hooper, M. M., Bradley, J. D., Bingham, C. O., 3rd, Weisman, M. H., Jackson, C. G., Lane, N. E., Cush, J. J., Moreland, L. W., Schumacher, H. R., Jr., Oddis, C. V., Wolfe, F., Molitor, J. A., Yocum, D. E., Schnitzer, T. J., Furst, D. E., Sawitzke, A. D., Shi, H., Brandt, K. D., Moskowitz, R. W., & Williams, H. J. (2006). Glucosamine, chondroitin sulfate, and the two in combination for painful knee osteoarthritis. *New England Journal of Medicine, 354*, 795–808. doi:10.1056/NEJMoa052771.

Corbett, M. S., Rice, S. J., Madurasinghe, V., Slack, R., Fayter, D. A., Harden, M., Sutton, A. J., Macpherson, H., & Woolacott, N. F. (2013). Acupuncture and other physical treatments for the relief of pain due to osteoarthritis of the knee: Network meta-analysis. *Osteoarthritis and Cartilage, 21*, 1290–1298. doi:10.1016/j.joca.2013.05.007.

Ebnezar, J., Nagarathna, R., Yogitha, B., & Nagendra, H. R. (2012). Effects of an integrated approach of hatha yoga therapy on functional disability, pain, and flexibility in osteoarthritis of the knee joint: A randomized controlled study. *Journal of Alternative and Complementary Medicine, 18*, 463–472. doi:10.1089/acm.2010.0320.

Eisenberg, D. M., Davis, R. B., Ettner, S. L., Appel, S., Wilkey, S., Van Rompay, M., & Kessler, R. C. (1998). Trends in alternative medicine use in the United States, 1990-1997: Results of a follow-up national survey. *Journal of the American Medical Association, 280*, 1569–1575.

Ernst, E. (2003). The safety of massage therapy. *Rheumatology, 42*, 1101–1106. doi:10.1093/rheumatology/keg306.

Evans, S., Moieni, M., Lung, K., Tsao, J., Sternlieb, B., Taylor, M., & Zeltzer, L. (2013). Impact of Iyengar yoga on quality of life in young women with rheumatoid arthritis. *Clinical Journal of Pain, 29*, 988–997. doi:10.1097/AJP.0b013e31827da381.

Evans, S., Moieni, M., Taub, R., Subramanian, S. K., Tsao, J. C., Sternlieb, B., & Zeltzer, L. K. (2010). Iyengar yoga for young adults with rheumatoid arthritis: Results from a mixed-methods pilot study. *Journal of Pain and Symptom Management, 39*, 904–913. doi:10.1016/j.jpainsymman.2009.09.018.

Field, T. (2014). Massage therapy research review. *Complementary Therapies in Clinical Practice, 20*(4), 224–229. doi:10.1016/j.ctcp.2014.07.002.

Field, T., Diego, M., Delgado, J., Garcia, D., & Funk, C. G. (2013). Rheumatoid arthritis in upper limbs benefits from moderate pressure massage therapy. *Complementary Therapies in Clinical Practice, 19*, 101–103. doi:10.1016/j.ctcp.2012.12.001.

Field, T., Diego, M., Hernandez-Reif, M., & Shea, J. (2007). Hand arthritis pain is reduced by massage therapy. *Journal of Bodywork and Movement Therapies, 11*, 21–24.

Field, T., Diego, M., & Solien-Wolfe, L. (2014). Massage therapy plus topical analgesic is more effective than massage alone for hand arthritis pain. *Journal of Bodywork and Movement Therapies, 18*, 322–325. doi:10.1016/j.jbmt.2013.12.002.

Gallagher, B., Tjoumakaris, F. P., Harwood, M. I., Good, R. P., Ciccotti, M. G., & Freedman, K. B. (2014). Chondroprotection and the prevention of osteoarthritis progression of the knee: A systematic review of treatment agents. *American Journal of Sports Medicine, 43*(3), 734–744. doi:10.1177/0363546514533777.

Garfinkel, M. S., Schumacher, H. R., Jr., Husain, A., Levy, M., & Reshetar, R. A. (1994). Evaluation of a yoga based regimen for treatment of osteoarthritis of the hands. *Journal of Rheumatology, 21*, 2341–2343.

Giordano, M., Capelli, L., & Chianese, U. (1975). The therapeutic activity of 1-(p-chlorobenzoyl)-5-methoxy-2-methylindole-3-acetic acid monohydrate glucosamide in rheumatoid arthritis (double blind trial). *Arzneimittel-Forschung, 25*, 435–437.

Grube, B., Grunwald, J., Krug, L., & Staiger, C. (2007). Efficacy of a comfrey root (Symphyti offic. radix) extract ointment in the treatment of patients with painful osteoarthritis of the knee: Results of a double-blind, randomised, bicenter, placebo-controlled trial. *Phytomedicine, 14*, 2–10. doi:10.1016/j.phymed.2006.11.006.

Han, A., Robinson, V., Judd, M., Taixiang, W., Wells, G., & Tugwell, P. (2004). Tai chi for treating rheumatoid arthritis. *Cochrane Database Systematic Review*, CD004849. doi:10.1002/14651858.CD004849.

Hawk, C., Ndetan, H., & Evans, M. W., Jr. (2012). Potential role of complementary and alternative health care providers in chronic disease prevention and health promotion: An analysis of National Health Interview Survey data. *Preventive Medicine, 54*, 18–22. doi:10.1016/j.ypmed.2011.07.002.

Henrotin, Y., Marty, M., & Mobasheri, A. (2014). What is the current status of chondroitin sulfate and glucosamine for the treatment of knee osteoarthritis? *Maturitas, 78*, 184–187. doi:10.1016/j.maturitas.2014.04.015.

Hochberg, M. C., Altman, R. D., April, K. T., Benkhalti, M., Guyatt, G., McGowan, J., Towheed, T., Welch, V., Wells, G., & Tugwell, P. (2012). American College of Rheumatology 2012 recommendations for the use of nonpharmacologic and pharmacologic therapies in osteoarthritis of the hand, hip, and knee. *Arthritis Care and Research, 64*, 465–474.

Hochberg, M., Chevalier, X., Henrotin, Y., Hunter, D. J., & Uebelhart, D. (2013). Symptom and structure modification in osteoarthritis with pharmaceutical-grade chondroitin sulfate: What's the evidence? *Current Medical Research and Opinion, 29*, 259–267. doi:10.1185/03007995.2012.753430.

Hoffer, L. J., Kaplan, L. N., Hamadeh, M. J., Grigoriu, A. C., & Baron, M. (2001). Sulfate could mediate the therapeutic effect of glucosamine sulfate. *Metabolism, 50*, 767–770. doi:10.1053/meta.2001.24201.

Jawahar, R., Yang, S., Eaton, C. B., McAlindon, T., & Lapane, K. L. (2012). Gender-specific correlates of complementary and alternative medicine use for knee osteoarthritis. *Journal of Women's Health, 21*, 1091–1099. doi:10.1089/jwh.2011.3434.

Kolasinski, S. L., Garfinkel, M., Tsai, A. G., Matz, W., Van Dyke, A., & Schumacher, H. R. (2005). Iyengar yoga for treating symptoms of osteoarthritis of the knees: A pilot study. *Journal of Alternative and Complementary Medicine, 11*, 689–693. doi:10.1089/acm.2005.11.689.

Laslett, L. L., & Jones, G. (2014). Capsaicin for osteoarthritis pain. *Progress in Drug Research, 68*, 277–291.

Lauche, R., Langhorst, J., Dobos, G., & Cramer, H. (2013). A systematic review and meta-analysis of tai chi for osteoarthritis of the knee. *Complementary Therapies in Medicine, 21*, 396–406. doi:10.1016/j.ctim.2013.06.001.

Lee, H. Y., Hale, C. A., Hemingway, B., & Woolridge, M. W. (2012). Tai Chi exercise and auricular acupressure for people with rheumatoid arthritis: An evaluation study. *Journal of Clinical Nursing, 21*, 2812–2822. doi:10.1111/j.1365-2702.2011.04058.x.

Lee, M. S., Lee, E. N., & Ernst, E. (2009). Is tai chi beneficial for improving aerobic capacity? A systematic review. *British Journal of Sports Medicine, 43*, 569–573. doi:10.1136/bjsm.2008.053272.

Lee, M. S., Pittler, M. H., Shin, B. C., & Ernst, E. (2008). Tai chi for osteoporosis: A systematic review. *Osteoporosis International, 19*, 139–146. doi:10.1007/s00198-007-0486-x.

Lee, M. S., Pittler, M. H., & Ernst, E. (2007). Tai chi for rheumatoid arthritis: Systematic review. *Rheumatology, 46*, 1648–1651. doi:10.1093/rheumatology/kem151.

Lee, M. S., Shin, B. C., & Ernst, E. (2008). Acupuncture for rheumatoid arthritis: A systematic review. *Rheumatology, 47*, 1747–1753. doi:10.1093/rheumatology/ken330.

Lee, J. A., Son, M. J., Choi, J., Jun, J. H., Kim, J. I., & Lee, M. S. (2014). Bee venom acupuncture for rheumatoid arthritis: A systematic review of randomised clinical trials. *BMJ Open, 4*, e006140. doi:10.1136/bmjopen-2014-006140.

Lee, Y. H., Woo, J. H., Choi, S. J., Ji, J. D., & Song, G. G. (2010). Effect of glucosamine or chondroitin sulfate on the osteoarthritis progression: A meta-analysis. *Rheumatology International, 30*, 357–363. doi:10.1007/s00296-009-0969-5.

Manheimer, E., Cheng, K., Linde, K., Lao, L., Yoo, J., Wieland, S., van der Windt, D. A., Berman, B. M., & Bouter, L. M. (2010). Acupuncture for peripheral joint osteoarthritis. *Cochrane Database Systematic Review*, CD001977. doi:10.1002/14651858.CD001977.pub2.

Manyanga, T., Froese, M., Zarychanski, R., Abou-Setta, A., Friesen, C., Tennenhouse, M., & Shay, B. L. (2014). Pain management with acupuncture in osteoarthritis: A systematic review and meta-analysis. *BMC Complementary and Alternative Medicine, 14*, 312. doi:10.1186/1472-6882-14-312.

Nakamura, H., Masuko, K., Yudoh, K., Kato, T., Kamada, T., & Kawahara, T. (2007). Effects of glucosamine administration on patients with rheumatoid arthritis. *Rheumatology International, 27*, 213–218. doi:10.1007/s00296-006-0197-1.

National Center for Complementary and Integrative Health. (2015). *Tai chi and qi gong*. Retrieved September 2, 2015, from https://nccih.nih.gov/health/taichi/introduction.htm?lang=en

National Center for Complementary and Integrative Health. (2015). *Complementary, alternative, or integrative health: What's in a name?*. Retrieved September 2, 2015, from https://nccih.nih.gov/health/integrative-health

Natural Standard. (2014a). *Glucosamine*. Retrieved November 19, 2014, from https://naturalmedicines.therapeuticresearch.com/databases/food,-herbs-supplements/g/glucosamine

Natural Standard. (2014b). *Chondroitin sulfate*. Retrieved November 14, 2014, from https://naturalmedicines.therapeuticresearch.com/databases/food,-herbs-supplements/professional.aspx?productid=744

Natural Standard. (2014c). *Arnica*. Retrieved November 21, 2014, from https://naturalmedicines.therapeuticresearch.com/databases/food,-herbs-supplements/a/arnica/professional.aspx

Natural Standard. (2014d). *Comfrey*. Retrieved November 21, 2014, https://naturalmedicines.therapeuticresearch.com/databases/food,-herbs-supplements/c/comfrey/professional.aspx

Park, J., McCaffrey, R., Dunn, D., & Goodman, R. (2011). Managing osteoarthritis: Comparisons of chair yoga, Reiki, and education (pilot study). *Holistic Nursing Practice, 25*, 316–326. doi:10.1097/HNP.0b013e318232c5f9.

Perlman, A. I., Ali, A., Njike, V. Y., Hom, D., Davidi, A., Gould-Fogerite, S., Milak, C., & Katz, D. L. (2012). Massage therapy for osteoarthritis of the knee: A randomized dose-finding trial. *PLoS One, 7*, e30248. doi:10.1371/journal.pone.0030248.

Perlman, A. I., Sabina, A., Williams, A. L., Njike, V. Y., & Katz, D. L. (2006). Massage therapy for osteoarthritis of the knee: A randomized controlled trial. *Archives of Internal Medicine, 166*, 2533–2538. doi:10.1001/archinte.166.22.2533.

Quandt, S. A., Chen, H., Grzywacz, J. G., Bell, R. A., Lang, W., & Arcury, T. A. (2005). Use of complementary and alternative medicine by persons with arthritis: Results of the National Health Interview Survey. *Arthritis and Rheumatism, 53*, 748–755. doi:10.1002/art.21443.

Robinson, A., & McGrail, M. R. (2004). Disclosure of CAM use to medical practitioners: A review of qualitative and quantitative studies. *Complementary Therapies in Medicine, 12*, 90–98. doi:10.1016/j.ctim.2004.09.006.

Roland, K. P., Jakobi, J. M., & Jones, G. R. (2011). Does yoga engender fitness in older adults? A critical review. *Journal of Aging and Physical Activity, 19*, 62–79.

Salazar, J., Bello, L., Chavez, M., Anez, R., Rojas, J., & Bermudez, V. (2014). Glucosamine for osteoarthritis: Biological effects, clinical efficacy, and safety on glucose metabolism. *Arthritis, 2014*, 432463. doi:10.1155/2014/432463.

Sawitzke, A. D., Shi, H., Finco, M. F., Dunlop, D. D., Bingham, C. O., 3rd, Harris, C. L., Harris, C. L., Singer, N. G., Bradley, J. D., Silver, D., Jackson, C. G., Lane, N. E., Oddis, C. V., Wolfe, F., Lisse, J., Furst, D. E., Reda, D. J., Moskowitz, R. W., Williams, H. J., & Clegg, D. O. (2008). The effect of glucosamine and/or chondroitin sulfate on the progression of knee osteoarthritis: A report from the glucosamine/chondroitin arthritis intervention trial. *Arthritis and Rheumatism, 58*, 3183–3191. doi:10.1002/art.23973.

Sawitzke, A. D., Shi, H., Finco, M. F., Dunlop, D. D., Harris, C. L., Singer, N. G., Bradley, J. D., , Silver, D., Jackson, C. G., Lane, N. E., Oddis, C. V., Wolfe, F., Lisse, J., Furst, D. E., Bingham, C. O., Reda, D. J., Moskowitz, R. W., Williams, H. J., & Clegg, D. O. (2010). Clinical efficacy and safety of glucosamine, chondroitin sulphate, their combination, celecoxib or placebo taken to treat osteoarthritis of the knee: 2-year results from GAIT. *Annals of the Rheumatic Diseases, 69*, 1459–1464. doi:10.1136/ard.2009.120469.

Sharma, M. (2014). Yoga as an alternative and complementary approach for arthritis: A systematic review. *Journal of Evidence-Based Complementary and Alternative Medicine, 19*, 51–58. doi:10.1177/2156587213499918.

Singh, V. K., Bhandari, R. B., & Rana, B. B. (2011). Effect of yogic package on rheumatoid arthritis. *Indian Journal of Physiology and Pharmacology, 55*, 329–335.

Taibi, D. M., & Vitiello, M. V. (2011). A pilot study of gentle yoga for sleep disturbance in women with osteoarthritis. *Sleep Medicine, 12*, 512–517. doi:10.1016/j.sleep.2010.09.016.

Telles, S., Naveen, K. V., Gaur, V., & Balkrishna, A. (2011). Effect of one week of yoga on function and severity in rheumatoid arthritis. *BMC Research Notes, 4*, 118. doi:10.1186/1756-0500-4-118.

Uhlig, T., Fongen, C., Steen, E., Christie, A., & Odegard, S. (2010). Exploring tai chi in rheumatoid arthritis: A quantitative and qualitative study. *BMC Musculoskeletal Disorders, 11*, 43. doi:10.1186/1471-2474-11-43.

Wandel, S., Juni, P., Tendal, B., Nuesch, E., Villiger, P. M., Welton, N. J., Reichenbach, S., & Trelle, S. (2010). Effects of glucosamine, chondroitin, or placebo in patients with osteoarthritis of hip or knee: Network meta-analysis. *British Medical Journal, 341*, c4675. doi:10.1136/bmj.c4675.

Wang, C. (2008). Tai Chi improves pain and functional status in adults with rheumatoid arthritis: Results of a pilot single-blinded randomized controlled trial. *Medicine and Sport Science, 52*, 218–229. doi:10.1159/000134302.

Wang, C., de Pablo, P., Chen, X., Schmid, C., & McAlindon, T. (2008). Acupuncture for pain relief in patients with rheumatoid arthritis: A systematic review. *Arthritis and Rheumatism, 59*, 1249–1256. doi:10.1002/art.24009.

Wayne, P. M., Berkowitz, D. L., Litrownik, D. E., Buring, J. E., & Yeh, G. Y. (2014). What do we really know about the safety of tai chi?: A systematic review of adverse event reports in randomized trials. *Archives of Physical Medicine and Rehabilitation, 95*(12), 2470–2483. doi:10.1016/j.apmr.2014.05.005.

Widrig, R., Suter, A., Saller, R., & Melzer, J. (2007). Choosing between NSAID and arnica for topical treatment of hand osteoarthritis in a randomised, double-blind study. *Rheumatology International, 27*, 585–591. doi:10.1007/s00296-007-0304-y.

Yan, J. H., Gu, W. J., Sun, J., Zhang, W. X., Li, B. W., & Pan, L. (2013). Efficacy of tai chi on pain, stiffness and function in patients with osteoarthritis: A meta-analysis. *PLoS One, 8*, e61672. doi:10.1371/journal.pone.0061672.

Yang, S., Dube, C. E., Eaton, C. B., McAlindon, T. E., & Lapane, K. L. (2013). Longitudinal use of complementary and alternative medicine among older adults with radiographic knee osteoarthritis. *Clinical Therapeutics, 35*, 1690–1702. doi:10.1016/j.clinthera.2013.09.022.

15 Enhancing Clinical Practice with Community-Based Self-Management Support Programs

Teresa J. Brady

Introduction

Beyond treatment of the presenting clinical issues, an essential challenge of working with people with arthritis in clinical practice is helping the individual develop the knowledge, skills, and confidence to manage their disease on a day-to-day basis. Typical patient–clinician interactions are time-limited and relatively infrequent in the context of diseases like arthritis that must be managed 24 h per day/7 days per week. However, clinicians can play a significant role in helping their patients become effective self-managers, which is becoming increasingly important in twenty-first century healthcare delivery.

This attention to self-management as a crucial part of high-quality chronic disease care is evident in the Institute of Medicine's (IOM) report on Crossing the Quality Chasm (Adams, Greiner, & Corrigan, 2004), the Chronic Care Model (Wagner, 1998), and even re-formulations of the definition of health (Huber et al., 2011). The IOM defined self-management as "the tasks the individual must undertake to live well with one or more chronic conditions" (Adams et al., 2004). The definition specifies that these tasks include having the confidence to deal with medical management, role management, and emotional management. The Chronic Care Model was developed to identify the key system changes necessary to transform the healthcare delivery system to better meet the challenges of caring for people with chronic diseases (Wagner, 1998). Provision of self- management support and use of community resources are two of the six dimensions of health system improvement articulated in the Chronic Care Model as essential for high-quality chronic disease care (Wagner, 1998). Huber and colleagues, who viewed the World Health Organization's definition of health ("a state of complete physical, mental, and social well-being and not merely the absence of disease") as counterproductive since it identifies people with chronic diseases as de facto "ill," proposed a refined definition of health as "the ability to adapt and self-manage" (Huber et al., 2011 p. 2).

Clinicians caring for people with arthritis can enhance their clinical practice by incorporating recommendations or referrals to self-management support programs, and strategies to foster patient commitment to participate, into their clinical routines. Use of evidence-based community self-management programs can be particularly advantageous because they have demonstrated improvements in both physical and psychological health status (Brady, Jernick, Hootman, & Sniezek, 2009). The purpose of this chapter is to describe why evidence-based

T.J. Brady, PhD (✉)
Arthritis Program, Centers for Disease Control and Prevention, 4770 Buford Hwy NE MS F-78, Atlanta, GA, 30341, USA
e-mail: Tob9@cdc.gov

P.M. Nicassio (ed.), *Psychosocial Factors in Arthritis*, DOI 10.1007/978-3-319-22858-7_15

community programs are an important adjunct to clinical care in arthritis, discuss specific types of community programs useful for people with arthritis, and identify strategies to incorporate these community programs into clinical practice and help people with arthritis commit to participating in these valuable community resources.

Why Evidence-Based Community Programs Are an Important Adjunct to Clinical Care in Arthritis

As alluded to above, good self-management is essential to good health outcomes in arthritis. The American College of Rheumatology's (ACR) 2012 guidelines for the treatment of osteoarthritis (OA) include a number of recommended treatment modalities, such as various forms of exercise, weight loss, or use of medications that can only be completed by the patient himself or herself (Hochberg et al., 2012). Similarly, the ACR guidelines for treating rheumatoid arthritis (RA) include recommendations for a number of treatment modalities that require daily participation by the patient (ACR Subcommittee on RA Guidelines, 2002). This need for the patients to be active participants in their daily care, or to be self-managers, has not diminished in this new era of biologic treatment in RA. In a 2014 qualitative study of patients with RA, Flurey and colleagues documented that even when the disease is stable, people with RA perceive the need to micromanage both their symptoms and their daily activities to accommodate their RA, and that they use self-management techniques to maintain that dynamic balance between life and RA (Flurey, Morris, Richards, Hughes, & Hewlett, 2014). Further, these self-management efforts intensify as RA flares threaten their carefully maintained balance (Flurey et al., 2014).

Clinicians working with patients with arthritis can play a key role helping their patients evolve into successful self-managers, through the self-management support they provide. The *National Public Health Agenda for Osteoarthritis 2010* (*OA Public Health Agenda*) slightly modified the IOM definition to define self-management *support* as "the systematic provision of education and supportive interventions by healthcare or other providers to strengthen patients' skills and confidence in managing their health problems, including regular assessment of progress and problems, goal setting, and problem-solving support" (Arthritis Foundation and Centers for Disease Control and Prevention, 2010). Clinicians can provide such self-management support in their routine clinical interactions, but rarely do busy clinicians have the luxury of time required to personally implement intensive behavior change interventions. Evidence-based intervention programs in the community can help fill this gap; many are designed to help people with arthritis acquire the knowledge, skills, and confidence to successfully manage their arthritis. These community-based programs include those focusing on physical activity, self-management education, and weight loss. Fostering participation in community-based self-management support programs with documented positive health outcomes is another form of self-management support that clinicians seeing patients with arthritis are well-positioned to provide (Brady, 2012).

The idea of referring to community programs is not foreign to many clinicians. Audience research with both primary care providers (PCPs) and physical therapists (PTs) noted that both groups routinely recommend community resources to their patients (Brady, Price, Ryan, Eidson, & Savage, 2009; Hefelfinger et al., 2014). Sixty percent of PCPs reported that they refer to community resources several times per week or more, and 56 % reported that they were aware of community resources for people with arthritis (Brady, Price, et al., 2009). Sixty-seven percent of PTs surveyed reported that they were aware of physical activity resources in their local community (Hefelfinger et al., 2014). However, when specific evidence-based, arthritis-appropriate physical activity or self-management education programs were described (Brady, Jernick et al., 2009), awareness fell to 20 % among PCPs (Brady, Price, et al., 2009) and 18 % (self-management education (SME) programs) and 40

% (PA programs) among PTs (Hefelfinger et al., 2014). As all of healthcare moves toward evidence-based practice, there are clear benefits to using what works—recommending those intervention programs with documented health benefits for people with arthritis. Further, audience research with people with arthritis found that a key reason people do not participate in SME programs is that they do not know they exist (Unpublished CDC Report)—clinician recommendation or referral can help fill this gap.

Types of Evidence-Based Self-Management Support Programs Useful for People with Arthritis

The ACR guidelines for OA (Hochberg et al., 2012) and RA (ACR Subcommittee on RA Guidelines, 2002) and the *OA Public Health Agenda* (Arthritis Foundation and Centers for Disease Control and Prevention, 2010) all identify physical activity, self-management education, and weight control as important self-management activities. While there have been a number of efficacy trials addressing these health behaviors, few interventions tested have developed the infrastructure to support widespread dissemination in communities across the country. The Centers for Disease Control and Prevention's (CDC) Arthritis Program has screened interventions to identify those that are arthritis-appropriate, have an adequate base of evidence supporting their health effects, and have the infrastructure (i.e., implementation guide, leaders manual, training, and technical assistance readily available) to support widespread dissemination (Brady, Jernick, et al., 2009). Six physical activity intervention programs and seven self-management education programs meet all of these criteria and are approved for dissemination by CDC-funded Arthritis Program grantees. Because these "packaged" (ready-to-use) interventions are available in multiple locations around the country, they are good resources for clinicians who want to enhance their clinical treatment with evidence-based intervention programs in the community.

Physical Activity Programs

Physical activity programs that meet the CDC Arthritis Program screening criteria are described in Table 15.1. The majority of physical activity programs that meet these criteria are small group programs—programs where 15–20 participants come together two to three times per week to exercise as a group. Most of the programs include multiple forms of exercise including flexibility, strengthening, aerobic conditioning, and balance activities. All can be modified to meet the capabilities of the individual participant. In 2011, Kelley and colleagues conducted a meta-analysis of 33 studies on the effects of community exercise programs among people with arthritis and found statistically significant and clinically meaningful improvements in pain (effect size 0.20) and function (effect size 0.34) (both intention-to-treat analyses) (Kelley, Kelley, Hootman, & Jones, 2011).

While the available programs have similar sets of exercises, they also have some important differences. The Arthritis Foundation Aquatic Program (AFAP) (Patrick et al., 2001) is performed in water, in contrast to the Arthritis Foundation Exercise Program (AFEP) (Callahan et al., 2008), EnhanceFitness (EF) (Wallace et al., 1998), and Fit & Strong! (F&S!) (Hughes et al., 2004), which are all done on land. Walk with Ease (WWE) (Callahan et al., 2011) focuses solely on walking, although it does include some warm-up stretching. Active Living Every Day (ALED) (Callahan et al., 2014) is a behavior change program focused on physical activity, but participants do not exercise in class. ALED class sessions focus on developing plans to incorporate exercise into daily routines and address barriers to regular exercise; all exercise is done outside of class.

Some of these more widely disseminated physical activity interventions, such as AFAP, AFEP, F&S!, and WWE, were all designed specifically for people with arthritis and include some educational components as well as the group exercise. In contrast, EF and ALED were developed to meet a more broad target population, but are also appropriate for people with arthritis.

While the majority of currently available physical activity programs require participants to meet together with a trained leader several times per week, WWE is designed to also accommodate self-directed participants—participants who conduct the program on their own by reading the book and gradually progressing the time or distance they walk. In an evaluation of both the group and self-directed formats of WWE, the participants in the self-directed WWE had 6-week improvements that were fairly equivalent to the group format and retained more of those benefits at 1 year follow-up than did the group participants (Callahan et al., 2011). Online tools are also available to support group and self-directed participants of WWE.

These physical activity programs are conveniently available at local fitness facilities, YMCAs, and community and senior centers. All of the physical activity programs identified in Table 15.1 are offered in multiple states across the country, although there is variability in availability. In 2014, EnhanceFitness was offered in more than 30 states, while Fit & Strong! was offered at multiple locations but in just three states (Illinois, North Carolina, and West Virginia). All of the small group exercise programs are led by trained instructors, with fitness or exercise training as well as 4–15 h of training in the specific intervention program. All of the interventions were developed at academic research centers or non-profit organizations, and all are offered at low cost (ranging from $2 to $3 dollars per session or $30 to $40 for an 8–12 week series of classes).

Self-Management Education Programs

The *OA Public Health Agenda*defines SME as interactive educational interventions specifically designed to enhance patient self-management. SME is patient-driven and focuses on building generalizable skills such as goal-setting, decision-making, problem-solving, and self-monitoring (Arthritis Foundation and Centers for Disease Control and Prevention, 2010). Self-management education differs from more traditional patient education in its focus on building those generalizable skills and helping people learn to solve the inevitable challenges of living with arthritis and make wise decisions about how to care for themselves, rather than a focus on disease information and compliance with healthcare professional directions (Bodenheimer, Lorig, Holman, & Grumbach, 2002). Seven SME interventions meet the criteria identified by the CDC Arthritis Program for interventions that are arthritis-appropriate, with an adequate evidence-base, and have the infrastructure to support widespread implementation (Brady, Jernick, et al., 2009). These programs are described in Table 15.2.

As with physical activity intervention programs, the majority of SME programs that met the CDC Arthritis Program screening criteria are small group programs, although not all of them require in-person meetings. The two prototype interventions are the Arthritis Self-Management Program (ASMP) (Lorig, Mazonson, & Holman, 1993) and the Chronic Disease Self-Management Program (CDSMP) (Lorig et al., 2001). The other programs are alternative delivery formats for these two seminal programs. All of these SME programs were developed at Stanford University and use enhancing self-efficacy, or confidence in ability to perform selected tasks, as the theoretical basis for behavior change (Lorig & Gonzalez, 1992).

ASMP is a 6-week small group in-person workshop for 15 people with arthritis; Programa de Manejo Personal de la Artritis (Lorig, Gonzalez, & Ritter, 1999) is a similar program developed to meet the needs of Spanish-speaking people with arthritis. Better Choices, Better Health for Arthritis (Lorig, Ritter, Laurent, & Plant, 2008) delivers the same content and utilizes similar processes as ASMP, but is delivered as a virtual group, meeting online for 6 weeks. The Arthritis Toolkit delivers the ASMP content in a self-study format and is available in English and Spanish (Goeppinger et al., 2009). The majority of studies of ASMP have examined the small group in-person delivery format; the alternative delivery formats have one to two studies each. A 2011 meta-analysis of 19 studies of the

Table 15.1 Physical activity programs meeting CDC arthritis program screening criteria

Program	Description	Evidence-base	Instructor qualifications	Availability	For information
Active Living Every Day (ALED)	Small group educational behavior change program focused on incorporating exercise into daily life	At 12 months:	One instructor per course	Available in nearly every state	www.activeliving.info
Developed by the Cooper Institute	All exercise done outside of class	↑ physical activity with no increase in arthritis symptoms. (Callahan et al., 2014)	Online preparatory course followed by 2-day web-based or in-person training. Competency test before certification	Online version available but no evaluation data available	Program locator:
Dissemination support provided by Active Living Partners	Offered as weekly class in 12 or 20 week series	↓ depression, perceived stress. (Baruth & Wilcox, 2011)			http://www.activeliving.info/TakeCourse.cfm
Arthritis Foundation Aquatic Program (AFAP)	Low impact water exercise program developed for people with arthritis	↑ flexibility, strength, and aerobic fitness. (Patrick et al., 2001)	Health and fitness staff or volunteers with fitness experience who complete online training	Available in multiple locations across the U.S.	www.aeawave.com
Developed by the Arthritis Foundation	Includes range of motion, muscle strengthening and conditioning exercise	Better outcomes among participants who attended 2+ classes per week. (Belza et al., 2002)			Program locator:
Dissemination support provided by Aquatic Exercise Association	Conducted in a warm water pool; offered 2–3 times per week in 8–12 week sessions or ongoing				www.arthritis.org
Arthritis Foundation Exercise Program (AFEP)	Low impact recreational exercise program developed for people with arthritis. Includes range of motion, strengthening, balance, and aerobic condition exercise. Includes a health education component	↑ self-efficacy, use of upper extremity	Health and fitness staff or volunteers with fitness experience who complete online training	Available in multiple locations across the U.S.	www.aeawave.com
Developed by the Arthritis Foundation	Offered 2–3 times per week in 8–12 week sessions or ongoing	↓ pain, fatigue (Callahan et al., 2008)			Program locator:
Dissemination support provided by Aquatic Exercise Association					www.arthritis.org

(continued)

Table 15.1 (continued)

Program	Description	Evidence-base	Instructor qualifications	Availability	For information
EnhanceFitness (EF)	Small group exercise program originally developed for older adults	↑ physical function	Certified fitness instructor with 12 h of specialized EF training	Available in more than 25 states	http://projectenhance.org/EnhanceFitness.aspx
Developed by the University of Washington	Includes flexibility, strengthening, balance, and conditioning exercise	↓ depression (Wallace et al., 1998)			Program locator:
Dissemination support provided by project enhance located at senior services	Offered three times per week on ongoing basis	↑ strength, mobility, self-rated health (Belza et al., 2006)			http://projectenhance.org/LocationMap.aspx
Fit & Strong! (F&S!)	Small group program that combines exercise and self-management education in each session. Developed for people with lower extremity osteoarthritis. Includes flexibility, strength training and aerobic working. Meets 3 times per week for 8 weeks. Concludes with participants developing a maintenance plan	↑ ability to exercise, adherence to exercise (Hughes et al., 2004)	Certified fitness instructor or physical therapist; 8 h of specialized training	Available in Illinois, North Carolina and west Virginia	http://www.fitandstrong.org/
Developed by the University of Illinois		↑ self-efficacy, strength, function			Program locator:
Dissemination support provided by the University of Illinois		↓ pain, stiffness (Seymour et al., 2009)			http://www.fitandstrong.org/about/locations_map.html
		↑ physical activity, strength, function			
		↓ pain, stiffness , depression, anxiety (Hughes et al., 2010)			

Walk with Ease (WWE)	Walking program designed for people with arthritis. Offered as small group instructor led program 3 times per week for 6 weeks or as a self-directed program. Includes educational modules on walking related topics	↑ strength, balance, walking pace, self-efficacy'	3–4 h of specialized online training. Must pass an online quiz to become certified	Available in many states; self-directed program can be done anywhere	http://www.arthritis.org/we-can-help/community-programs/walk-with-ease/
Developed by the University of North Carolina	Online tools available to support participants	↓ pain, stiffness, fatigue, disability			Program locator:
Dissemination support provided by the Arthritis Foundation		More benefits maintained at 12 months in self-directed format (Callahan et al., 2011)			www.arthritis.org
					Online tools: http://www.arthritistoday.org/tools-and-resources/walk-with-ease-program/walk-with-ease-modules.php

Table 15.2 Self-management education programs meeting CDC arthritis program screening criteria

Program	Description	Evidence-base	Instructor qualifications	Availability	For information
Arthritis Self-Management Program (ASMP)	Interactive in-person small group workshop offered for 2–2.5 h per week for 6 weeks. Focuses on healthy behaviors such as physical activity, cognitive stress management, and communication with health care providers and generalizable skills such as problem-solving, decision-making, and action planning. Developed specifically for people with arthritis and all participants have arthritis	Meta-analysis of 19 studies demonstrated	Pair of leaders, preferably at least one who has arthritis; successful completion of CDSMP 4.5 day training followed by 4 h online arthritis-specific cross-training	Organizations in 15–20 states are licensed to offer ASMP; some are using CDSMP instead	http://patienteducation.stanford.edu/programs/asmp.html
Developed by Stanford University		↑ self-efficacy, cognitive symptom management			Program locator:
Dissemination support provided by Stanford University		↓ depression, anxiety, health distress and fatigue, all sustained at 12 months			http://patienteducation.stanford.edu/organ/asmpsites.html
		↑ exercise present at 6 months but not sustained at 12 months (Brady et al., 2010)			
The Arthritis Toolkit (Toolkit)	Same content as the ASMP provided in a self-study format. Toolkit includes a self-assessment to direct user to most relevant content, The Arthritis Helpbook, tip sheets to address common problems, exercise and relaxation CDs. Available in English or Spanish	↑ self-efficacy, role function	No leader required	Available by mail order nationwide	https://www.bullpub.com/catalog/the-arthritis-toolkit/
Developed by Stanford University		↓ pain, fatigue, disability, depression, health distress (Goeppinger et al., 2009)			Program locator:
Disseminated by Bull Publishing					Order toolkit through Bull Publishing
Better Choices, Better Health (BCBH)	Interactive online small group workshop covering the same content as the in-person CDSMP	↑ stretch/strength exercise	Experience as a CDSMP leader, additional training to moderate online discussions	Available to members of contracted organizations	http://www.ncoa.org/improve-health/chronic-conditions/better-choices-better-health.html
Developed by Stanford University		↓ pain, fatigue, health distress, shortness of breath (Lorig et al., 2006)			Program locator:
Disseminated by National Council on Aging/Canary Health					Information available through contracted organizations.

Better Choices, Better Health for Arthritis (BCBH-A)	Interactive online small group workshop covering the same content as the in-person ASMP	↑ self-efficacy, self-reported health	Experience as a CDSMP leader, additional training to moderate online discussions	Available nationwide	http://www.ncoa.org/improve-health/chronic-conditions/better-choices-better-health.html
Disseminated by National Council on Aging/Canary Health		↓ pain, disability, health distress, all sustained at 12 months (Lorig et al., 2008)			Program locator:
					http://www.arthritistoday.org/arthritis-self-management-program/
Chronic Disease Self-Management Program (CDSMP)	Interactive in-person small group workshop offered for 2–2.5 h per week for 6 weeks. Focuses on healthy behaviors such as physical activity, cognitive stress management, and communication with health care providers and generalizable skills such as problem-solving, decision-making, and action planning. Developed for people with a variety of chronic conditions; participants can have a variety of chronic conditions	Meta-analysis of 18 studies demonstrated	Pair of leaders, preferably at least one who has a chronic condition; 4.5 day training program	Organizations licensed to offer the program in all 50 states in the United States and well as internationally	http://patienteducation.stanford.edu/programs/cdsmp.html
Developed by Stanford University		↑ self-efficacy, cognitive symptom management, aerobic exercise			Program locator:
Dissemination support provided by Stanford University		↓ depression, health distress, social/role limitations, pain, shortness of breath, all sustained at 12 months (Brady et al., 2013)			www.restartliving.org
CDSMP Tool Kit for Active Living (CDSMP Toolkit)	Same content as the CDSMP provided in a self-study format. Toolkit includes a self-assessment to direct user to most relevant content, living a healthy life with chronic conditions book, tip sheets to address common problems, exercise and relaxation CDs	↑ communication with doctor, self-rated health, muscle strength/stretch	No leader required	Available by mail order nationwide	https://www.bullpub.com/catalog/Chronic-Disease-Self-Management-Program-Tool-Kit-for-Active-Living
Developed by Stanford University		↓ depression, role limitations, unhealthy days (Lorig et al., 2015)			Program locator:
Disseminated by Bull Publishing					Order toolkit through Bull Publishing

(continued)

Table 15.2 (continued)

Program	Description	Evidence-base	Instructor qualifications	Availability	For information
Programa de Manejo Personal la Artritis	Same content and format as ASMP, delivered in Spanish, developed to be culturally and linguistically appropriate for people of Hispanic origin	↑ self-efficacy, exercise, self-reported health	Pair of leaders, preferably at least one who has a arthritis; 4.5 day training program conducted in Spanish	Organizations in five states (Florida, Massachusetts, Minnesota, Rhode Island, Wisconsin,) and several Spanish-speaking countries licensed to offer the program	http://patienteducation.stanford.edu/programs_spanish/asmpesp.html
Developed by Stanford University		↓ pain, disability, depression, all sustained at 12 months (Lorig et al., 1999)			Program locator:
Dissemination support provided by Stanford University					http://patienteducation.stanford.edu/organ/asmpsitesesp.html
Tomando Control de su Salud (Tomando)	Same content and format as CDSMP, delivered in Spanish, developed to be culturally and linguistically appropriate for people of Hispanic origin	↑ self-efficacy, self-reported health	Pair of leaders, preferably at least one who has a arthritis; 4.5 day training program conducted in Spanish	Organizations licensed to offer the program in all 50 states in the United States as well as internationally in Spanish-speaking countries	http://patienteducation.stanford.edu/programs_spanish/tomando.html
Developed by Stanford University		↓ pain, disability, health distress, all sustained at 12 months (Lorig et al., 2003)			Program locator:
Dissemination support provided by Stanford University					www.restartliving.org

small group in-person ASMP found small to moderate improvements in self efficacy, psychological health status, and selected health behaviors at 4–6-month follow-up, and most improvements persisted at 9–12-month follow-up. Fatigue and functional disability showed small improvements at 4–6 months, but these improvements were not maintained at 9–12-month follow-up (Brady, O'Colmain, Mobley, Greenberg, & Murphy, 2010).

CDSMP is similar in content and processes to ASMP, but has the advantage of addressing participants with a variety of health conditions (Lorig et al., 2001). CDSMP is based on two key premises: that people with chronic diseases have similar challenges in problem-solving and decision-making and need to learn generic skills to address these challenges, and that many people with chronic diseases have more than one chronic condition. Forty-seven percent of people with arthritis have at least one other chronic condition (Murphy, Bolen, Helmick, & Brady, 2009) and 28 % of all adult Americans have two or more chronic conditions (Anderson, 2010).

Similar to ASMP, CDSMP is also available in a variety of delivery formats. While the CDSMP is a small group in-person workshop, Tomando Control de su Salud (Lorig, Ritter, & Gonzàlez, 2003) is the culturally appropriate parallel course developed for a Spanish-speaking population. Better Choices, Better Health is the online virtual group version of CDSMP (Lorig, Ritter, Laurent, & Plant, 2006). A self-study version of CDSMP is also available (Lorig, Ritter, Moreland, & Laurent, 2015). Also similar to ASMP, the majority of studies of CDSMP have examined the small group in-person delivery format, while the evaluations of other delivery formats are limited to one to two studies each. A 2011 meta-analysis of 18 studies of the small group in-person CDSMP demonstrated small to moderate improvements in psychological health (self-efficacy, depression, and health distress) and selected health behaviors (cognitive symptom management and aerobic exercise) at 4–6-month follow-up that persisted at 12-month follow-up. Improvements in stretching/strengthening exercise and pain emerged at the 12-month follow-up (Brady et al., 2013).

CDSMP is the most widely disseminated of these SME programs and is currently available in almost every state in the United States as well as various countries across the world. For example, in the period 2010–2012, more than 100,000 participants completed CDSMP offered through Aging Network affiliated organizations alone (Ory et al., 2013). The availability of online virtual workshops and the self-study formats provides easy access for people anywhere in the country to participate in SME programs. Availability of the small group in-person ASMP has declined with the growth of CDSMP, but the online and self-study delivery formats are still readily accessible for those who prefer an arthritis-specific SME program. Studies comparing the health outcomes of CDSMP with ASMP among people with arthritis have shown equivocal results (Goeppinger et al., 2007; Lorig, Ritter, & Plant, 2005), so one program is not preferred over the other in terms of health benefits for people with arthritis.

These SME programs are offered in local health care and community settings and are generally low cost—less than $50 for a 6-week workshop. Both self-study toolkits are available for less than $50 as well. The small group programs are each led by two trained leaders, one of whom is a person with arthritis or chronic disease, all of whom have completed a 4.5 day training session.

Weight Loss Programs

Despite the importance of weight control in the management of osteoarthritis of the hip and knee, and a few limited clinical trials of weight loss interventions (Messier et al., 2004), there are no widely disseminated arthritis-specific weight loss interventions in the community. In qualitative formative research on the use of community-based programs for arthritis management, PCPs specifically mentioned commercial weight loss programs as common referrals (Brady, Price, et al., 2009). A 2014 cost-effectiveness analysis of medications and commercial weight loss programs concluded Weight Watchers was the best value in terms of cost per weight lost or quality-adjusted life year saved (Finkelstein & Kruger, 2014). Weight Watchers also has an impressive distribution system with over 40,000 meetings weekly across the world and over 10,000 trained leaders, all of whom have lost weight on the program. Weight Watchers identifies itself as a behavior change program focused on healthy eating, behavior modification, and physical activity. An online version of Weight Watchers is also available http://www.weightwatchersinternational.com/phoenix.zhtml?c=130178&p=irol-IRHome.

Integrating Community-Based Programs into Clinical Practice

Integrating community-based self-management support programs into clinical practice requires identifying which patients are appropriate for community-based programs, and how to effectively encourage patients to participate in and commit to these programs.

Identifying Patients Appropriate for Community-Based Programs

Physical Activity: The Guidelines for Physical Activity for all Americans, issued by the U.S. Department of health and Human Services, recommend that all Americans perform 150 min of moderate physical activity each week (US Department of Health and Human Services, 2008). However, only 26 % of people with arthritis meet that recommendation and 44 % of people with arthritis are inactive—that is do not participate in any leisure time physical activity for a minimum of 10 min (Shih, Hootman, Kruger, & Helmick, 2006). Some people with arthritis may be able to increase their physical activity by simply being informed of the guidelines and encouraged to be more physically active, but the majority of patients are likely to require additional structured support.

People with arthritis face the same barriers to physical activity that people without arthritis do, as well as some arthritis-specific barriers, including pain or fear of pain, not being able to find an exercise they can do and not being sure of what exercise is safe for them to do (Wilcox et al., 2006). Arthritis-appropriate physical activity programs, such as those described in Table 15.1, can address these barriers.

Self-Management Education: One of the most robust findings from evaluations of self-management education programs is the positive changes in self-efficacy or confidence in ability to manage symptoms (Brady et al., 2010, 2013). Self-efficacy is correlated with health status such as mental and physical well-being (Lefebvre et al., 1999) and predicts health behaviors such as physical activity, healthy eating, and coping skills (Taal, Rasker, Seydel, & Wiegman, 1993). Self-management education can serve as the catalyst to help people become active self-managers. Any patient who is not taking active control of his or her health could likely benefit from a self-management education program. Reeves and colleagues demonstrated that those patients with lower self-efficacy and health-related quality of life at baseline experienced greater health benefits from participation in CDSMP than did those with higher baseline scores (Reeves et al., 2008).

Weight Loss: Patients who are overweight and struggle to lose weight are obvious candidates for structured weight loss programs. Sixty-seven percent of people with arthritis are overweight or obese (Shih et al., 2006), but only 41 % of overweight or obese adults with arthritis have been told by their clinician to lose weight (Do, Hootman, Helmick, & Brady, 2011).

Strategies to Effectively Encourage Patients to Participate in Community-Based Programs

At a minimum, clinicians can enhance their clinical practice by referring their patients to, or recommending their patients attend, physical activity, self-management education, or weight loss program in the community. Murphy and colleagues reported that people who receive a healthcare provider referral are 18 times more likely to attend than those who do not receive a provider referral (Murphy et al., 2007). However, that same analysis documented that only half of the people who receive the referral actually attend the program (Murphy et al., 2007). Additional strategies, beyond just making the recommendation, can help patients evolve into more active self-managers and receive the benefits available from these community-based self-management support programs.

Although most clinicians do not have time in their limited patient encounters to implement complex behavioral interventions, provider counseling techniques borrowed from the addictions and smoking cessation literature are gaining recognition as useful means of providing chronic disease self-management support and have been used to support self-management behaviors such as increasing physical activity or losing weight (Brady, 2012; Lin, O'Connor, Whitlock, & Beil, 2010; Pearson, Mattke, Shaw, Ridgely, & Wiseman, 2007).

The American College of Preventive Medicine recommends the use of the 5 A's model of behavioral counseling to strengthen providers' approaches to encouraging their patients to become more physically active (Jacobson et al., 2005). The 5 A's model includes a sequence of five pragmatic steps to elicit and foster behavior change (Glasgow, Goldstein, Ockene, & Pronk, 2004). Jay and colleagues surveyed obese patients on their physician's use of 5 A techniques. Patients who received more 5 A techniques had higher motivation and change intentions in a dose–response relationship—each additional technique was associated with greater odds of being motivated to lose weight and greater intentions to exercise or eat better (Jay, Gillespie, Schlair, Sherman, & Kalet, 2010). The 5 As are outlined in Table 15.3.

Similarly, motivational interviewing (MI) emerged from addictions counseling and is also being used to support self-management in patients with chronic disease. MI is a patient-centered yet directive form of counseling to promote behavior change by focusing on the patient's own perceptions and motivations and to foster behavior change by surfacing and addressing their ambivalence about the change (Miller and Rollnick, 2002). Key principles of MI are outlined in Table 15.3.

MI has been used in a variety of health behaviors. In a meta-analysis of controlled clinical trials of MI, Burke and colleagues demonstrated that MI-based interventions had a moderate effect (0.53 effect size) on diet and exercise behaviors (Burke, Arkowitz, & Menchola, 2003). Pollack and colleagues demonstrated in an observational study that patients whose physician used MI-consistent behaviors in their weight counseling lost significantly more weight than those whose physician used MI-inconsistent behaviors (3.1 lb loss versus 0.4 lb gain) (Pollack et al., 2010). A meta-analysis of MI used in medical settings found significant improvement in weight control, increasing physical activity, intention to change, and confidence in approaching change when dealing with chronic conditions (Lundahl et al., 2013). Ranatunga and colleagues reported no difficulties in using MI in their academic rheumatology clinic as part of their approach for providing self-management support (Ranatunga et al., 2010).

A third approach to behavioral counseling, called Brief Action Planning (BAP), is emerging; it combines the behavior counseling techniques of motivational interviewing with evidence-based constructs from behavior change literature, specifically goal setting, action planning, and self-efficacy (Gutnick et al., 2014). BAP focuses on three core questions and is designed to help patients shape an action plan, assess their confidence in their ability to complete their plan, and negotiate a mutually agreeable follow-up plan to check progress. More details on BAP are available in Table 15.3. BAP was designed in part to serve as a quick alternative to behavioral counseling strategies that require more extensive training to acquire the required skills and that take longer to implement in clinical practice. Although there are no data yet on the effects of BAP, clinicians using this approach have found it useful and feasible to fit into a brief clinical encounter (Gutnick et al., 2014).

All of the behavioral counseling techniques described have some common elements, specifi-

Table 15.3 Behavioral counseling techniques

Technique	5A's	Motivational interviewing	Brief action planning
Background	Developed in smoking cessation	Developed in addictions counseling	Developed for clinical settings
Description	Sequence of five pragmatic steps:	Four basic principles of motivational interviewing:	Three key questions discussed with the patient:
	• Assess: assess current beliefs and behaviors related to behavior change, and once plan is established, assess confidence in ability to achieve plan	• Express empathy through reflective listening	• Is there anything you would like to do for your health in the next 1–2 weeks?
	• Advise: offer specific personalized information on health risk and need for behavior change	• Develop discrepancy between patient's goals and current behavior (to highlight importance of change)	• How confident are you, on a scale of 0–10, about carrying out your plan?
	• Agree: through a collaborative process, negotiate a mutually agreed upon action plan	• Roll with patient resistance rather than opposing it (avoiding arguments or direct confrontation)	• Would it be helpful to set up a time to check in to discuss how you are coming with your plan?
	• Assist: provide resources to support patient in achieving their plan	• Support self-efficacy and optimism (Burke et al., 2003)	Five core skills:
	• Arrange: Arrange to follow up to assess and support progress in achieving plan (Glasgow et al., 2004)		• Offering a behavioral menu
			• Developing a SMART plan
			• Eliciting a commitment statement
			• Problem solving when low confidence rating
			• Follow-up/progress check (Gutnick et al., 2014)
For more information	http://www.ahrq.gov/professionals/clinicians-providers/guidelines-recommendations/tobacco/5steps.html	http://www.motivationalinterviewing.org/	www.centreCMI.ca

cally building a collaborative partnership, asking permission before educating, starting from the patient's current position, arranging follow-up, and striving for repeated small successes, rather than a single large behavior change. All of the approaches described can be used to elicit patient goals, such as increasing physical activity, losing weight, or learning new pain management strategies, and these goals can be achieved by their participation in a community-based self-management support program. Rather than just didactically recommending a community program to a patient, follow-though is likely to be better when the recommendation is positioned as a means for the patient to achieve his or her own goal.

In addition, all of these behavioral counseling techniques will alter the dynamics of the patient–healthcare provider interaction. Rather than the interaction being dominated by clinician assessment questions and treatment recommendation, use of the 5 A's, MI, or BAP will necessitate a more collaborative dialogue between patient and clinician. Bodenheimer and colleagues define self-management support in just that way, as both a set of techniques and strategies to help patients choose health behaviors, and as a fundamental transformation of the patient–caregiver relationship into a collaborative partnership (Bodenheimer, MacGregor, & Sharifi, 2005).

Conclusion

Acquiring skills and confidence to appropriately self-manage their condition is an essential task for people with arthritis. Clinicians can facilitate that process through the self-management support they provide, not only in their clinical interactions, but in their recommending and facilitating participation in community-based physical activity, self-management education, and weight control programs. There is a reasonably large number of evidence-based physical activity and self-management education interventions available, with increasing numbers of community sites offering the intervention. Particularly for self-management education, there are also online and self-study programs that can serve people who do not have the accessibility or inclination to attend a small-group in-person program. However, it is not enough to simply recommend a community-based program; clinicians can play a valuable role in using behavioral counseling techniques to foster their patients' commitment to participate in a program that can help them achieve their personal goals.

Disclaimer The findings and conclusions in this commentary are those of the author and do not necessarily represent the official position of the Centers for Disease Control and Prevention.

References

Adams, K., Greiner, A. C., & Corrigan, J. M. (Eds.). (2004). Report of a summit. The 1st annual crossing the quality chasm summit—A focus on communities. Washington, DC: National Academies Press.

American College of Rheumatology Subcommittee on Rheumatoid Arthritis Guidelines. (2002). Guidelines for the management of rheumatoid arthritis. *Arthritis and Rheumatism, 46*(2), 328–346.

Anderson, G. (2010). *Chronic care: Making the case for ongoing care*. Princeton, NJ: Robert Woods Johnson Foundation. Retrieved from www.rwjf.org/files/research/50968chronic.care.chartbook.pdf

Arthritis Foundation, & Centers for Disease Control and Prevention. (2010). *National Public Health Agenda for Osteoarthritis. 2010*. Atlanta: Arthritis Foundation. Retrieved from http://www.arthritis.org/media/Ad%20Council%20101/OA_Agenda_2010.pdf

Baruth, M., & Wilcox, S. (2011). Effectiveness of two evidence-based programs in participants with arthritis: Findings from the active for life initiative. *Arthritis Care & Research, 63*(7), 1038–1047.

Belza, B., Shumway-Cook, A., Phelan, E. A., Williams, B., Snyder, S. J. (2006). The effects of a community-based exercise program on function and health in older adults: The EnhanceFitness program. *Journal of Applied Gerontology, 25*(4), 291–306.

Belza, B., Topolski, T., Kinne, S., Patrick, D. L., Ramsey, S. D. (2002). Does adherence make a difference? Results from a community-based aquatic exercise program. *Nursing Research, 51*(5), 285–291.

Bodenheimer, T., Lorig, K., Holman, H., & Grumbach, K. (2002). Patient self management of chronic disease in primary care. *Journal of the American Medical Association, 288*, 2469–2475.

Bodenheimer, T., MacGregor, K., & Sharifi, C. (2005). *Helping patients manage their chronic conditions*. Published by the California HeathCare Foundation, Oakland, CA.

Brady, T. J. (2012). Strategies to support self-management in osteoarthritis. *American Journal of Nursing, 112*, S54–S60. doi:10.1097/01.NAJ.0000412653.56291.

Brady, T. J., Jernick, S. L., Hootman, J. M., & Sniezek, J. E. (2009). Public health interventions for arthritis: Expanding the toolbox of evidence-based interventions. *Journal of Women's Health, 18*(12), 1905–1917.

Brady, T. J., Murphy, L., O'Colmain, B. J., Beauchesne, D., Daniels, B., Greenberg, M., House, M., Chervin, D. (2013). A meta-analysis of health status, health behaviors, and health care utilization outcomes of the chronic disease self-management program. *Preventing Chronic Disease, 10*, 120112.

Brady, T., O'Colmain, B., Mobley, B., Greenberg, M., & Murphy, L. (2010). A meta-analytic assessment of the effects of stanford's small group english version of the arthritis self management program. *Arthritis and Rheumatism, 62*(Suppl 10), 2062. doi:10.1002/art.29827.

Brady, T., Price, S., Ryan, C., Eidson, P., & Savage, T. (2009). Engaging providers to recommend community-based self management programs to their patients: Results from a survey of primary care practices. *Arthritis and Rheumatism, 60*, S759.

Burke, B. L., Arkowitz, H., & Menchola, M. (2003). The efficacy of motivational interviewing: A meta-analysis of controlled clinical trials. *Journal of Consulting and Clinical Psychology, 71*(5), 843–861.

Callahan, L., Cleveland, R., Shreffler, R., Hootman, J., Mielenz, T., Schoster, B. (2014). Evaluation of active living every day in adults with arthritis. *Journal of Physical Activity & Health, 11*(2), 285–295.

Callahan, L. F., Mielenz, T., Freburger, J., Shreffler, J., Hootman, J., Brady, T., Schwartz, T. (2008). A randomized controlled trial of the people with arthritis can exercise program: Symptoms, function, physical activity, and psychosocial outcomes. *Arthritis Care & Research, 59*(1), 92–101.

Callahan, L. F., Shreffler, J., Altpeter, M., Schoster, B., Hootman, J., Houenou, L. O., Martin, K. R., Schwartz, T. A. (2011). Evaluation of group and self-directed formats of the Arthritis Foundation's Walk With Ease Program. *Arthritis Care & Research, 63*(8), 1098–1107.

Do, B. T., Hootman, J. M., Helmick, C. G., & Brady, T. J. (2011). Monitoring healthy people 2010 arthritis management objectives: Self-management education and clinician counseling for weight loss and exercise. *Annals of Family Medicine, 9*(2), 136–141.

Finkelstein, E. A., & Kruger, E. (2014). Meta- and cost-effectiveness analysis of commercial weight loss strategies. *Obesity, 22*(9), 1942–1951. doi:10.1002/oby.20824.

Flurey, C. A., Morris, M., Richards, P., Hughes, R., & Hewlett, S. (2014). It's like a juggling act: Rheumatolid arthritis patient perspectives on daily life and flare while on current treatment regimes. *Rheumatology, 53*, 696–703. doi:10.1093/rheumatology/ket416.

Glasgow, R. E., Goldstein, M. G., Ockene, J. K., & Pronk, N. P. (2004). Translating what we have learned into practice: Principles and hypotheses for interventions addressing multiple behaviors in primary care. *American Journal of Preventive Medicine, 27*(2S), 88–101.

Goeppinger, J., Armstrong, B., Schwartz, T., Ensley, D., Brady, T. (2007). Self-management education for persons with arthritis: Managing comorbidity and eliminating health disparities. *Arthritis and Rheumatism, 57*(6), 1081–1088.

Goeppinger, J., Lorig, K. R., Ritter, P. L., Mutatkar, S., Villa, F., Gizlice, Z. (2009). Mail-delivered arthritis self-management tool kit: A randomized trial and longitudinal followup. *Arthritis and Rheumatism, 61*(7), 867–875.

Gutnick, D., Reims, K., Davis, C., Gainforth, H., Jay, M., & Cole, S. (2014). Brief action planning to facilitate behavior change and support patient self-management. *Journal of Clinical Outcomes Management, 1*, 17–29.

Hefelfinger, J., Brady, T., Berktold, J., Goldstein, M., Bonilla, E., Brick, M., …, Cowen, P. (2014). Reaching out to physical therapists: Results of a survey on physical therapists preferences for learning about evidence-based community programs. *Arthritis & Rheumatology 66*(10 Suppl), S882–S883.

Hochberg, M. C., Altman, R. D., April, K. T., Benkhalti, M., Guyatt, G., McGowan, J., …, Tugwell, P. (2012). American College of Rheumatology 2012 recommendations for the use of nonpharmacologic and pharmacologic therapies in osteoarthritis of the hand, hip, and knee. *Arthritis Care and Research, 64*, 465–474.

Huber, M., Knottnerous, J. A., Green, L., van der Horst, H., Leonard, B., Lorig, K., … Smid, H. (2011). How should we define health? *British Medical Journal, 343*, d4163. doi:10.1136/bmj.d4163.

Hughes, S. L., Seymour, R. B., Campbell, R., Pollack, N., Huber, G., Sharma, L. (2004). Impact of the fit & strong! Intervention on older adults with osteoarthritis. *Gerontologist, 44*(2), 217–228.

Hughes, S. L., Seymour, R. B., Campbell, R. T., Huber, G., Desai, P., Chang, J. H. (2010). Fit and strong!: Bolstering maintenance of physical activity among older adults with lower-extremity osteoarthritis. *American Journal of Health Behavior, 34*(6), 750–763.

Jacobson, D. M., Strohecker, L., Compton, M. T., Katz, D. L. (2005). Physical activity counseling in adult primary care. *American Journal of Preventive Medicine, 29*, 158–162.

Jay, M., Gillespie, C., Schlair, S. S., Sherman, S., & Kalet, A. (2010). Physicians' use of the 5 As in counseling obese patients: Is the quality of counseling associated with patients' motivation and intention to lose weight? *BMC Health Services Research, 10*, 159. doi:10.1186/1472-6963-10-159.

Kelley, G. A., Kelley, K. S., Hootman, J. M., & Jones, D. L. (2011). Effects of community-deliverable exercise on pain and physical function in adults with arthritis and other rheumatic diseases: A meta-analysis. *Arthritis Care & Research, 63*(1), 79–93.

Lefebvre, J. C., Keefe, F. J., Affleck, G., Raezer, L. B., Starr, K., Caldwell, D. S., Tennen, H. (1999). The relationship of arthritis self-efficacy to daily pain, daily mood, and daily pain coping in rheumatoid arthritis patients. *Pain, 80*, 425–435.

Lin, J. S., O'Connor, E., Whitlock, E. P., & Beil, T. (2010). Behavioral counseling to promote physical activity and a healthful diet to prevent cardiovascular disease in adults: A systematic review for the US Preventive Services Task Force. *Annals of Internal Medicine, 153*, 736–750.

Lorig, K., & Gonzales, V. (1992). The integration of theory with practice: A 12 year case study. *Health Eduation Quarterly, 19*, 355–368.

Lorig, K., Gonzalez, V. M., & Ritter, P. (1999). Community-based Spanish language arthritis education program: A randomized trial. *Medical Care, 37*, 957–963.

Lorig, K., Mazonson, P., & Holman, H. R. (1993). Evidence suggesting that health education for self-management in patients with chronic arthritis has sustained health benefits while reducing health care costs. *Arthritis and Rheumatism, 36*(4), 439–446.

Lorig, K. R., Ritter, P. L., & Gonzàlez, V. M. (2003). Hispanic chronic disease self-management: A randomized community-based outcome trial. *Nursing Research, 62*(6), 361–369.

Lorig, K., Ritter, P. L., Laurent, D. D., & Plant, K. (2006). Internet-based chronic disease self-management: A randomized trial. *Medical Care, 44*(11), 964–971.

Lorig, K. R., Ritter, P. L., Laurent, D. D., & Plant, K. (2008). The internet-based arthritis self management program: A one year randomized trial for patients with arthritis or fibromyalgia. *Arthritis and Rheumatology, 57*, 1009–1017.

Lorig, K., Ritter, P. L., Moreland, C., & Laurent, D. D. (2015). Can a box of mailed materials achieve the triple aim of health care? The mailed chronic disease self management toolkit study.

Lorig, K., Ritter, P. L., & Plant, K. (2005). A disease-specific self-help program compared with a generalized chronic disease self-help program for arthritis patients. *Arthritis and Rheumatology, 53*(6), 950–957.

Lorig, K. R., Ritter, P., Stewart, A. L., Sobel, D. S., Brown, B. W., Bandura, A., Gonzales, V. M., Laurent, D. D., Holman, H. R. (2001). Chronic Disease Self-Management Program: 2-year health status and health care utilization outcomes. *Medical Care, 39*(11), 1217–1223.

Lundahl, B., Moleni, T., Burke, B. L., Butters, R., Tollefson, D., Butler, C., & Rollnick, S. (2013). Motivational interviewing in medical care settings: A systematic review and meta-analysis of randomized controlled trials. *Patient Education and Counseling, 93*(2), 157–168

Messier, S. P., Loeser, R. F., Miller, G. D., Morgan, T. M., Rejeski, W. J., Sevick, M. A., ... Williamson, J. D. (2004). Exercise and dietary weight loss in overweight and obese older adults with knee osteoarthritis. *Arthritis and Rheumatism, 50*, 1501–1510.

Miller, W. R., & Rollnick, S. (2002). *Motivational interviewing: Preparing people for change*. New York, NY: The Guilford Press.

Murphy, L., Bolen, J., Helmick, C. G., & Brady, T. J. (2009, February). *Comorbidities are very common among people with arthritis*. Poster 43. 20th national conference on chronic disease prevention and control, CDC. http://www.cdc.gov/arthritis/data_statistics/comorbidities.htm

Murphy, L., Theis, K., Brady, T., Hootman, J., Helmick, C., Bolen, J., Sacks J. (2007). A health care provider's recommendation is the most influential factor in taking an arthritis self-management course: A national perspective from the Arthritis Conditions and Health Effects Survey. *Arthritis and Rheumatism, 56*(9), S307–S308.

Ory, M. G., Smith, M. L., Patton, K., Lorig, K., Zenker, W., & Whitelaw, N. (2013). Self-management at the tipping point: Reaching 100,000 Americans with evidence-based programs. *Journal of the American Geriatrics Society, 61*(5), 821–823.

Patrick, D. L., Ramsey, S. D., Spencer, A. C., Kinne, S., Belza, B., Topolski, T. D. (2001). Economic evaluation of aquatic exercise for persons with osteoarthritis. *Medical Care, 39*(5), 413–424.

Pearson, M. L., Mattke, S., Shaw, R., Ridgely, M. S., & Wiseman, S. H. (2007, November). Patient self-management support programs: An evaluation. Final Contract Report (Prepared by RAND Health under Contract No. 282-00-0005). Rockville, MD: Agency for Healthcare Research and Quality. AHRQ Publication No. 08-0011.

Pollack, K. I., Alexander, S. C., Coffman, C. J., Tulsky, J. A., Lyna, P., Dolor, R. J., ... Ostby, T. (2010). Physician communication techniques and weight loss in adults: Project CHAT. *American Journal of Preventive Medicine, 39*, 321–328.

Ranatunga, S., Myers, S., Redding, S., Scaife, S. L., Francis, M. D., & Francis, M. L. (2010). Introduction of the chronic care model into an academic rheumatology clinic. *Quality Safety in Health Care Journal, 19*, e48. doi:10.1136/qshc2009.035030.

Reeves, D., Kennedy, A., Fullwood, C., Bower, P., Gardner, C., Gately, C., ... Rogers, A. (2008). Predicting who will benefit from an Expert Patients Programme self management course. *British Journal of General Practice, 58*, 198–203.

Seymour, R. B., Hughes, S. L., Campbell, R. T., Huber, G. M., Desai, P. (2009). Comparison of two methods of conducting the Fit & Strong! program. *Arthritis and Rheumatism, 61*(7), 876–884.

Shih, M., Hootman, J. M., Kruger, J., & Helmick, C. G. (2006). Physical activity in men and women with arthritis, National Health Interview Survey, 2002. *American Journal of Preventive Medicine, 30*(5), 385–393.

Taal, E., Rasker, J. J., Seydel, E. R., & Wiegman, O. (1993). Health status, adherence with health recommendations, self-efficacy and social support in patients with rheumatoid arthritis. *Patient Education and Counseling, 20*, 63–76.

Unpublished CDC Report. (2005). *The value proposition of self management education*. A focus group report to The Centers for Disease Control and Prevention. Unpublished report by Fleishman Hillard.

US Department of Health and Human Services. (2008). *Physical activity guidelines for Americans*. Retrieved from http://www.health.gov/PAGuidelines/

Wagner, E. H. (1998). Chronic disease management: What will it take to improve care for chronic illness? *Effective Clinical Practice, 1*(1), 2–4.

Wallace, J. I., Buchner, D. M., Grothaus, L., Leveille, S., Tyll, L., LaCroix, A. Z., Wagner, E. H. (1998). Implementation and effectiveness of a community-based health promotion program for older adults. *Journal of Gerontology: Medical Sciences, 53*(4), M301–M306.

Wilcox, S., Der Ananian, C., Abbott, J., Vrazel, J., Ramsey, C., Sharpe, P. A., & Brady, T. (2006). Perceived exercise barriers, enablers, and benefits among exercising and nonexercising adults with arthritis: Results from a qualitative study. *Arthritis and Rheumatism, 55*(4), 616–627.

The Nature, Efficacy, and Future of Behavioral Treatments for Arthritis

16

Perry M. Nicassio and Desiree R. Azizoddin

Background and Evolution of Behavioral Approaches for Arthritis

The Development of Health Psychology and Behavioral Medicine

Since behavioral interventions have played a prominent role in the management of chronic disease for many years, it is important to consider the historical and theoretical factors that have contributed to their relevance and importance to arthritis. The evolution and development of the allied fields of health psychology and behavioral medicine have contributed significantly to the emergence of behavioral and psychosocial interventions for chronic disease and the management of arthritis (Nicassio & Smith, 1995). While these fields are overlapping and synergistic, they are paradigmatically distinct. The discipline of health psychology refers to the application of psychological principles and techniques to understanding the effects of psychological processes on the manifestations of disease, the prevention of illness, the promotion of adaptive health practices, the management of chronic illness, and the examination of the healthcare system (Belar, 1997; Taylor, 1990). In contrast, behavioral medicine is interdisciplinary in focus, reflecting the integrated contributions of medicine, psychology, social science, allied health, and public health to the prevention of disease, the promotion of adaptive health practices, and the treatment of disease (Buse & Andrasik, 2009). Since the inception of these fields in the late 1970s, new paradigms and approaches for treating patients with a variety of health problems have been developed and tested, creating a broadening awareness of the importance of these fields and their value in research, patient education, and disease management. Health psychology and behavioral medicine continue to have an important impact on healthcare delivery and treatment of chronic disease through the adoption of the biopsychosocial model and its emphasis on understanding the unique circumstances of patients who may be diagnosed with the same medical condition.

In concert with the increased interest in, and growth, of these fields, researchers began to study how psychosocial processes affect the adjustment of patients with arthritis, along with the impact of arthritis on emotional well-being and functional outcomes such as disability and quality of life. Early research on the role of helplessness, perceptions of control over arthritis, and social support confirmed the importance of such factors in understanding depression, pain, and arthritis-

P.M. Nicassio, PhD (✉)
Department of Psychiatry, School of Medicine, University of California, Los Angeles, CA, USA
e-mail: pnicassio@mednet.ucla

D. Azizoddin, MA
Department of Psychology, Loma Linda University, Loma Linda, CA, USA

P.M. Nicassio (ed.), *Psychosocial Factors in Arthritis*, DOI 10.1007/978-3-319-22858-7_16

related disability (e.g., Brown & Nicassio, 1987; Brown, Wallston, & Nicassio, 1989; Nicassio & Smith, 1995; Stein, Wallston, & Nicassio, 1988). Investigators have also focused on how patients' strategies for coping with pain may affect many of these same outcomes (Brown & Nicassio, 1987; Rosentiel & Keefe, 1983, see Chap. 3, this volume). Research has examined the effects of many of these same factors on health outcomes in other illnesses such as diabetes, cancer, kidney disease, and heart disease (Christensen & Ehlers, 2002; Faul, Jim, Williams, Loftus, & Jacobsen, 2010; Fok, Chair, & Lopez, 2005; Glasgow, Toobert, & Gillette, 2001; Muehrer & Becker, 2005; Paschalides et al., 2004; Rose, Fliege, Hildebrandt, Schirop, & Burghard, 2002; Sarenmalm, Ohlen, Ode, & Gaston-johansson, 2008; Shimbo, Davidson, Haas, Fuster, & Badimon, 2005; Sloan et al., 2012; Tully, Baker, Turnbull, Winefield, & Knight, 2009).

Importantly, since variables such as helplessness, coping, and social support were considered to be potentially modifiable, the premise that behavioral interventions could be developed to address them was embraced and subsequently explored empirically. Accordingly, over the last three decades, a significant body of clinical trials research has demonstrated the efficacy of behavioral interventions across a range of diseases and health problems (Abbott et al., 2014; Anderson & Taylor, 2014; Davidson et al., 2006; Goyer et al., 2013; Hart et al., 2012; Linden & Girgis, 2012; Linden, Phillips, & Leclerc, 2007; Montgomery et al., 2014; Newell, Sanson-Fisher, & Savolainen, 2002; Ott, 2002; Sharma & Haider, 2013; Somers, Wren, & Shelby, 2012). This research has provided confirmation of the scientific and clinical value of behavioral interventions and the need for behavioral interventions to reach populations who are likely to benefit from their dissemination and application in clinical and community settings.

Emergence of Social Learning Theory as a Dominant Theoretical Paradigm

The advent of social learning theory has also contributed to our understanding of the dynamic influences between psychosocial and biological influences on health outcomes and subsequently to the development of behavioral interventions for chronic illness (Bandura, 1991, 2001; Bandura & Adams, 1977; Rosenstock, Strecher, & Becker, 1988). Self-efficacy, a key tenet of this framework, refers to the degree of certainty that an individual has regarding whether he or she can perform a specific behavior that will lead to a desired outcome. The application of self-efficacy theory to arthritis has led to many important findings. For example, self-efficacy has proven to be an important construct in understanding whether arthritis patients will cope adaptively with their pain, manage their activity level, and engage in other adaptive health behaviors (Lorig, Chastain, Ung, Shoor, & Holman, 1989). Self-efficacy may be viewed as a form of "illness cognition." Illness cognitions provide a "window" into patients' subjective meaning of their illness and health related to subsequent health behaviors. Accordingly, social learning theory has illustrated the importance of understanding the central role of patients' beliefs in their illness experience, their interpretation of symptoms, their coping mechanisms, and their response to treatment. It has also established the theoretical and empirical foundation for clinical interventions such as cognitive behavior therapy that address distortions in thinking that may lead to maladaptive coping and negative health outcomes.

In some instances, patients' experience with illness may be discordant with objective medical findings and recommended treatment practices. For example, theoretically efficacious treatments may not lead to improvement if patients lack self-efficacy in their ability to implement them in their daily lives. This is particularly true of behavioral interventions whose efficacy depends largely on the performance of learned skills. Self-efficacy theory also applies to medical and allied health interventions (e.g., physical therapy, nursing) that promote adherence to medications and other self-initiated behaviors (e.g., exercise, improved eating). Thus, many behavioral interventions for arthritis have focused on the development of self-efficacy as a principal clinical target under the assumption that self-efficacy will contribute to effective management practices that will lead to beneficial changes in clinical outcomes such as pain, mood, and disability (Marks, Allegrante, & Lorig, 2005).

Limitations of Disease-Modifying Drugs

Behavioral interventions have represented an important complement to the use of pharmacological treatments for arthritis whose focus is to reduce inflammation and dampen disease activity. Importantly, many studies over the last decade have confirmed the efficacy of new biologic agents in the amelioration of disease activity in arthritis (Gartlehner, Hansen, Jonas, & Lohr, 2006; Singh et al., 2012). While biological agents have been successful in dampening the inflammatory response, the efficacy of these medications is variable across patients, and in some instances, they may increase other health risks due to their suppression of the immune system (e.g., Nurmohamed & Dijkmans, 2005). Importantly, non-pharmacological treatment approaches have the potential to reduce dependency on medications that pose such problems. In this regard, it has been found that behavioral interventions have contributed to significant clinical improvement in patients who are receiving standard medical treatment that may involve the prescription of biologic agents and other disease-modifying drugs (Kiecolt-Glaser, McGuire, Robles, & Glaser, 2002; Miller & Cohen, 2001; Zautra et al., 2008). In clinical trials, behavioral interventions have been compared with control groups in which patients continue to participate in their standard medical regimens under the care of their rheumatologists. This has been necessary since the withholding of medical treatment from patients with active disease would heighten health risks and, therefore, raise ethical concerns about patient safety.

Importantly, behavioral interventions have been shown to have incremental scientific and clinical value, an effect over and above the impact of pharmacological treatments. That has represented a rigorous standard to achieve in research as patients may already be getting optimal care. Additional information on the efficacy of behavioral interventions will be presented later in this chapter. It is a standard, however, that health psychology and behavioral medicine researchers and clinicians embrace since they are invested in developing treatment approaches that complement standard, effective medical practices and procedures.

Early Research on Mind-Body Treatments

The research on mind-body techniques such as relaxation training, meditation, and biofeedback that began in the 1960s and 1970s has provided a foundation for their incorporation into behavioral treatment programs for arthritis. Relaxation training methods have proven to reduce pain and emotional distress in a variety of patient populations (Astin, Shapiro, Eisenberg, & Forys, 2003; Carroll & Seers, 1998; Kwekkeboom & Gretarsdottir, 2006; Morone & Greco, 2007). Biofeedback has demonstrated that feedback about the intensity of a physiological response (e.g., muscle tension) provides the basis for learning to modulate the direction of the response and subsequently to its control (Hauri, 1981). Collectively, these techniques have shown that patients have the ability to mitigate distressing symptoms and the potential to exert a measure of control over important health outcomes, chiefly on their own, or with minimal guidance from medical providers and other healthcare practitioners (Budzynski, Stoyva, Adler, & Mullaney, 1973; Clemens et al., 2000; Flor & Birbaumer, 1993; Newton-John, Spence, & Schotte, 1995). Thus, there has been an important evidence-based, empirical rationale for their inclusion in treatment programs for arthritis.

Behavioral treatments based on mind-body approaches have also played a significant role in the development of other treatment strategies that promote the learning of new skills and a philosophy of patient self-empowerment and independence. This philosophy is embodied in community-based interventions and complementary treatments (see Chaps. 14 and 15, this volume) that have become increasingly popular to arthritis patients who are interested in exploring new ways to promote their health and emotional well-being. The appeal of such interventions to patients provides added momentum for continued changes in the healthcare system due to their "organic" nature and their "patient centeredness" philosophy. As patients take more responsibility for their healthcare, their roles and communication patterns with physicians may undergo change as they become less dependent on healthcare providers for the management of their medical circumstances. As a result, the relationship between patients and rheumatologists becomes more collaborative in nature, leading to medical decision-making that reflects the needs and values of arthritis sufferers in conjunction with the opinions of the medical team.

Efficacy of Behavioral Interventions

What is generally known about the effectiveness of behavioral interventions in ameliorating arthritis symptoms and preventing adverse health outcomes? Considerable research over the past three decades has been conducted to evaluate their efficacy. Related issues concern understanding the magnitude of the effects of behavioral interventions on important clinical criteria and whether behavioral interventions are having an impact on improving patients' well-being and making a difference in patients' daily lives. Two meta-analyses have explored the efficacy of behavioral interventions for arthritis in clinical trials research. The meta-analyses have adopted rigorous inclusion criteria and have covered a wide range of behavioral modalities (see Dixon, Keefe, Scipio, Perry, & Abernethy, 2007; Knittle, Maes, & de Gucht, 2010). In a broad sense, they have included studies that have espoused a self-management approach, many of which have incorporated key elements of social learning theory principles and self-efficacy. The meta-analyses have examined the effects of behavioral interventions on a number of clinical outcomes, including pain, disability, various indices of psychosocial functioning, and emotional distress.

The review by Dixon et al. (2007) addressed the efficacy of behavioral interventions that focused on pain management. Their review included a range of behavioral modalities administered in both individual and group format; cognitive-behavioral therapy (CBT), emotional disclosure, hypnosis, pain-coping skills training, psychodynamic therapy, biofeedback, and stress management. Both RA and OA patients and 27 RCT's were included in the review. Compared to controls, behavioral interventions led to significant improvement, evidenced by the following effect sizes for pain (.18), anxiety (28), depression (=.21), psychological disability (.25), physical disability (.15), active coping (.72), pain self-efficacy (18), and joint swelling (=.35).

The review by Knittle et al. (2010) from the Netherlands evaluated 27 randomized controlled trials and only included patients with RA. A unique focus of this meta-analysis was to determine whether interventions based on self-regulation theory (SRT) would improve physical activity, which had not been addressed in the Dixon et al. review. Investigators rated each intervention for the inclusion of the following strategies; goal setting, planning, self-monitoring, feedback, and relapse prevention. Their review only included individual face-to-face interactions between patients and healthcare providers. Behavioral interventions led to significant improvement with effect sizes of .45 for physical activity, .18 for pain, .32 for disability, .23 for depressive symptoms, and .17 for anxiety. At follow-up (2–14 months), the effect size for physical activity was .36, for pain, .13, for disability, .15, and for depression, .32. Their review did not include data on the efficacy of behavioral interventions for disease activity.

The findings from the two meta-analyses reflected substantial concordance. First, behavioral interventions led to improvement across a range of clinical outcomes. Improvement was found in pain, psychological distress, and functional domains in both reviews. Second, the magnitude of improvement was modest. Third, behavioral interventions led to improvement in coping, activity level, and self-efficacy. Fourth, the reviews did not find that behavioral interventions reduced inflammation or arthritis-related biomarkers.

It is important to note that behavioral interventions may have "ripple effects" (Wilson, 2015). "Ripple effects" occur when a behavioral intervention that focuses on one primary domain has effects on other outcomes. "Ripple effects" have important implications for the health of populations since changes in exercise habits and diet, for example, may promote positive changes in a variety of health outcomes and prevent health risk. With respect to arthritis, it appears that a similar phenomenon also occurs. For example, the Dixon et al. (2007) review showed that interventions that targeted pain also improved functional outcomes and depression. The same pattern of findings was reported by Knittle et al. (2010). There are two plausible explanations for "ripple effects" in behavioral intervention research for arthritis. One is that since pain, disability, and psychological distress are correlated with each other, and that improvement in one area may lead to change in another. Importantly, these outcomes may not only be correlated, but causally linked with each other as well. Behavioral interventions for pain, for example, may contribute to less disability and depression or vice versa (Fig. 16.1).

The other is that behavioral interventions promote a common core of principles or strategies that have general significance and have separate effects on several different clinical outcomes simultaneously. In this scenario, teaching patients to cope actively with their arthritis pain may contribute directly to improving pain, disability, and psychological distress (Fig. 16.2).

While the magnitude of the effects of behavioral interventions tends to be modest, their potential public health impact could still be significant. Small effect sizes may translate into meaningful gains on a population level if thousands of patients have access to behavioral interventions in clinic settings or through community intervention programs. There are other examples in the literature supporting the efficacy of brief interventions administered through primary care settings (Cape, Whittington, Buszewicz, Wallace, & Underwood, 2010; Erickson, Gerstle, & Feldstein, 2005) to promote adaptive behavioral

Fig. 16.1 Hypothetical model postulating linkages between behavioral intervention, pain, disability, and depression

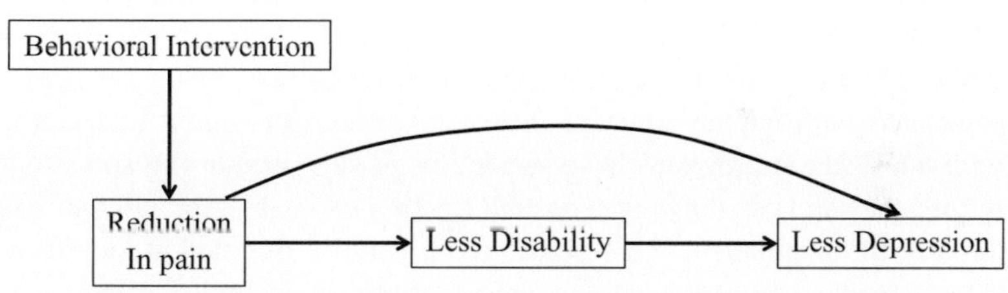

Hypothetical model postulating linkages between behavioral intervention, pain, disability, and depression

Fig. 16.2 Hypothetical model illustrating independent effect of active coping on pain, disability, and depression

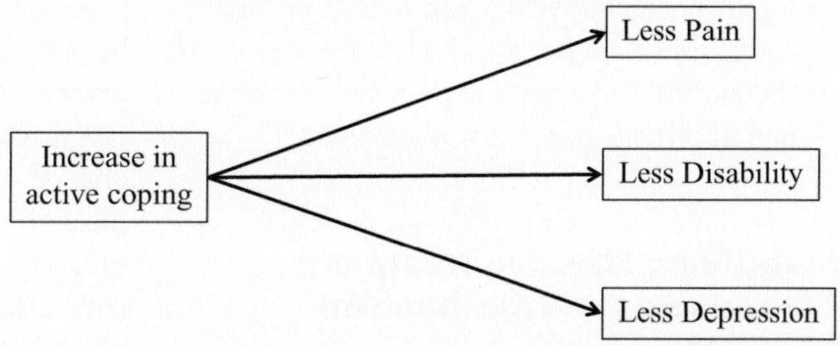

Hypothetical model illustrating independent effect of active coping on pain, disability, and depression

changes that have a public health impact. Increasing patient access to effective treatments is a major public health challenge and also a significant issue for patients who are struggling with managing debilitating arthritis symptoms.

Accordingly, the question of whether behavioral interventions are making a difference in patients' lives is more difficult to answer for the following reasons: (1) patients may have limited access to behavioral interventions, (2) patients may have difficulties with the "uptake" of behavioral interventions or the learning of needed skills, or (3) patients may experience difficulty in applying skills on a daily basis. Community self-management approaches have represented an attempt to deliver easily consumable interventions to arthritis patients proximal to their living environments (see Brady this volume, Bodenheimer, Lorig, Holman, & Grumbach, 2002; Lorig, Gonzalez, & Ritter, 1999; Lorig & Holman, 2003; Lorig, Lubeck, Kraines, Seleznick, & Holman, 1985) and have had a significant impact in the enhancement of patient well-being. These programs not only promote greater education and knowledge about arthritis management, they also engender meaningful social interaction and support that reduces the social isolation and loneliness associated with having arthritis. However, while such intervention programs have yielded positive results, they still can only reach a small fraction of the arthritis population. We would have a better idea if behavioral interventions are improving patients' lives if they were promoted and integrated in arthritis clinics where the vast majority of arthritis patients receive their clinical care. At this juncture, there is evidence that psychosocial issues are not identified or addressed in rheumatology settings (Sleath et al., 2008), decreasing the likelihood that behavioral approaches to management will be considered or implemented.

Identifying Effective Treatment Components and Mechanisms of Action

Behavioral interventions for arthritis have frequently been "omnibus" in nature. Omnibus interventions are comprised of many different treatment elements and require the acquisition of several skills on the part of patients. Interventions for pain, for example, have included such elements as rational restructuring, activity pacing, relaxation training, increasing social support, and engaging in pleasurable activities and events (Dixon et al., 2007; Radojevic, Nicassio, & Weisman, 1992). The inclusion of several treatment elements in clinical trials research may reflect the expectation that teaching patients several skills is a more effective way of enhancing the potency of interventions instead of relying on more streamlined, targeted approaches that focus on a limited set of treatment skills or strategies. However, the risk of omnibus approaches is that interventions may become saturated, making it problematic for patients to master a range of skills and apply them on a consistent basis. The uptake or learning of aspects of the interventions and resulting impacts becomes more difficult as complexity of the interventions increases (Ingersoll & Cohen, 2008; Stone et al., 2001; Vermeire, Hearnshaw, Van Royen, & Denekens, 2001). Adherence to, and performance of, learned skills may also be compromised as patient demands increase (Barlett 2002). Furthermore, the inclusion of several elements in behavioral treatment interventions has made it difficult to isolate the specific components that are responsible for clinical improvement. Future research directed at identifying active treatment elements in multifaceted treatment packages would fill an important gap in the behavioral intervention literature. Doing so will also contribute to the efficiency of delivering psychosocial care.

There is also a need for understanding the mechanisms of action underlying the efficacy of behavioral treatment approaches for arthritis pain and disease activity. Figure 16.3 illustrates potential mechanisms that may contribute to clinical change. Behavioral interventions may work through a number of potential pathways either individually or in concert with one another. They may also be correlated or causally related with one another.

Behavioral interventions may contribute to improvements in patients' beliefs or appraisals of their health. They may promote increases in self-efficacy or reductions in negative beliefs such as

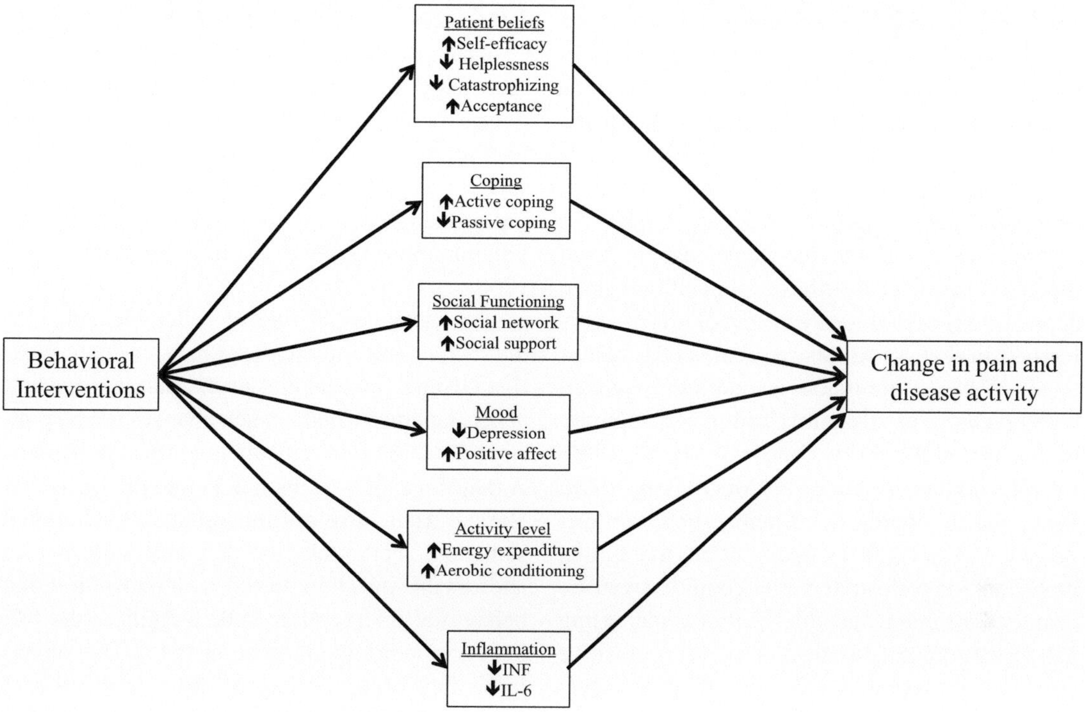

Fig. 16.3 Potential mediators of behavioral interventions

helplessness or catastrophizing. Most behavioral interventions based on social learning theory principles have attempted to foster healthier illness appraisals that promote a sense of optimism and agency in patients. Recently, investigators have shown increased interest in mindfulness approaches that foster acceptance and a nonjudgmental awareness about health (Grossman, Niemann, Schmidt, & Walach, 2004; Hofmann, Sawyer, Witt, & Oh, 2010; Nyklíček, Hoogwegt, & Westgeest, 2015; Rosenzweig, Greeson, Reibel, Green, & Jasser, 2009). Changes in patients' beliefs have been linked to a range of outcomes, including less pain, improved mood, and decreased disease activity (Carrico & Antoni, 2008; Irwin et al., 2015; McCracken & Turk, 2002; McCracken & Vowles, 2008; Turk & Okifuji, 2002). Reductions in helplessness and catastrophizing, in turn, have been shown to contribute to adaptive coping (Cabib, Campus, & Colelli, 2012; Evers, Kraaimaat, Van Riel, & De Jong, 2002; Hannibal & Bishop, 2014; Hewlett et al., 2011).

Importantly, behavioral interventions may promote changes in patients' coping mechanisms for their pain by increasing active coping and reducing passive or avoidant coping strategies. Greater active coping and less passive coping have been shown to be consistently related to reductions in pain and improvements in mood in a range of pain populations (Higgins, Bailey, LaChapelle, Harman, & Hadjistavropoulos, 2014; McCracken & Turk, 2002).

Behavioral interventions also may target mechanisms for increasing the social network size and quality of support of patients. Social support has been associated with positive health outcomes in both OA and RA patient populations (Ethgen et al., 2004; Evers et al., 2002; Holtzman, Newth, & Delongis, 2004; Krol, Sanderman, & Suurmeijer, 1993; Zyrianova, 2006). Many behavioral interventions are rendered in a group format that promotes a supportive, interactive atmosphere. Social support interventions build on that foundation by incorporating specific strategies for increasing support and effective social integration.

Some behavioral interventions have addressed social support by including a family member in the intervention (Radojevic et al., 1992) to facilitate the performance of behavioral skills in the patient or by enhancing communication skills around pain and related issues (Cegela, McClure, Marinelli, & Post, 2000; Keefe et al., 2004).

Behavioral interventions have also targeted mood disturbance in arthritis populations since depression is a common symptom of arthritis sufferers (Lin et al., 2003; Sharpe et al., 2001; Zautra et al., 2008). Depression is commonly linked with greater pain, disability, and disease activity in patients with arthritis (Baqar & Moore, 1990; Fifield, Tennen, Reisine, & McQuillan, 1998; Peck, Smith, Ward, & Milano, 1989; Sharpe, Sensky, & Allard, 2001). Interventions to improve mood include such strategies as cognitive restructuring to promote healthier beliefs, increasing daily pleasurable activities, or savoring positive emotions to promote gains in positive affect through mindfulness practices.

Interventions for arthritis may also include strategies to increase activity level and energy expenditure through structured aerobic exercise, walking, or by reducing sedentary behavior (see Chap. 13; Knittle et al., 2010). Behavioral interventions for pain often include strategies for pacing of activity that combines periods of energy exertion and rest (Gatchel & Turk, 1996; Murphy, Lyden, Smith, Dong, & Koliba, 2010). Activity pacing can be integrated with other approaches such as relaxation during periods of rest or emotional savoring while patients engage in pleasurable activity.

Inflammation is the underlying cause of joint pain and swelling in RA and also may exacerbate fatigue, sleep disturbance, and depression (Belza, Henke, Yelin, Epstein, & Gilliss, 1993; Bergman et al., 2009; Davis et al., 2008; Drewes, 1999; Lee et al., 2009; Stebbings, Herbison, Doyle, Treharne, & Highton, 2010). There is some evidence that behavioral interventions in other chronic diseases may lead to reduced inflammation and positive alterations in immune functioning (Antoni et al., 2000; Balagopal et al., 2005; Irwin, Wang, Campomayor, Collado-Hidalgo, & Cole, 2006; Miller, Ancoli-Israel, Bower, Capuron, & Irwin, 2008; Miller & Cohen, 2001; Thornton, Andersen, Schuler, & Carson, 2009; Zautra et al., 2008). Theoretically, behavioral interventions for arthritis should have similar salutary effects on inflammation. Evidence attesting to the effects of behavioral interventions on inflammation, however, is limited (Zautra et al., 2008).

However, despite the considerable evidence that behavioral interventions may promote positive changes in potential mediators, it is unclear at this juncture whether such changes are responsible for the improvements in clinical outcomes. A major reason for this gap in knowledge is that clinical trials have not incorporated mediational statistical methodologies that are necessary to address this question. In order for a mediator of a behavioral intervention to be identified, the following conditions must be met: (1) The behavioral intervention has to affect the clinical outcome, (2) The behavioral intervention has to lead to change in the mediator, (3) The mediator must be related to the clinical outcome, and (4) for full mediation, the effect of the behavioral intervention becomes non-significant after the contribution of the mediating variable is taken into account (Baron & Kenny, 1986). Partial mediation occurs when the pathway from the behavioral intervention to the clinical outcome remains significant after controlling for the mediating variable. Frameworks also can be adopted that incorporate a multiple mediation approach in which the effects of two or more mediators are analyzed simultaneously (Preacher & Hayes, 2008a, 2008b). Multiple mediation strategies may be particularly appropriate for analyzing the effects of behavioral interventions since they commonly target more than one mechanism for improvement.

While identifying mechanisms provides an explanation of why behavioral interventions are effective, there are other benefits to identifying mechanisms as well. A key advantage is that behavioral interventions may increase their efficiency by focusing more directly on mediators that are critical to change. Potential mediators that do not show a relationship with outcomes may be deemphasized in favor of those that have a clinical impact. Another advantage is that other approaches may be developed or implemented that focus on the mediator. Rather than fostering allegiance to a particular theoretical approach or model, new treatments can be developed that focus directly on altering the underlying mechanisms involved. For example, independent of traditional behavioral interventions that are primarily based on social learning theory, there could be other strategies (e.g., complementary medicine techniques, exercise, physical therapy) that target self-efficacy, increase active coping, foster social support, or improve mood. Greater knowledge and application of these mediational frameworks may thus lead to increased treatment efficiencies by promoting rational integration between treatments, mediators, and clinical outcomes.

Integration of Behavioral Treatments in Rheumatology

The Council of Academic Health Centers for Integrative Medicinehas advocated for the adoption of an integrative medicine model in the management of chronic disease. Kligler and Chesney (2014) note that this organization has defined integrative medicine in the following way:

> "Integrative medicine is the practice of medicine that reaffirms the importance of the relationship between practitioner and patient, focuses on the whole person, is informed by evidence, and makes use of all therapeutic approaches, healthcare professionals, and disciplines to achieve optimal health and healing."

Behavioral interventions fall under the integrative medicine rubric to the extent that they are evidence-based, are holistic in nature, and promote a collaborative relationship between patients and practitioners. The implementation of this framework in arthritis care represents both a challenge and opportunity in the effort to improve the quality of life of arthritis sufferers. Key questions emerge regarding the dissemination of behavioral treatments and their integration into clinical practice.

Dissemination

The RE-AIM (Reach, Effectiveness, Adoption, Implementation, Maintenance) model borrowed from public health has provided impetus for examining the translational impact of behavioral interventions in clinical and community settings (Gaglio, Shoup, & Glasgow, 2013). Reach refers to the absolute number of individuals who are willing to participate in an initiative; effectiveness refers to the impact of the initiative on clinical outcomes; adoption involves the number of settings and intervention agents who are willing to initiate a program; implementation refers to the degree of fidelity on the part of intervention agents to elements of a program protocol; maintenance involves the degree to which a program becomes institutionalized or part of the institution's routine organizational practices. While the RE-AIM framework has had a major impact on the dissemination of interventions to increase physical activity (Dzewaltowski, Estabrooks, & Glasgow, 2004), it also is relevant to examining the potential expansion and integration of behavioral interventions in arthritis clinics and community settings. The RE-AIM framework provides a conceptual background for addressing the logistical issues involved in integrative care. In many instances, the mechanisms for integration can be challenging and difficult due to obstacles that are inherent in the healthcare system. Access to care problems, time constraints during medical visits, and lack of personnel resources in the clinic setting to incorporate behavioral interventions may all be operative to various degrees and interfere with integrated treatment (Nicassio, 2008).

Mechanisms of Integration

There are different models for examining the integration of behavioral treatments in arthritis care. An essential prerequisite is that members of the healthcare team (e.g., rheumatologists, allied health professionals, behavioral medicine specialists) have a mutual understanding of the need to adopt a biopsychosocial model of care and to embrace its relevance in working with clinic patients. Agreement on the importance of the model will facilitate communication among healthcare providers and between healthcare providers and patients. It will provide a foundation for the coordination and implementation of behavioral interventions and their role in medical care. After embracing the importance of behavioral interventions and their clinical value, healthcare providers face the challenge of how to integrate them in the clinic.

Referral-based frameworks involve the provision of behavioral medicine services by a specialist who functions in a different environment and is independent of the rheumatology clinic. Referrals are made to a specialist with expertise in pain management, the treatment of depression, or other psychosocial issues. This traditional model of providing psychosocial care makes integration more difficult since patients may be reticent to see an outside specialist. Also, communication between the rheumatologist and behavioral medicine professional may become problematic and interfere with coordination of treatments. This model still may achieve some success, however, if patients do, in fact, receive effective care from the specialist. Referral-based models are common in medical practice with its increased specialization and compartmentalization of care. Despite its drawbacks, it is the model that has the greatest familiarity among rheumatologists and other medical providers.

A superior model for integration involves the provision of behavioral treatments in the rheumatology setting. In this form of integration, behavioral treatments are "embedded" into the clinical environment. This could be accomplished in the following ways. First, the behavioral medicine specialist may function as part of the rheumatology team. The specialist could perform psychosocial evaluations and screenings, and work with individual patients to manage their pain and other problems that impact their arthritis. The specialist could provide feedback to the rheumatologist that would facilitate treatment planning and medical decision-making. This model of care has had a positive impact in primary care and oncology settings (Fisher & Dickinson, 2014; Guo et al., 2013; Holland, 2004; Jacobsen & Wagner, 2012; Kearney, Post, Pomerantz, & Zeiss, 2014; Miller, Petterson, Burke, Phillips, & Green, 2014; Villareal et al., 2006).

If it isn't feasible to have a behavioral medicine specialist in the rheumatology clinic, other alternatives may still be possible for the integration of behavioral medicine services. Allied health professionals such as nurses or physical therapists who work in the same setting as rheumatologists have the potential to implement behavioral treatments during the course of their interactions with patients. Behavioral treatments for pain, for example, can be brief and efficiently implemented. Manualized treatment applications exist that are suitable for use by professionals without formal training in behavioral medicine. Another alternative is that rheumatologists themselves take responsibility for implementing behavioral interventions with support from the allied health professionals. While time constraints may interfere with the feasibility of this option, behavioral treatments may have high credibility to patients when rendered by rheumatologists. The two aforementioned approaches would require expansion of the roles of allied health professionals and rheumatologists. Education and training on behavioral approaches would be necessary through continuing education and support from professional organizations. Increasing the capacity of rheumatology health professionals to render behavioral treatments could also be addressed through more frequent consultation with behavioral medicine specialists.

Summary

There are significant opportunities for the growth and relevance of behavioral treatments for arthritis. Behavioral treatments have an established history in the treatment of chronic disease and the amelioration of patient suffering. Clinical trials research has established their efficacy in reducing pain, psychological distress, and disability. Further research is needed to address their mechanisms of action, shedding light on why they are effective. The increased impact of behavioral treatments for arthritis will depend on the adoption of models that will facilitate their dissemination and application in clinical care in order to expand their reach. Behavioral medicine specialists and rheumatology health professionals are both invested in providing optimal care to arthritis patients. They must form a closer academic and clinical partnership in order to achieve this important goal.

References

Abbott, R. A., Whear, R., Rodgers, L. R., Bethel, A., Thompson Coon, J., Kuyken, W., … Dickens, C. (2014). Effectiveness of mindfulness-based stress reduction and mindfulness based cognitive therapy in vascular disease: A systematic review and meta-analysis of randomised controlled trials. *Journal of Psychosomatic Research, 76*(5), 341–351. doi:10.1016/j.jpsychores.2014.02.012.

Anderson, L., & Taylor, R. S. (2014). Cardiac rehabilitation for people with heart disease : An overview of Cochrane systematic reviews (Review). *Cochrane Database Systematic Review,* (12), CD011273.

Antoni, M. H., Cruess, S., Cruess, D. G., Kumar, M., Lutgendorf, S., Ironson, G., … Schneiderman, N. (2000). Cognitive-behavioral stress management reduces distress and 24-hour urinary free cortisol output among symptomatic HIV-infected gay men. *Annals of Behavioral Medicine, 22*(1), 29–37. doi:10.1007/BF02895165.

Astin, J. A., Shapiro, S. L., Eisenberg, D. M., & Forys, K. L. (2003). Mind-body medicine: State of the science, implications for practice. *The Journal of the American Board of Family Practice, 16*(2), 131–147. doi:10.3122/jabfm.16.2.131.

Balagopal, P., George, D., Patton, N., Yarandi, H., Roberts, W. L., Bayne, E., & Gidding, S. (2005). Lifestyle-only intervention attenuates the inflammatory state associated with obesity: A randomized controlled study in adolescents. *The Journal of Pediatrics, 146(3),* 342–348. doi:10.1016/j.jpeds.2004.11.033.

Bandura, A. (1991). Social cognitive theory of self-regulation. *Organizational Behavior and Human Decision Processes, 50,* 248–287.

Bandura, A. (2001). Social cognitive theory: An agentic perspective. *Annual Review of Psychology, 52*(1), 1–26.

Bandura, A., & Adams, N. E. (1977). Analysis of self-efficacy theory of behavioral change. *Cognitive Therapy and Research, 1*(4), 287–310. doi:10.1007/BF01663995.

Baqar, H. A., & Moore, S. T. (1990). Arthritis disability, depression, and life satisfaction among black elderly people. *Health & Social Work, 15*(4), 253–260. doi:10.1093/hsw/15.4.253.

Barlett, J. A. (2002). Addressing the challenges of adherence. *Journal of Acquired Immune Deficiency Syndrome, 29,* S2–S10.

Baron, R. M., & Kenny, D. A. (1986). The moderator-mediator variable distinction in social psychological research: Conceptual, strategic, and statistical considerations. *Journal of Personality and Social Psychology, 51,* 1173–1182. doi:10.1037/0022-3514.51.6.1173.

Belar, C. D. (1997). Clinical health psychology: A specialty for the 21st century. *Health Psychology, 16*(5), 411–416.

Belza, B. L., Henke, C. J., Yelin, E. H., Epstein, W. V., & Gilliss, C. L. (1993). Correlates of fatigue in older adults with rheumatoid arthritis. *Nursing Research, 42*(2), 93–99. doi:10.1097/00006199-199303000-00006.

Bergman, M. J., Shahouri, S. S., Shaver, T. S., Anderson, J. D., Weidensaul, D. N., Busch, R. E., … Wolfe, F. (2009). Is fatigue an inflammatory variable in rheumatoid arthritis (RA)? Analyses of fatigue in RA, osteoarthritis, and fibromyalgia. *Journal of Rheumatology, 36*(12), 2788–2794. doi:10.3899/jrheum.090561.

Bodenheimer, T., Lorig, K., Holman, H., & Grumbach, K. (2002). Patient self-management of chronic disease in primary care. *The Journal of the American Medical Association, 288*(19), 2469–2475. doi:10.1001/jama.288.19.2469.

Brown, G. K., & Nicassio, P. M. (1987). Development of a questionnaire for the assessment of active and passive coping strategies in chronic pain patients. *Pain, 31*(1), 53–64. doi:10.1016/0304-3959(87)90006-6.

Brown, G. K., Wallston, K. A., & Nicassio, P. M. (1989). Social support and depression in rheumatoid arthritis: A one-year prospective study. *Journal of Applied Social Psychology, 19*(14), 1164–1181. doi:10.1111/j.1559-1816.1989.tb01245.

Budzynski, T. H., Stoyva, J. M., Adler, C. S., & Mullaney, D. J. (1973). EMG biofeedback and tension headache: A controlled outcome study. *Psychosomatic Medicine, 35*(6), 484–496.

Buse, D. C., & Andrasik, F. (2009). Behavioral medicine for migraine. *Neurologic Clinics, 27*(2), 445–465. doi:10.1016/j.ncl.2009.01.003.

Cabib, S., Campus, P., & Colelli, V. (2012). Learning to cope with stress: Psychobiological mechanisms of stress resilience. *Reviews in the Neurosciences, 23*(5–6), 659–672. doi:10.1515/revneuro-2012-0080.

Cape, J., Whittington, C., Buszewicz, M., Wallace, P., & Underwood, L. (2010). Brief psychological therapies for anxiety and depression in primary care: Meta-analysis and meta-regression. *BMC Medicine, 8*(38), 1–13. doi:10.1186/1741-7015-8-38.

Carrico, A. W., & Antoni, M. H. (2008). The effects of psychological interventions on neuroendocrine hormone regulation and immune status in HIV-positive persons: A review of randomized controlled trials. *Psychosomatic Medicine, 70*(5), 575.

Carroll, D., & Seers, K. (1998). Relaxation for the relief of chronic pain: A systematic review. *Journal of Advanced Nursing, 27*(3), 476–487.

Cegela, D. J., McClure, L., Marinelli, T. M., & Post, D. M. (2000). The effects of communication skills training in patients' participation during medical interviews. *Patient Education and Counseling, 41*(2), 209–222. doi:10.1016/S0738-3991(00)00093-8.

Christensen, A. J., & Ehlers, S. L. (2002). Psychological factors in end-stage renal disease: An emerging context for behavioral medicine research. *Journal of Consulting and Clinical Psychology, 70*(3), 712–724. doi:10.1037/0022-006X.70.3.712.

Clemens, J. Q., Nadler, R. B., Schaeffer, A. J., Belani, J., Albaugh, J., & Bushman, W. (2000). Biofeedback, pelvic floor re-education, and bladder training for male chronic pelvic pain syndrome. *Urology, 56*(6), 951–955.

Davidson, K. W., Kupfer, D. J., Bigger, J. T., Califf, R. M., Carney, R. M., Coyne, J. C., … Suls, J. M. (2006). Assessment and treatment of depression in patients with cardiovascular disease: National Heart, Lung, and Blood Institute Working Group Report. *Psychosomatic Medicine, 68*(5), 645–650. doi:10.1097/01.psy.0000233233.48738.22.

Davis, M. C., Zautra, A. J., Younger, J., Motivala, S. J., Attrep, J., & Irwin, M. R. (2008). Chronic stress and regulation of cellular markers of inflammation in rheumatoid arthritis; implications for fatigue. *Brain, Behavior, and Immunity, 22*(1), 24–32.

Dixon, K. E., Keefe, F. J., Scipio, C. D., Perry, L. M., & Abernethy, A. P. (2007). Psychological interventions for arthritis pain management in adults: A meta-analysis. *Health Psychology, 26*(3), 241–250.

Drewes, A. M. (1999). Pain and sleep disturbances with special reference to fibromyalgia and rheumatoid arthritis. *Rheumatology, 38*(11), 1035–1038.

Dzewaltowski, D. A., Estabrooks, P. A., & Glasgow, R. E. (2004). The future of physical activity behavior change research: What is needed to improve translation of research into health promotion practice? *Exercise and Sport Sciences Reviews, 32*(2), 57–63. doi:10.1097/00003677-200404000-00004.

Erickson, S. J., Gerstle, M., & Feldstein, S. W. (2005). Brief interventions and motivational interviewing with children, adolescents, and their parents in pediatric health care settings: A review. *Archives of Pediatrics & Adolescent Medicine, 159*(12), 1173–1180. doi:10.1001/archpedi.159.12.1173.

Ethgen, O., Vanparijs, P., Delhalle, S., Rosant, S., Bruyère, O., & Reginster, J. Y. (2004). Social support and health-related quality of life in hip and knee osteoarthritis. *Quality of Life Research, 13*(2), 321–330.

Evers, A. W., Kraaimaat, F. W., Geenen, R., Jacobs, J. W., & Bijlsma, J. W. (2003). Pain coping and social support as predictors of long-term functional disability and pain in early rheumatoid arthritis. *Behaviour Research and Therapy, 41*(11), 1295–1310.

Evers, A. W. M., Kraaimaat, F. W., Van Riel, P. L. C. M., & De Jong, A. J. L. (2002). Tailored cognitive-behavioral therapy in early rheumatoid arthritis for patients at risk: A randomized controlled trial. *Pain, 100*(1–2), 141–153. doi:10.1016/S0304-3959(02)00274-9.

Faul, L. A., Jim, H. S., Williams, C., Loftus, L., & Jacobsen, P. B. (2010). Relationship of stress management skill to psychological distress and quality of life in adults with cancer. *Psycho-Oncology, 19*(1), 102–109. doi:10.1002/pon.1547.

Fifield, J., Tennen, H., Reisine, S., & McQuillan, J. (1998). Depression and the long-term risk of pain, fatigue, and disability in patients with rheumatoid arthritis. *Arthritis and Rheumatism, 41*(10), 1851–1857. doi:10.1002/1529-0131(199810)41:10<1851::AID-ART18>3.0.CO;2-I.

Fisher, L., & Dickinson, W. P. (2014). Psychology and primary care: New collaborations for providing effective care for adults with chronic health conditions. *The American Psychologist, 69*(4), 355–363. doi:10.1037/a0036101.

Flor, H., & Birbaumer, N. (1993). Comparison of the efficacy of electromyographic biofeedback, cognitive-behavioral therapy, and conservative medical interventions in the treatment of chronic musculoskeletal pain. *Journal of Consulting and Clinical Psychology, 61*(4), 653–658. doi:10.1037/0022-006X.61.4.653.

Fok, S. K., Sek Ying, C., & Violeta, L. (2005). Sense of coherence, coping and quality of life following a critical illness. *Issues and Innovations in Nursing Practice, 49*(2), 173–181.

Gaglio, B., Shoup, J. A., & Glasgow, R. E. (2013). The RE-AIM framework: A systematic review of use over time. *American Journal of Public Health, 103*(6), e1–e9. doi:10.2105/AJPH.2013.301299.

Gartlehner, G., Hansen, R. A., Jonas, B. L., & Lohr, H. N. (2006). The comparative efficacy and safety of biologics for the treatment of rheumatoid arthritis: A systematic review and meta-analysis. *The Journal of Rheumatology, 33*(12), 2398–2408.

Gatchel, R. J., & Turk, D. C. (1996). *Activity-rest cycling. Psychological approaches to pain management—a practitioner's handbook* (pp. 272–274). New York, NY: Guilford.

Glasgow, R. E., Toobert, D. J., & Gillette, C. D. (2001). Psychosocial barriers to diabetes self-management and quality of life. *Diabetes Spectrum, 14*(1), 33–41. doi:10.2337/diaspect.14.1.33.

Goyer, L., Dufour, R., Janelle, C., Blais, C., L'Abbé, C., Raymond, E., … Larochelle, P. (2013). Randomized controlled trial on the long-term efficacy of a multifaceted, interdisciplinary lifestyle intervention in reducing cardiovascular risk and improving lifestyle in patients at risk of cardiovascular disease. *Journal of Behavioral Medicine, 36*(2), 212–224. doi:10.1007/s10865-012-9407-3.

Grossman, P., Niemann, L., Schmidt, S., & Walach, H. (2004). Mindfulness-based stress reduction and health benefits: A meta-analysis. *Journal of Psychosomatic Research, 57*(1), 35–43.

Guo, Z., Tang, H.-Y., Li, H., Tan, S.-K., Feng, K.-H., Huang, Y.-C., … Jiang, W. (2013). The benefits of psychosocial interventions for cancer patients undergoing radiotherapy. *Health and Quality of Life Outcomes, 11*(121), 1–12. doi:10.1186/1477-7525-11-121.

Hannibal, K. E., & Bishop, M. D. (2014). Chronic stress, cortisol dysfunction, and pain: A psychoneuroendocrine rationale for stress management in pain rehabilitation. *Physical Therapy, 94*(12), 1816–1825.

Hart, S. L., Hoyt, M. A., Diefenbach, M., Anderson, D. R., Kilbourn, K. M., Craft, L. L., … Stanton, A. L. (2012). Meta-analysis of efficacy of interventions for elevated depressive symptoms in adults diagnosed with cancer. *Journal of the National Cancer Institute, 104*(13), 990–1004. doi:10.1093/jnci/djs256.

Hauri, P. (1981). Treating psychophysiologic insomnia with biofeedback. *Archives of General Psychiatry, 38*(7), 752–758. doi:10.1001/archpsyc.1981.01780320032002.

Hewlett, S., Ambler, N., Almeida, C., Cliss, A., Hammond, A., Kitchen, K., … Pollock, J. (2011). Self-management of fatigue in rheumatoid arthritis: A randomised controlled trial of group cognitive-behavioural therapy. *Annals of the Rheumatic Diseases, 70*(6), 1060–1067. doi:10.1136/ard.2010.144691.

Higgins, N. C., Bailey, S. J., LaChapelle, D. L., Harman, K., & Hadjistavropoulos, T. (2014). Coping styles, pain expressiveness, and implicit theories of chronic pain. *Journal of Psychology, 14*, 1–14. doi:10.1080/00223980.2014.977759.

Hofmann, S. G., Sawyer, A. T., Witt, A. A., & Oh, D. (2010). The effect of mindfulness-based therapy on anxiety and depression: A meta-analytic review. *Journal of Consulting and Clinical Psychology, 78*(2), 169–183. doi:10.1037/a0018555.

Holland, J. C. (2004). IPOS sutherland memorial lecture: An international perspective on the development of psychosocial oncology: Overcoming cultural and attitudinal barriers to improve. *Psycho-Oncology, 13*, 445–459.

Holtzman, S., Newth, S., & Delongis, A. (2004). The role of social support in coping with daily pain among patients with rheumatoid arthritis. *Journal of Health Psychology, 9*(5), 677–695.

Ingersoll, K. S., & Cohen, J. (2008). The impact of medication regimen factors on adherence to chronic treatment: A review of literature. *Journal of Behavioral Medicine, 31*(3), 213–224. doi:10.1007/s10865-007-9147-y.The.

Irwin, M. R., Olmstead, R., Breen, E. C., Witarama, T., Carrillo, C., Sadeghi, N., … Cole, S. (2015). Cognitive behavioral therapy and tai chi reverse cellular and genomic markers of inflammation in late life insomnia: A randomized controlled trial. *Biological Psychiatry*, 1–9. doi:10.1016/j.biopsych.2015.01.010.

Irwin, M. R., Wang, M., Campomayor, C. O., Collado-Hidalgo, A., & Cole, S. (2006). Sleep deprivation and activation of morning levels of cellular and genomic markers of inflammation. *Archives of Internal Medicine, 166*(16), 1756–1762. doi:10.1001/archinte.166.16.1756.

Jacobsen, P. B., & Wagner, L. I. (2012). A new quality standard: The integration of psychosocial care into routine cancer care. *Journal of Clinical Oncology, 30*(11), 1154–1159. doi:10.1200/JCO.2011.39.5046.

Kearney, L. K., Post, E. P., Pomerantz, A. S., & Zeiss, A. M. (2014). Applying the interprofessional patient aligned care team in the Department of Veterans Affairs: Transforming primary care. *The American Psychologist, 69*(4), 399–408. doi:10.1037/a0035909.

Keefe, F. J., Blumenthal, J., Baucom, D., Affleck, G., Waugh, R., Caldwell, D. S., … Lefebvre, J. (2004). Effects of spouse-assisted coping skills training and exercise training in patients with osteoarthritic knee pain: A randomized controlled study. *Pain, 110*(3), 539–549.

Kiecolt-Glaser, J. K., McGuire, L., Robles, T. F., & Glaser, R. (2002). Psychoneuroimmunology and psychosomatic medicine: Back to the future. *Psychosomatic Medicine, 64*(1), 15–28. doi:10.1097/00006842-200201000-00004.

Kligler, B., & Chesney, M. (2014). Academic health centers and the growth of integrative medicine. *JNCI Monographs, 2014*(50), 292–293. doi:10.1093/jncimonographs/lgu039.

Knittle, K., Maes, S., & de Gucht, V. (2010). Psychological interventions for rheumatoid arthritis: Examining the role of self-regulation with a systematic review and meta-analysis of randomized controlled trials. *Arthritis Care & Research, 62*(10), 1460–1472. doi:10.1002/acr.20251.

Krol, B., Sanderman, R., & Suurmeijer, T. P. (1993). Social support, rheumatoid arthritis and quality of life: Concepts, measurement and research. *Patient Education and Counseling, 20*(2–3), 101–120. doi:10.1016/0738-3991(93)90125-G.

Kwekkeboom, K. L., & Gretarsdottir, E. (2006). Systematic review of relaxation interventions for pain. *Journal of Nursing Scholarship, 38*(3), 269–277. doi:10.1111/j.1547-5069.2006.00113.x.

Lee, Y. C., Chibnik, L. B., Lu, B., Wasan, A. D., Edwards, R. R., Fossel, A. H., … Karlson, E. W. (2009). The relationship between disease activity, sleep, psychiatric distress and pain sensitivity in rheumatoid arthritis: A cross sectional study. *Arthritis Research & Therapy, 11*(5), R160. doi:10.1186/ar2842.

Lin, E. H. B., Katon, W., Von Korff, M., Tang, L., Williams, J. W., Kroenke, K., … Langston, C. (2003). Effect of improving depression care on pain and functional outcomes among older adults with arthritis. *The Journal of American Medical Association, 290*(18), 2428–2429.

Linden, W., & Girgis, A. (2012). Psychological treatment outcomes for cancer patients: What do meta-analyses tell us about distress reduction? *Psycho-Oncology, 21*, 343–350. doi:10.1002/pon.2035.

Linden, W., Phillips, M. J., & Leclerc, J. (2007). Psychological treatment of cardiac patients: A meta-analysis. *European Heart Journal, 28*(24), 2972–2984. doi:10.1093/eurheartj/ehm504.

Lorig, K., Chastain, R. L., Ung, E., Shoor, S., & Holman, H. R. (1989). Development and evaluation of a scale to measure perceived self-efficacy in people with arthritis. *Arthritis and Rheumatism, 32*(1), 37–44. doi:10.1002/anr.1780320107.

Lorig, K., Gonzalez, V. M., & Ritter, P. (1999). Community-based Spanish language arthritis education program: A randomized trial. *Medical Care, 37*(9), 957–963.

Lorig, K. R., & Holman, H. (2003). Self-management education: History, definition, outcomes, and mechanisms. *Annals of Behavioral Medicine, 26*(1), 1–7. doi:10.1207/S15324796ABM2601_01.

Lorig, K., Lubeck, D., Kraines, R. G., Seleznick, M., & Holman, H. R. (1985). Outcomes of self-help education for patients with arthritis. *Arthritis and Rheumatism, 28*(6), 680–685. doi:10.1002/art.1780280612.

Marks, R., Allegrante, J. P., & Lorig, K. (2005). A review and synthesis of research evidence for self-efficacy-enhancing interventions for reducing chronic disability: Implications for health education practice (part II). *Health Promotion Practice, 6*(2), 148–156. doi:10.1177/1524839904266792.

McCracken, L. M., & Turk, D. C. (2002). Behavioral and cognitive-behavioral treatment for chronic pain: Outcome, predictors of outcome, and treatment process. *Spine, 27*(22), 2564–2573. doi:10.1097/01.BRS.0000032130.45175.66.

McCracken, L. M., & Vowles, K. E. (2008). A prospective analysis of acceptance of pain and values-based action in patients with chronic pain. *Health Psychology, 27*(2), 215.

Miller, A. H., Ancoli-Israel, S., Bower, J. E., Capuron, L., & Irwin, M. R. (2008). Neuroendocrine-immune mechanisms of behavioral comorbidities in patients with cancer. *Journal of Clinical Oncology, 26*(6), 971–982. doi:10.1200/JCO.2007.10.7805.

Miller, G. E., & Cohen, S. (2001). Psychological interventions and the immune system: A meta-analytic review and critique. *Health Psychology, 20*(1), 47–63. doi:10.1037/0278-6133.20.1.47.

Miller, B. F., Petterson, S., Burke, B. T., Phillips, R. L., & Green, L. A. (2014). Proximity of providers: Colocating behavioral health and primary care and the prospects for an integrated workforce. *The American Psychologist, 69*(4), 443–451. doi:10.1037/a0036093.

Montgomery, G. H., David, D., Kangas, M., Green, S., Sucala, M., Bovbjerg, D. H., … Schnur, J. B. (2014). Randomized controlled trial of a cognitive-behavioral therapy plus hypnosis intervention to control fatigue in patients undergoing radiotherapy for breast cancer. *Journal of Clinical Oncology*, *32*, 1–7. doi:10.1200/JCO.2013.49.3437.

Morone, N. E., & Greco, C. M. (2007). Mind-body interventions for chronic pain in older adults: A structured review. *Pain Medicine, 8*(4), 359–375. doi:10.1111/j.1526-4637.2007.00312.x.

Muehrer, R. J., & Becker, B. N. (2005). Life after transplantation: New transitions in quality of life and psychological distress. *Seminars in Dialysis, 18*(2), 124–131. doi:10.1111/j.1525-139X.2005.18214.x.

Murphy, S. L., Lyden, A. K., Smith, D. M., Dong, Q., & Koliba, J. F. (2010). Effects of a tailored activity pacing intervention on pain and fatigue for adults with osteoarthritis. *American Journal of Occupational Therapy, 64*(6), 869–876. doi:10.5014/ajot.2010.09198.

Newell, S. A., Sanson-Fisher, R. W., & Savolainen, N. J. (2002). Systematic review of psychological therapies for cancer patients: Overview and recommendations for future research. *Journal of the National Cancer Institute, 94*(23), 558–584.

Newton-John, T. R. O., Spence, S. H., & Schotte, D. (1995). Pergamon cognitive-behavioural therapy versus E M G biofeedback in the treatment of chronic low back pain. *Behaviour Research and Therapy, 33*(6), 691–697.

Nicassio, P. M. (2008). The problem of detecting and managing depression in the rheumatology clinic. *Arthritis Care and Research, 59*(2), 155–158. doi:10.1002/art.23348.

Nicassio, P. M., & Smith, T. W. (1995). *Managing chronic illness: A biopsychosocial perspective*. Washington, DC: American Psychological Association.

Nurmohamed, M. T., & Dijkmans, B. A. (2005). Efficacy, tolerability and cost effectiveness of disease-modifying antirheumatic drugs and biologic agents in rheumatoid arthritis. *Drugs, 65*(5), 661–694. Retrieved from http://www.scopus.com/inward/record.url?eid=2-s2.0-16444377894&partnerID=40&md5=7d636b80c41c57f565e80710a20ade1f

Nyklíček, I., Hoogwegt, F., & Westgeest, T. (2015). Psychological distress across twelve months in patients with rheumatoid arthritis: The role of disease activity, disability, and mindfulness. *Journal of Psychosomatic Research, 78*(2), 162–167. doi:10.1016/j.jpsychores.2014.08.004.

Ott, M. J. (2002). Complementary and alternative therapies in cancer symptom management. *Cancer Practice, 10*(3), 162–166.

Paschalides, C., Wearden, A. J., Dunkerley, R., Bundy, C., Davies, R., & Dickens, C. M. (2004). The associations of anxiety, depression and personal illness representations with glycaemic control and health-related quality of life in patients with type 2 diabetes mellitus. *Journal of Psychosomatic Research, 57*(6), 557–564. doi:10.1016/j.jpsychores.2004.03.006.

Peck, J. R., Smith, T. W., Ward, J. R., & Milano, R. (1989). Disability and depression in rheumatoid arthritis. A multi-trait, multi-method investigation. *Arthritis and Rheumatism, 32*(9), 1100–1106.

Preacher, K. J., & Hayes, A. F. (2008a). Asymptotic and resampling strategies for assessing and comparing indirect effects in multiple mediator models. *Behavior Research Methods, 40*(3), 879–891.

Preacher, K. J., & Hayes, A. F. (2008b). Contemporary approaches to assessing mediation in communication research. In A. F. Hayes, M. D. Slater, & L. B. Snyder (Eds.), *The SAGE sourcebook of advanced data analysis methods for communication research* (pp. 13–54). Thousand Oaks, CA: Sage Publications.

Radojevic, V., Nicassio, P. M., & Weisman, M. H. (1992). Behavioral intervention with and without family support for rheumatoid arthritis. *Behavior Therapy, 23*, 13–30.

Rose, M., Fliege, H., Hildebrandt, M., Schirop, T., & Burghard, F. K. (2002). The network of psychological variables in patients with diabetes and their importance for quality of life and metabolic control. *Diabetes Care, 25*(1), 35–42. doi:10.2337/diacare.25.1.35.

Rosenstock, I. M., Strecher, V. J., & Becker, M. H. (1988). Social learning theory and the Health Belief Model. *Health Education Quarterly, 15*(2), 175–183. doi:10.1177/109019818801500203.

Rosentiel, A. K., & Keefe, F. J. (1983). The use of coping strategies in chronic low back pain patients: Relationship to patient characteristics and current adjustment. *Pain, 17*(1), 33–34. doi:10.1016/0304-3959(83)90125-2.

Rosenzweig, S., Greeson, J. M., Reibel, D. K., Green, J. S., Jasser, S. A., & Beasley, D. (2009). Mindfulness-based stress reduction for chronic pain conditions: Variation in treatment outcomes and role of home meditation practice. *Journal of Psychosomatic Research, 68*(1), 29–36. doi:10.1016/j.jpsychores.2009.03.010.

Sarenmalm, E. K., Ohlen, J., Ode, A., & Gaston-johansson, F. (2008). Experience and predictors of symptoms, distress and health-related quality of life over time in postmenopausal women with recurrent breast cancer. *Psycho-Oncology, 505*, 497–505. doi:10.1002/pon.

Sharma, M., & Haider, T. (2013). Yoga as an alternative and complementary treatment for patients with low back pain: A systematic review. *Journal of Evidence-Based Complementary & Alternative Medicine, 19*(1), 51–58. doi:10.1177/2156587212458693.

Sharpe, L., Sensky, T., & Allard, S. (2001). The course of depression in recent onset rheumatoid arthritis: The predictive role of disability, illness perceptions, pain and coping. *Journal of Psychosomatic Research, 51*(6), 713–719. doi:10.1016/S0022-3999(01)00266-5.

Sharpe, L., Sensky, T., Timberlake, N., Ryan, B., Brewin, C. R., & Allard, S. (2001). A blind, randomized, controlled trial of cognitive-behavioural intervention for patients with recent onset rheumatoid arthritis: Preventing psychological and physical morbidity. *Pain, 89*(2–3), 275–283. doi:10.1016/S0304-3959(00)00379-1.

Shimbo, D., Davidson, K. W., Haas, D. C., Fuster, V., & Badimon, J. J. (2005). Negative impact of depression on outcomes in patients with coronary artery disease: Mechanisms, treatment considerations, and future directions. *Journal of Thrombosis and Haemostasis, 3*, 897–908.

Singh, J. A, Furst, D. E., Bharat, A., Curtis, J. R., Kavanaugh, A. F., Kremer, J. M., … Saag, K. G. (2012). 2012 update of the 2008 American College of Rheumatology recommendations for the use of disease-modifying antirheumatic drugs and biologic agents in the treatment of rheumatoid arthritis. *American College of Rheumatology, 64*(5), 625–39. doi:10.1002/acr.21641.

Sleath, B., Chewning, B., De Vellis, B. M., Weinberger, M., De Vellis, R. F., Tudor, G., & Beard, A. (2008). Communication about depression during rheumatoid arthritis patient visits. *Arthritis Care and Research, 59*(2), 186–191. doi:10.1002/art.23347.

Sloan, J. A., Zhao, X., Novotny, P. J., Wampfler, J., Garces, Y., Clark, M. M., & Yang, P. (2012). Relationship between deficits in overall quality of life and non-small-cell lung cancer survival. *Journal of Clinical Oncology, 30*(13), 1498–1504. doi:10.1200/JCO.2010.33.4631.

Somers, T. J., Wren, A. A., & Shelby, R. A. (2012). The context of pain in arthritis: Self-efficacy for managing pain and other symptoms. *Current Pain and Headache Reports, 16*(6), 502–508. doi:10.1007/s11916-012-0298-3.

Stebbings, S., Herbison, P., Doyle, T. C. H., Treharne, G. J., & Highton, J. (2010). A comparison of fatigue correlates in rheumatoid arthritis and osteoarthritis: Disparity in associations with disability, anxiety and sleep disturbance. *Rheumatology, 49*(2), 361–367. doi:10.1093/rheumatology/kep367.

Stein, M. J., Wallston, K. A., & Nicassio, P. M. (1988). Factor structure of the arthritis helplessness index. *Journal of Rheumatology, 15*(3), 427–432.

Stone, V. E., Hogan, J. W., Schuman, P., Rompalo, A. M., Howard, A. A., Korkontzelou, C., & Smith, D. K. (2001). Antiretroviral regimen complexity, self-reported adherence, and HIV patients' understanding of their regimens: Survey of women in the HER study. *Journal of Acquired Immune Deficiency Syndrome, 28*, 124–131.

Taylor, S. E. (1990). Health psychology: The science and the field. *American Psychologist, 45*(1), 40–50.

Thornton, L. M., Andersen, B. L., Schuler, T. A., & Carson, W. E. (2009). A psychological intervention reduces inflammatory markers by alleviating depressive symptoms: Secondary analysis of a randomized controlled trial. *Psychosomatic Medicine, 71*(7), 1–21. doi:10.1097/PSY.0b013e3181b0545c.A.

Tully, P. J., Baker, R. A., Turnbull, D. A., Winefield, H. R., & Knight, J. L. (2009). Negative emotions and quality of life six months after cardiac surgery: The dominant role of depression not anxiety symptoms. *Journal of Behavioral Medicine, 32*(6), 510–522. doi:10.1007/s10865-009-9225-4.

Turk, D. C., & Okifuji, A. (2002). Psychological factors in chronic pain: Evolution and revolution. *Journal of Consulting and Clinical Psychology, 70*(3), 678–690. doi:10.1037/0022-006X.70.3.678.

Vermeire, E., Hearnshaw, H., Van Royen, P., & Denekens, J. (2001). Patient adherence to treatment: Three decades of research. A comprehensive review. *Journal of Clinical Pharmacy and Therapeutics, 26*(5), 331–342. doi:10.1046/j.1365-2710.2001.00363.x.

Villareal, D. T., Miller, B. V., Banks, M., Fontana, L., Sinacore, D. R., & Klein, S. (2006). Effect of lifestyle intervention on metabolic coronary heart disease risk factors in obese older adults. *The American Journal of Clinical Nutrition, 84*(6), 1317–1323.

Wilson, D. K. (2015). Behavior matters: The relevance, impact, and reach of behavioral medicine. *Annals of Behavioral Medicine, 49*, 1–9.

Zautra, A. J., Davis, M. C., Reich, J. W., Nicassario, P., Tennen, H., Finan, P., … Irwin, M. R. (2008). Comparison of cognitive behavioral and mindfulness meditation interventions on adaptation to rheumatoid arthritis for patients with and without history of recurrent depression. *Journal of Consulting and Clinical Psychology, 76*(3), 408–421. doi:10.1037/0022-006X.76.3.408.

Zyrianova, E., Kelly, B. D., Gallagher, C., McCarthy, C. Molloy, M. G., Sheehan, J., & Dinan, T. G. (2006). Depression and anxiety in rheumatoid arthritis: The role of perceived social support. *Irish Journal of Medical Science, 175*(2), 32–26.

Index

P.M. Nicassio (ed.), *Psychosocial Factors in Arthritis*, DOI 10.1007/978-3-319-22858-7

MIX
Papier aus verantwortungsvollen Quellen
Paper from responsible sources
FSC® C105338

If you have any concerns about our products,
you can contact us on
ProductSafety@springernature.com

In case Publisher is established outside the EU,
the EU authorized representative is:
Springer Nature Customer Service Center GmbH
Europaplatz 3, 69115 Heidelberg, Germany

Printed by Libri Plureos GmbH
in Hamburg, Germany